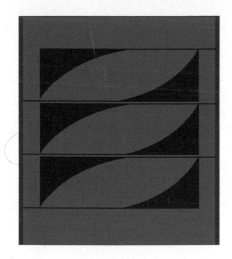

# SURGICAL EXPOSURES IN

# ORTHOPAEDICS

## The Anatomic Approach

# Stanley Hoppenfeld, M.D.

Clinical Professor of Orthopaedic Surgery,
Albert Einstein College of Medicine;
Bronx, New York

Attending Physician, Jack D. Weiler Hospital
of the Albert Einstein College of Medicine,
Montefiore Hospital and Medical Center
Bronx, New York

# Piet deBoer, M.A., F.R.C.S.

Consultant Orthopaedic Surgeon, University of
Hull and York Medical School, York, England

Associate Professor, St. George's Medical School,
Grenada

Visiting Professor, University of Mississippi
Medical School, Jackson, Mississippi

Educational Consultant, AO International, Davos,
Switzerland


*In collaboration with* **Richard Hutton**
*Illustrated by* **Hugh A. Thomas**

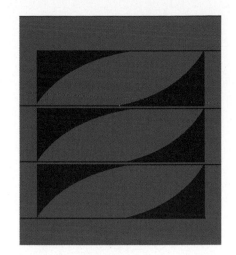

# SURGICAL EXPOSURES IN
# ORTHOPAEDICS

## The Anatomic Approach

**Stanley Hoppenfeld**
**Piet deBoer**

**Illustrations by Hugh A. Thomas**

*Third Edition*

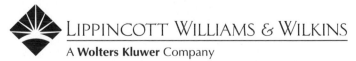

LIPPINCOTT WILLIAMS & WILKINS
A **Wolters Kluwer** Company

Philadelphia · Baltimore · New York · London
Buenos Aires · Hong Kong · Sydney · Tokyo

*Acquisitions Editor:* Robert Hurley
*Developmental Editor:* Eileen Wolfberg
*Production Manager:* Toni Ann Scaramuzzo
*Production Editor:* Michael Mallard
*Manufacturing Manager:* Ben Rivera
*Cover Designer:* Karen Quigley
*Compositor:* Lippincott Williams & Wilkins Desktop Division
*Printer:* Quebecor World Taunton

© 2003 by LIPPINCOTT WILLIAMS & WILKINS
530 Walnut Street
Philadelphia, PA 19106 USA
LWW.com

**Library of Congress Cataloging-in-Publication Data**
Hoppenfeld, Stanley, 1934-
    Surgical exposures in orthopaedics : the anatomic approach / Stanley Hoppenfeld, Piet DeBoer ; illustrations by Hugh A. Thomas.—3rd ed.
        p. ; cm.
    Includes bibliographical references and index.
    ISBN-13: 978-0-7817-4228-3
    ISBN-10: 0-7817-4228-5
    1. Orthopedic surgery. 2. Anatomy, Surgical and topographical. I. DeBoer, Piet. II. Title.
    [DNLM: 1. Orthopedic Procedures.  WE 168 H798s 2003]
    RD732.H66 2003
    617.4′7—dc21

                                                                    2003047511

Care has been taken to confirm the accuracy of the information presented and to describe generally accepted practices. However, the authors, editors, and publisher are not responsible for errors or omissions or for any consequences from application of the information in this book and make no warranty, expressed or implied, with respect to the currency, completeness, or accuracy of the contents of the publication. Application of this information in a particular situation remains the professional responsibility of the practitioner.

The authors, editors, and publisher have exerted every effort to ensure that drug selection and dosage set forth in this text are in accordance with current recommendations and practice at the time of publication. However, in view of ongoing research, changes in government regulations, and the constant flow of information relating to drug therapy and drug reactions, the reader is urged to check the package insert for each drug for any change in indications and dosage and for added warnings and precautions. This is particularly important when the recommended agent is a new or infrequently employed drug.

Some drugs and medical devices presented in this publication have Food and Drug Administration (FDA) clearance for limited use in restricted research settings. It is the responsibility of the health care provider to ascertain the FDA status of each drug or device planned for use in their clinical practice.

10 9 8 7 6 5

# Dedication

To my wife Norma,
my sons Jon-David,
Robert, and Stephen,
and my parents Agatha and David,
all in their own special way have made my life full
and made this book possible.
S.H.

To Suzanne, Katy, James, Jan,
and all the other members of my family.
P.deB.

# Preface

Since its publication in 1984, *Surgical Exposures in Orthopaedics—The Anatomic Approach* has been the standard textbook for surgical approaches in orthopaedics and traumatology, regularly consulted by trainees as well as by experienced surgeons throughout the world. Its enduring success is evidence that it continues to meet a need in the practice of orthopaedics and traumatology. Why, then, a third edition?

The field of orthopaedics continues to evolve at a rapid rate. The previous edition introduced the concept of preserving blood supply and minimizing soft-tissue damage in fracture surgery in order to preserve the biological envelope of the injured bone as much as possible. In this edition we introduce three minimal access approaches to allow the surgeon to perform intramedullary nailing of the femur, tibia, and humerus. Again, we emphasize that "you should make every effort to preserve the soft-tissue attachments of the bone wherever possible. Only expose what you actually need to see to ensure an adequate surgical procedure."

A significant development in the field has been the enormous increase in arthroscopic procedures, which have largely replaced open operations within the knee joint. Arthroscopy of the shoulder joint similarly is a rapidly developing approach. Therefore, this new edition introduces arthroscopic approaches to these joints—specifically the anteromedial and anterolateral approaches to the knee joint, and the anterior and posterior approaches to the shoulder joint, which allow the surgeons to examine the joint and have proved acceptable to large numbers of surgeons for some time.

Although arthroscopic procedures have largely superseded open procedures and surgery in the developed world, surgeons still need to incorporate the classic surgical approaches to the knee. These approaches and knowledge of their underlying anatomy are useful when a surgeon has to deal with an open wound with associated ligament damage or when operating in countries where arthroscopy is not readily available.

The third edition also contains changes in the section on acetabular approaches, particularly in the posterior approach to the acetabulum, which has become the standard approach for these complex and challenging injuries.

In addition, full color has been added to all the illustrations, enhancing their attractiveness as well as their verisimilitude.

*Piet deBoer*
*Stanley Hoppenfeld*

# Preface to the Second Edition

How do you make a good book better, in a radically changing orthopaedic environment? By keeping to basics and heeding the requests of our fellow surgeons who have written to us over these past nine years, since the publication of the first edition.

The emphasis on the concept of internervous planes remains a hallmark of the book. The basic principle of "do not cut round structures" is further reinforced by adding color to the nerves, arteries and veins, which enhances the clinical dimensions of the illustrations.

New surgical approaches have been added, such as the anterolateral approach to the shoulder, the anterolateral approach to the tibia, and an improved lateral approach to the hip.

A whole new section on approaches to the acetabulum and pelvis is presented. The chapter is enriched with numerous original detailed surgical and anatomic drawings.

A new chapter on safe routes for percutaneous insertion of external fixators into the long bones is offered. The illustrations with their insets provide three-dimensional clarity and location of the important neurovascular structures.

Although anatomy has clearly not changed in the past nine years, more emphasis has been given to the preservation of the blood supply to the bone during orthopaedic surgery. This concept is of particular importance in fracture surgery where the blood supply to the bone has often been disrupted by the original injury. Preservation of blood supply is achieved by maintaining the soft tissue envelope of the bone. The approaches described in this book necessarily describe exposure of the whole anatomical site; the illustrations demonstrate this. In clinical practice you will often only need part of the approach described. You should make every effort to preserve the soft tissue attachments of the bone wherever possible. Do not fall into the trap of stripping bone extensively to allow complete exposure of all sides of a fracture; dead bone does not unite in the fracture situation. Only expose what you actually need to see to ensure an adequate surgical procedure. The concept of "biological fixation" of fractures relies on these principles.

*Stanley Hoppenfeld, M.D.*
*Piet deBoer, M.A., F.R.C.S.*

# Preface to the First Edition

It has often been said that successful orthopaedic procedures are based on a simple principle: Get to bone and stay there." *Surgical Exposures in Orthopaedics: The Anatomic Approach*, the product of an anatomy course for orthopaedic surgeons that has been run at the Albert Einstein College of Medicine for the past 15 years, expands on the principle. The book explains the techniques of commonly used orthopaedic approaches and relates the regional anatomy of the area relevant to the approach.

Safety in surgery depends on knowledge of anatomy and technical skill. The two go hand in hand; one is useless without the other. Surgical skill can be learned only by practical experience under expert supervision. But the knowledge that underlies it must come from both book and dissection.

Structurally, this book is divided into 11 chapters, each dealing with a particular area of the body. The most commonly performed approaches are described; we have omitted approaches designed only for one specific procedure—they are best understood in the original papers of those who first described them. Nevertheless, the vast majority of orthopaedic procedures can be safely and successfully accomplished through the approaches we have included.

Orthopaedics is a rapidly evolving field. New procedures are appearing at a prodigious rate; some are discarded in a comparatively short time. Thus, any book that concerns itself with the specifics of operative surgery inevitably becomes dated, sometimes even before publication. To avoid this problem, we have concentrated on getting to the bone or joint concerned, and not on what to do after. When applicable, we have included references to individual surgical procedures but without incorporating their details into our textbook.

The key to *Surgical Exposures in Orthopaedics* is a consistent organization throughout (*see* Table 1). Each approach is explained; then the relevant surgical anatomy of the area is discussed. When one or more approaches share anatomy, they are grouped together, with the relevant anatomical section at the end. The idea is for the surgeon to read the approach and anatomy sections together before attempting a given procedure, because once the anatomical principles of a procedure are fully understood, the logic of an approach becomes clear.

## SURGICAL APPROACHES

The crucial element in successful surgical approaches is exploiting *internervous planes*. These planes lie between muscles—muscles supplied by different nerves. Internervous planes are helpful mainly because they can be used along their entire length without either of the muscles involved being denervated. These approaches can generally be extended to expose adjacent structures. Virtually all the classic *extensile* approaches to bone use internervous planes—a concept first described by A. K. Henry, who believed that if the key to operative surgery is surgical anatomy, then the key to surgical anatomy is the internervous plane.

The approach sections are structured as follows.

The introduction to each approach describes indications and points out the major advantages or disadvantages of the proposed surgery. Significant dangers are also outlined in this section.

## Table 1. Chapter Outline

The *position of the patient* is critical to clear, full exposures, as well as to the comfort of the operating surgeon.

Surgical *landmarks* form the basis for any incision; they are described with instructions on how to find them. The *incision* follows these key landmarks. Although the incisions described are generally straight, many surgeons prefer to use curved or zigzag incisions because they heal with less tension than do equivalent straight incisions.

The approaches often allow exposure of the whole length of a bone; usually, only part of an exposure is required for any given operation.

The surgical dissection has been divided into *superficial* and *deep surgical dissections* for teaching purposes to reinforce the concept that each layer must be developed fully before the next layer is dissected. Adequate exposure depends on a systematic and deliberate technique that exploits each plane completely before deeper dissection begins.

The *dangers* of each approach are listed under four headings: nerves, vessels, muscles and tendons, and special points. The dangers are described, along with how to avoid them.

The approach section concludes with a description of *how to enlarge the approach*. All too often, the surgeon discovers that the incised exposure is inadequate. There are two ways in which the exposure can be enlarged: *Local measures* include extending skin incisions, repositioning retractors, detaching muscles, or even adjusting the light source; and *extensile measures* are ways in which an approach can be extended to include adjacent bony structures. In approaches through internervous planes, extensile measures may permit the exposure of the entire length of the bone.

## ANATOMICAL SECTIONS

The anatomy of each approach begins with a brief overview of the muscular anatomy, along with the arrangement of the neurovascular structures.

The anatomy of the *landmarks* relates these structures to their surroundings. The anatomy of the *skin incision* describes the angle between the incision and the natural lines of skin cleavage first described by Langer—a relationship that may influence the size and prominence of the resultant scar. Nevertheless, the site of a skin incision must be determined largely by safety and effectiveness and not by cosmetic considerations. Skin incisions generally avoid cutting major cutaneous nerves; where they might, the danger is clearly stated.

The *anatomy of the superficial and deep surgical dissection* discusses the regional anatomy encountered during the approaches—not only the anatomy of the plane to be used but also that of adjacent structures that may appear if the surgeon strays out of plane. Perhaps the greatest value of knowing topographical anatomy is in cases of trauma, where the surgeon may explore wounds with confidence, aware of the potential dangers created by any given wound. Relevant clinical information on the anatomical structures is offered, but a comprehensive clinical picture is beyond the scope of this book. The origins, insertions, actions, and nerve supplies of relevant muscles are listed in legends under the muscles' illustrations.

The anatomical and surgical illustrations are drawn from the surgeon's point of view whenever possible, with the patient on the operating table, so that the surgeon can see exactly how the approach must look when he operates.

The anatomical terms used in *Surgical Exposures in Orthopaedics* are generally those used in modern anatomical textbooks. Terms now in orthopaedic usage sometimes differ from them; when that occurs (for instance, with the flexor retinaculum/transverse carpal ligament), both terms are given. Variation also occurs in usage on either side of the Atlantic; we have used those terms on which the authors (one American and one English) have reached consensus.

It has been said that all of orthopaedic surgical approaches can be reduced to one line: "Avoid cutting round structures." This book has been written to tell you how.

*Stanley Hoppenfeld, M.D.*
*Piet deBoer, M.A., F.R.C.S.*

# Acknowledgments

This book reflects the accumulated experience of many people over many decades. We should like to thank those in particular who helped us during the writing of this book.

**To Richard Hutton,**
my long-term friend and editor, who adds organization and reality to our writings. His love of the English language is reflected in this book.

**To Hugh Thomas,**
my long-term friend and medical illustrator, who added clarity to the book by his imaginative original illustrations, which reflect anatomic knowledge and clinical detail. In preparing the artwork for *Surgical Exposures in Orthopaedics: The Anatomic Approach*, he managed to draw beautifully on two continents.

**To Ray Coomaraswamy, M.D.,**
for his help and guidance in writing the transabdominal and thoracotomy approaches to the spine. He has furthered his life experience by becoming a psychiatrist.

**To David M. Hirch, M.D.,**
for his detailed, expert review of the chapter on the hip and for his guidance in its presentation and clinical details.

**To Barnard Kleiger, M.D.,**
for reviewing the chapters on the tibia and fibula and on the foot and ankle. He has been a source of inspiration to us during these years. We miss him.

**To Roy Kulick, M.D.,**
for reviewing the chapter on the hand several times and for giving it that little extra to help its clinical tone.

**To Martin Levy, M.D.,**
for his multiple reviews of the chapter on the knee for his valuable suggestions and clarity of thought.

**To Eric Radin, M.D.,**
for reviewing parts of our book in its early stages, encouraging us, and making valuable suggestions.

**To Arthur Sadler, M.D.,**
for his review of the chapter on the femur.

**To Leonard Seimon, M.D.,**
for reviewing the medial approach to the hip and sharing his unusual surgical experiences with us.

**To Neil Cobelli, M.D.,**
Chairman of the Department of Orthopaedic Surgery at the Montefiore Medical Center and Director of Orthopaedic Surgery of the Albert Einstein College of Medicine, for his continued interest in teaching anatomy and surgical approaches to the resident staff.

**To Jerry Sosler, M.D.,**
for demonstrating and reviewing the retroperitoneal approach to the spine and his positive suggestions.

**To Morton Spinner, M.D.,**
for reviewing the chapters on the elbow and forearm, helping us with clinical details, and for sharing a lifetime of clinical and surgical experience.

**To Keith Watson, M.D.,**
for reviewing the chapter on the shoulder.

**To the British Fellows,**
who visit the Albert Einstein College of Medicine from St. Thomas Hospital in England each year. Each has made a major contribution to the educational program and to our Anatomy course: *Clive Whaley, Robert Jackson, David Grubel-Lee, David Reynolds, Roger Weeks, Fred Heatley, Peter Johnson, Richard Foster, Kenneth Walker, Maldwyn Griffith, John Patrick, Paul Allen, Paul Evans, Robert Johnson, Martin Knight, Robert Simonis*, and *David Dempster.*

**To the Anatomy Department of the Albert Einstein College of Medicine—in particular.**

**To France Baker-Cohen,**
who worked closely with us in establishing the course each year, and whom we miss

**and to Michael D'Alessandro,**
who has kept the rooms and cadaver material for us.

**To Dr. M. Bull,**
**Dr. E. M. Chisholm,**
and the Examiners of the primary fellowship in London, who convinced me that topographical anatomy was worth learning.

**To Ronald Furlong,**
**Eric Denman,**
**and David Reynolds,**
for their efforts in teaching me and others operative surgery.

**To Marianne Broadbent,**
**Ken Peel,**
and the nursing staff and ODAs at York District Hospital and the Purey Cust Nuffield Hospital, York, for making surgery not only possible and safe, but also for their endless good humor, which makes surgery a pleasure.

To the operating staff and technicians of Princess Margaret Hospital, Swindon and St. Thomas Hospital, London—and especially

**Jim Lovegrove,**
for making surgery possible.

**To Alan Apley,**
not only for providing the model for teaching, but also for writing a book that teaches.

**To Professor Kinmonth,**
**Fred Heatley,**
**Malcolm Morrison,**
**and John Wilkinson,**
for their generous help during my own orthopaedic training.

To the fellow physicians who have participated in teaching the Anatomy course over these many years: *Uriel Adar, M.D., Russell Anderson, M.D., Mel Adler, M.D., Martin Barschi, M.D., Robert Dennis, M.D., Michael DiStefano, M.D., Henry Ergas, M.D., Aziz Eshraghi, M.D., Madgi Gabriel, M.D., Ralph Ger, M.D., Ed Habermann, M.D., Armen Haig, M.D., Steve Harwin, M.D., John Katonah, M.D., Ray Koval, M.D., Luc Lapommaray, M.D., Al Larkins, M.D., Mark Lazansky, M.D., Shelly Manspeizer, M.D., Mel Manin, M.D., David Mendes, M.D., Basil Preefer, M.D., Leela Rangaswamy, M.D., Ira Rochelle, M.D., Art Sadler, M.D., Jerry Sallis, M.D., Eli Sedlin, M.D., Lenny Seimon, M.D., Dick Selznick, M.D., Ken Seslowe, M.D., Rashmi Sheth, M.D., Bob Shultz, M.D., Richard Seigel, M.D., Norman Silver, M.D., Irvin Spira, M.D., Moe Szporn, M.D., Richard Stern, M.D., Jacob Teladano, M.D., Alan Weisel, M.D.,* and *Charles Weiss, M.D.*

To the residents who have participated in the Orthopaedic Anatomy course at the "Einstein," who have been a continual course of stimulation and inspiration.

**To Muriel Chaleff,**
who spent many hours helping to organize the Orthopaedic Anatomy course at the Albert Einstein College of Medicine. We owe her a great debt of gratitude for the kindness she has shown.

**To Leon Strong,**
my first Professor of Anatomy in Medical School for a stimulating introduction to anatomy.

**To Emanuel Kaplan, M.D.,**
whose great fund of anatomy and comparative anatomy was passed on to many of us while we were residents. His presence is still felt.

**To Herman Robbins, M.D.,**
for his professional support and teaching of anatomy during the many sessions held in the library of the old Hospital for Joint Diseases.

**To Dr. and Mrs. N. A. Shore,**
my long-term friends, who had a positive effect on my medical writings and clinical practice. We greatly miss them.

**To Mr. Abraham Irvings,**
my long-term friend and accountant, who kept the financial records, helping to make this book possible.

**To Ruth Gottesman,**
for making reading possible for all through her great endeavors at the Albert Einstein College of Medicine, Fisher Landau Center for the Treatment of Learning Disabilities.

**To David "Sandy" Gottesman,**
in appreciation of his friendship and professional dissection of the marketplace.

**To Marie Capizzuto,**
my long-term secretary and friend, for her professional help in making this book possible.

**To Frank Ferrieri,**
my long-term friend, in appreciation of his help. His loss is greatly felt.

**To Mary Kearney,**
my secretary, for help in communicating with the J. B. Lippincott Company and mailing and calling, and calling, and calling! We miss her.

**To Tracy Davis,**
for English editing of the Third Edition.

**To Barbara Ferrari,**
for her friendship, positive suggestions, and typing the Third Edition of our book.

To our secretarial staff, and **Mary Ann Becchetti,** who took hours out of their busy schedules to type, retype, retype, and retype the text until it was perfect.

**To J. Stuart Freeman, Jr.,**
former Senior Editor at Lippincott Williams & Wilkins, who has befriended me over these years and has been a source of positive suggestions and inspiration.

**To Robert Hurley,**
Executive Editor at Lippincott Williams & Wilkins, in appreciation of his friendship and professional help in structuring the Third Edition.

**To Eileen Wolfberg,**
Developmental Editor at Lippincott Williams & Wilkins, in appreciation of her detailed work in keeping the production and editing of this book on track and for her good humor at all times.

To the professional staff at Lippincott Williams & Wilkins, for their help in producing this book. Special thanks to *Michael Mallard*, Production Editor, *Toni Ann Scaramuzzo*, Acting Director of the Production Department and Production Manager, *Diane Farrell*, Senior Desktop Editor, who did the page layout, and *Diana Andrews*, Art Director, for giving form and shape to the book.

# Contents

## Chapter Eleven   The Tibia and Fibula   569

## Chapter Twelve   The Ankle and Foot   607

## Chapter Thirteen   Approaches for External Fixation   677

# Introduction: Orthopaedic Surgical Technique

Surgical technique in orthopaedics varies from surgeon to surgeon; the more experienced the surgeon, the fewer instruments he uses and the simpler his technique becomes. Certain principles, however, remain constant. They are listed below as they apply to each surgical section.

The *position of the patient* is fundamental to any approach; it is always worth taking time to ensure that the patient is in the best position and that he is secured so that he cannot move during the procedure. Operating tables are well padded, but certain bony prominences—such as the head of the fibula and greater trochanter—are not. These prominences must always be padded adequately to prevent skin breakdown and nerve entrapment during surgery. Patients who are prone must have suitable padding placed under their pelvis, chest, head, and nose to allow respiration during surgery. Many different systems ensure adequate ventilation of the patient; bolsters placed longitudinally under the side of the patient are probably the best. Ventilation of the prone patient must be adequate before surgery, since repositioning of the patient during surgery is difficult and almost inevitably contaminates the sterile field.

The surgeon should be comfortable during surgery, with the patient placed at the correct height for the surgeon's size or the table low enough to allow him to operate sitting down.

In surgery on the limbs, a tourniquet is often used to create a bloodless field, making identification of vital structures easier and expediting surgery.

To apply the tourniquet, empty the limb of blood, either by elevating it for 3 to 5 minutes or by applying a soft rubber compression bandage. The tourniquet should be padded with a soft dressing to prevent the wrinkles (and blisters) that inevitably occur when the skin is pinched. The tourniquet may be applied to the upper arm or thigh. Both of these areas are well muscled; the major nerves are protected from compression of the tourniquet. The inflated pressure of the tourniquet should be about 275 mm Hg in the upper limb and 450 mm Hg in the lower limb, depending on the circumference of the limb. Test the tourniquet by inflating it *before* applying it to the patient. In children, inflate the tourniquet to 50% above their systolic pressure. In hypertensive patients, inflate it 50% more than their systolic pressure. Finally, do not leave the tourniquet inflated for longer than 1 hour in the upper limb and 1½ hours in the lower limb to minimize risk; do not use tourniquets when the peripheral circulation of the patient is suspect or in the presence of sickle cell disease.

Partial exsanguination of the limb, which can be achieved after 2 minutes of elevation, leaves blood in the venous structures. It makes for a bloodier field during surgery but does make it easier to identify neurovascular bundles—something of immense value in, for example, lateral meniscectomy, where it is safer to identify and to coagulate the lateral inferior geniculate artery than to cut it accidentally, learning about it only after the tourniquet has been deflated. Deflate the tourniquet before closure to identify and to coagulate major bleeding points.

The *landmarks* are critical to the planning of any incision. It is often convenient to mark them on the skin with methylene blue to ensure that the skin incision lines up with them.

All skin incisions heal with the formation of scar tissue, which contracts with time. For this reason, skin incisions should not cross flexion creases at 90°; cutting perpendicular to flexion creases can cause contractures to develop over the involved joints. That is why incisions that cross major flexion creases are usually curved to traverse the crease at about 60°.

The techniques of the *superficial and deep surgical* dissections are the province of practical experience, not book knowledge. However, two techniques are frequently referred to in the book.

Subperiosteal dissection protects vital structures that lie near the bone, helping to prevent their damage by instruments. The rule holds true, but vital structures often lie on the periosteum itself: the posterior interosseous nerve, for instance, lies on the periosteum of the neck of the radius. The radial nerve lies on the periosteum on the back of the humerus. In these cases subperiosteal dissection must be strictly subperiosteal, something that may not be possible if the periosteum is damaged in case of fracture. The periosteum normally detaches easily from the bone except at sites of muscle or ligament attachments where it may adhere strongly. Blunt dissection may be difficult or impossible at the sites of insertion. Note that the periosteum of children is thicker than that of adults, more easily defined, and less adherent to bone. In fracture surgery subperiosteal dissection is rarely indicated except in the region of the proximal radius and the center of the humeral shaft. Subperiosteal stripping will destroy the periosteal supply of blood to the bone and if extensive will devitalize the fracture site. In such cases periosteal stripping is only permissible to allow accurate reduction of the fracture. The more experienced the surgeon becomes the less soft tissue damage he will need to create to allow accurate visualization and reduction of the fracture.

The second technique is that of detaching muscle from bone. Remember to strip *into* the *acute angle* that fibers make with the bone to which they attach. This is perhaps clearest in the fibula: To detach the peroneal muscles, pass an elevator from distal to proximal; to detach the interosseous membrane, where fibers run in a different direction, strip from proximal to distal.

Exposures can be improved in two ways. *Local measures* enhance the immediate exposure. *Extensile measures* allow the surgeon to expose adjacent bony structures. It is vital to appreciate that not all approaches are extensile: Specialized approaches should be used only in cases where the pathology is accurately pinpointed and where the surgeon does not have to expose any adjacent structures. Inadequate exposure is one of the most common causes of surgical failure. If the surgeon is in difficulty, one of the first things he should try is to improve the exposure either by local or by extensile means.

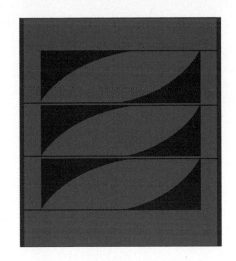

# SURGICAL EXPOSURES IN

# ORTHOPAEDICS

## The Anatomic Approach

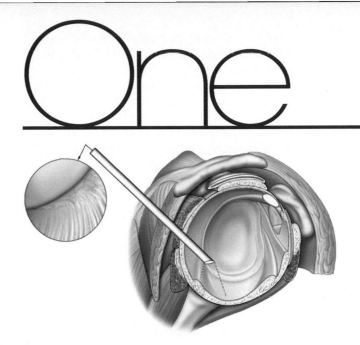

# One

# The Shoulder

The shoulder is the most mobile joint in the body. It is surrounded by two sleeves of muscle: the outer sleeve, or deltoid muscle; and the inner sleeve, or rotator cuff, which is critical for the stability of the joint. The two most common shoulder pathologies that necessitate surgery are instability, such as recurrent anterior dislocation of the shoulder (see Fig. 1-26), and degenerative lesions of the rotator cuff.

Six surgical approaches are described in this chapter: anterior, anterolateral, lateral, minimal access approach to the proximal humerus, posterior, and arthroscopic. Of these, the anterior approach is the "work-horse" incision of the shoulder, providing excellent exposure of both the joint and its anterior coverings. The anterolateral approach is used mainly to expose the subacromial structures, especially the rotator cuff. The lateral approach also exposes the rotator cuff; its lower half can be used to provide limited access to the upper end of the humerus. The minimal access approach to the proximal humerus is useful only for intramedullary nailing of humeral shaft fractures. The posterior approach, which is used rarely, is effective for treating recurrent posterior dislocations. The arthroscopic approaches to the shoulder (anterior and posterior) provide excellent visualization of the internal structures of the joint.

The surgical anatomy of the area is divided into three sections: anterior, anterolateral, and posterior. A description of each area is found immediately after its respective operative section in this chapter.

# Anterior Approach

The anterior surgical approach offers good wide exposure of the shoulder joint, allowing repairs to be made of its anterior, inferior, and superior coverings. Among its many uses, the anterior approach permits the following:

1. Reconstruction of recurrent dislocations[1-6]
2. Drainage of sepsis
3. Biopsy and excision of tumors
4. Repair or stabilization of the tendon of the long head of the biceps[7]
5. Shoulder arthroplasties, which usually are inserted through modified anterior incisions[8]

The anterior approach is notorious for the amount of bleeding that occurs from skin and subcutaneous tissues during superficial dissection. The bleeding must be controlled before the deeper layers are dissected. Failure to do so may obscure important anatomic structures and endanger their integrity.

## Position of the Patient

Place the patient in a supine position on the operating table. Wedge a sandbag under the spine and medial border of the scapula to push the affected side forward while allowing the arm to fall backward, opening up the front of the joint (Fig. 1-1). Elevate the head of the table 30° to 45° to reduce venous pressure, and thereby decrease bleeding, and to allow the blood to drain away from the operative field during surgery. If a headrest is used, make sure that it is padded properly to prevent the development of a pressure sore on the occiput. Drape the arm free because it will have to be moved during the approach.

## Landmarks and Incision

### Landmarks

*Coracoid Process.* At the deepest point in the clavicular concavity, the surgeon should drop his or her fingers distally about 1 in. from the anterior edge of the clavicle and press laterally and posteriorly in an oblique line until the coracoid process is felt. The process faces anterolaterally; because it lies deep under the cover of the pectoralis major, it can be felt only by firm palpation.

*Deltopectoral Groove.* The deltopectoral groove is easier to see than to feel, especially in thin patients. The cephalic vein, which runs in the groove, sometimes is visible.

### Incisions

The anterior aspect of the shoulder can be approached through either of two skin incisions.

*Anterior Incision.* Make a 10- to 15-cm straight incision, following the line of the deltopectoral groove. The incision should begin just above the coracoid process (Fig. 1-2).

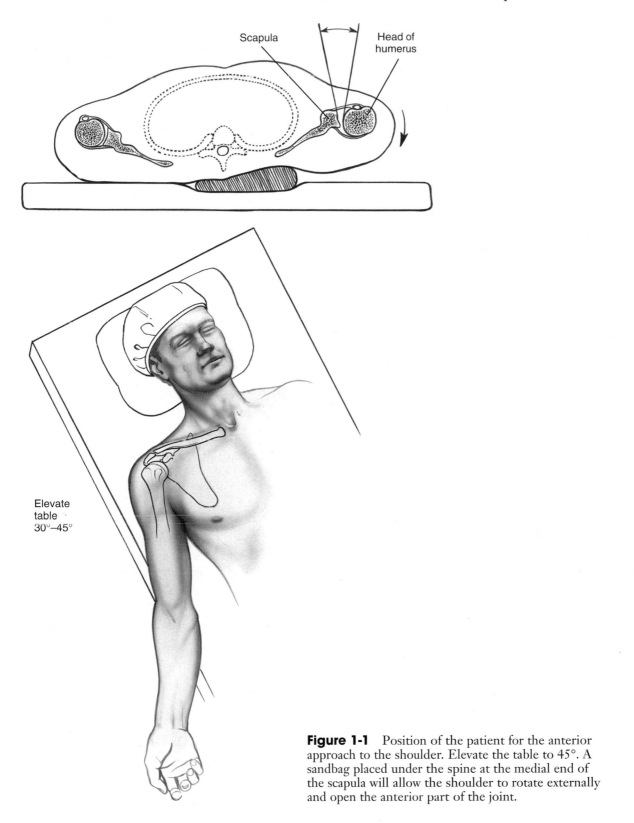

Scapula

Head of
humerus

Elevate
table
30°–45°

**Figure 1-1**  Position of the patient for the anterior
approach to the shoulder. Elevate the table to 45°. A
sandbag placed under the spine at the medial end of
the scapula will allow the shoulder to rotate externally
and open the anterior part of the joint.

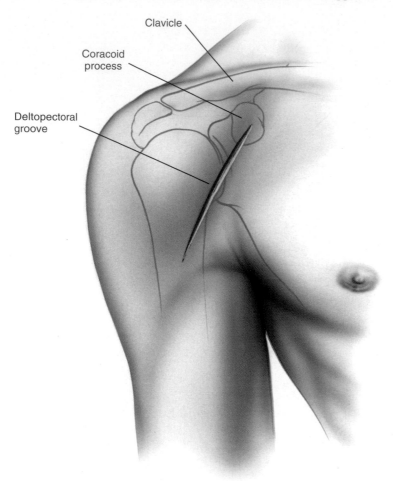

Clavicle

Coracoid
process

Deltopectoral
groove

**Figure 1-2**  Make a straight incision in the deltopectoral groove, starting at the level of the coracoid process.

***Axillary Incision.*** With the patient supine, abduct the shoulder 90° and rotate it externally. Mark the anterior axillary skin fold with a sterile pen. Make a vertical incision 8 to 10 cm long, starting at the midpoint of the anterior axillary fold and extending posteriorly into the axilla.[9] The skin flaps should be undermined extensively with a finger, especially superiorly in the area of the deltopectoral groove, using the cephalic vein as a guide to ensure correct position in the vertical plane. Retract the skin flaps upward and laterally so that the incision comes to lie over the deltopectoral groove (Figs. 1-3 and 1-4).

The axillary incision has a significant cosmetic advantage over the anterior incision, both because it is hidden in the axilla and because the resulting scar is covered by hair. In addition, the suture line remains free from tension while it heals; thus, the scar has little opportunity to spread. The only situation in which this incision may be contraindicated is when, in extremely muscular patients, the skin flaps cannot be moved enough to allow adequate exposure of the muscular structures that lie in front of the shoulder. If adequate exposure cannot be obtained through the axillary incision, it should be extended superiorly into the deltopectoral groove.

## Internervous Plane

The internervous plane lies between the deltoid muscle, which is supplied by the axillary nerve, and the pectoralis major muscle, which is supplied by the medial and lateral pectoral nerves (Fig. 1-5).

## Superficial Surgical Dissection

Find the deltopectoral groove, with its cephalic vein (Fig. 1-6). Retract the pectoralis major medially and the deltoid laterally, splitting the two muscles apart. The vein may be retracted either medially or laterally. Taking a small cuff of deltoid with the vein may reduce the number of bleeding tributaries that require ligation, but it leaves a small amount of denervated muscle. For that reason, it is not recommended as a routine practice.

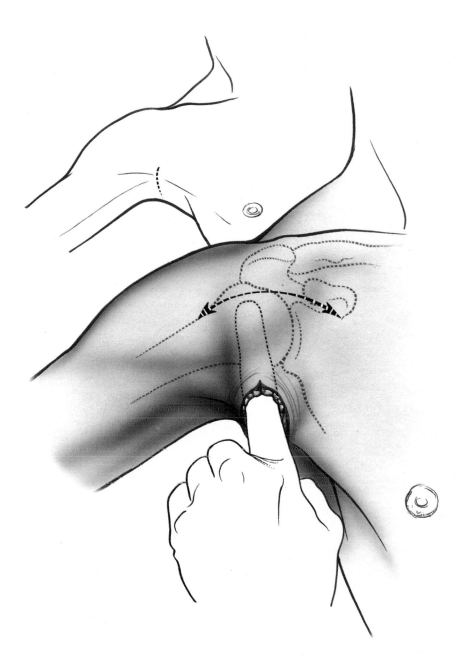

**Figure 1-3** Make an incision in the axilla. Dissect subcutaneously to mobilize skin.

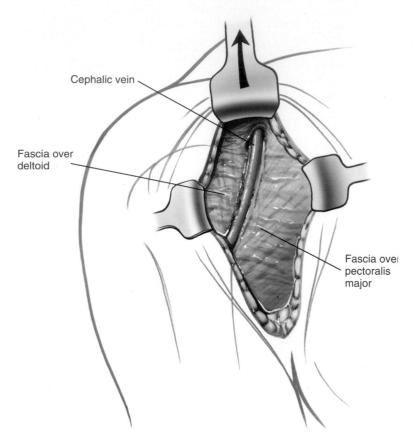

Cephalic vein

Fascia over deltoid

Fascia over pectoralis major

**Figure 1-4**   Retract the axillary incision cephalad to expose the cephalic vein and the deltopectoral groove.

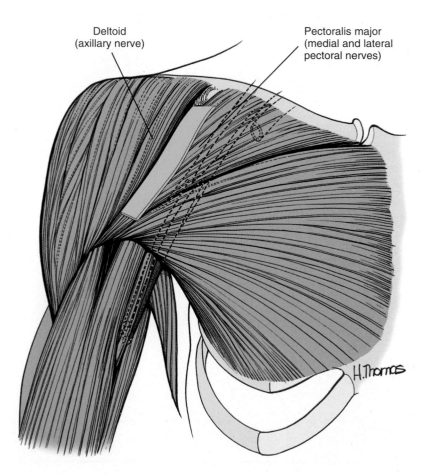

Deltoid (axillary nerve)

Pectoralis major (medial and lateral pectoral nerves)

H. Thomas

**Figure 1-5**   The internervous plane lies between the deltoid muscle (axillary nerve) and the pectoralis major muscle (medial and lateral pectoral nerves).

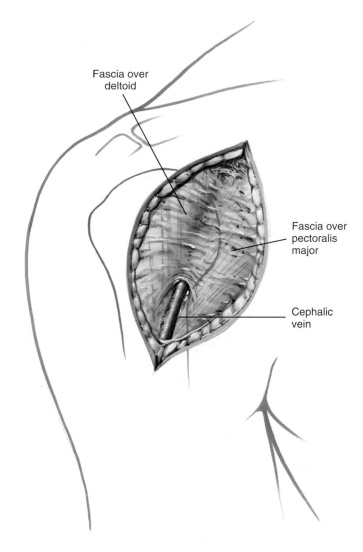

Fascia over deltoid

Fascia over pectoralis major

Cephalic vein

**Figure 1-6** Develop the groove between the fascia overlying the pectoralis major and the fascia overlying the deltoid. The cephalic vein will be of help in locating the groove.

## Deep Surgical Dissection

The short head of the biceps (which is supplied by the musculocutaneous nerve) and the coracobrachialis (which is supplied by the musculocutaneous nerve) must be displaced medially before access can be gained to the anterior aspect of the shoulder joint. Simple medial retraction after division of the overlying fascia may be enough for procedures such as the Magnuson-Stack subscapularis tendon advancement[3] or the Putti-Platt subscapularis[2] and capsule imbrication, but if more exposure is necessary, or if the coracoid process is to be transposed,[5] the two muscles can be detached with the tip of the coracoid process. To release them, detach the tip of the coracoid process with an osteotome. The bone can be replaced later either with a screw or with sutures. If a screw is used, the coracoid process must be drilled and tapped before the osteotomy is carried out. Otherwise, the small piece of coracoid may split during drilling, and anatomic reduction can be obtained only with extreme difficulty (Figs. 1-7 and 1-8).

The axillary artery is surrounded by the cords of the brachial plexus, which lie behind the pectoralis minor muscle. Abduction of the arm causes these neurovascular structures to become tight and brings them close to the tip of the coracoid and the operative site. Therefore, the arm should be kept adducted while work is being done around the coracoid process (Fig. 1-9).[1]

Retract the coracoid (with its attached muscles) medially. Divide the fascia that fans out from the conjoined tendons of the coracobrachialis and the short head of the biceps on the lateral side of the coracobrachialis—the safe side of the muscle, because the musculocutaneous nerve enters the coracobrachialis on its medial side. Use care in retracting the coracoid with its attached muscles; overzealous downward retraction can cause a neurapraxia of the musculocutaneous nerve. If the coracoid process is left intact, the attached coracoid muscles protect the nerve from traction injury (Fig. 1-10).

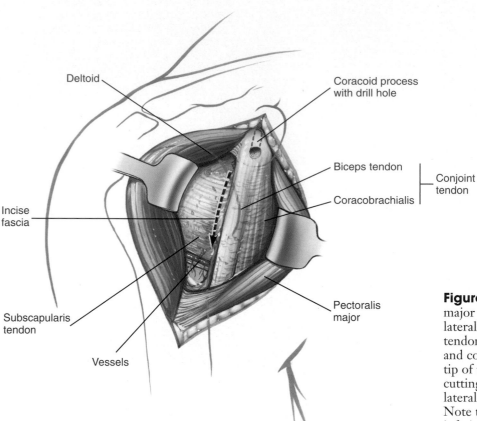

Deltoid

Coracoid process
with drill hole

Biceps tendon ⎫
                 ⎬ Conjoint
Coracobrachialis ⎭ tendon

Incise
fascia

Subscapularis
tendon

Vessels

Pectoralis
major

**Figure 1-7**   Retract the pectoralis major medially and the deltoid laterally to expose the conjoined tendon of the short head of the biceps and coracobrachialis muscle. Drill the tip of the coracoid process before cutting it. Incise the fascia on the lateral aspect of the conjoint tendon. Note the leash of vessels at the inferior end of the subscapularis muscle.

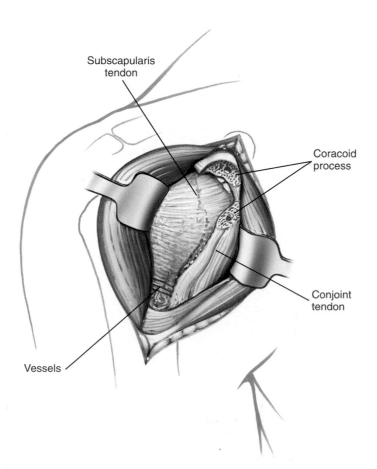

Subscapularis
tendon

Coracoid
process

Conjoint
tendon

Vessels

**Figure 1-8**   Cut through the predrilled coracoid process. Retract the conjoint tendon medially to give greater exposure to the subscapularis tendon.

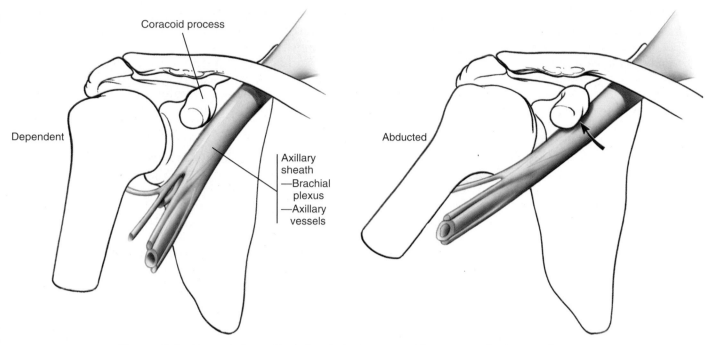

**Figure 1-9** Protect the axillary sheath during coracoid osteotomy by having the arm in the dependent position; abduction of the arm will draw the sheath against the coracoid process.

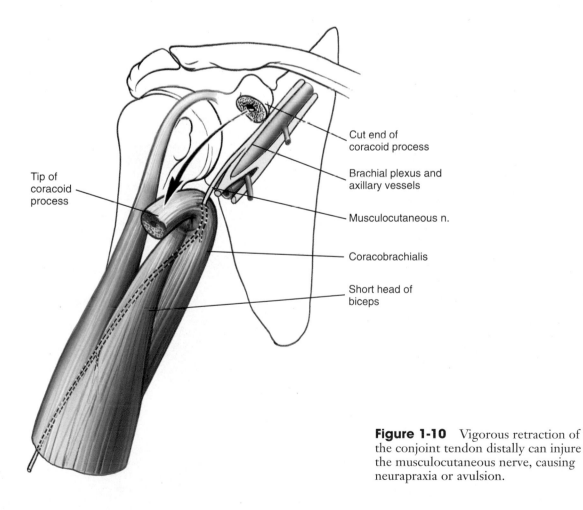

**Figure 1-10** Vigorous retraction of the conjoint tendon distally can injure the musculocutaneous nerve, causing neurapraxia or avulsion.

Beneath the conjoined tendons of the coraco-brachialis and the short head of the biceps lie the transversely running fibers of the subscapularis muscle, which forms the only remaining anterior covering of the shoulder joint capsule (Fig. 1-11).[1] As the muscle crosses the glenoid cavity, a bursa separates it from the joint capsule; that bursa may communicate with the shoulder joint. In cases of multiple anterior dislocations, adhesions often exist between the muscle and the joint capsule, making it difficult, if not impossible, to find the layer between the two. Apply external rotation to the arm to stretch the subscapularis, bringing the muscle belly into the wound and making its superior and inferior borders easier to define. External rotation of the humerus also increases the distance between the subscapularis and the axillary nerve as it disappears below the lower border of the muscle (see Fig. 1-11).

The most easily identified landmarks on the inferior border of the subscapularis are a series of small vessels that run transversely and often require ligation or cauterization. The vessels run as a triad: a small artery with its two surrounding venae comitantes, one above and one below the artery (Fig. 1-12). The superior border of the subscapularis muscle is indistinct and blends in with the fibers of the supraspinatus muscle.

Pass a blunt instrument between the capsule and the subscapularis, moving upward (see Fig. 1-12). Tag the muscle belly with stay sutures to prevent it from disappearing medially when it is cut and to allow easy reattachment of the muscle to its new insertion onto the humerus. Then divide the subscapularis 1 in. from its insertion onto the lesser tuberosity of the humerus (Fig. 1-13). Note that some of its muscle fibers insert onto the joint capsule itself; the capsule frequently may be opened inadvertently when the muscle is divided, because the two layers cannot always be defined.

Alternatively, rotate the shoulder internally and identify the insertion of the tendon of the subscapularis onto the humerus. Detach this insertion with a small flake of bone using a fine osteotome. This will allow more lateral reattachment of the muscle in a prepared channel in the bone, using staples.

Incise the capsule longitudinally to enter the joint wherever the selected repair must be performed. Each type of repair has its own specific location for incision (Fig. 1-14).

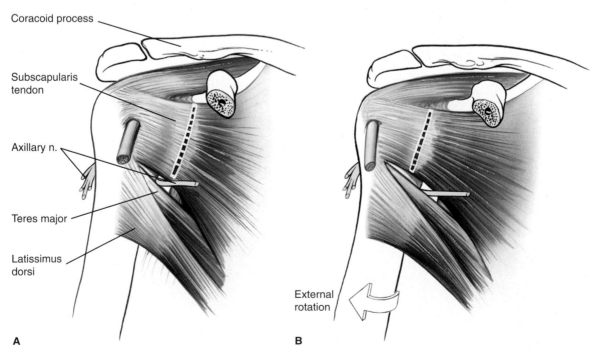

Coracoid process

Subscapularis tendon

Axillary n.

Teres major

Latissimus dorsi

External rotation

A

B

**Figure 1-11**  **(A)** The subscapularis muscle lies in the deep part of the wound. It is to be incised perpendicular to its fibers, close to its tendon. The axillary nerve passes anteroposteriorly through the quadrangular space. **(B)** External rotation of the arm during incision into the subscapularis tendon will draw the point of incision away from the axillary nerve.

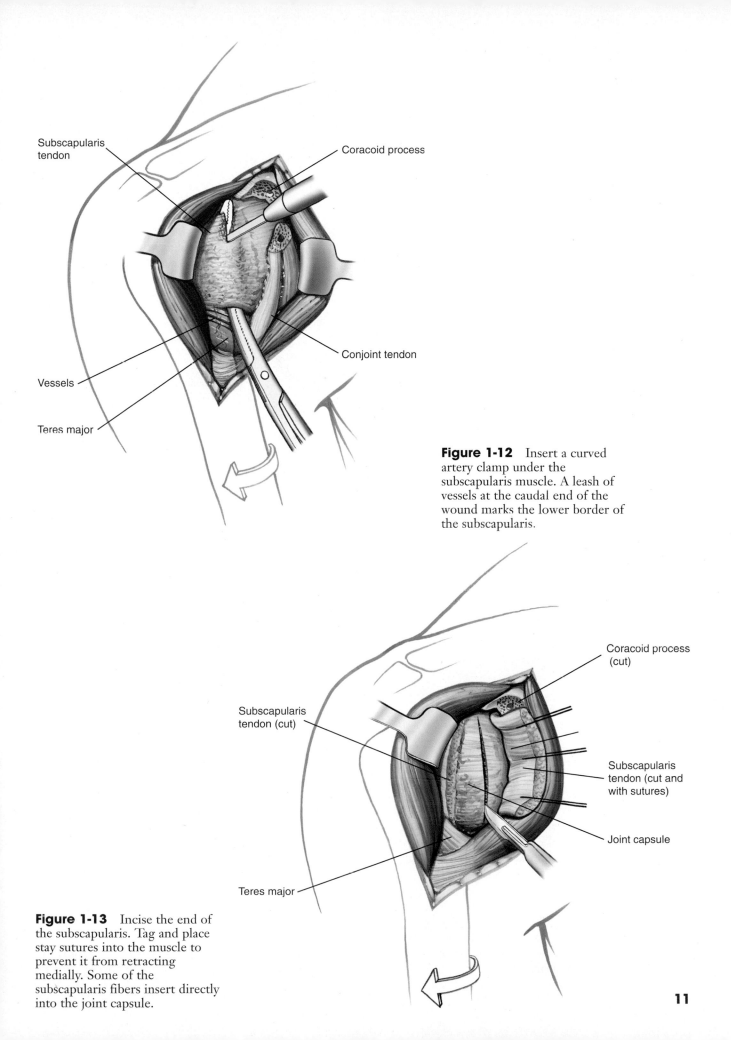

Subscapularis tendon

Coracoid process

Subscapularis tendon

Vessels

Teres major

Conjoint tendon

**Figure 1-12** Insert a curved artery clamp under the subscapularis muscle. A leash of vessels at the caudal end of the wound marks the lower border of the subscapularis.

Coracoid process (cut)

Subscapularis tendon (cut)

Subscapularis tendon (cut and with sutures)

Joint capsule

Teres major

**Figure 1-13** Incise the end of the subscapularis. Tag and place stay sutures into the muscle to prevent it from retracting medially. Some of the subscapularis fibers insert directly into the joint capsule.

**11**

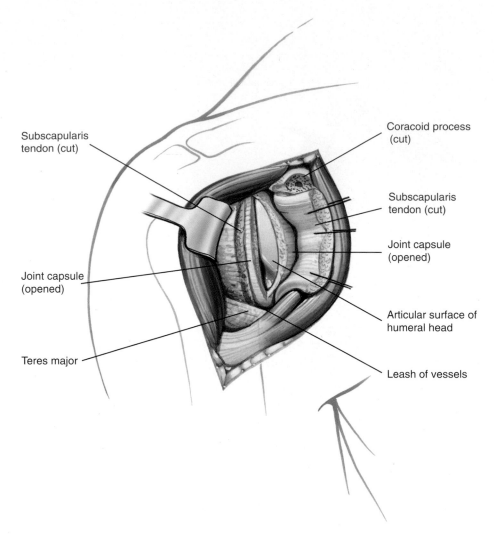

**Figure 1-14** Incise the joint capsule longitudinally to expose the humeral head and the glenoid cavity.

## Dangers

### Nerves

The **musculocutaneous nerve** enters the body of the coracobrachialis about 5 to 8 cm distal to the muscle's origin at the coracoid process. Because the nerve enters the muscle from its medial side, all dissection must remain on the lateral side of the muscle. Great care should be taken not to retract the muscle inferiorly, to avoid stretching the nerve and causing paralysis of the elbow flexors (see Fig. 1-10).

### Vessels

The **cephalic vein** should be preserved, if possible, although ligation leads to few problems. A traumatized cephalic vein should be ligated to prevent the slight danger of thromboembolism.

## How to Enlarge the Approach

### Local Measures

The exposure can be enlarged in the following four ways:

1. Extend the skin incision superiorly by curving it laterally along the lower border of the clavicle. Detach the deltoid from its origin on the outer surface of the clavicle for 2 to 4 cm to permit better lateral retraction of the muscle (Fig. 1-15). Unfortunately, because reattaching the deltoid may be difficult, this maneuver is not recommended for routine use. If further deltoid retraction is required, it may be best to detach part of the muscle's insertion onto the humerus.

2. Lengthen the skin incision inferiorly along the deltopectoral groove to separate the pectoralis major

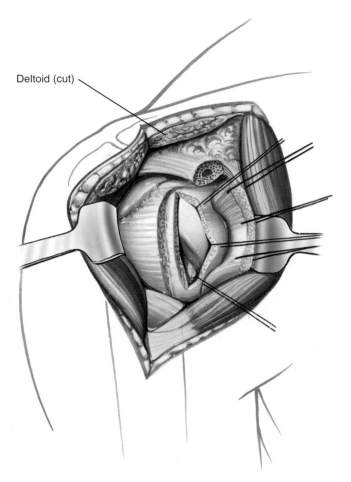

Deltoid (cut)

**Figure 1-15**   Remove the origins of the deltoid from the anterior portion of the clavicle to expose the joint further proximally. Identify the coracoacromial ligament.

from the deltoid further inferiorly and to improve the exposure without having to detach the deltoid origin.

3. Use a suitable retractor (such as the Bankart skid) for the humeral head. A humeral head retractor is the key to excellent exposure of the inside of the glenoid fossa once the joint has been opened (Fig. 1-16).

4. Rotate the shoulder internally and externally to bring different elements of the anterior shoulder coverings into view.

## Extensile Measures

*Proximal Extension.* To expose the brachial plexus and axillary artery, and to gain control of arterial bleeding from the axillary artery, extend the skin incision superomedially, crossing the middle third of the clavicle. Next, dissect the middle third of the

clavicle subperiosteally and perform osteotomy of the bone, removing the middle third. Cut the subclavius muscle, which runs transversely under the clavicle. Retract the trapezius superiorly and the pectoralis major and pectoralis minor inferiorly to reveal the underlying axillary artery and the surrounding brachial plexus (Fig. 1-17). Take care not to damage the musculocutaneous nerve, which is the most superficial nerve in the brachial plexus.

*Distal Extension.* The approach can be extended into an anterolateral approach to the humerus.

Extend the skin incision down the deltopectoral groove, then curve it inferiorly, following the lateral border of the biceps. Deep dissection consists of moving the biceps brachii medially to reveal the underlying brachialis, which then can be split along the line of its fibers to provide access to the humerus. For details of this approach, see Chapter 2.

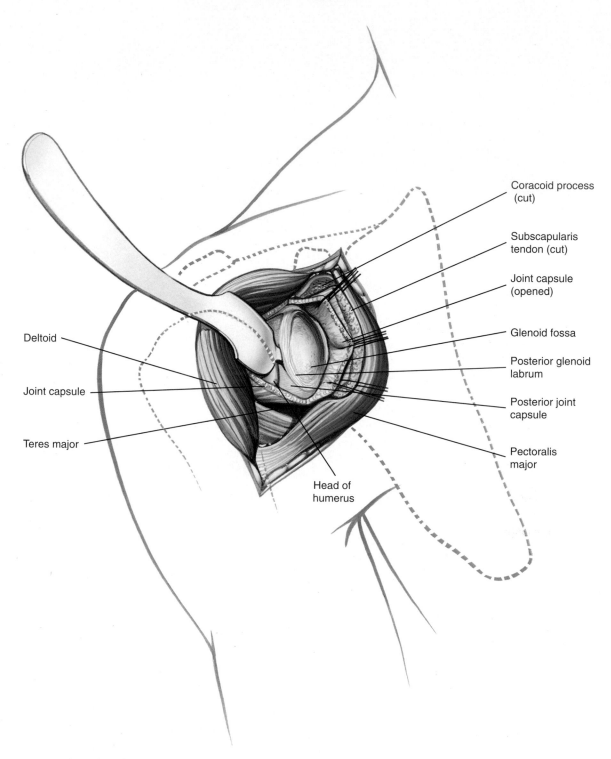

Coracoid process (cut)

Subscapularis tendon (cut)

Joint capsule (opened)

Glenoid fossa

Posterior glenoid labrum

Posterior joint capsule

Pectoralis major

Deltoid

Joint capsule

Teres major

Head of humerus

**Figure 1-16**   A Bankart skid is used to retract the humeral head to expose the glenoid cavity and its labrum.

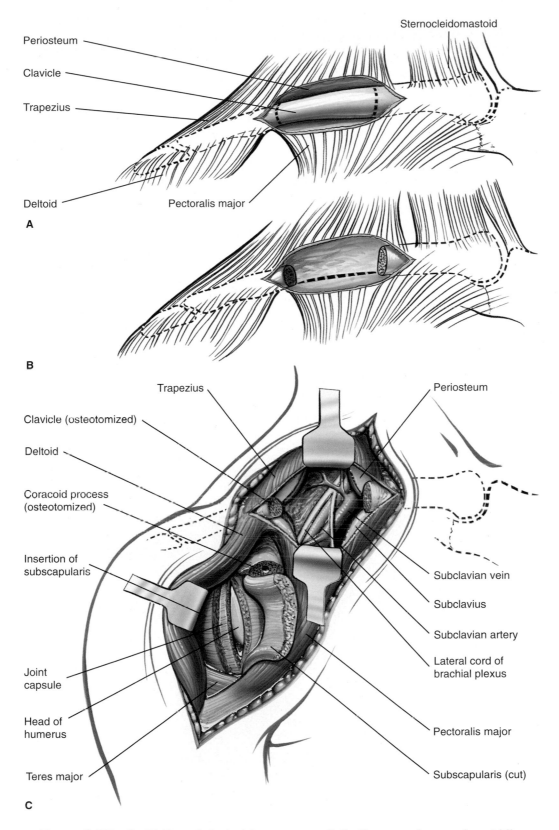

**Figure 1-17** **(A, B)** Extend the incision superomedially. Expose and resect the middle third of the clavicle subperiosteally. **(C)** Expose the brachial plexus and axillary artery.

# Applied Surgical Anatomy of the Anterior Approach

## Overview

All approaches to the shoulder involve penetrating the two muscular coverings, or sleeves, over the joint. The outer sleeve is the deltoid muscle. The inner sleeve is the rotator cuff, which consists of four muscles: the supraspinatus, infraspinatus, teres minor, and subscapularis (Fig. 1-18).

Anteriorly, gaining access to the shoulder joint involves reflecting the outer sleeve laterally and incising the inner sleeve, specifically the subscapularis.

The deltoid, together with the pectoralis major and the latissimus dorsi (the two great muscles of the axillary fold), supplies most of the power that is required for shoulder movement. The muscles of the inner sleeve all can act as prime movers of the humerus, but their most important action is to control the humeral head within the glenoid cavity while the other muscles are carrying out major movements.

The supraspinatus has a key role as a prime mover of the humerus in initiating abduction. The teres minor and infraspinatus muscles are the only important external rotators of the shoulder. Pathology of this joint nearly always is associated with this inner group of muscles; their function is critical not only to the coordination of joint movement, but also to the stability of the shoulder joint itself. Degenerative lesions of the rotator cuff are common.

A third group of muscles intervenes between the two muscular sleeves when the joint is approached from the front. These muscles (the short head of the

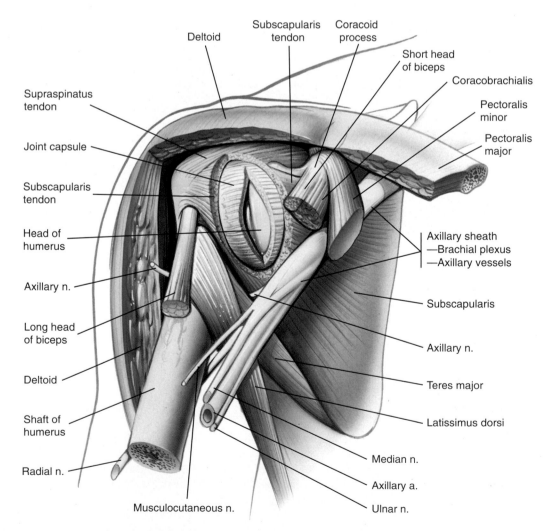

**Figure 1-18** Anatomy of the anterior portion of the shoulder.

biceps, the coracobrachialis, and the pectoralis minor) require medial retraction for exposure of the inner sleeve. They all are attached to the coracoid process (see Fig. 1-18).

## Landmarks and Incision

### Landmarks

The *coracoid process of the scapula* is an accessible bony protuberance that lies at the upper end of the deltopectoral groove and is the landmark for incisions based on that groove. It also is a critical landmark for injections and arthroscopic examinations of the shoulder joint. Hook shaped, the coracoid process sometimes is described as resembling a crow's beak, as is implied by its name, corax. The tip of the coracoid process projects forward, laterally, and inferiorly toward the glenoid cavity. Therefore, it is palpated best by posterior and medial pressure. Be aware that palpation of the coracoid process often is painful; therefore, tenderness over this site is not diagnostic of local pathology. Attached to the coracoid process are the five clinically important structures described below (Fig. 1-19).

*Coracoacromial Ligament.* The tough, fibrous coracoacromial ligament is triangular and connects the horizontal portion of the coracoid process to the tip of the acromion. It is one of the few ligaments that connects two parts of the same bone. The coracoid process, the acromion, and the coracoacromial ligament form the coracoacromial arch.

*Conoid and Trapezoid Ligaments.* The conoid and trapezoid ligaments are extremely strong. The conoid ligament, which resembles an inverted cone, extends upward from the upper surface of the knuckle of the coracoid process to the undersurface of the clavicle. The trapezoid ligament runs from the upper surface of the coracoid process and extends superiorly and laterally to the trapezoid ridge on the undersurface of the clavicle. These two structures are the main accessory ligaments of the acromioclavicular joint. They are extremely difficult to repair in cases of acromioclavicular dislocation and, once they are torn, are difficult to identify as individual structures. This structure may be implicated in the pathology of the impingement syndrome. The function of the coracoacromial ligament is unclear. Resection of the coracoacromial ligament, which is frequently carried out in subacromial decompression, does not appear to be associated with significant long-term clinical problems.

*Conjoined Tendons of the Coracobrachialis and Biceps Brachii.* See Figure 1-22.

*Pectoralis Minor Muscle.* See Applied Surgical Anatomy of the Anterior Approach in this chapter.

### Incision

Because a skin incision that runs down the deltopectoral groove cuts almost transversely across the cleavage lines of the skin, it often leaves a broad and ugly scar. An incision in the axilla runs with the cleavage line of the skin and leaves a much more narrow

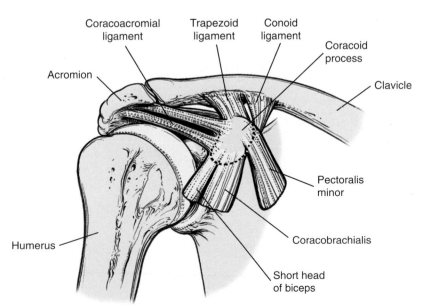

**Figure 1-19** Five clinically important structures are attached to the coracoid process.

scar. The latter scar is almost invisible, because it is hidden in the axillary fold and is covered by hair.

## Superficial Surgical Dissection

Three major structures are involved in the superficial surgical dissection of the anterior approach to the shoulder joint: the deltoid muscle laterally, the pectoralis major muscle medially, and the cephalic vein, which lies between them in the deltopectoral groove (Fig. 1-20).

### Deltoid Muscle

The anterior fibers of the deltoid muscle run parallel to each other, without fibrous septa between them. Because sutures placed in this kind of muscle fiber tend to tear out, it is difficult to reattach the deltoid to the clavicle. Sutures must be placed through the full thickness of the muscle, including its fascial coverings, to effect a strong reattachment. The attach-ment should be protected from active stress for 4 weeks to allow for adequate healing.

The anterior portion of the deltoid can be dener-vated only if the entire anterior part of the muscle is stripped and retracted vigorously in a lateral direc-tion (Fig. 1-21).

### Pectoralis Major Muscle

The two nerve supplies of the pectoralis major allow the muscle to be split without the loss of innervation to either part, making possible muscle transfers such as the Clark procedure, in which the distal part of the muscle is separated from the proximal part and is inserted into the biceps tendon in the arm (see Fig. 1-21).[10]

### Cephalic Vein

The cephalic vein drains into the axillary vein after passing through the clavipectoral fascia. On occasion, it may be absent. Few complications result from its ligation (see Fig. 1-20).

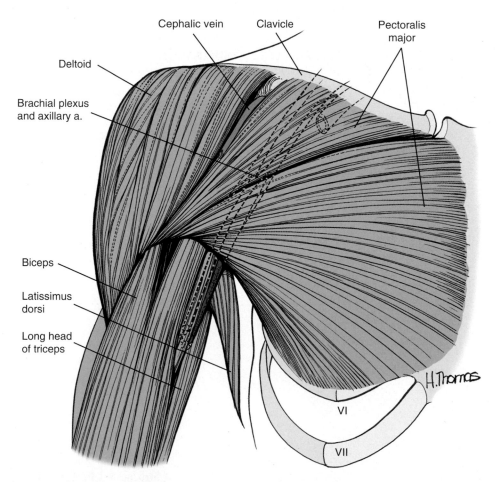

**Figure 1-20** The superficial anatomy of the anterior shoulder, revealing the deltopectoral groove and the neurovascular bundle.

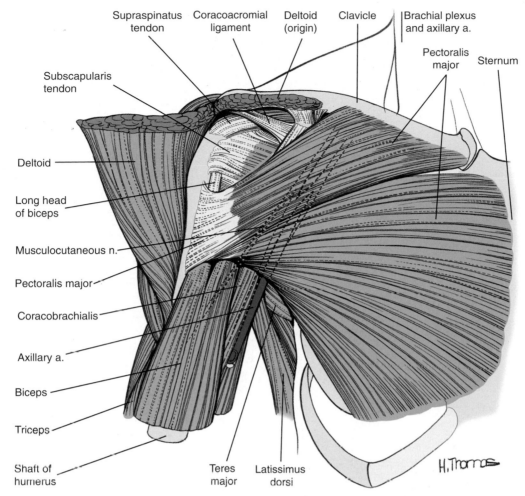

Subscapularis tendon

Supraspinatus tendon

Coracoacromial ligament

Deltoid (origin)

Clavicle

Brachial plexus and axillary a.

Pectoralis major

Sternum

Deltoid

Long head of biceps

Musculocutaneous n.

Pectoralis major

Coracobrachialis

Axillary a.

Biceps

Triceps

Shaft of humerus

Teres major

Latissimus dorsi

H. Thomas

**Figure 1-21** The anterior portion of the deltoid has been resected from its origin, revealing the insertion of the pectoralis major muscle and the subscapularis tendon, supraspinatus tendon, and coracoacromial ligament.

## Deep Surgical Dissection

The coracobrachialis and the short head of the biceps brachii share a common origin from the tip of the coracoid process. They also share a common nerve supply, the musculocutaneous nerve. These muscles form an intermediate layer during the surgical approach (Fig. 1-22).

### Coracobrachialis Muscle

The coracobrachialis muscle is largely vestigial and has little function. Extremely variable in size, it is the counterpart in the arm of the adductors in the thigh.

The coracobrachialis used to have three heads of origin. The musculocutaneous nerve passes between two of the original heads, which now are fused during development. Its course represents one of the few instances in which a nerve appears to pass through a

muscle. When a nerve does this, it always is passing between two heads of origin (see Fig. 1-22).

### Biceps Brachii Muscle

The tendon of the long head of the biceps is an anatomic curiosity; it is one of only two tendons to pass through a synovial cavity. The joint capsule of the shoulder is incomplete inferiorly, so the tendon can escape under the transverse ligament. From there, it runs in the bicipital groove of the humerus. It is easy to palpate the tendon in the groove as long as the arm is rotated externally (see Fig. 1-24). The biceps tendon is a common site of inflammatory changes, partly because it is capable of tremendous excursion, moving some 6 cm between full abduction and full adduction of the shoulder. This continual movement may produce attrition between the ten-

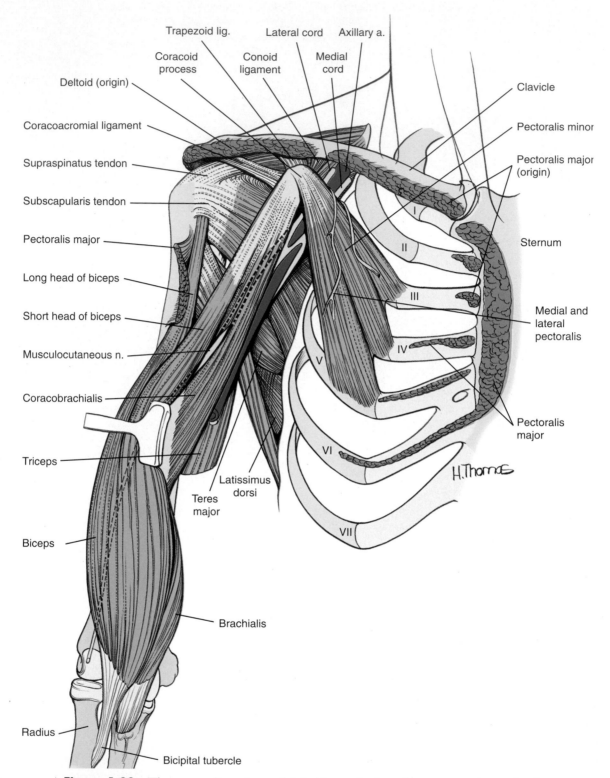

**Figure 1-22**    The pectoralis major and deltoid muscles have been removed completely, revealing the two heads of the biceps tendon, the rotator cuff, the coracoacromial ligament, and the neurovascular bundle.

don and the bicipital groove. The tendon also may rupture, producing a characteristic change in the contour of the muscle.

The biceps can slip medially out of the bicipital groove. This dislocation usually is painful,[11] although it sometimes is found during postmortem examinations of individuals who have had no known shoulder symptomatology.[12]

Considerable variability exists in the depth of the bicipital groove and in the angle that its medial wall makes with its floor.[13] Shallow grooves with flat medial walls may be predisposed to such tendon dislocation. Nevertheless, the transverse humeral ligament (retinaculum), which is the chief stabilizer for the tendon, must be ruptured before the tendon can be displaced.

## Pectoralis Minor Muscle

The only surgical importance of the pectoralis minor muscle lies in its neurovascular relations. The second part of the axillary artery and the cords of the brachial plexus lie directly behind the muscle and below the coracoid process (see Fig. 1-22).

## Subscapularis Muscle

The deep layer of the dissection is formed by the subscapularis muscle, which covers the shoulder joint capsule.

The subscapularis, which is the anterior portion of the rotator cuff, inserts partly into the capsule of the joint. The muscle tendon undergoes degeneration in the same way as do other muscles of the rotator cuff, but to a lesser extent. The problem rarely is severe or symptomatic, because there are other internal rotators of the shoulder and the loss of subscapularis action is not functionally disabling. The subscapularis may be stretched in cases of anterior dislocations of the shoulder or it may be contracted as a result of previous surgery.[13]

The subscapularis limits external rotation, helping to prevent anterior dislocations; it also may block anterior dislocation physically because of its size and its position in front of the shoulder joint. Because the two subscapular nerves enter the subscapularis medially, incising it 2.5 cm from its insertion does not denervate the muscle (Fig. 1-23).

Superiorly, the muscle is connected intimately to the supraspinatus. The plane of cleavage between the two muscles, which represents a true internervous plane between the suprascapular and subscapular nerves, may be difficult to define, especially near the insertions of the muscles. The tendon of the long head of the biceps corresponds to the interval between the muscles and can be used as a surgical guideline to that interval.

## Shoulder Joint Capsule

The shoulder joint has an enormous range of motion. The capsule is loose and redundant, particularly inferiorly and anteriorly. The area of the fibrous capsule itself is about twice the surface area of the humeral head (see Fig. 1-23). Anteriorly, the capsule is attached to the scapula via the border of the glenoid labrum and the bone next to it. The anterior part of the capsule usually has a small gap that allows the synovial lining of the joint to communicate with the bursa underlying the subscapularis.[14,15] This bursa extends across the front of the neck of the scapula toward the coracoid process (Fig. 1-24; see Fig. 1-36).

Posteriorly and inferiorly, the capsule is attached to the border of the labrum. A second gap may exist at this point to allow communication between the synovial lining of the joint and the infraspinatus bursa.

The fibrous capsule inserts into the humerus around the articular margins of the neck, except inferiorly, where the insertion is 1 cm below the articular margin. The capsule bridges the gap across the bicipital groove, forming a structure known as the transverse ligament. The long head of the biceps enters the joint beneath this ligament (see Fig. 1-24).

The shoulder joint capsule receives reinforcement from all four muscles of the rotator cuff. Further reinforcement is provided by the three glenohumeral ligaments, which appear as thickenings in the capsule. These ligaments are extremely difficult to identify during open surgery, but are usually obvious in arthroscopic procedures. They appear to be of no clinical relevance (see Figs. 1-70A and 1-72A).

## Synovial Lining of the Shoulder Joint

The synovial membrane, which is attached around the glenoid labrum, lines the capsule of the joint. The membrane usually communicates with the subscapularis bursa and, occasionally, with the infraspinatus bursa (see Figs. 1-24 and 1-36). It envelopes the tendon of the long head of the biceps within the shoulder joint. The synovium forms a tubular sleeve that permits the tendon to glide back and forth during abduction and adduction of the arm. Therefore, the tendon is anatomically intracapsular, but extrasynovial (Fig. 1-25; see Fig. 1-36).

## Glenoid Labrum

The glenoid labrum is a triangular, fibrocartilaginous structure that rings the glenoid cavity (see Fig. 1-25). The joint capsule attaches to it superiorly, inferiorly, and posteriorly. Anteriorly, the attachment depends on the presence or absence of the synovial recess running across the scapular neck (subscapularis

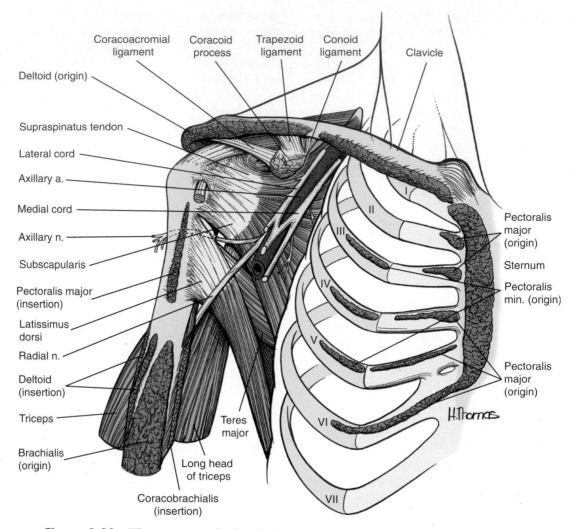

Coracoacromial ligament    Coracoid process    Trapezoid ligament    Conoid ligament    Clavicle

Deltoid (origin)

Supraspinatus tendon

Lateral cord

Axillary a.

Medial cord

Axillary n.

Subscapularis

Pectoralis major (insertion)

Latissimus dorsi

Radial n.

Deltoid (insertion)

Triceps

Brachialis (origin)

Teres major

Long head of triceps

Coracobrachialis (insertion)

Pectoralis major (origin)

Sternum

Pectoralis min. (origin)

Pectoralis major (origin)

H. Thomas

**Figure 1-23**    The neurovascular bundle lying on the subscapularis is revealed. The axillary nerve exists through the quadrangular space, and the radial nerve exists through the triangular space.

**Deltoid.** *Origin.* Anterior border of lateral third of clavicle. Outer border of acromion and inferior lip of crest of scapular spine. *Insertion.* Deltoid tubercle of humerus. *Action.* Abduction of shoulder. Anterior fibers act as flexors of shoulder; posterior fibers act as extensors of shoulder. *Nerve supply.* Axillary nerve.

**Pectoralis Major.** *Origin.* From two heads. Clavicular head: from medial half of clavicle. Sternocostal head: from manubrium and body of sternum, upper six costal cartilages, and aponeurosis of external oblique. *Insertion.* Lateral lip of bicipital groove of humerus. *Action.* Adduction of arm. *Nerve supply.* Medial and lateral pectoral nerves. (A separate branch of the lateral pectoral groove supplies the clavicular fibers.)

**Coracobrachialis.** *Origin.* Tip of coracoid process. *Insertion.* Middle of medial border of humerus. *Action.* Weak flexor of arm and weak adductor of arm. *Nerve supply.* Musculocutaneous nerve.

**Biceps Brachii.** *Origin.* Short head from tip of coracoid process. Long head from supraglenoid tubercle of scapula. *Insertion.* Bicipital tuberosity of radius. *Action.* Flexor of elbow. Supinator of forearm. Weak flexor of shoulder. *Nerve supply.* Musculocutaneous nerve.

**Pectoralis Minor.** *Origin.* Outer borders of third, fourth, fifth, and sixth ribs. *Insertion.* Coracoid process of scapula. *Action.* Lowers lateral angle of scapula. Protracts scapula. *Nerve supply.* Medial pectoral nerve.

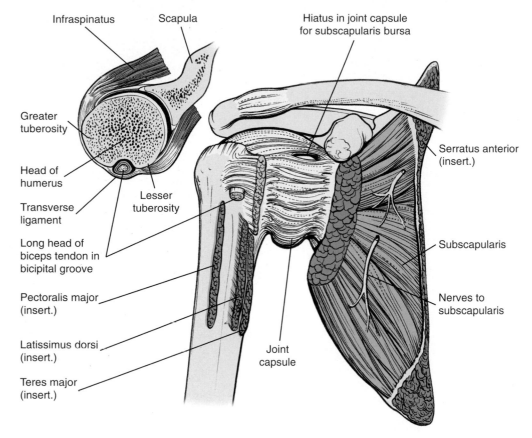

Figure 1-24 labels:

Infraspinatus

Scapula

Hiatus in joint capsule for subscapularis bursa

Greater tuberosity

Head of humerus

Transverse ligament

Lesser tuberosity

Long head of biceps tendon in bicipital groove

Pectoralis major (insert.)

Latissimus dorsi (insert.)

Teres major (insert.)

Joint capsule

Serratus anterior (insert.)

Subscapularis

Nerves to subscapularis

**Figure 1-24**  The fibrous joint capsule inserts into the humerus around the articular margin of the neck. Inspect inferiorly where it inserts below that articular margin. The capsule bridges the gap across the bicipital groove, forming a structure known as the transverse ligament.

**Subscapularis.** *Origin.* Medial four fifths of anterior surface of scapula. *Insertion.* Lesser tuberosity of humerus. *Action.* Internal rotator of humerus. *Nerve supply.* Upper and lower subscapularis nerves.

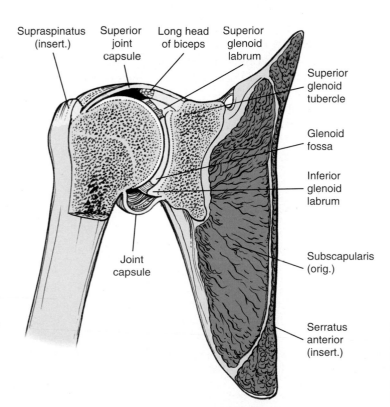

Figure 1-25 labels:

Supraspinatus (insert.)

Superior joint capsule

Long head of biceps

Superior glenoid labrum

Superior glenoid tubercle

Glenoid fossa

Inferior glenoid labrum

Joint capsule

Subscapularis (orig.)

Serratus anterior (insert.)

**Figure 1-25**  Cross section of the joint. The joint capsule is redundant inferiorly to allow abduction. The long head of the biceps tendon traverses the joint. The tendon is surrounded by synovium and, therefore, is anatomically intracapsular but extrasynovial.

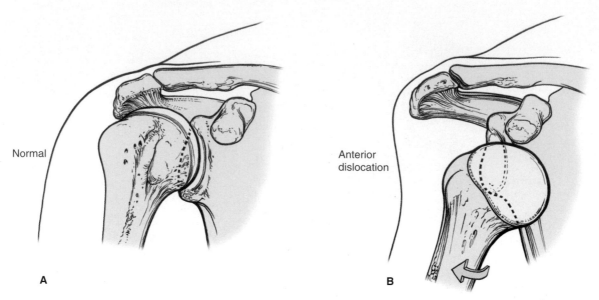

**Figure 1-26** **(A)** The normal relationship of the humerus to the glenoid cavity. **(B)** Anterior dislocation of the humerus.

bursa; see Fig. 1-36); the presence of the synovial recess leaves a gap in the attachment of the glenoid to the scapula (see Fig. 1-24).

It is the detachment of the glenoid labrum anteriorly that creates the Bankart lesion in cases of recurrent anterior dislocation of the shoulder (Fig. 1-26).

## Dangers

### Nerves

The **musculocutaneous nerve** is a branch of the lateral cord of the brachial plexus. It supplies the coracobrachialis, biceps brachii, and brachialis muscles, and terminates as the upper lateral cutaneous nerve of the forearm (see Figs. 1-10 and 1-22).

The nerve passes through the coracobrachialis, entering the muscle from its medial side about 8 cm

below the tip of the coracoid process. The nerve rarely is cut during surgery, but a neurapraxia resulting from excessive retraction can occur.

When the arm is abducted, the musculocutaneous nerve becomes the most superficial nerve structure in the axillary bundle. Therefore, it is the most common nerve structure to be injured in types of trauma such as fractures and fracture repairs of the clavicle. Damage to the nerve appears as a paralysis of the flexors of the elbow.

### Vessels

The **second part of the axillary artery** lies inferior to the coracoid process under cover of the pectoralis minor muscle. It may be damaged if the arm is not kept adducted while work is being performed on the coracoid process (see Figs. 1-9 and 1-23).

# Anterolateral Approach

The anterolateral approach to the shoulder offers excellent exposure of the acromioclavicular joint and the underlying coracoacromial ligament and supraspinatus tendon. Its uses include the following:

1. Anterior decompression of the shoulder[16]
2. Repair of the rotator cuff
3. Repair or stabilization of the long head of a biceps tendon

4. Excision of osteophytes from the acromioclavicular joint

The use of arthroscopic subacromial decompression has reduced the use of this approach in the treatment of impingement syndrome and for some cases of rotator cuff repair. The approach, however, remains clinically relevant in large numbers of cases involving extensive degenerative disease of the rotator cuff.

## Position of the Patient

Place the patient in the supine position on the operating table, with a sandbag under the spine and medial border of the scapula to push the affected side forward (see Fig. 1-1). Elevate the head of the table 45°. Apply surgical drapes in such a way that the limb can be moved easily during the operation. This allows different structures to be brought into view.

## Landmarks and Incision

### Landmarks

***Coracoid Process.*** Palpate the coracoid process 1 in. from the anterior end of the clavicle just inferior to the deepest point of the clavicular concavity.

***Acromion.*** Palpate the acromion at the shoulder summit.

### Incision

Make a transverse incision that begins at the anterolateral corner of the acromion and ends just lateral to the coracoid process (Fig. 1-27).

## Internervous Plane

No internervous plane is available for use. The deltoid muscle is detached at a point well proximal to its nerve supply, which, therefore, is not in danger.

## Superficial Surgical Dissection

Deepen the incision through the subcutaneous fat to the deep fascia. Numerous small vessels will be divided. Coagulate these meticulously to ensure adequate visualization of the deeper structures. Incise the deep fascia in the line of the skin incision (Fig. 1-28). Palpate the acromioclavicular joint. If the approach is to be used for a subacromial decom-

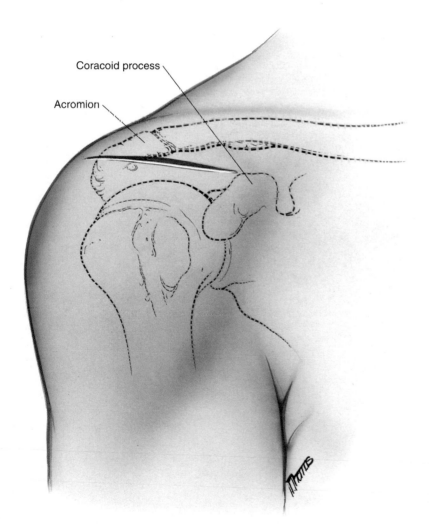

Coracoid process

Acromion

**Figure 1-27** Make a transverse incision beginning at the anterolateral corner of the acromion, ending just lateral to the coracoid process.

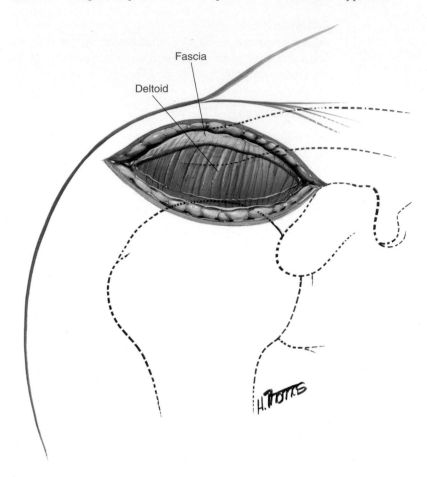

**Figure 1-28** Incise the deep fascia in the line of the skin incision to reveal the underlying deltoid muscle.

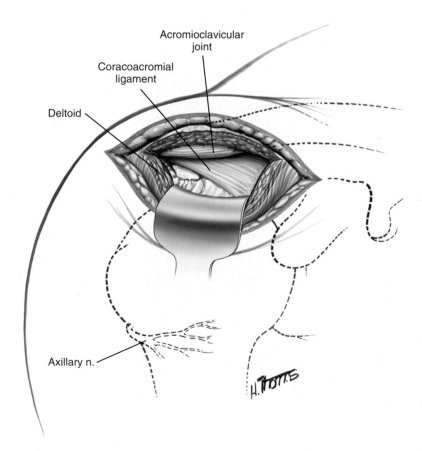

**Figure 1-29** Detach the deltoid from the acromioclavicular joint and 1 cm of the anterior aspect of the acromion.

pression and access to the rotator cuff is not required, detach the fibers of the deltoid that arise from the acromioclavicular joint and continue this detachment by sharp dissection laterally to expose 1 cm of the anterior aspect of the acromion (Fig. 1-29). Bleeding will be encountered during this dissection as a result of the division of the acromial branch of the coracoacromial artery. This must be coagulated. Do not detach more of the deltoid than is necessary because reattachment is difficult and extensive stripping of the deltoid from the acromion may be associated with poor long-term results of surgery.

If the approach is to be used for repairs of the rotator cuff, split the deltoid muscle in the line of its fibers starting at the acromioclavicular joint. Extend this split 5 cm down from the acromioclavicular joint (Fig. 1-30). Insert stay sutures in the apex of the split to prevent the muscle from splitting inadvertently further down during retraction and damaging the axillary nerve. Continue the dissection as for sub-

acromial decompression by detaching the fibers of the deltoid that arise from the acromioclavicular joint, and, as before, continue this detachment by sharp dissection laterally to expose 1 cm of the anterior aspect of the acromion. Retract the split edges of the deltoid muscle to reveal the underlying coracoacromial ligament.

## Deep Surgical Dissection

Detach the coracoacromial ligament from the acromion, either by sharp dissection or by removing it with a block of bone from the undersurface of the acromion. Detach the medial end of the coracoacromial ligament just proximal to the coracoid process and excise the ligament. The supraspinatus tendon with its overlying subacromial bursa now is revealed. Rotate the head of the humerus to expose different portions of the rotator cuff (Fig. 1-31). Full external rotation will reveal the long head of the biceps tendon in its groove.

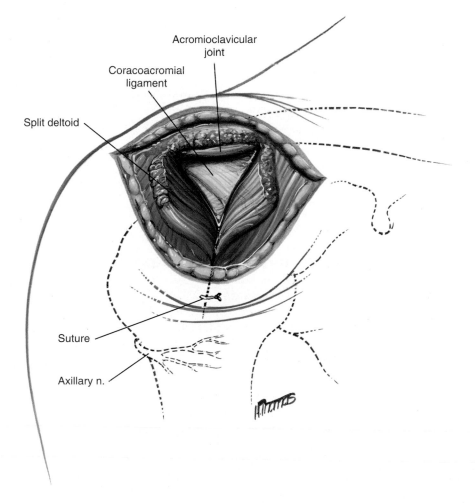

**Figure 1-30** Split the deltoid muscle in the line of its fibers for 5 cm.

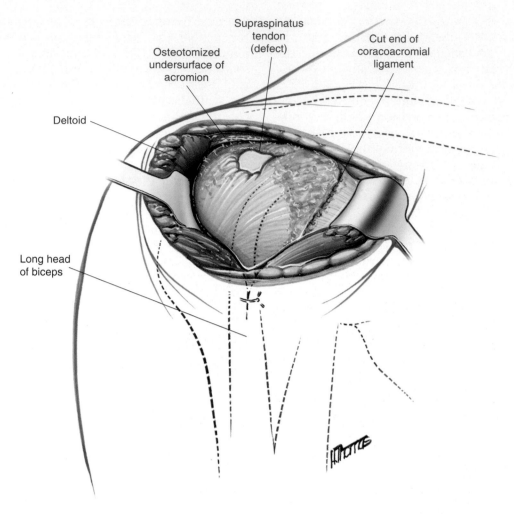

**Figure 1-31** Resect the coracoacromial ligament with a block of bone from the undersurface of the acromion to reveal the underlying subacromial bursa and supraspinatus tendon.

## Dangers

### Nerves
The **axillary nerve** runs transversely across the deep surface of the deltoid muscle about 7 cm below the tip of the acromion. Splitting the deltoid below this level may damage the nerve. Inserting the stay suture in the apex of the deltoid split will prevent this possibility.

### Vessels
The acromial branch of the coracoacromial artery that runs immediately under the deltoid muscle will be divided during the superficial surgical dissection. Unless bleeding from this site is controlled, it will be very difficult to identify deeper structures, which may cause inadvertent deviation from the proper surgical plane.

## How to Enlarge the Approach

### Local Measures
Because reattaching the deltoid to its insertion is so difficult, extensive detachment of this muscle is not recommended, even though it does facilitate the exposure.

### Extensile Measures
Because this approach does not operate in an internervous plane, no useful extensions, either proximal or distal, are possible.

## Lateral Approach

The lateral approach provides limited access to the head and surgical neck of the humerus. It is not a classically extensile approach, because it is limited distally by the traverse of the axillary nerve over the deep surfaces of the deltoid muscle. It can be extended usefully in a proximal direction to reveal the entire length of the supraspinatus muscle. Because the approach cannot be extended distally, its use in fracture surgery is reserved for fractures of the surgical neck and tuberosities of the humerus. Most distal fractures need to be approached through the anterior approach to the shoulder.

The uses of the lateral approach include the following:

1. Open reduction and internal fixation of displaced fractures of the greater tuberosity of the humerus
2. Open reduction and internal fixation of humeral neck fractures
3. Removal of calcific deposits from the subacromial bursa
4. Repair of the supraspinatus tendon
5. Repair of the rotator cuff

### Position of the Patient

Place the patient in a supine position, with the affected arm at the edge of the table. Elevate the head of the table to reduce venous pressure and operative bleeding (Fig. 1-32). A sandbag should be placed under the patient's shoulder.

### Landmarks and Incision

#### Landmark

The *acromion* is rectangular. Its bony dorsum and lateral border are easy to palpate on the outer aspect of the shoulder.

#### Incision

Make a 5-cm longitudinal incision from the tip of the acromion down the lateral aspect of the arm (Fig. 1-33).

### Internervous Plane

There is no true internervous plane; the lateral approach involves splitting the deltoid muscle.

### Superficial Surgical Dissection

Split the deltoid muscle in the line of its fibers from the acromion downward for 5 cm. Insert a suture at the inferior apex of the split to help prevent it from extending accidentally, with consequent axillary nerve damage, as the exposure is worked on (Figs. 1-34 and 1-35).

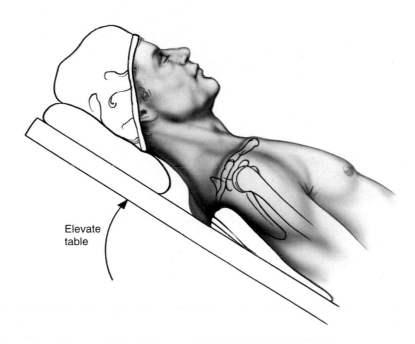

Elevate table

**Figure 1-32** Position of the patient on the operating table for the lateral approach to the shoulder. Elevate the table 45°. Place a sandbag under the shoulder to lift it off the operating table.

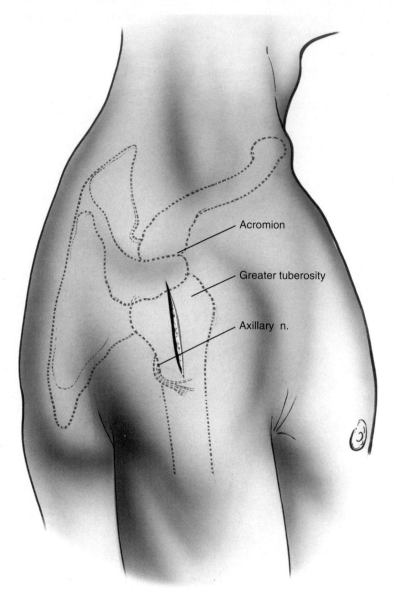

Acromion

Greater tuberosity

Axillary n.

**Figure 1-33**   Make a 5-cm longitudinal incision from the tip of the acromion down the lateral aspect of the arm.

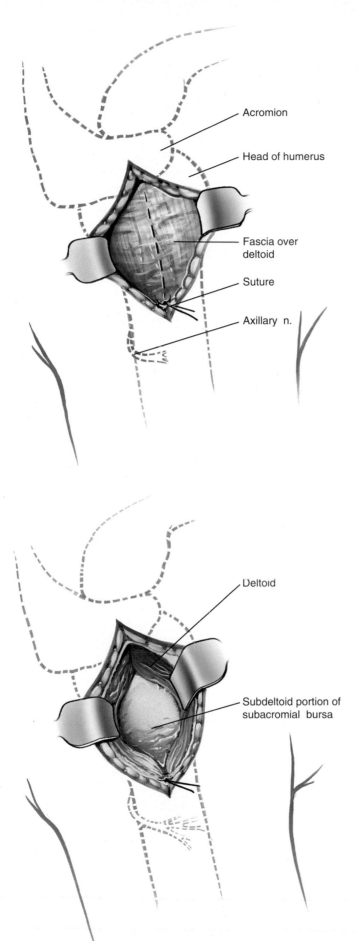

Acromion

Head of humerus

Fascia over
deltoid

Suture

Axillary n.

**Figure 1-34** Split the deltoid muscle in line with its
fibers and insert a stay suture at the inferior apex of
the split to prevent it from extending distally and
causing axillary nerve damage.

Deltoid

Subdeltoid portion of
subacromial bursa

**Figure 1-35** Expose the subdeltoid portion of the
subacromial bursa by retracting the deltoid muscle
anteriorly and posteriorly.

## Deep Surgical Dissection

The lateral aspect of the upper humerus and its attached rotator cuff lie directly under the deltoid muscle and the subacromial bursa (Fig. 1-36). In fractures of the neck of the humerus, the bare ends of bone usually appear at this point without further dissection.

Small tears of the supraspinatus muscle also can be reached through this approach. Most defects in the supraspinatus muscle are large, however. Some surgical procedures require that the whole supraspinatus be mobilized so that the muscle can be advanced and the tendon repaired (Fig. 1-37).

In the upper part of the wound, the exposed subacromial bursa must be incised longitudinally to provide access to the upper lateral portion of the head of the humerus (see Fig. 1-36).

## Dangers

### Nerves

The **axillary nerve** leaves the posterior wall of the axilla by penetrating the quadrangular space. Then it winds around the humerus with the posterior circumflex humeral arteries (see Figs. 1-34 and 1-39). The nerve enters the deltoid muscle posteriorly from its deep surface, about 7 cm below the tip of the acromion. From that point, its fibers spread anteriorly. Because of the nerve's course, the dissection cannot be extended farther in an inferior direction without denervating that portion of the deltoid muscle that is located anterior to the muscle split.

## How to Enlarge the Approach

### Extensile Measures

*Proximal Extension.* Extend the incision superiorly and medially across the acromion and parallel to the upper margin of the spine of the scapula, about 1 cm above it along the lateral two thirds of the scapular spine.[17]

Incise the trapezius muscle parallel to the spine of the scapula and about 1 cm above it. Retract the mus-

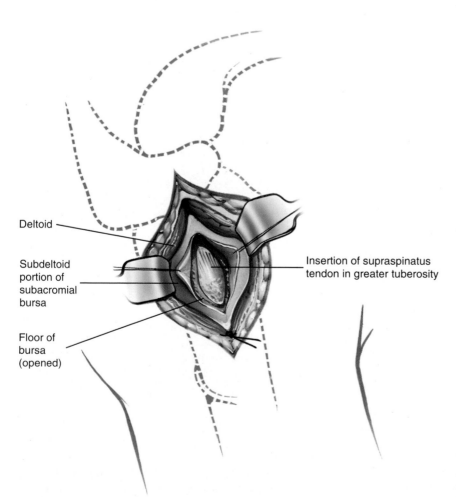

Deltoid

Subdeltoid portion of subacromial bursa

Floor of bursa (opened)

Insertion of supraspinatus tendon in greater tuberosity

**Figure 1-36**   Incise the bursa to reveal the insertion of the supraspinatus tendon into the greater tuberosity.

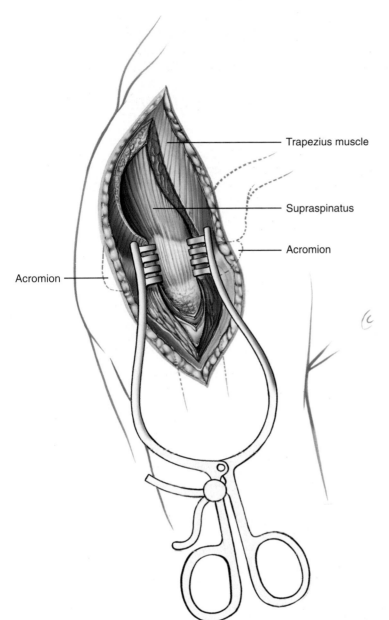

Trapezius muscle

Supraspinatus

Acromion

Acromion

**Figure 1-37** To expose the entire supraspinatus muscle, cut the acromion and split the trapezius muscle to reveal the underlying supraspinatus muscle belly and tendon. The entire muscle can be advanced and the tendon repaired.

cle superiorly to reveal the supraspinatus and its fascial covering.

Incise the fascia overlying the supraspinatus in the line of the skin incision to expose the muscle.

Split the acromion in the line of the skin incision, using an osteotome.

Retract the two parts of the acromion with a self-retaining retractor. The entire length of the supraspinatus, from its origin in the supraspinous fossa to its insertion onto the greater tuberosity of the humerus, now is exposed (Fig. 1-37; see Fig. 1-40). Take great care to reconstruct the divided acromion during closure.

# Applied Surgical Anatomy of the Anterolateral and Lateral Approaches

## Overview

Two muscular sleeves cover the lateral aspect of the shoulder joint: the outer sleeve consists of the lateral portion of the deltoid muscle, and the inner sleeve is the supraspinatus tendon (part of the rotator cuff) (Figs. 1-38 and 1-39).

## Landmarks and Incision

### Landmark

The **acromion,** which is the lateral continuation of the spine of the scapula, is the summit of the shoulder, overhanging the greater tuberosity of the humerus. Muscles either insert onto it or take origin

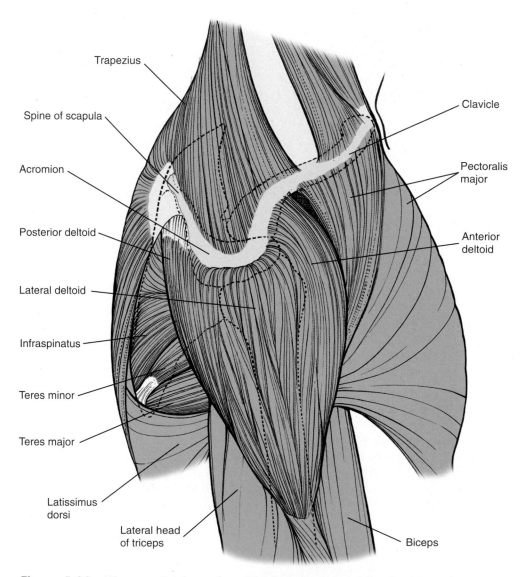

**Figure 1-38**    The superficial muscles of the lateral aspects of the shoulder. The muscles take origin from or insert into the acromion and the spine of the scapula, but do not cross them.

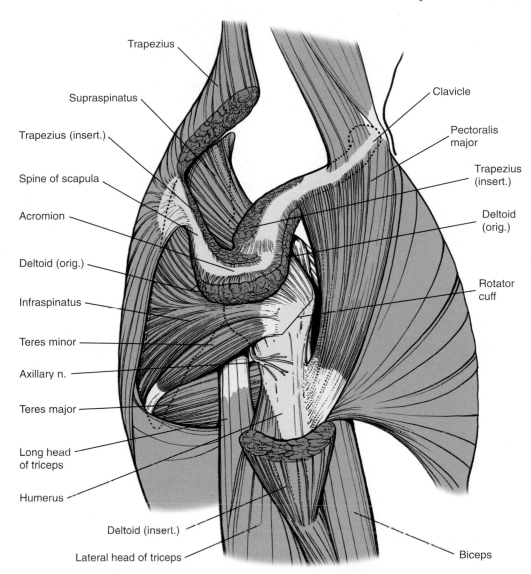

Trapezius

Supraspinatus

Trapezius (insert.)

Spine of scapula

Acromion

Deltoid (orig.)

Infraspinatus

Teres minor

Axillary n.

Teres major

Long head
of triceps

Humerus

Deltoid (insert.)

Lateral head of triceps

Clavicle

Pectoralis
major

Trapezius
(insert.)

Deltoid
(orig.)

Rotator
cuff

Biceps

**Figure 1-39** Portions of the deltoid and trapezius have been removed to reveal the underlying rotator cuff and the axillary nerve, usually beneath the teres minor in the quadrangular space.

from it, but no muscle crosses it. Thus, it is partially subcutaneous and can be palpated (see Fig. 1-38).

### Incision
Because the lateral skin incision crosses the lines of cleavage in the skin almost transversely, it is likely to leave a broad scar.

## Superficial Surgical Dissection

Superficial surgical dissection involves splitting the fibers of the deltoid muscle. Proximal extension of the approach to expose the supraspinatus involves

splitting the fibers of the trapezius muscle (see Fig. 1-37).

### Deltoid Muscle
The lateral approach affects the portion of the deltoid muscle that arises from the lateral border of the acromion. The lateral deltoid consists of oblique fibers arising in a multipennate fashion from tough tendinous bands that originate from the acromion. These bands actually mark the bone with a series of notches. Similar bands arise from the insertion of the muscle onto the humerus halfway down the lateral border; the muscle fibers arising from these

tendinous bands interdigitate in a herringbone pattern.

This multipennate arrangement provides the deltoid muscle with maximum strength, although it limits the degree to which it can contract. Nevertheless, despite the arrangement of the fibers, it is relatively easy to split the muscle in a longitudinal fashion. The tough tendinous bands also prevent excessive damage to the muscle when it is split during surgery (Fig. 1-40).

Whether the deltoid muscle should be detached from the acromion still is in question, because reattachment is difficult and often unsuccessful.[18] An acromial osteotomy and subsequent reattachment of the bone, with the muscle still attached to it, may be the best solution, although acromial nonunion may occur because the anterior and posterior portions of the deltoid tend to pull apart the site subjected to osteotomy.

### Trapezius Muscle

See the section regarding the posterior approach to the cervical spine.

### Axillary Nerve

See the sections regarding dangers in the lateral approach to the shoulder.

### Coracoid Branch of the Coracoacromial Artery

The coracoid branch of the coracoacromial artery is a tributary of the acromiothoracic artery, which arises from the second part of the axillary artery. Running immediately deep to the insertion of the deltoid muscle to the acromioclavicular joint, it is coagulated easily.

### Subacromial (Subdeltoid) Bursa

The subacromial bursa separates the two sleeves of muscle that cover the lateral aspect of the shoulder joint. It helps them glide past each other and protects the rotator cuff (the inner sleeve) from the hard overlying bone and ligamentous complex—the acromial process (acromion), the coracoacromial ligament (which spans the gap between the coracoid process and the acromion), and the coracoid process of the scapula. Because the bursa lies between the

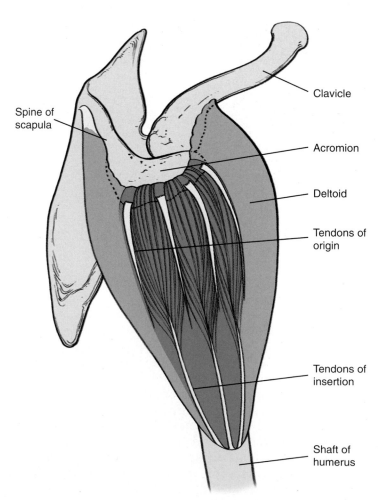

Spine of scapula

Clavicle

Acromion

Deltoid

Tendons of origin

Tendons of insertion

Shaft of humerus

**Figure 1-40**  The multipennate arrangement of the muscle fibers of the middle portion of the deltoid muscle.

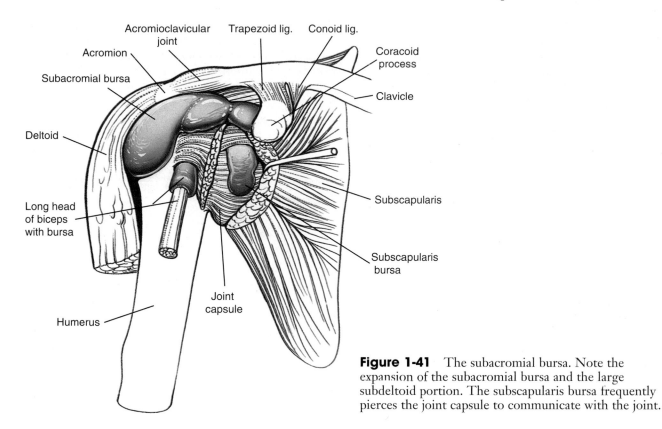

**Figure 1-41** The subacromial bursa. Note the expansion of the subacromial bursa and the large subdeltoid portion. The subscapularis bursa frequently pierces the joint capsule to communicate with the joint.

supraspinatus and deltoid muscles, and between the supraspinatus and coracoacromial ligaments, it is called both the subacromial bursa and the subdeltoid bursa (Figs. 1-41 and 1-42).

The bursa is a large structure, extending anteriorly from beneath the coracoid process. At this point, it provides lubrication between the conjoined tendons of the coracobrachialis and biceps brachii muscles, and the underlying subscapularis muscle.

The bursa ordinarily does not communicate with the shoulder joint. Rupture of the supraspinatus tendon, however, can cause the two synovial-lined cavities to join; an arthrogram of the shoulder can reveal this communication (Fig. 1-43).[19,20]

With the arm in the dependent position, the bursa lies under the deltoid muscle and the coracoacromial ligament. When the arm is abducted, the bursa retreats under the cover of this ligament. At this point, the patient feels pain if there is inflammation of the bursa, mainly because the bursa is compressed between the undersurface of the acromion and the humeral head (Fig. 1-44). Paradoxically, there is no tenderness on the lateral aspect of the shoulder in this position, because the bursa now is protected from palpation completely by the coracoacromial ligament. When the arm is

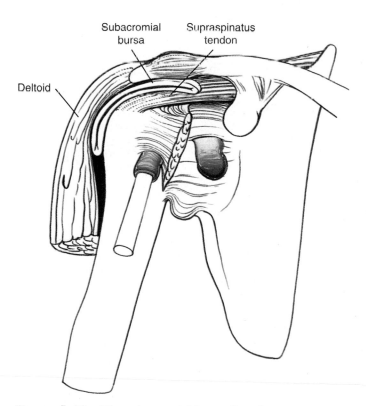

**Figure 1-42** The subacromial bursa directly protects the supraspinatus tendon from the bone and ligamentous complex that covers it.

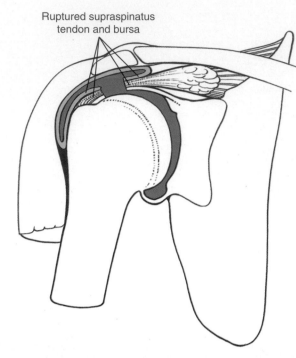

Ruptured supraspinatus
tendon and bursa

**Figure 1-43**    Rupture of the supraspinatus tendon allows direct communication between the joint and the subacromial bursa. An arthrogram of the shoulder will reveal this communication, helping to establish the diagnosis of a torn rotator cuff.

adducted again, the pain disappears, because the bursa no longer is compressed between the ligament and the supraspinatus. Tenderness on palpation may be elicited on the lateral aspect of the shoulder below the acromion, however, because the bursa now is accessible. Passive extension of the shoulder also brings the bursa out anteriorly from beneath the acromion and makes it palpable.

## Deep Surgical Dissection and Its Dangers

### Supraspinatus Muscle

The supraspinatus, which is a multipennate muscle, passes laterally beneath the coracoacromial ligament. The muscle is the frequent site of degenerative changes and frank tears. Degeneration in its tendon invokes an inflammatory response in the overlying subacromial bursa, and most cases of subacromial bursitis probably reflect pathology in the muscle.[21] The close relationship of the supraspinatus to the coracoacromial ligament may result in mechanical abrasion between the two structures during abduction of the arm, causing degeneration of the tendon. The subacromial bursa minimizes this tendency (see Figs. 1-42 and 1-46).

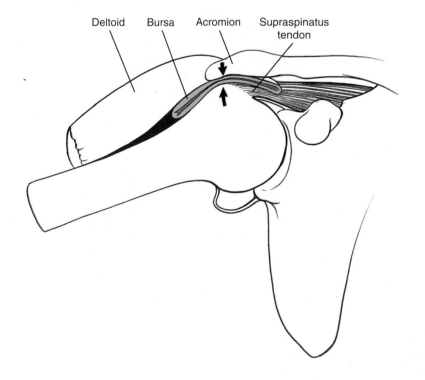

Deltoid    Bursa    Acromion    Supraspinatus
tendon

**Figure 1-44**    Abduction of the arm can impinge the subacromial bursa between the greater tuberosity and the undersurface of the acromion and coracoacromial ligament.

When the arm is by the patient's side, the supraspinatus tendon takes a 90° turn over the humeral head before its insertion, putting the blood supply to the tendon on a stretch. Vascular insufficiency may result, which is another possible cause of degenerative change.[22]

Regardless of the mechanism of degeneration, about one fourth of all individuals who reach 65 years of age rupture their supraspinatus tendon.[23] Patients with complete ruptures of the supraspinatus are unable to abduct their arms without adopting such trick movements as a shrug mechanism. If patients with a ruptured supraspinatus lower the affected arm slowly from the vertical, they lose control of it at about 30° and it drops suddenly to their side.

The suprascapular nerve is a branch of the upper trunk of the brachial plexus; it enters the muscle on its deep surface. Some methods of repairing tears of the supraspinatus tendon involve mobilizing the entire muscle belly and advancing it laterally to take tension off the suture line of the repair.[17] Take great care in mobilizing the supraspinatus muscle from its fossa, to avoid damaging its nerve (Fig. 1-45).

## Impingement Syndrome

Abduction of the arm may pinch the supraspinatus muscle between the head of the humerus and the arch created by the acromion and the coracoacromial ligament. The anatomy of the acromion varies considerably from individual to individual, and certain acromial shapes have been associated with an impingement syndrome. Performing an acromioplasty and cutting the coracoacromial ligament may provide relief in some patients with impingement syndrome. This procedure can be carried out by an open operation (see Anterolateral Approach to the Shoulder) or by arthroscopic techniques.

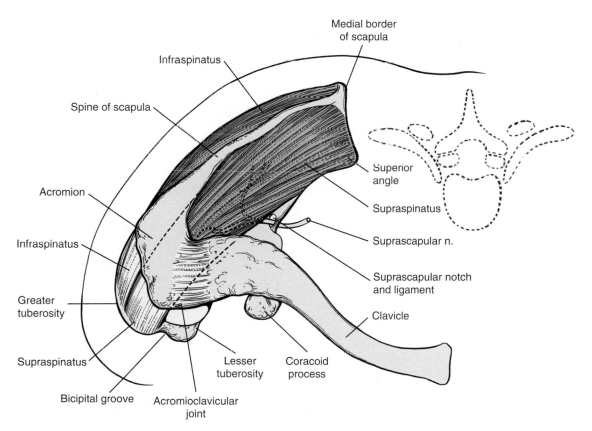

**Figure 1-45** Superior view of the shoulder, showing the rotator cuff and the acromioclavicular joint. The suprascapular nerve supplies the supraspinatus and infraspinatus muscles after passing through the suprascapular notch and ligament.

**Supraspinatus.** *Origin.* Medial three fourths of supraspinous fossa of scapula. *Insertion.* Upper facet of greater tuberosity of humerus. *Action.* Initiates abduction of shoulder. *Nerve supply.* Suprascapular nerve.

## Special Anatomic Points

The acromioclavicular joint is a synovial joint between the lateral end of the clavicle and the medial border of the acromion. The lateral end of the clavicle is higher than the acromion; the joint can be palpated by pushing medially against the thickness at the end of the clavicle.

The acromioclavicular joint contains a fibrocartilaginous meniscus, which usually is incomplete; the meniscus may be displaced during traumatic subluxation of the joint (Fig. 1-46B).

The two most common disease processes affecting the acromioclavicular joint are acromioclavicular dislocations and acromioclavicular arthritis. In cases of acromioclavicular dislocation, it is important to remember that the major accessory ligaments of the joint from the coracoid process to the undersurface of the clavicle are some distance from

it. They cannot be repaired, but they can, and should, be replaced if the joint is to be rendered stable. Acromioclavicular arthritis commonly is associated with the development of inferior osteophytes, which are a contributing factor to cases of impingement syndromes.

The joint is exposed easily by way of a superior approach because it is essentially subcutaneous. The insertions of the trapezius and deltoid muscles to the superior surface of the clavicle are confluent; however, the two muscles are separated easily by subperiosteal dissection (Fig. 1-47). In cases of acromioclavicular dislocation, however, this dissection will have been done for you and the distal end of the clavicle often lies in a subcutaneous position.

The joint may also be approached from its anterior surface (see Anterolateral Approach to the Shoulder).

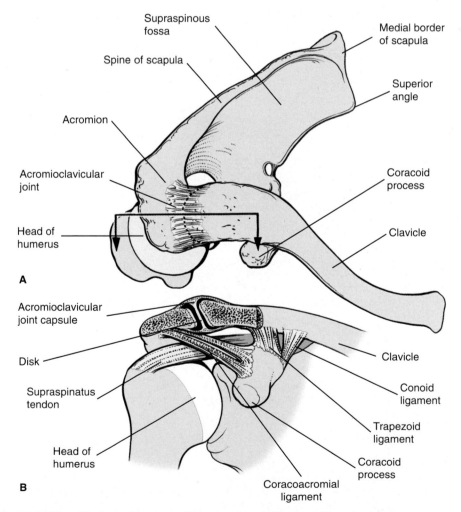

**Figure 1-46** **(A)** Superior view of the shoulder joint, revealing the bone structure and acromioclavicular joint capsule. **(B)** Cross section of anterior view of the shoulder, revealing the acromioclavicular joint and meniscus, as well as the supraspinatus tendon and its relationship to the coracoacromial ligament.

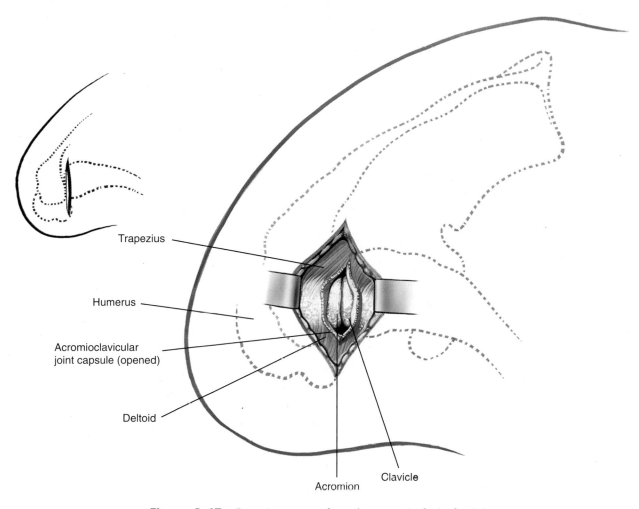

Trapezius

Humerus

Acromioclavicular
joint capsule (opened)

Deltoid

Clavicle

Acromion

**Figure 1-47** Superior approach to the acromioclavicular joint.

## Posterior Approach

The posterior approach offers access to the posterior and inferior aspects of the shoulder joint.[24] It rarely is needed, but can be used in the following instances:

1. Repairs in cases of recurrent posterior dislocation or subluxation of the shoulder[25,26]
2. Glenoid osteotomy[27]
3. Biopsy and excision of tumors
4. Removal of loose bodies in the posterior recess of the shoulder
5. Drainage of sepsis (the approach allows dependent drainage with the patient in the normal position in bed)
6. Treatment of fractures of the scapula neck, particularly those in association with fractured clavicles (floating shoulder)

7. Treatment of posterior fracture dislocations of the proximal humerus

### Position of the Patient

Place the patient in a lateral position on the edge of the operating table, with the affected side uppermost. Drape him or her to allow independent movement of the arm (Fig. 1-48). Stand behind the patient and take care that the ear is not folded accidentally under the head.

### Landmarks and Incision

#### Landmarks

The **acromion** and the **spine of the scapula** form one continuous arch. The spine of the scapula extends

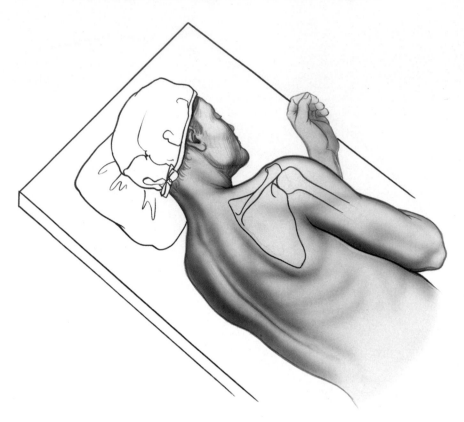

**Figure 1-48**  Position of the patient on the operating table for the posterior approach to the shoulder. Drape the involved arm to allow for independent motion.

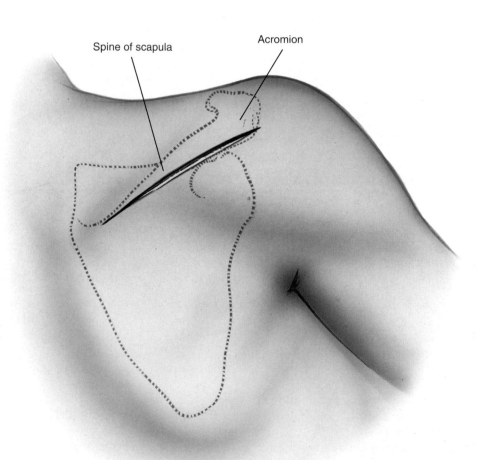

**Figure 1-49**  Make a linear incision over the entire length of the scapular spine, extending to the posterior corner of the acromion. You may choose to curve the medial end of the incision distally to enhance the exposure.

obliquely across the upper four fifths of the dorsum of the scapula and ends in a flat, smooth triangle at the medial border of the scapula. It is easy to palpate.

### Incision

Make a linear incision along the entire length of the scapular spine, extending to the posterior corner of the acromion (Fig. 1-49).

## Internervous Plane

The internervous plane lies between the teres minor muscle, which is supplied by the axillary nerve, and the infraspinatus muscle, which is supplied by the suprascapular nerve (Fig. 1-50).

## Superficial Surgical Dissection

Identify the origin of the deltoid on the scapular spine and detach the muscle from this origin. The plane between the deltoid muscle and the underlying infraspinatus muscle may be difficult to find, mainly because there is a tendency to look for it too close to bone and to end up stripping the infraspinatus off the scapula. The plane is easier to locate at the lateral end of the incision. Once it has been found, it is not difficult to develop if the deltoid is retracted inferiorly and the infraspinatus is exposed (Fig. 1-51). Note that the plane also is an internervous plane, because the deltoid is supplied by the axillary nerve and the infraspinatus is supplied by the suprascapular nerve.

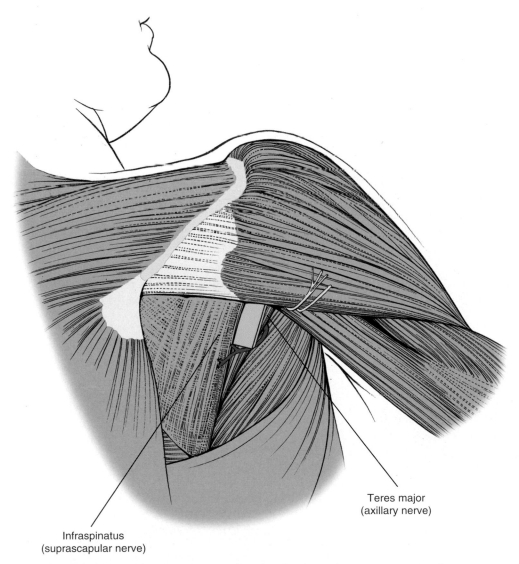

Infraspinatus
(suprascapular nerve)

Teres major
(axillary nerve)

**Figure 1-50** The internervous plane lies between the teres minor (axillary nerve) and the infraspinatus (suprascapular nerve).

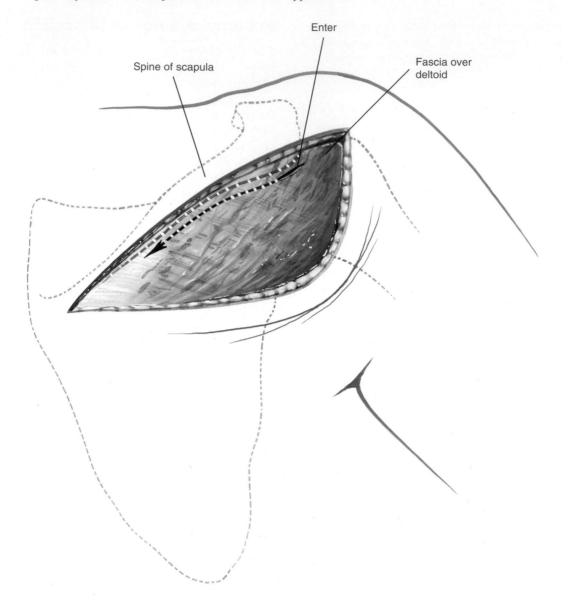

**Figure 1-51**  Identify the origin of the deltoid muscle, the spine of the scapula, and the attachment from its origin. Begin detaching the muscle from the lateral to the medial point.

## Deep Surgical Dissection

Identify the internervous plane between the infraspinatus and teres minor muscles, and develop it by blunt dissection, using a finger. This important plane is difficult to define (Fig. 1-52). Retract the infraspinatus superiorly and the teres minor inferiorly to reach the posterior regions of the glenoid cavity and the neck of the scapula (Fig. 1-53). The posteroinferior corner of the shoulder joint capsule now is exposed. To explore the joint, incise it longitudinally, close to the edge of the scapula (Figs. 1-54 and 1-55).

## Dangers

### Nerves

The **axillary nerve** runs through the quadrangular space beneath the teres minor. Because a dissection carried out inferior to the teres minor can damage

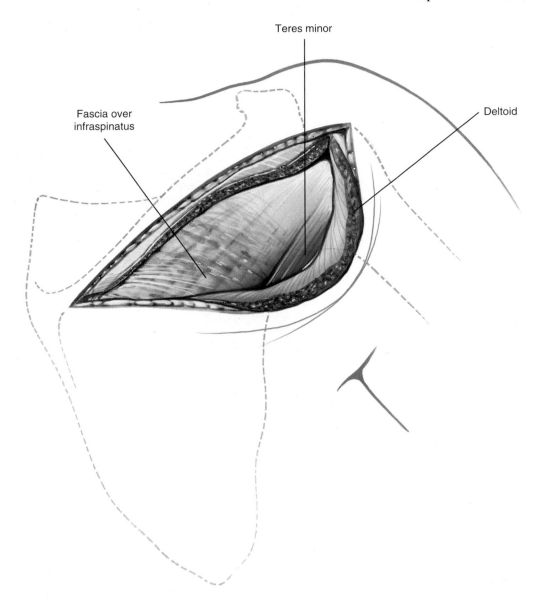

Teres minor

Fascia over
infraspinatus

Deltoid

**Figure 1-52**   Identify the internervous plane between the infraspinatus and teres minor. Note that it is difficult to define.

the axillary nerve, it is critical to identify the muscular interval between the infraspinatus and teres minor muscles, and to stay within that interval.

The **suprascapular nerve** passes around the base of the spine of the scapula as it runs from the supraspinous fossa to the infraspinous fossa. It is the nerve supply for both the supraspinatus and infraspinatus muscles. The infraspinatus must not be retracted forcefully too far medially during the approach because a neurapraxia may result from stretching the nerve around the unyielding lateral edge of the scapular spine (see Fig. 1-59).

**Vessels**

The **posterior circumflex humeral artery** runs with the axillary nerve in the quadrangular space beneath the inferior border of the teres minor muscle. Damage to this artery leads to hemorrhaging that is difficult to control. This danger can be avoided by staying in the correct intermuscular plane (see Fig. 1-58).

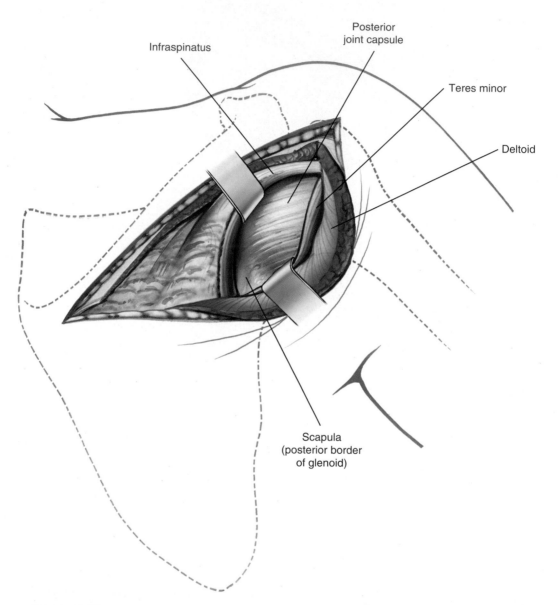

**Figure 1-53**    Retract the infraspinatus superiorly and the teres minor inferiorly to reach the posterior aspect of the joint capsule of the shoulder.

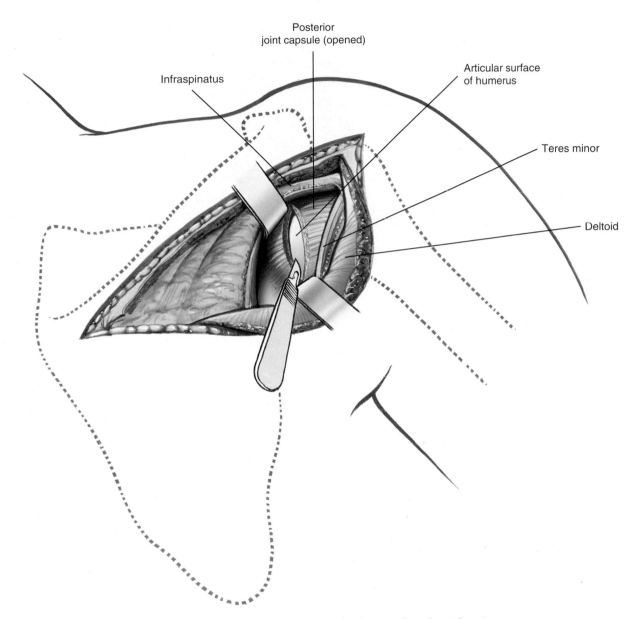

**Figure 1-54** Incise the joint capsule close to the glenoid cavity.

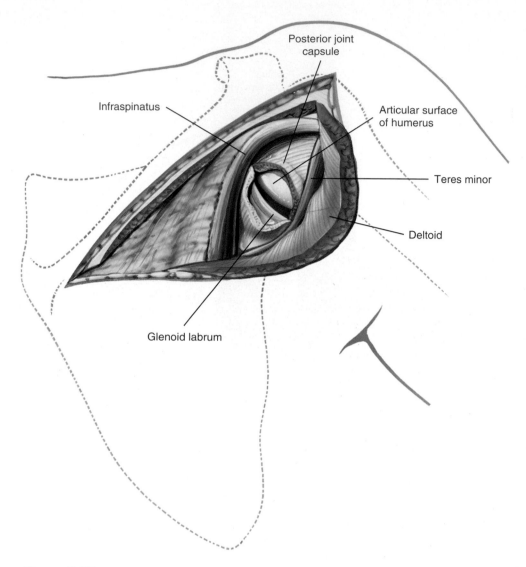

**Figure 1-55**    Retract the joint capsule to reveal the posterior regions of the glenoid cavity, the neck of the scapula, and the head of the humerus.

# How to Enlarge the Approach

## Local Measures

To gain better exposure of the deep layer of muscles, split the detached deltoid muscle at the lateral edge of the wound. To gain better access to the posterior aspect of the shoulder joint, detach the infraspinatus 1 cm from its insertion onto the greater tuberosity of the humerus. Retract the muscle medially, taking care not to damage the suprascapular nerve, which enters the undersurface of the muscle just below the spine of the scapula. Such an exposure is necessary for correct placement of a posterior bone block (Fig. 1-56).

## Extensile Measures

The incision cannot be extended usefully. Its sole function is to provide access to the posterior aspect of the shoulder joint.

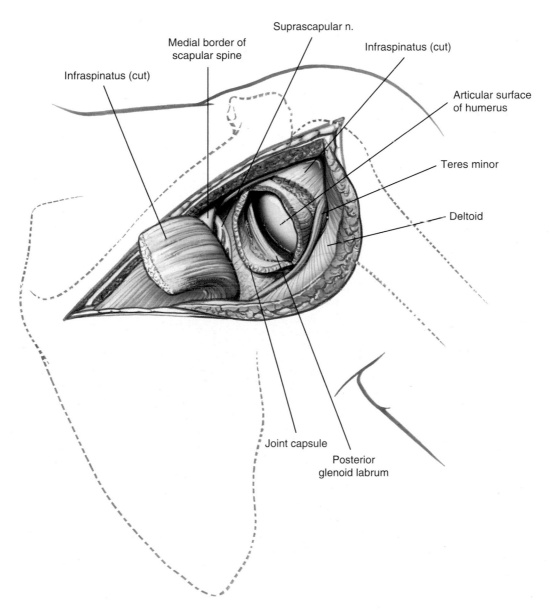

**Figure 1-56**  To gain greater exposure of the joint, cut the infraspinatus muscle close to its attachment to the humerus and retract it medially. Be careful to retract the muscle gently to avoid stretching the suprascapular nerve, which enters the muscle on its undersurface.

# Applied Surgical Anatomy of the Posterior Approach

## Overview

The posterior aspect of the shoulder, similar to the anterior and lateral aspects, is covered by two muscular sleeves. The posterior part of the deltoid muscle forms the outer sleeve of muscle, as it does for all other approaches to the shoulder joint. The inner sleeve consists of two muscles of the rotator cuff, the infraspinatus and the teres minor (Figs. 1-57 and 1-58).

## Landmark and Incision

### Landmark

The *spine of the scapula* is a thick, bony ridge projecting from the back of the blade of the scapula. Its base runs almost horizontally, and its free lateral border curves forward to form the acromion. The spine separates the supraspinous fossa from the infraspinous fossa. The trapezius muscle inserts into it from

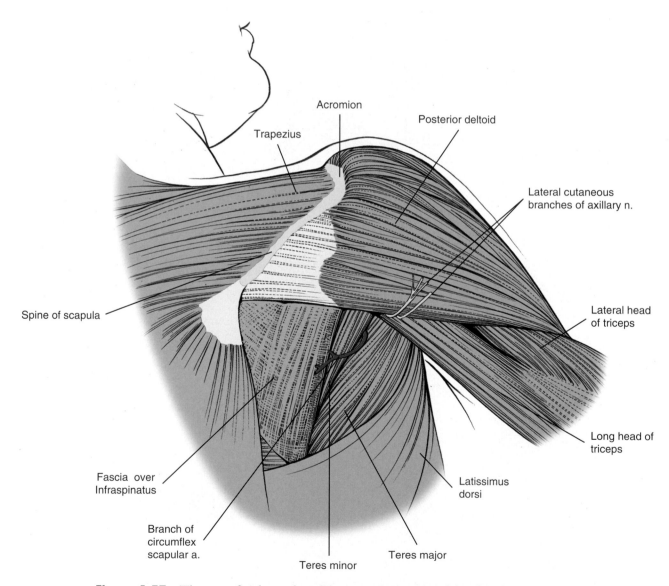

**Figure 1-57**   The superficial muscles of the posterior aspect of the shoulder. The posterior portion of the deltoid as it takes origin from the spine of the scapula is aponeurotic, and the plane between it and the underlying infraspinatus is difficult to identify.

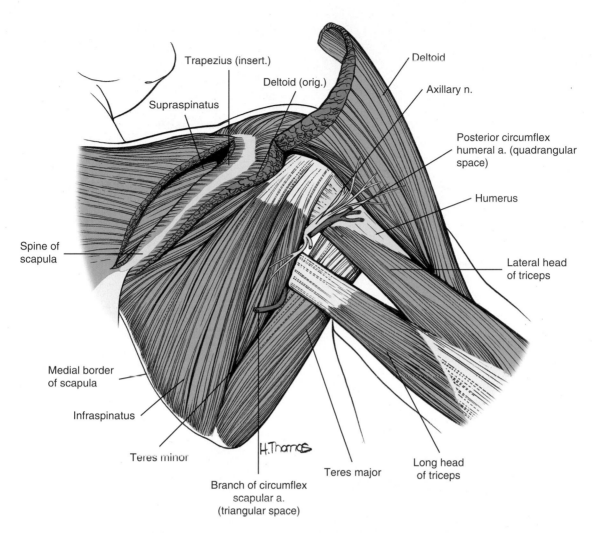

**Figure 1-58** The posterior portion of the deltoid is detached from the spine of the scapula, revealing the infraspinatus, teres minor, and teres major muscles, as well as the long and lateral heads of the triceps muscle. The boundaries of the quadrangular space are, superiorly, the lower border of the teres minor; laterally, the surgical neck of the humerus; medially, the long head of the triceps; and, anteriorly, the upper border of the teres major. Through this space run the axillary nerve and the posterior circumflex humeral artery.

**Infraspinatus.** *Origin.* Medial three fourths of infraspinous fossa of scapula. *Insertion.* Central facet on greater tuberosity of humerus. *Action.* Lateral rotator of humerus. *Nerve supply.* Suprascapular nerve.
**Teres Minor.** *Origin.* Axillary border of scapula. *Insertion.* Lowest facet on greater tuberosity of humerus. *Action.* Lateral rotator of humerus. *Nerve supply.* Axillary nerve.

above; part of the deltoid muscle originates from its inferior border (see Fig. 1-57).

### Incision

Because the transverse skin incision runs across the lines of cleavage of the skin, the resultant scar usually is broad. A vertical incision at the lateral end of the scapular spine is more cosmetic, but provides poor exposure of the joint.

## Superficial Surgical Dissection

In the posterior approach, only those fibers of the deltoid muscle that arise from the spine of the scapula are detached. Because the fibers are straight and blend intimately with the periosteum of the scapula, the muscle can be removed subperiosteally. During closure, the good, tough tissue that remains attached to the muscle provides an excellent anchor for sutures, in contrast to the anterior and lateral portions of the muscle. Drill holes may need to be placed through the spine, however, to anchor the muscular sutures.

## Deep Surgical Dissection

The deep dissection in this approach lies between the infraspinatus and teres minor muscles (see Fig. 1-58).

### Infraspinatus Muscle

The fibers of the infraspinatus muscle are multipennate; numerous fibrous intramuscular septa give attachment to them.

The infraspinatus forms its tendon just before crossing the back of the shoulder joint; a small bursa lies between the muscle and the posterior aspect of the scapular neck to help the tendon glide freely over the bone. The muscle also inserts into the capsule of the shoulder joint, mechanically increasing the capsule's strength (Fig. 1-59).

### Teres Minor Muscle

The teres minor runs side by side with the infraspinatus. Its fibers run parallel with one another, in contrast to the multipennate fibers of the infraspinatus; this difference may help in identification of the interval between the two muscles.

The axillary nerve enters the muscle from its inferior border. The superior border (the boundary between the infraspinatus and teres minor muscles),

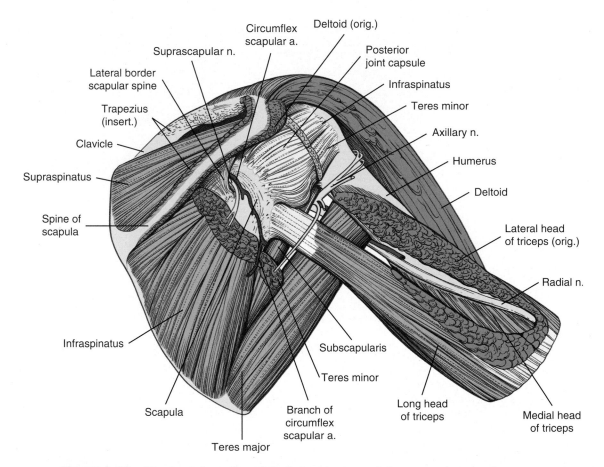

**Figure 1-59** The lateral portion of the infraspinatus and the teres minor has been removed to reveal the joint capsule. The suprascapular nerve and the circumflex scapular artery are seen curving medially and distally around the lateral border of the spine of the scapula. The axillary nerve is seen emerging through the quadrangular space and splitting into many branches. The medial branch splits to supply the teres minor muscle. The radial nerve is seen crossing through the triangular space and entering the spiral groove in the upper portion of the humerus. The triangular space is formed superiorly by the lower border of the teres major muscle, medially by the long head of the triceps, and laterally by the shaft of the humerus.

therefore, is the safe side of the muscle and a true internervous plane (see Fig. 1-58).

## Dangers

### Axillary Nerve

The **axillary nerve** is a branch of the posterior cord of the brachial plexus. It runs down along the posterior wall of the axilla on the surface of the subscapularis, far from the incision made in that muscle during the anterior approach to the shoulder (see Fig. 1-23). The nerve then runs through the quadrangular space, where it touches the surgical neck of the humerus. At that point, it can be damaged easily by surgery, by fractures of the surgical neck of the humerus, or by anterior dislocation of the shoulder.

The boundaries of the quadrangular space differ when viewed from the front and from the back (see Fig. 1-58).

*Posterior View.* The boundaries from the posterior view are as follows: superiorly, the lower border of the teres minor; laterally, the surgical neck of the humerus; medially, the long head of the triceps; and inferiorly, the upper border of the teres major.

*Anterior View.* The boundaries from the anterior view are as follows: superiorly, the subscapularis; laterally, the surgical neck of the humerus; medially, the long head of the triceps; and inferiorly, the upper border of the teres major (see Fig. 1-23).

The axillary nerve disappears beneath the lower border of the subscapularis and, after traversing the quadrangular space, emerges in the back of the shoulder beneath the lower border of the teres minor. The posterior circumflex humeral vessels run with it (see Fig. 1-58).

Dissections carried out above the teres minor do not damage the axillary nerve; however, if the dissection strays out of the correct plane and below the teres minor, the axillary nerve can be damaged. Because the axillary nerve is the sole nerve supply to the deltoid muscle, any damage to it is serious.

Within the quadrangular space, the axillary nerve divides into two branches after giving off a twig to the shoulder joint. The deep branch enters and supplies the deep surface of the deltoid (see Fig. 1-58). The superficial branch supplies the teres minor muscle and sends a cutaneous branch to the lateral aspect of the upper arm, namely, the upper lateral cutaneous nerve of the arm, which supplies the skin over the insertion of the deltoid muscle (see Fig. 1-57).

The upper lateral cutaneous nerve of the arm is of clinical importance in cases of traumatic axillary nerve palsy following, for instance, an acute anterior dislocation of the shoulder. Examination of the paralyzed deltoid and teres minor muscles may be difficult because of the pain that follows this injury. Diminution of sensation over the insertion of the deltoid is good presumptive evidence of the presence of an axillary nerve palsy.

The axillary nerve is the best example of Hilton's law, which states that the motor nerve to a muscle tends to send a branch to the joint that the muscle moves and another branch to the skin over the joint.[28] Pain in the shoulder is perceived via the axillary nerve and, therefore, may be referred to the cutaneous distribution of that nerve.

### Radial Nerve

The radial nerve, which is the other major branch of the posterior cord of the brachial plexus, leaves the axilla by passing backward through a triangular space that is defined superiorly by the lower border of the teres major, laterally by the shaft of the humerus, and medially by the long head of the triceps (see Figs. 1-58 and 1-59).

The odds of endangering the radial nerve by this approach are remote. It cannot be damaged during the posterior approach to the shoulder unless the correct plane is deviated from substantially, below not only the teres minor but the teres major as well.

### Circumflex Scapular Vessels

Yet another triangular space exists when the inner sleeve of shoulder muscles is viewed from the back. Its boundaries are as follows: superiorly, the lower border of the teres minor; laterally, the long head of the triceps; and inferiorly, the upper border of the teres major (see Fig. 1-58).

This triangular space contains the circumflex scapular vessels, which form part of the extremely rich blood supply to the scapula. Dissection carried out between the teres minor and teres major muscles may damage these vessels, causing profuse hemorrhage that is difficult to control (see Fig. 1-58). Because the scapula has such a rich blood supply, fractures of the scapula are often associated with profuse blood loss. The hematoma is constrained within the fascia surrounding the scapula muscles and is not obvious. Potential blood loss from a fractured scapula always must be considered during vascular assessment of a polytraumatized patient.

# Arthroscopic Approaches to the Shoulder

## General Principles of Arthroscopy

Visualization of anatomic structures in open surgical approaches is straightforward. If a given structure is not visible, it may be exposed by extending the incision, thus expanding the surgical approach. By contrast, visualization of structures in arthroscopic approaches is achieved by using a telescope. The most commonly used arthroscope is angulated 30° at its tip so that the view obtained shows the structures that are 30° from the long axis of the arthroscope and not the structures that are directly in front of the scope. This is the arthroscope described in this book (Fig. 1-60, *inset*).

Angled scopes are required because the bony structure of the joint allows the arthroscope to be placed only in certain positions. The use of an angled scope allows the surgeon to see "around the corner"

and thereby greatly increases the view obtained within any joint.

Visualization of structures using an arthroscope can be achieved in several ways. Moving the scope forward or backward (advancing or withdrawing it) will reveal structures in front of or behind the original view (see Fig. 1-60). Keep the following important points in mind during arthroscopic use:

1. Because the scope is angled 30° from its axis, it is not possible to zoom in on an object merely by advancing the scope.
2. Rotating the arthroscope will reveal a series of views angled at 30° from the axis of the scope (Fig. 1-61).
3. Angling the scope will change the direction of the view (Fig. 1-62). You will not be able to visualize those structures directly in front of the arthroscope unless you angle it.

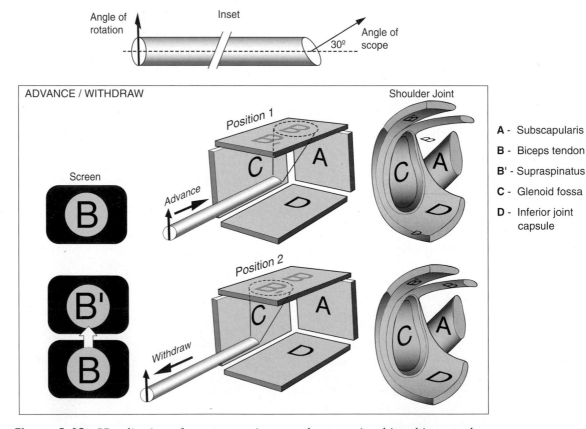

**Figure 1-60**   Visualization of structures using an arthroscope is achieved in several ways. Moving the arthroscope forward and backward (advancing or withdrawing) will show you structures in front of or behind your original view. Withdrawing the arthroscope from Position 1 to Position 2 changes the view from B to B'. Because the tip of the scope is angled at 30° from its axis, it is not possible to zoom in on an object merely by advancing the scope.

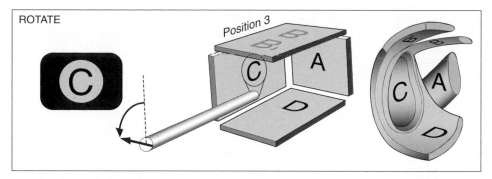

**Figure 1-61**   Rotating the scope will provide a series of views at angles of 30° from the axis of the scope. Rotating the arthroscope 90° counterclockwise from Position 2 to Position 3 changes the view from B′ to C.

4. It is possible to change the view by moving the joint while leaving the arthroscope in the same position. This maneuver is vital for full inspection of any joint.

## Posterior and Anterior Approaches

The shoulder is a large ball and shallow socket joint with a generous capsule that allows a large range of movement in all planes. Therefore, the anatomy of the joint makes it ideal for arthroscopic approaches. However, the shoulder is covered by thick layers of muscles, and this can make arthroscopic approaches somewhat difficult (Figs. 1-63 and 1-64). Neurovascular structures also are potentially at risk in arthroscopic approaches to the shoulder. The presence of the main neurovascular bundle antero-inferior to the joint limits anterior approaches. Other neurovascular structures may also be at risk if the entry portals are inaccurately positioned (see Dangers).

Arthroscopy of the shoulder is indicated for the following:

1. Arthroscopic subacromial decompression for chronic rotator cuff tendonitis
2. Treatment of partial thickness tears of the rotator cuff
3. Treatment of tears of the glenoid labrum
4. Treatment of degenerative disease of the acromio-clavicular joint
5. Removal of loose bodies
6. Treatment of osteochondritis dissecans
7. Synovectomy

Numerous arthroscopic portals have been described in shoulder arthroscopy surgery. The posterior portal is the one most commonly used for diagnostic purposes. It is nearly always used in conjunction with the anterior portal. The combination of these approaches allows the use of the arthroscope along with arthroscopic instrumentation. Usually the arthroscope is inserted via the posterior portal, and instruments are inserted via the anterior portal. However, either portal can be used for either purpose. These two approaches are described in this section.

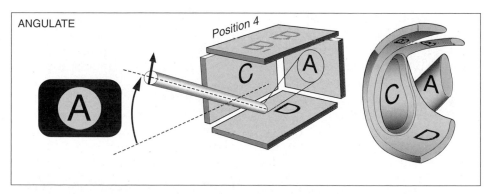

**Figure 1-62**   Angling the scope changes the direction of the view. It is the only way to be able to visualize those structures directly in front of the scope. Angling the arthroscope from Position 2 to Position 4 changes the view from B′ to A.

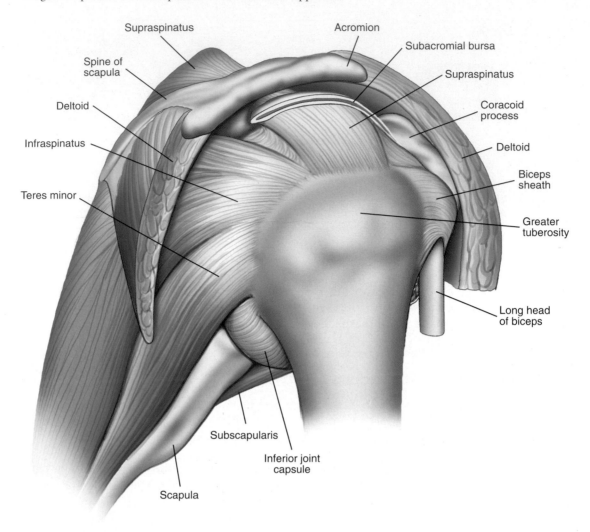

**Figure 1-63**   Anatomy of the shoulder joint. Lateral view of the right shoulder with the lateral aspect of deltoid muscle removed, showing the thick muscular covering of the joint.

## Position of the Patient

Place the patient supine on the operating table. Elevate the upper half of the table 60°. Position the patient so that the operative shoulder is off the edge of the table, allowing access to both sides of the shoulder (Fig. 1-65). Prep and drape the arm so that it can be freely manipulated during arthroscopy. This position, known as the beach chair position,[7] reduces venous pressure around the shoulder and reduces bleeding. Arm traction is useful in arthroscopic subacromial decompression but is not necessarily for diagnostic arthroscopy.

## Landmarks and Incision

The shoulder is surrounded on all sides by thick muscular coverings (see Figs. 1-38 and 1-63). The joint line cannot be palpated, therefore arthroscopic approaches rely on landmarks distant from the joint.

### Landmarks

The *acromion* and the *spine of the scapula* form one continuous arch. The bony dorsum and lateral aspect of the acromion are easy to palpate on the outer aspect of the shoulder (see Figs. 1-38, 1-40, and 1-46*A*).

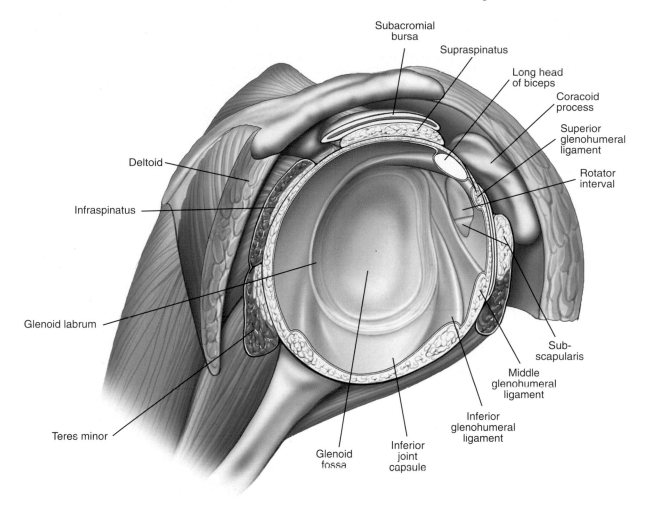

Figure 1-64   Lateral view of glenoid cavity with the humeral head removed.

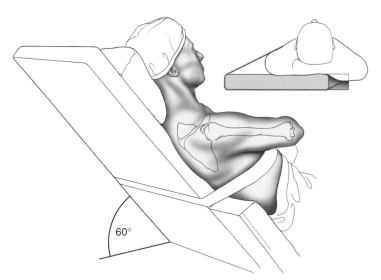

**Figure 1-65**   Position of the patient for arthroscopy. Elevate the upper half of the table 60°. Position the patient so that the operative shoulder is off the edge of the table, allowing access to both sides of the shoulder. This is known as the "beach chair" position.[7]

To identify the *coracoid process*, drop your fingers distally about 1 in. from the anterior edge of the lateral one-third of the clavicle. Press laterally and posteriorly in an oblique line until you feel the coracoid process.

### Incisions

*Posterior.* Make an 8-mm stab incision 2 cm inferior and 1 cm medial to the posterolateral tip of the acromion (Fig. 1-66).

*Anterior.* Make an 8-mm stab incision halfway between the tip of the coracoid process and the anterior aspect of the acromion (Fig. 1-67).

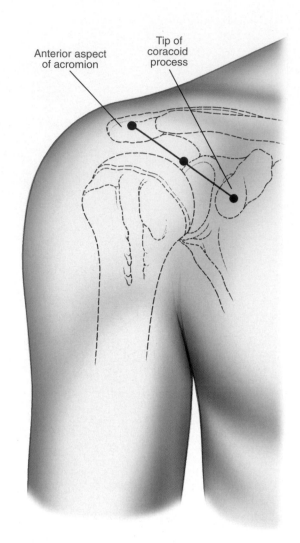

**Figure 1-67** Anterior incision. Make an 8-mm stab incision halfway between the tip of the coracoid process and the anterior aspect of the acromion.

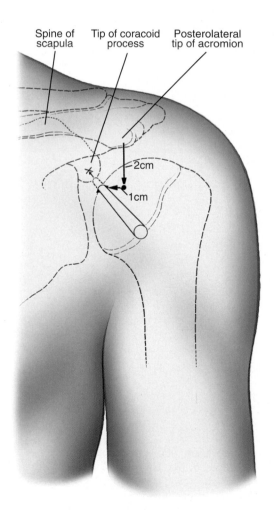

**Figure 1-66** Posterior incision. Make an 8-mm stab incision 2 cm inferior and 1 cm medial to the posterior lateral tip of the acromion.

## Internervous Plane

### Posterior
The internervous plane lies between the teres minor muscle (supplied by the axillary nerve) and the infraspinatus muscle (supplied by the suprascapular nerve) (see Fig. 1-63).

### Anterior
The internervous plane lies between the pectoralis major muscle (supplied by the medial and lateral pectoral nerves) and the deltoid (supplied by the axillary nerve) (see Fig. 1-5).

## Surgical Dissection

### Posterior

Place your finger on the coracoid process. Insert the trochar and arthroscopic sheath through the posterior skin incision, aiming the tip of the arthroscope toward your finger (Fig. 1-68). You will enter the glenohumeral joint at a point just above its equator. Although, in theory, the arthro-scope may penetrate the rotator cuff between the infraspinatus and teres minor, the scope usually traverses through the substance of the infraspinatus (see Fig. 1-68).

### Anterior

Two techniques are possible. The safest technique is to insert the arthroscope through the posterior por-

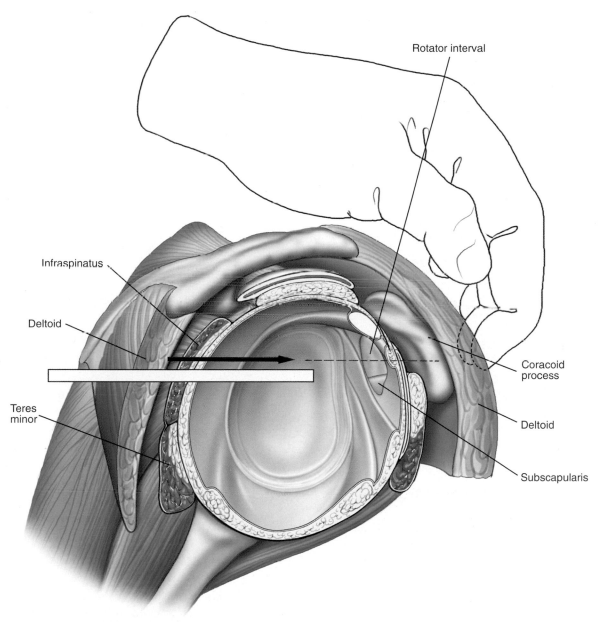

**Figure 1-68** Posterior insertion of the arthroscope. Place your finger on the coracoid process. Insert the trochar and arthroscopic sheath through the posterior skin incision, aiming the tip of the arthroscope toward your finger.

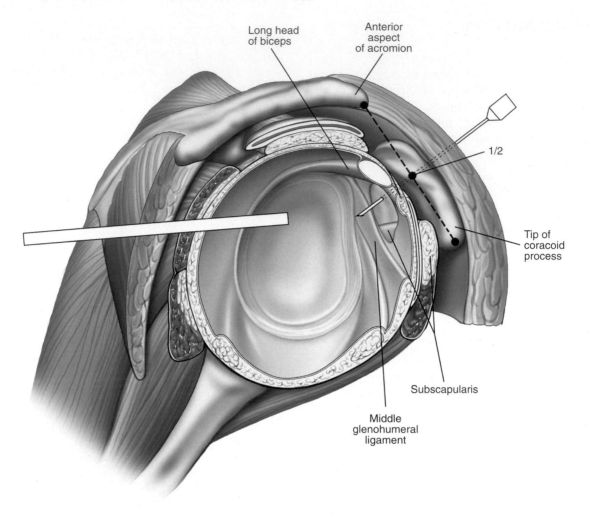

Long head
of biceps

Anterior
aspect
of acromion

1/2

Tip of
coracoid
process

Subscapularis

Middle
glenohumeral
ligament

**Figure 1-69** Anterior insertion of the arthroscope. Insert an arthroscope through the posterior portal to allow you to visualize the anterior capsule of the shoulder joint. Next, insert a long hypodermic needle through the anterior skin incision and enter the joint under direct vision of the scope.

tal to allow you to visualize the anterior capsule of the shoulder joint. Next insert a long hypodermic needle through the anterior skin incision and enter the joint under direct vision of the arthroscope. This will ensure that you enter the joint in a correct and safe position (Fig. 1-69).

# Arthroscopic Exploration of the Shoulder Joint through the Posterior Portal

## Order of Scoping

1. Insert a 30° arthroscope through the posterior incision (see Fig. 1-66).
2. Identify the biceps tendon and its origin as it runs from superior to inferior (Fig. 1-70A,B, View 1).
3. Next, rotate the arthroscope superiorly to allow visualization of the supraspinatus (Fig. 1-70A,B, View 2). The supraspinatus lies posterior to the biceps tendon.
4. To visualize infraspinatus and teres minor you will need to rotate not only the arthroscope but also the humeral head (Fig. 1-71A,B, View 3).
5. Next, note the anterior triangle of the shoulder, formed by the biceps tendon, the superior edge of the subscapularis, and the glenoid (Fig. 1-72A,B, View 4; see Fig. 1-70A,B, View 1). This triangle

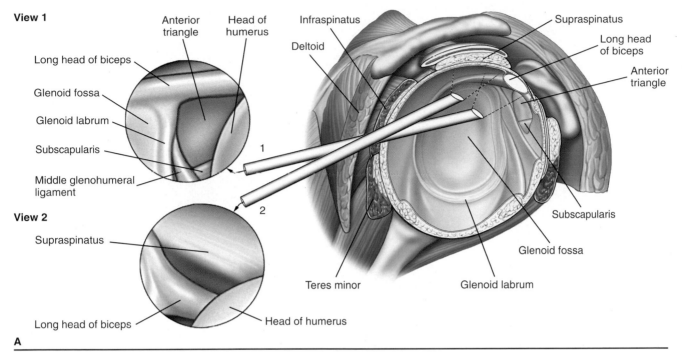

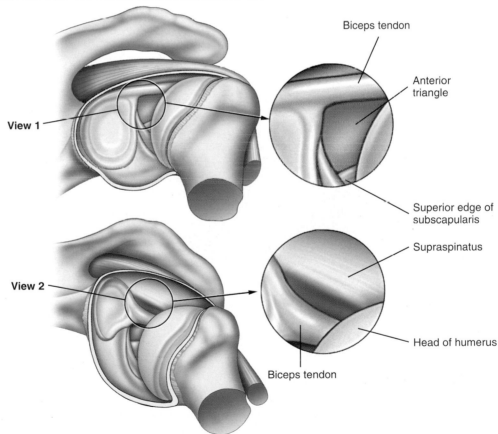

**Figure 1-70** **(A)** Lateral view of the shoulder joint with the scope in place **(right)**, correlated with their respective arthroscopic views **(left)**. View 1: Insert the arthroscope through a posterior approach and identify the biceps tendon. Identify the long head of biceps as it runs superiorly to its origin. Note the position of the arthroscope in the joint and the view obtained. View 2: Rotate the arthroscope superiorly to visualize the rotator cuff. Observe the supraspinatus portion of the rotator cuff. **(B)** Overall views of the shoulder joint seen from the direction of the arthroscope in Views 1 and 2 **(left)**, correlated with their respective arthroscopic views **(right)**.

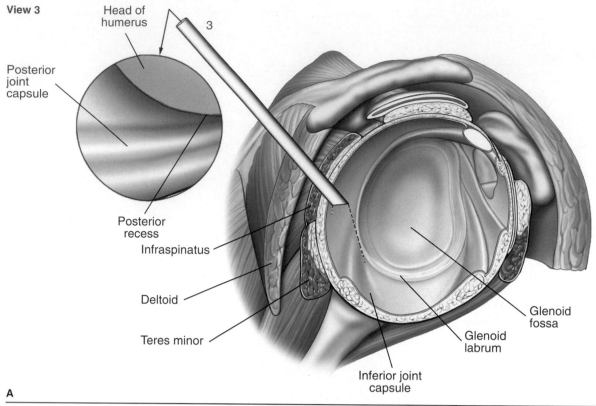

**A**

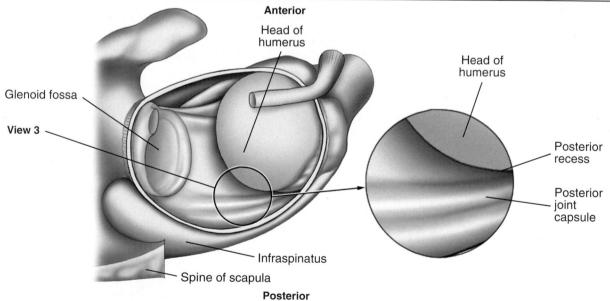

**B**

**Figure 1-71**    (**A**) Lateral view of the shoulder joint with the scope in place (**right**), correlated with its arthroscopic view (**left**). View 3: Rotate the arthroscope to look inferiorly and identify the inferior portion of the rotator cuff (infraspinatus and teres minor). Rotate the humeral head to visualize the infraspinatus tendon. (**B**) Overall view of the shoulder joint seen from the direction of the arthroscope in View 3 (**left**), correlated with its arthroscopic view (**right**).

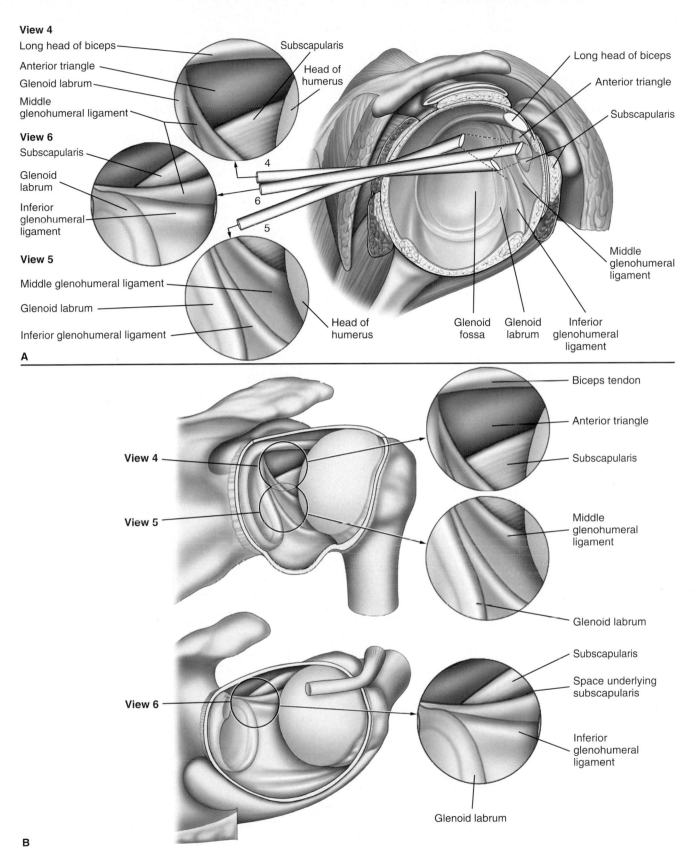

**View 4**
Long head of biceps
Anterior triangle
Glenoid labrum
Middle
glenohumeral ligament

Subscapularis
Head of
humerus

**View 6**
Subscapularis
Glenoid
labrum
Inferior
glenohumeral
ligament

**View 5**
Middle glenohumeral ligament
Glenoid labrum
Inferior glenohumeral ligament

Head of
humerus

Long head of biceps
Anterior triangle
Subscapularis

Middle
glenohumeral
ligament

Glenoid
fossa
Glenoid
labrum
Inferior
glenohumeral
ligament

**A**

View 4

View 5

View 6

Biceps tendon
Anterior triangle
Subscapularis

Middle
glenohumeral
ligament

Glenoid labrum

Subscapularis
Space underlying
subscapularis

Inferior
glenohumeral
ligament

Glenoid labrum

**B**

**Figure 1-72** **(A)** Lateral views of the shoulder joint with the scope in place **(right)**, correlated with their respective arthroscopic views **(left)**. View 4: Advance the arthroscope anteriorly and identify the anterior triangle. Observe the anterior triangle formed by the biceps tendon, the superior edge of subscapularis, and the glenoid labrum. View 5: Pass the arthroscope to the upper margin of the glenoid and rotate the arthroscope inferiorly. Observe the anterior gleno-humeral complex. View 6: Pass the arthroscope anteriorly and then rotate it to allow you to look inferiorly. Observe the space underlying the subscapularis. Direct the arthroscope inferiorly and then rotate it to look posteriorly. **(B)** Overall views of the shoulder joint seen from the direction of the scope in Views 4, 5, and 6 **(left)**, correlated with their respective arthroscopic views **(right)**.

marks the safe spot for entry through the anterior portal (see Fig. 1-69).

6. Pass the arthroscope to the upper anterior margin of the glenoid and rotate the scope inferiorly to allow examination of the anterior glenohumeral complex (Fig. 1-72*A,B*, View 5). You may need to apply a distraction force to the shoulder at that time, or alternatively use a 70° rather than a 30° telescope.

7. Pass the arthroscope anteriorly into the anterior triangle and rotate the scope so as to allow you to look inferiorly into a space underlying the subscapularis (Fig. 1-72*A,B*, View 6). This space is a frequent site for loose bodies.

8. Next, redirect the arthroscope inferiorly and rotate the telescope posteriorly to allow access to the posterior recess of the shoulder (Fig. 1-73*A,B*, View 7; see Fig. 1-71). Visualization of the humeral head and glenoid are easily accomplished through the posterior portal. Careful manipulation of the shoulder is required to visualize the whole of the articular surface.

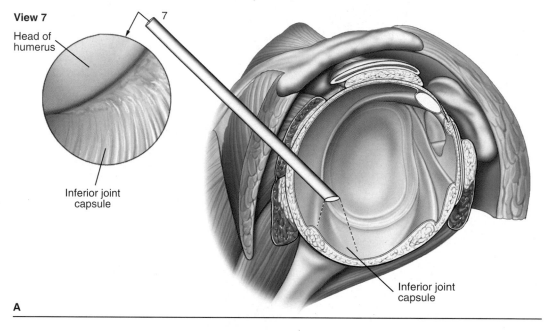

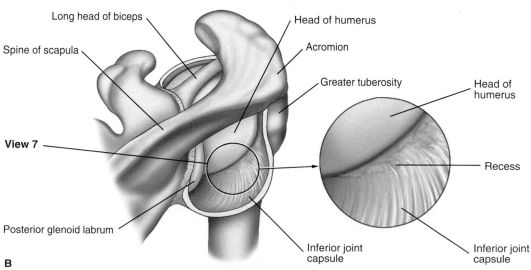

**Figure 1-73** **(A)** Lateral view of the shoulder joint with the scope in place **(right)**, correlated with its arthroscopic view **(left)**. View 7: Direct the arthroscope inferiorly and then rotate it to look posteriorly. Observe the posterior recess of the shoulder. **(B)** Overall view of the shoulder joint seen from the direction of the arthroscope in View 7 **(left)**, correlated with its arthroscopic view **(right)**.

# Dangers

## Nerves

***Posterior.*** The *axillary nerve* leaves the posterior wall of the axilla by penetrating the quadrangular space. It winds around the humerus running on the deep surface of the deltoid muscle, about 7 cm below the tip of the acromion (see Figs. 1-23, 1-33, 1-39, and 1-58). If the posterior portal is correctly located with regard to the posterolateral tip of the acromion, this portal should lie about 3 cm superior to the nerve. Only a very inferiorly placed incision will endanger the nerve.

The *suprascapular nerve*, the nerve supplied to both the supraspinatus and infraspinatus, runs around the base of the spine of the scapula as it runs from the supraspinatus fossa to the infraspinatus fossa (see Figs. 1-45 and 1-59). This nerve is at risk if the posterior portal is made too medially. The correctly positioned portal is approximately 2 cm lateral to the nerve.

***Anterior.*** The *axillary nerve* may be in danger as it traverses along the deep surface of the deltoid from superiorly placed incisions.

The *musculocutaneous nerve*, the nerve supply of the flexor muscles of the upper arm, enters those muscles some 2 cm to 8 cm distal to the tip of the coracoid process. The nerve, therefore, is unlikely to be damaged by a portal made superior and lateral to the level of the coracoid process (see Figs. 1-10, 1-18, and 1-22).

## Vessels

The *cephalic vein* runs superficially between the deltoid and pectoralis major muscle. It can only be damaged from incisions made too laterally.

The acromial branches of the *thoraco-acromial artery* lie along the medial side of the coraco-acromial ligament and will not be endangered through the classic anterior portal. Branches of the artery will, however, be damaged by more superior approaches used to enter the subacromial space.

# How to Enlarge the Approach

To use the *posterior portal* to access the subacromial space, withdraw the arthroscope from the shoulder; using the same skin incision, redirect the scope more superiorly to run on the underside of the acromion. To do this you will need to create a separate arthroscopic penetration of the deltoid muscle. Access to the subacromial space is often difficult due to disease processes, especially of the subacromial bursa. Con-tinuous traction is indicated. Bleeding is frequently encountered.

The *anterior portal* cannot be extended.

## REFERENCES

1. BANKART ASB: The pathology and treatment of recurrent dislocation of the shoulder joint. Br J Surg 26:23, 1938
2. OSMOND-CLARKE H: Habitual dislocation of the shoulder: the Putti-Platt operation. J Bone Joint Surg [Br] 30:19, 1948
3. MAGNUSON PB, STACK JK: Recurrent dislocation of the shoulder. JAMA 123:889, 1943
4. BOYD HB, HUNT HL: Recurrent dislocation of the shoulder: the staple capsulorrhaphy. J Bone Joint Surg [Am] 47:1514, 1965
5. HELFET AJ: Coracoid transplantation for recurring dislocation of the shoulder. J Bone Joint Surg [Br] 40:198, 1958
6. ROWE CARTER R, PATEL O, SOUTHMARD WW: Bankart procedure: long-term end result study. J Bone Joint Surg [Am] 60:1, 1978
7. FROIMSON AI, OH I: Keyhole tenodesis of biceps origin at the shoulder. Clin Orthop 112:245, 1975
8. NEER CS II: Prosthetic replacement of the humeral head: indications and operative technique. Surg Clin North Am 43:1581, 1963
9. LESLIE JT Jr, RYAN TJ: The anterior axillary incision to approach the shoulder joint. J Bone Joint Surg [Am] 44:193, 1962
10. CLARK JMP: Reconstruction of biceps brachii by pectoral muscle transplantation. Br J Surg 34:180, 1946
11. MEYER AW: Spontaneous dislocation and destruction of tendon of long head of biceps brachii: fifty-nine instances. Arch Surg 17:493, 1928
12. MEYER AW: Chronic functional lesions of the shoulder. Arch Surg 35:646, 1937
13. HITCHCOCK HH, BECHTOL CO: Painful shoulder: observations on the role of the tendon of the long head of the biceps brachii in its causation. J Bone Joint Surg [Am] 30:263, 1948
14. DE PALMA AF, CALLERT G, BENNETT GA: Variational anatomy and degenerative lesions of the shoulder joint. Instr Course Lect 6:255, 1949
15. HORWITZ MT, TOCANTINS LM: An anatomical study of the role of the long thoracic nerve and the related scapular bursa in the pathogenesis of local paralysis of the serratus anterior muscle. Anat Rec 71:375, 1938
16. NEER CS II: Anterior acromioplasty for the chronic impingement syndrome in the shoulder. J Bone Joint Surg [Am] 54:41, 1972
17. DEBEVRE J, PATTE D, ELMEUK E: Repair of rupture of the rotator cuff of the shoulder, with a note on the advancement of the supraspinatus muscle. J Bone Joint Surg [Br] 47:36, 1965
18. DE PALMA AF: Surgery of the shoulder. Philadelphia, JB Lippincott Co, 1950
19. PRESTO BJ, JACKSON JP: Investigation of shoulder disability by arthrography. Clin Radiol 28:259, 1977
20. KERWEIN GA, ROSEBERG B, SNEED WR Jr: Arthrographic studies of the shoulder joint. J Bone Joint Surg [Am] 39:1267, 1957
21. BOSWORTH DM: Supraspinatus syndrome: symptomatology, pathology and repair. JAMA 117:422, 1941
22. RATHBUN JB, MACNAB I: The microvascular pattern of the rotator cuff. J Bone Joint Surg [Br] 52:540, 1970
23. WILSON CLL, DUFF GL: Pathologic studies of degeneration and rupture of the supraspinatus tendon. Arch Surg 47:121, 1943
24. ROWE R, VEE LBK: A posterior approach to the shoulder joint. J Bone Joint Surg 26:580, 1944
25. ITINDENACH JCR: Recurrent posterior dislocation of the shoulder. J Bone Joint Surg 29:582, 1947
26. BOYD HB, SISK TD: Recurrent posterior dislocation of the shoulder. J Bone Joint Surg [Am] 54:779, 1972
27. SCOTT DJ Jr: Treatment of recurrent posterior dislocation of the shoulder by glenoplasty: report of three cases. J Bone Joint Surg [Am] 49:471, 1967
28. HILTON J: Lectures on rest and pain. In: Joint innervation: reflex control of muscles activating joints, 6th ed. London, 1950:156

## SELECTED BIBLIOGRAPHY

ANDREWS JR, TIMMERMAN LA: Diagnostic and operative arthroscopy. Philadelphia, WB Saunders, 1997

LAURENCIN CT, DEUTSCH A, O'BRIEN FJ ET AL: The supero-lateral portal for arthroscopy of the shoulder. Arthroscopy 10:255, 1994

MARTIN DR, GARTH WP: Results of arthroscopic debridement of glenoid-labral tears. Am J Sports Med 23:447, 1995

MATTHEWS LS, LABUDDLE JK: Arthroscopic treatment of synovial diseases of the shoulder. Orthop Clin North Am 24:101, 1993

OLSEWISKI JM, DE PEW AD: Arthroscopic sub-acromial decompression and rotator cuff debridement for stage II and stage III impingement. Arthroscopy 10:61, 1994

PAULOS LE, FRANKLIN JL: Arthroscopic shoulder decompression development and application. Am J Sports Med 18:359, 1990

SKYHAR MJ, ALTCHEK DW, WARREN RF ET AL: Shoulder arthroscopy with the patient in the beach chair position. Arthroscopy 4:256, 1988

WOOLFE EM: Anterior portals in shoulder arthroscopy. Arthroscopy 5:201, 1989

ZVIJAC JE, LEVY HJ, LEMAK LJ: Arthroscopic sub-acromial decompression in the treatment of full thickness rotator cuff: a 3- to 6-year follow-up. Arthroscopy 10:518, 1994

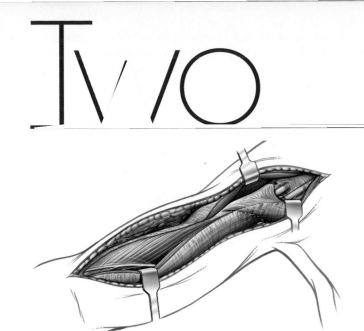

# The Humerus

Operations on the humerus are relatively infrequent and generally involve the open reduction and internal fixation of fractures. All approaches to the humerus are potentially dangerous because the major nerves and vessels at this site run much closer to the bone than they do elsewhere in the body; the axillary, radial, and ulnar nerves all have a direct relationship to the humerus. Of these structures, the radial nerve is at greatest risk during exposure of the humeral shaft (see Fig. 2-27).

Four approaches to the humerus are described in this chapter: the anterior approach, the anterolateral approach to the distal humerus, the posterior approach, and the lateral approach to the distal humerus. Of these, the anterior and posterior approaches are the most versatile, providing access to large portions of bone. The anterolateral approach to the distal humerus is extensile both proximally and distally, but this facility rarely is required. The lateral approach to the distal humerus is a strictly local approach to the common extensor origin and adjacent structures. Because the key surgical structure of the area (the radial nerve) courses down the arm in both the anterior and posterior compartments, the surgical anatomy of the humerus is described in a single section of this chapter, immediately after the description of the operative approaches.

## Anterior Approach

The anterior approach exposes the anterior surface of the shaft of the humerus.[1-3] Normally, only a portion of the approach is needed for any one procedure. As in all approaches to the humerus, the radial nerve is the structure at greatest risk during surgery.

The uses of the anterior approach include the following:

1. Internal fixation of fractures of the humerus
2. Osteotomy of the humerus
3. Biopsy and resection of bone tumors
4. Treatment of osteomyelitis

### Position of the Patient

Place the patient supine on the operating table, with the arm on an arm board, abducted about 60°. Tilt the patient away from the affected arm to reduce bleeding. Most surgeons prefer to sit facing the patient's axilla, with the surgical assistant on the

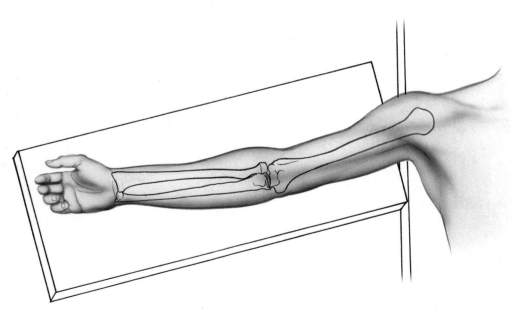

**Figure 2-1**   Place the patient supine on the operating table. Place his or her arm on an arm board and abduct the arm about 60°.

opposite side of the arm. Do not use a tourniquet; it will only get in the way (Fig. 2-1).

## Landmarks and Incision

### Landmarks

Palpate the *coracoid process* of the scapula immediately below the junction of the middle and outer thirds of the clavicle (Fig. 2-2, *inset*).

Palpate the long head of the *biceps brachii* as it crosses the shoulder and runs down the arm. The lateral border of its freely moving muscular belly lies on the anterior surface of the arm.

### Incision

Begin a longitudinal incision over the tip of the coracoid process of the scapula. Run it distally and laterally in the line of the deltopectoral groove to the insertion of the deltoid muscle on the lateral aspect of the humerus, about halfway down its shaft. From there, the incision should be continued distally as far as necessary, following the lateral border of the biceps muscle. The incision should be stopped about 5 cm above the flexion crease of the elbow (see Fig. 2-2).

## Internervous Plane

The anterior approach makes use of two different internervous planes (Fig. 2-3*A*). Proximally, the plane lies between the deltoid muscle (which is supplied by the axillary nerve) and the pectoralis major muscle (which is supplied by the medial and lateral pectoral nerves). Distally, the plane lies between the medial fibers of the brachialis muscle (which is supplied by the musculocutaneous nerve) medially and the lateral fibers of the brachialis muscle (which is supplied by the radial nerve) laterally (see Fig. 2-3*B*).

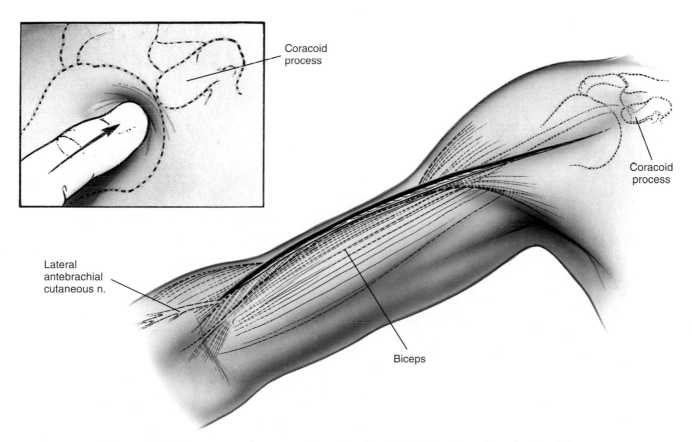

**Figure 2-2**   For an anterior approach, make a longitudinal incision from the tip of the coracoid process distally in line with the deltopectoral groove and continue along the lateral aspect of the shaft of the humerus. Extend the incision as far distally as necessary, stopping about 5 cm above the flexion crease of the elbow. Palpate the coracoid process in a lateral to medial direction *(inset)*.

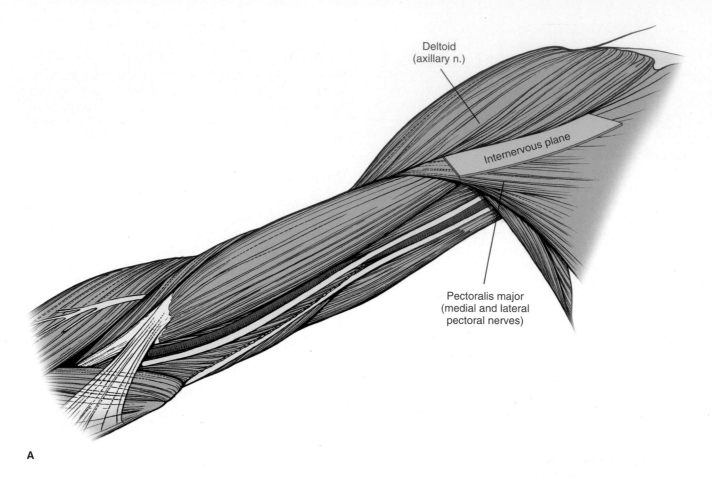

A

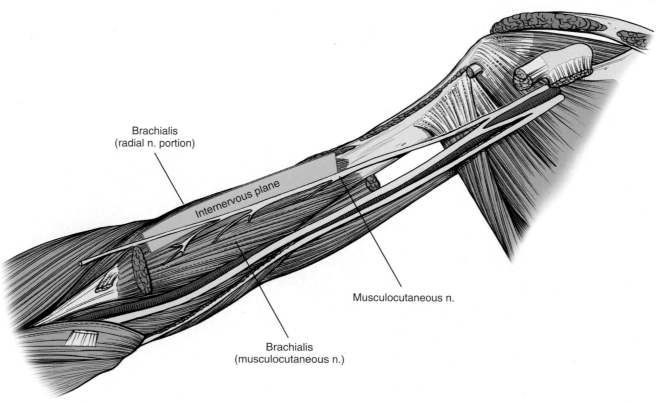

B

**Figure 2-3** Internervous plane. **(A)** Proximally, the plane lies between the deltoid (axillary nerve) and the pectoralis major (medial and lateral pectoral nerves). **(B)** Distally, the plane lies between the medial fibers of the brachialis (musculocutaneous nerve) medially and the lateral fibers of the brachialis (radial nerve) laterally.

## Superficial Surgical Dissection

### Proximal Humeral Shaft

Identify the deltopectoral groove, using the cephalic vein as a guide (Fig. 2-4, *inset*), and separate the two muscles, retracting the cephalic vein either medially with the pectoralis major or laterally with the deltoid, whichever is easier. Develop the muscular interval distally down to the insertion of the deltoid into the deltoid tuberosity and the insertion of the pectoralis major into the lateral lip of the bicipital groove (see Fig. 2-4). Take care when retracting the deltoid; overzealous use of the retractor may paralyze the anterior half of the muscle by causing a compression injury to the axillary nerve.

### Distal Humeral Shaft

Incise the deep fascia of the arm in line with the skin incision. Identify the muscular interval between the biceps brachii and the brachialis. Develop the interval by retracting the biceps medially. Beneath it lies the anterior aspect of the brachialis, which cloaks the humeral shaft (Fig. 2-5; see Fig. 2-4).

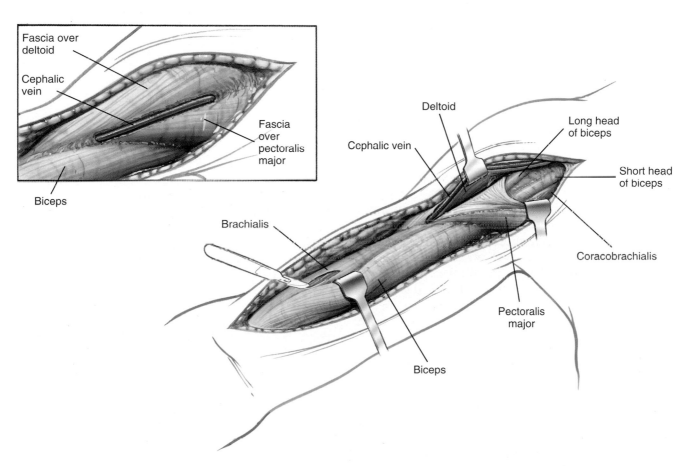

**Figure 2-4** Identify the deltopectoral groove, using the cephalic vein as a guide *(inset)*. Develop the muscular interval down to the insertion of the deltoid into the deltoid tuberosity and the insertion of the pectoralis major into the lateral bicipital groove. Distally, incise the deep fascia in line with the skin incision to identify the interval between the biceps brachii and the brachialis.

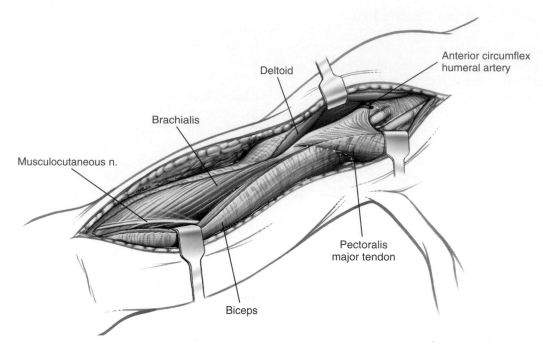

**Figure 2-5**    Retract the biceps medially, being careful to identify the musculocutaneous nerve. Proximally, identify the anterior circumflex humeral artery as it crosses the field of dissection in a medial to lateral direction.

## Deep Surgical Dissection

### Proximal Humeral Shaft

To expose the upper part of the shaft of the humerus, incise the periosteum longitudinally just lateral to the insertion of the tendon of the pectoralis major. Continue the incision proximally, staying lateral to the tendon of the long head of the biceps. The anterior circumflex humeral artery crosses the field of dissection in a medial to lateral direction and must be ligated (see Fig. 2-5). To expose the bone fully, you may need to detach part or all of the insertion of the pectoralis major muscle from the lateral lip of the bicipital groove of the humerus (Fig. 2-6). This must be done subperiosteally. Only detach the minimum amount of soft tissue to allow accurate visualization and reduction of the fracture. Try to preserve as much soft-tissue attachment as possible. If you need to dissect further around the bone, this dissection should remain in a strictly subperiosteal plane to avoid damage to the radial nerve, which lies in the spiral groove of the humerus and crosses the back of the middle third of the bone in a medial to lateral direction (Fig. 2-7).

In extreme proximal humeral fractures, especially comminuted fractures, the head and anatomic neck of the humerus may need to be exposed. To accomplish this, the subscapularis muscle must be divided, with care taken to coagulate the triad of vessels that runs along the lower border of that muscle (Fig. 2-8; see Fig. 1-12).

### Distal Humeral Shaft

Split the fibers of the brachialis longitudinally along its midline to expose the periosteum on the anterior surface of the humeral shaft. Incise the periosteum longitudinally in line with the muscle dissection and strip the brachialis off the anterior surface of the bone. Try to preserve as much soft-tissue attachment as possible. To make the task easier, flex the elbow to take tension off the brachialis. The bone is now exposed (see Fig. 2-6).

## Dangers

### Nerves

The **radial nerve** is vulnerable at the following two points:

1. In the spiral groove on the back of the middle third of the humerus. Minimize the danger by dissecting muscle from bone strictly in a subperiosteal plane without straying onto the posterior surface of the bone (see Figs. 2-7 and 2-31). Remember that the radial nerve may be damaged by drills, taps, or screws that are inserted anteroposteriorly when anterior plates are being applied in the middle third of the bone.

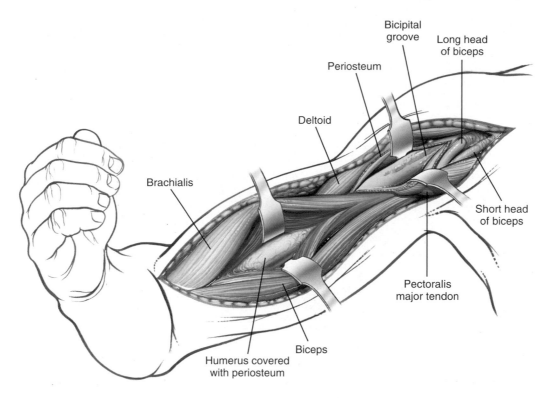

**Figure 2-6** Proximally, detach the insertion of the pectoralis major from the lateral bicipital groove and then continue dissection subperiosteally to expose the upper portion of the humerus. Distally, split the fibers of the brachialis to expose the periosteum of the anterior humerus. Incise the periosteum, and strip the brachialis off the bone. Flexion of the elbow will take tension off the brachialis, making the exposure easier.

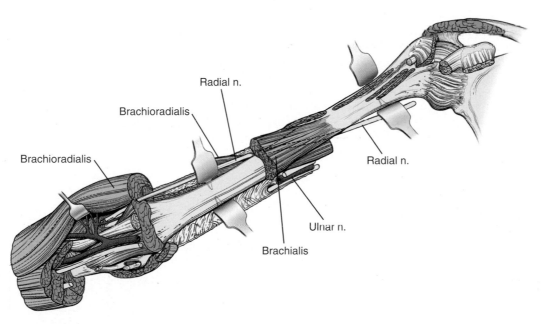

**Figure 2-7** The radial nerve is vulnerable at two points as it courses along the humerus: one, in the spiral groove, and two, as it pierces the lateral intermuscular septum to run between the brachioradialis and the brachialis.

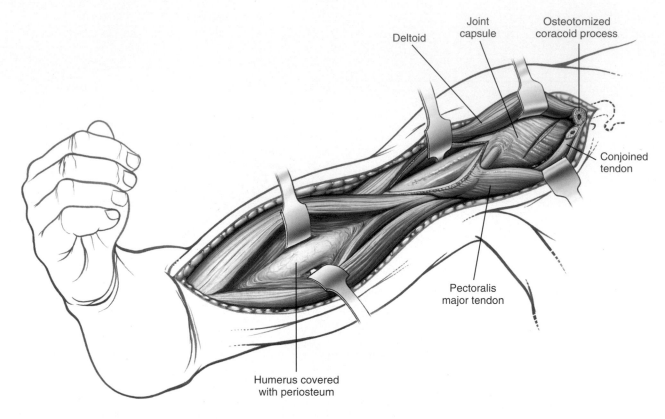

**Figure 2-8**  Proximal extension of the exposure. Using the deltopectoral interval, cut the tip of the coracoid and incise the subscapularis to provide an anterior approach to the shoulder.

2. In the anterior compartment of the distal third of the arm. At this point, the nerve has pierced the lateral intermuscular septum and lies between the brachioradialis and brachialis muscles (see Fig. 2-40). To avoid damaging the nerve, split the brachialis along its midline; the lateral portion of the muscle then serves as a cushion between the retractors that are being used in the exposure and the nerve itself (see Figs. 2-7 and 2-31).

The **axillary nerve,** which runs on the underside of the deltoid muscle, may be damaged as a result of a compression injury caused by overly vigorous retraction of the muscle. Care should be taken when the retractors are being positioned on the deltoid to avoid injuring the nerve (see Fig. 2-4).

### Vessels
The **anterior circumflex humeral vessels** cross the operative field in the interval between the pectoralis major and deltoid muscles in the upper third of the arm. Because cutting these vessels cannot be avoided, they should be ligated or subjected to diathermy (see Figs. 2-5 and 2-6).

## How to Enlarge the Approach

### Local Measures
Flexion of the elbow relaxes both the brachialis and the biceps brachii, facilitating retraction of these muscles.

### Extensile Measures

*Proximal Extension.* Because the anterior approach uses the deltopectoral interval, its upper end can be modified easily into an anterior approach to the shoulder (see Fig. 2-8).

*Distal Extension.* The anterior approach cannot be extended distally.

# Anterolateral Approach to the Distal Humerus

The anterolateral approach exposes the distal fourth of the humerus. Its major advantage over the brachialis-splitting anterior approach is that it can be extended both distally and proximally, whereas the brachialis-splitting approach cannot be extended distally. Its uses include the following:

1. Open reduction and internal fixation of fractures
2. Exploration of the radial nerve in the distal part of the arm

## Position of the Patient

Place the patient supine on the operating table, with the arm lying on an arm board and abducted about 60°. Exsanguinate the limb either by elevating it for 3 minutes or by applying a soft rubber bandage; then apply a tourniquet in as high a position as possible (see Fig. 2-1).

## Landmarks and Incision

### Landmarks
The landmarks in this approach include the *biceps brachii* muscle (see Applied Surgical Anatomy of the Anterior Approach in Chapter 1) and the *flexion crease of the elbow.*

### Incision
Make a curved longitudinal incision over the lateral border of the biceps, starting about 10 cm proximal to the flexion crease of the elbow. Follow the contour of the muscle, ending the incision just above the flexion crease of the elbow (Fig. 2-9).

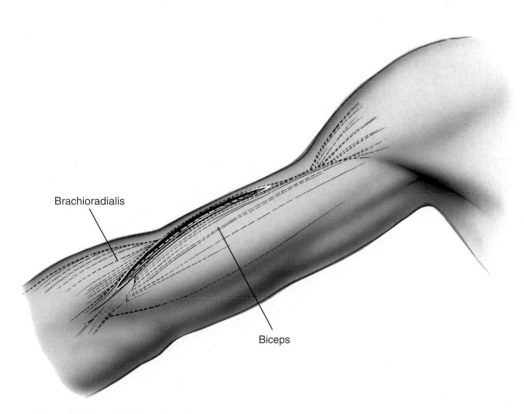

Brachioradialis

Biceps

**Figure 2-9**   The incision for the anterior lateral approach. Make a curved longitudinal incision over the lateral border of the biceps, starting about 10 cm proximal to the flexion crease of the elbow. End the incision just above the flexion crease.

## Internervous Plane

There is no true internervous plane, because both the brachioradialis muscle and the lateral half of the brachialis muscle are supplied by the radial nerve proximal to the area of the incision. Proximal extension of the incision may denervate part of the brachialis, but this is of no clinical significance, because the radial nerve supply to the brachialis is minor and, probably, only proprioceptive. For this reason, the plane is both safe and extensile. Care should be taken during dissection down to the deep fascia; the lateral cutaneous nerve of the forearm runs roughly in the line of approach and should be retracted clear of the incision, in conjunction with the biceps (Figs. 2-10 and 2-11).

## Superficial Surgical Dissection

Incise the deep fascia of the arm in line with the skin incision and identify the lateral border of the biceps (see Fig. 2-10). Retract the biceps medially to reveal the brachialis and brachioradialis (see Fig. 2-11). Next, identify the interval between these muscles just above the elbow, incise the deep fascia over them in line with the intermuscular interval, and develop the intermuscular plane (Fig. 2-12). Find the radial nerve between the two muscles at the level of the elbow joint by exploring this oblique intermuscular plane gently with a finger. This is the easiest point at which to find the nerve. (The elbow is the point at which the radial nerve should be identified in all surgery performed in this general area.) Retract the brachioradialis laterally and the brachialis and biceps medially. Trace the radial nerve proximally until it pierces the lateral intermuscular septum.

## Deep Surgical Dissection

Carefully avoiding the radial nerve and staying on its medial side, incise the lateral border of the brachialis muscle longitudinally, cutting down to bone (Fig. 2-13). Incise the periosteum of the anterolateral aspect of the humerus longitudinally and retract the brachialis medially, lifting it off the anterior aspect of the bone by subperiosteal dissection. The anterior aspect of the distal humeral shaft now is exposed.

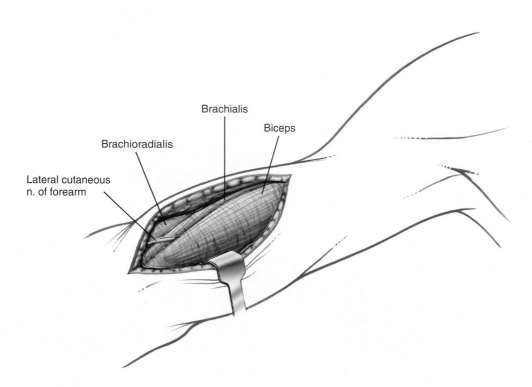

**Figure 2-10** There is no true internervous plane, but both the brachioradialis and the lateral half of the brachialis are supplied well proximal to the incision by the radial nerve. The sensory branch of the musculocutaneous nerve, the lateral cutaneous nerve of the forearm (lateral antebrachial cutaneous nerve), is seen emerging between the biceps and brachialis muscles.

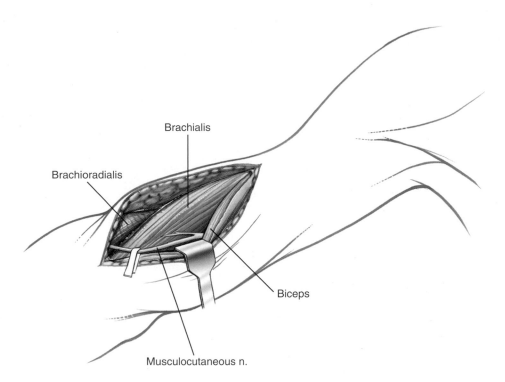

**Figure 2-11** Retract the biceps medially. Identify the lateral cutaneous nerve of the forearm (the sensory continuation of the musculocutaneous nerve) and retract it with the biceps. Identify the interval between the brachialis and the brachioradialis.

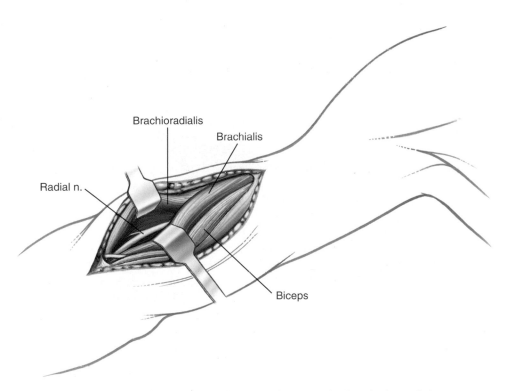

**Figure 2-12** Develop the intermuscular plane between the brachialis and the brachioradialis. Identify the radial nerve between the two muscles. Retract the brachioradialis laterally and the brachialis and biceps medially. Then trace the radial nerve proximally until it pierces the lateral intermuscular septum.

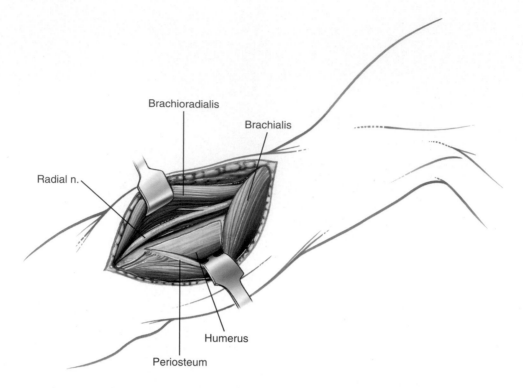

**Figure 2-13** Incise the periosteum of the anterolateral aspect of the humerus, and retract the brachialis and the periosteum medially to expose the anterior aspect of the distal shaft of the humerus.

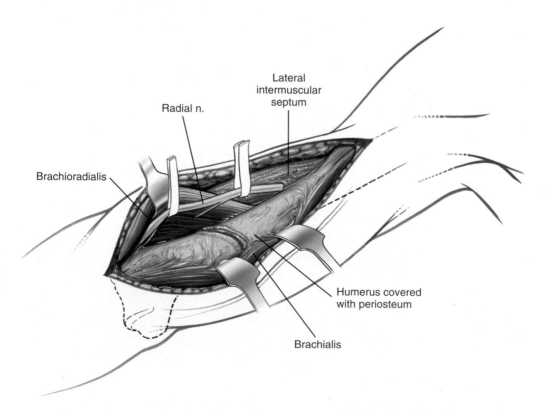

**Figure 2-14** The incision can be extended proximally by developing the plane between the brachialis and the lateral head of the triceps. The radial nerve is seen piercing the intermuscular septum. Posterior dissection may endanger the nerve as it passes through the spiral groove unless the dissection is kept below the periosteum.

## Dangers

### Nerves

The **radial nerve** must be identified and preserved before any incision is made through the substance of the brachialis muscle.

## How to Enlarge the Approach

### Extensile Measures

*Proximal Extension.* The incision can be extended proximally (although this rarely is required) by developing the plane between the brachialis medially and the lateral head of the triceps posterolaterally. Stripping brachialis from the front of the anterior aspect of the humerus exposes the bone. Care must be taken, however, if the dissection is taken further pos-

teriorly as posterior dissection may endanger the radial nerve as it passes in the spiral groove. If the approach is therefore extended posteriorly, a subperiosteal plane must be used. The disadvantage of soft-tissue stripping of the bone is in this case outweighed by the need to reduce the risk of damage to the radial nerve (Fig. 2-14).

*Distal Extension.* The anterolateral approach may be extended into an anterior approach to the elbow by continuing the skin incision distally and developing a plane between the brachioradialis muscle (which is supplied by the radial nerve) and the pronator teres muscle (which is supplied by the median nerve). Care should be taken to avoid the lateral cutaneous nerve of the forearm (the continuation of the musculocutaneous nerve), which emerges along the lateral side of the biceps tendon (see Anterolateral Approach in Chapter 3).

# Posterior Approach

The midline posterior approach to the humerus is classically extensile, providing excellent access to the lower three fourths of the posterior aspect of the humerus.[1] As is true for all other approaches to the humerus, the posterior approach is complicated by the vulnerability of the radial nerve, which spirals around the back of the bone. The uses of this surgical approach include the following:

1. Open reduction and internal fixation of fractures of the humerus. In fractures in which the radial nerve is damaged, this incision exposes the nerve as it traverses the back of the humerus.
2. Treatment of osteomyelitis
3. Biopsy and excision of tumors
4. Treatment of nonunion of fractures
5. Exploration of the radial nerve in the spiral groove
6. Insertion of retrograde humeral nails

## Position of the Patient

Two positions of the patient are possible during surgery: a lateral position on the operating table with

the affected side uppermost (Fig. 2-15*A*) or a prone position on the operating table with the arm abducted 90° (Fig. 2-15*B*). A sandbag should be placed under the shoulder of the side to be operated on, and the elbow should be allowed to bend and the forearm to hang over the side of the table. A tourniquet should not be used because it will get in the way.

## Landmarks and Incision

### Landmarks

The *acromion* is a rectangular bony prominence that forms the summit of the shoulder.

The *olecranon fossa* should be palpated at the distal end of the posterior aspect of the arm. Precise palpation is difficult, because the fossa is filled with fat and covered by a portion of the triceps muscle and aponeurosis. The fossa is filled by the olecranon when the elbow is extended.

### Incision

Make a longitudinal incision in the midline of the posterior aspect of the arm, from 8 cm below the acromion to the olecranon fossa (Fig. 2-16).

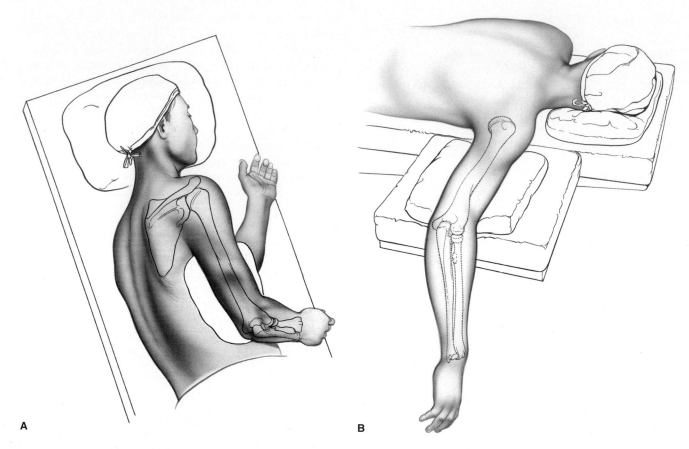

**A**

**B**

**Figure 2-15** Position of the patient for the approach to the upper arm in either the **(A)** lateral or **(B)** prone position.

## Internervous Plane

There is no true internervous plane; dissection involves separating the heads of the triceps brachii muscle, all of which are supplied by the radial nerve. Because the nerve branches enter the muscle heads relatively near their origin and run down the arm in the muscle's substance, splitting the muscle longitudinally does not denervate any part of it. In addition, the medial head (which is the deepest head) has a dual nerve supply consisting of the radial and ulnar nerves; splitting the medial head longitudinally does not denervate either half (see Fig. 2-35).

## Superficial Surgical Dissection

Incise the deep fascia of the arm in line with the skin incision (Fig. 2-17).

The key to superficial dissection lies in understanding the anatomy of the triceps muscle. This muscle has two layers. The outer layer consists of two heads: the lateral head arises from the lateral lip of the spiral groove, and the long head arises from the infraglenoid tubercle of the scapula. The inner layer consists of the third head, the medial (or deep) head, which arises from the whole width of the posterior aspect of the humerus below the spiral groove all the way down to the distal fourth of the bone. The spiral groove contains the radial nerve; thus, the radial nerve actually separates the origins of the lateral and medial heads (see Fig. 2-35).

To identify the gap between the lateral and long heads, begin proximally, above the point at which the two heads fuse to form a common tendon (Fig. 2-18). Proximally, develop this interval between the

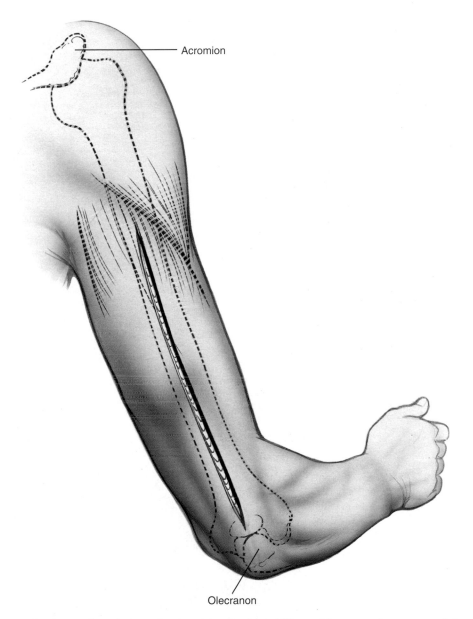

Acromion

Olecranon

**Figure 2-16**   Make a longitudinal incision in the midline of the posterior aspect of the arm, from 8 cm below the acromion to the olecranon fossa.

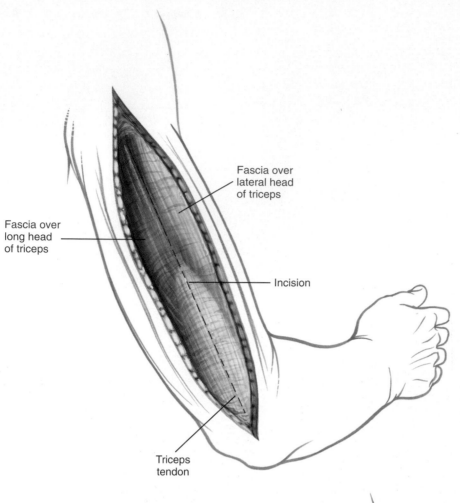

Fascia over
lateral head
of triceps

Fascia over
long head
of triceps

Incision

Triceps
tendon

**Figure 2-17** Incise the deep fascia of the arm in line with the skin incision.

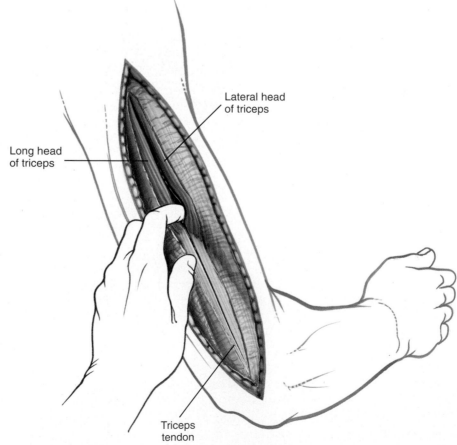

Lateral head
of triceps

Long head
of triceps

Triceps
tendon

**Figure 2-18** Identify the gap between the lateral and long heads of the triceps muscle.

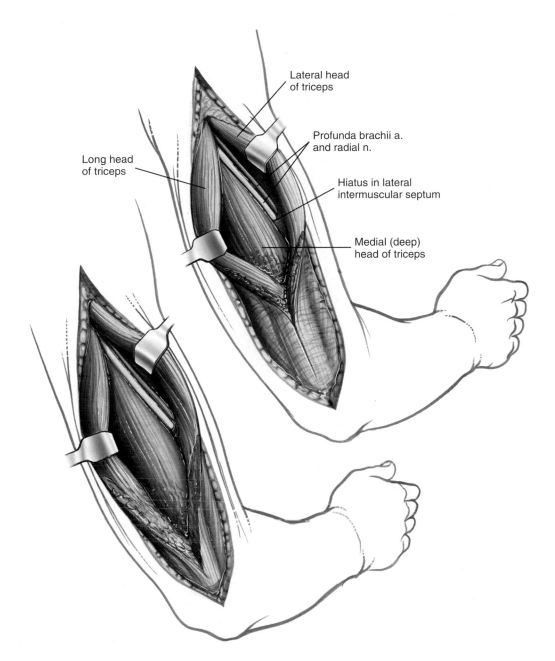

Lateral head
of triceps

Profunda brachii a.
and radial n.

Long head
of triceps

Hiatus in lateral
intermuscular septum

Medial (deep)
head of triceps

**Figure 2-19**   Proximally develop the interval between the two heads by blunt dissection, retracting the lateral head laterally and the long head medially. Distally split their common tendon along the line of the skin incision by sharp dissection. Identify the radial nerve and the accompanying profunda brachii artery.

heads by blunt dissection, retracting the lateral head laterally and the long head medially. Distally, the muscle will need to be divided by sharp dissection along the line of the skin incision (Fig. 2-19; see Fig. 2-34). Many small blood vessels cross the muscle at this level; these need to be coagulated individually.

## Deep Surgical Dissection

The medial head of the triceps muscle lies below the other two heads; the radial nerve runs just proximal to it in the spiral groove (see Fig. 2-19). Incise the medial head in the midline, continuing the dissection down to the periosteum of the humerus. Then, strip

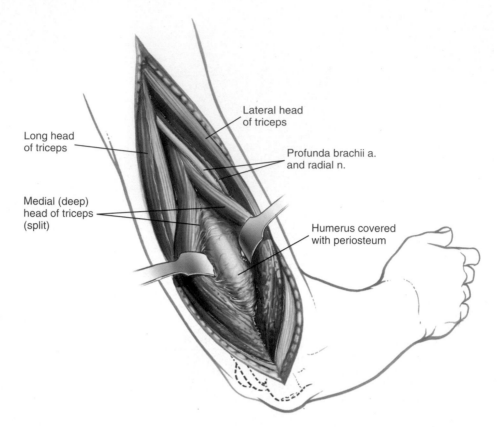

**Figure 2-20**    Incise the medial head of the triceps in the midline. Strip the muscle off the bone subperiosteally. The radial nerve, which runs just proximal to the origin of the muscle in the spiral groove, must be identified and preserved. The muscle must be stripped from the bone below the level of the periosteum to avoid damaging the ulnar nerve, which pierces the medial intermuscular septum. Preserve as much soft-tissue attachment to the bone as possible.

the muscle off the bone by subperiosteal dissection (Fig. 2-20). The plane of operation must remain in a subperiosteal location to avoid damaging the ulnar nerve, which pierces the medial intermuscular septum as it passes in an anterior to posterior direction in the lower third of the arm (see Figs. 2-20 and 2-36). Detach as little soft tissue as possible to preserve blood supply to the zone of injury.

## Dangers

### Nerves

The radial nerve is vulnerable in the spiral groove. Once it is identified, however, the nerve is safe. To avoid problems, never continue the dissection down to bone in the proximal two thirds of the arm until the nerve has been identified positively (see Fig. 2-19).

The ulnar nerve lies deep to the medial head of the triceps in the lower third of the arm and may be damaged if that muscle is elevated off the humerus in anything but a subperiosteal plane (see Fig. 2-36).

### Vessels

The profunda brachii artery lies with the radial nerve in the spiral groove and is similarly vulnerable (see Fig. 2-19).

## How to Enlarge the Approach

### Extensile Measures

*Proximal Extension.* The bone cannot be exposed effectively above the spiral groove using the posterior approach. At this point, the deltoid muscle (which is the outer layer of the musculature) also crosses the operative field. More proximal exposures should be accomplished by the anterior route.

*Distal Extension.* The skin incision can be extended distally over the olecranon; deepening the approach provides access to the elbow joint via an olecranon osteotomy (see Posterior Approach in Chapter 3; Fig. 2-21).

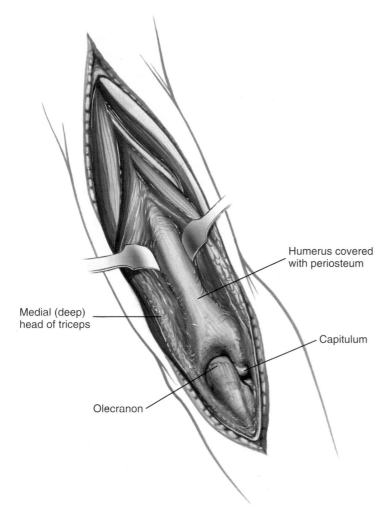

Humerus covered
with periosteum

Medial (deep)
head of triceps

Capitulum

Olecranon

**Figure 2-21**   The incision can be extended
distally over the olecranon to give access to the
elbow joint via an olecranon osteotomy. Proximal
extension cannot be used effectively above the spiral
groove because of the position of the radial nerve.

# Lateral Approach to the Distal Humerus

The lateral approach exposes the lateral epicondyle
and the origin of the wrist extensors. Its uses include
the following:

1. Open reduction and internal fixation of fractures
   of the lateral condyle
2. Surgical treatment of tennis elbow[4]

The lateral approach does not afford access to the
lateral portion of the elbow joint except by extension.
The joint itself should be accessed by the posterior,
posterolateral, or anterolateral approach.

## Position of the Patient

Place the patient supine on the operating table, with
the arm lying across the chest. Exsanguinate the arm
either by elevating it for 3 minutes or by applying a
soft, thin rubber bandage or exanguinator. Then,
apply a tourniquet (Fig. 2-22).

## Landmarks and Incision

### Landmarks

Palpate the *lateral epicondyle* on the lateral aspect of
the distal arm. It is the smaller of the two epicondyles.

The *lateral supracondylar ridge of the humerus* is
defined better and longer than is the medial supracondylar ridge. It extends almost to the deltoid
tuberosity (Fig. 2-23).

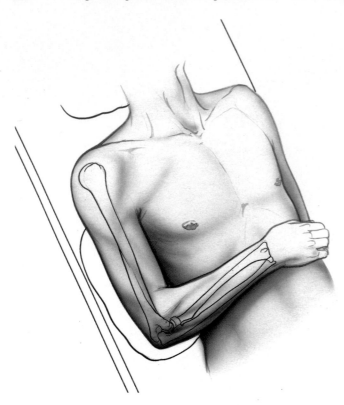

**Figure 2-22**    Position of the patient on the operating table. Place the patient supine on the operating table with the arm lying across the chest.

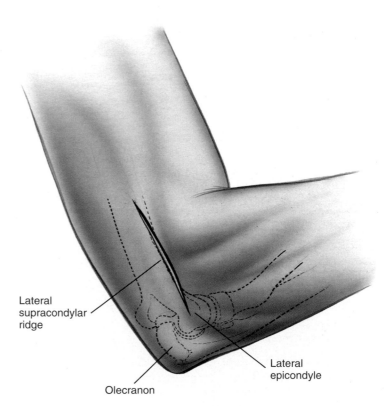

**Figure 2-23**    Make a straight or curved incision over the lateral supracondylar ridge of the elbow.

Lateral supracondylar ridge

Lateral epicondyle

Olecranon

## Incision

Make a 4- to 6-cm curved or straight incision on the lateral aspect of the elbow over the lateral supracondylar ridge (see Fig. 2-23).

## Internervous Plane

There is no true internervous plane, because both the triceps and the brachioradialis muscles are supplied by the radial nerve. Because the nerve supplies these muscles well proximal to the area of the surgical approach, however, the plane between them can be exploited distally without fear of damaging the nerve supply to either muscle (Fig. 2-24*A*).

## Superficial Surgical Dissection

Incise the deep fascia in line with the skin incision (see Fig. 2-24*B*). Define the plane between the brachioradialis, which originates from the lateral supra-

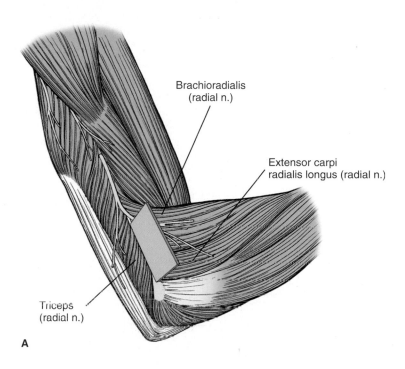

Brachioradialis (radial n.)

Extensor carpi radialis longus (radial n.)

Triceps (radial n.)

**A**

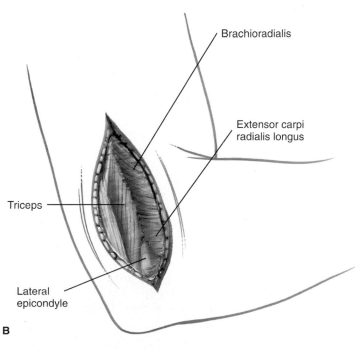

Brachioradialis

Extensor carpi radialis longus

Triceps

Lateral epicondyle

**B**

**Figure 2-24** (A, B) Intermuscular plane between the triceps and brachioradialis muscles. Both are supplied by the radial nerve proximal to the incision.

condylar ridge, and the triceps, and cut between these muscles down to bone, reflecting the brachioradialis anteriorly and the triceps posteriorly (Fig. 2-25; see Fig. 2-38).

## Deep Surgical Dissection

Identify the common extensor origin as it arises from the lateral epicondyle of the humerus (see Fig. 2-25). If further exposure of the bone is required, reflect the triceps off the back of the humerus. Release the extensor origin if a better view of the lateral epicondyle is needed (Fig. 2-26).

## Dangers

### Nerves

The radial nerve pierces the lateral intermuscular septum in the distal third of the arm. It is safe as long as the approach is not extended proximally (Fig. 2-27; see Fig. 2-40).

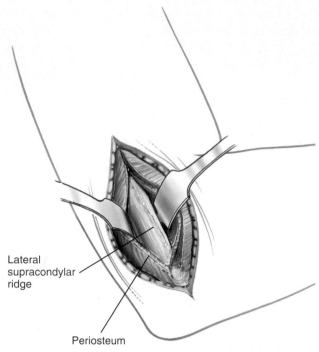

**Figure 2-25**   Incise the deep fascia in line with the skin incision. Define the plane between the brachioradialis and the triceps muscle and make an incision between them down onto the lateral supracondylar ridge. Reflect the brachioradialis anteriorly and the triceps posteriorly.

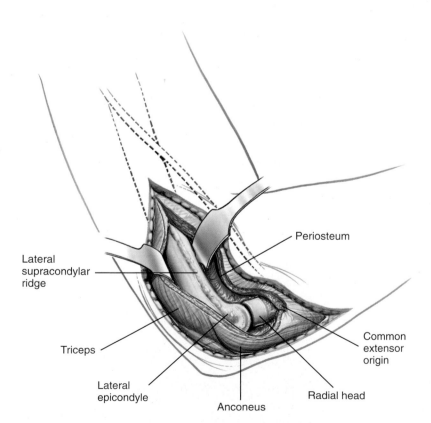

**Figure 2-26**   The incision may be extended to expose the radial head by using the internervous plane between the anconeus (radial nerve) and the extensor carpi ulnaris (posterior interosseous nerve). The common extensor origin is detached and reflected anteriorly. The triceps also may be reflected more posteriorly. Proximal extension is not possible because of the course of the radial nerve.

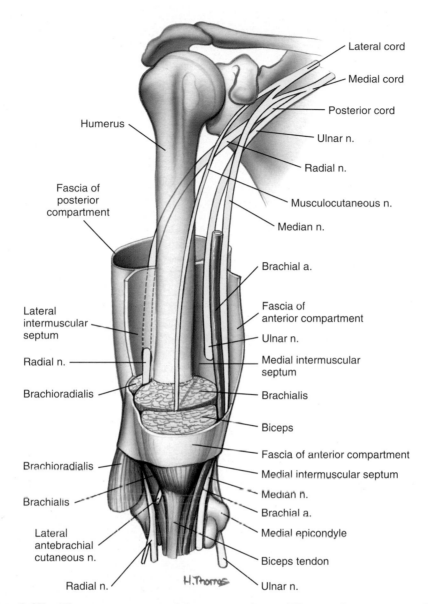

**Figure 2-27** The compartments of the arm are shown. The muscles are removed partially to show the course of the radial, ulnar, and median nerves as they run down the arm. The relationships of the nerves to the compartments and septa are seen.

## How to Enlarge the Approach

### Extensile Measures

***Proximal Extension.*** Proximal extension is not possible, because the radial nerve crosses the proposed line of dissection.

***Distal Extension.*** The lateral approach can be extended to the radial head only by using the intra-muscular plane between the anconeus muscle (which is supplied by the radial nerve) and the extensor carpi ulnaris muscle (which is supplied by the posterior interosseous nerve; see Posterior Approach to the Radius in Chapter 4 and Fig. 2-26). This approach cannot be extended further distally due to the presence of the posterior interosseous nerve winding round the neck of the proximal radius.

# Applied Surgical Anatomy of the Arm

## Overview

The critical neurovascular structures in surgery of the arm do not stay neatly in one operative field, but cross from compartment to compartment as they course down the arm. Therefore, it is easiest to view the anatomy of the arm as consisting of two major muscle compartments, flexor and extensor, that share responsibility for three major nerves and arteries (see Fig. 2-27).

## Muscle Compartments

1. The *anterior flexor compartment* contains three muscles: the coracobrachialis, the biceps brachii, and the brachialis. Two are flexors of the elbow; all are supplied by the musculocutaneous nerve.
2. The *posterior extensor compartment* consists of one muscle, the triceps brachii, which is supplied by the radial nerve. In the distal two thirds of the arm, the muscle compartments are separated by lateral and medial intermuscular septa.

## Nerves

1. The *radial nerve*, which is the key surgical landmark in the arm, is the continuation of the posterior cord of the brachial plexus. It begins behind the axillary artery at the shoulder, runs along the posterior wall of the axilla (on the subscapularis, latissimus dorsi, and teres major muscles), and then passes through the triangular space between the long head of the triceps muscle and the shaft of the humerus beneath the teres major muscle. In the arm, the nerve lies in the spiral groove on the posterior aspect of the humerus between the lateral and medial (deep) heads of the triceps muscle. After crossing the back of the humerus and giving off branches to the lateral head and the lateral part

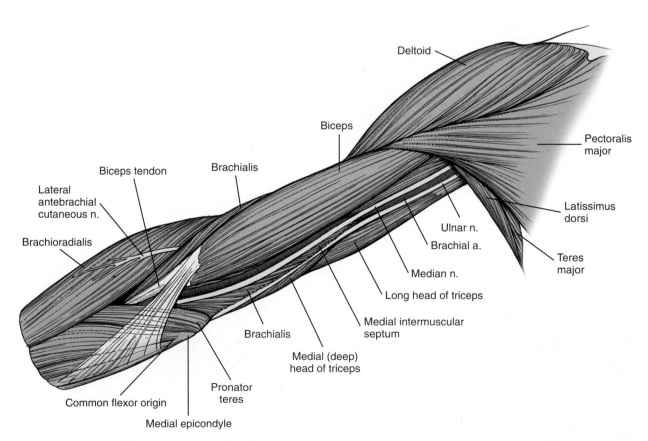

**Figure 2-28**  Superficial layer of muscles of the arm. Note the course of the brachial artery and the median and ulnar nerves. The brachial artery starts medial to the median nerve. In the distal part of the arm, it moves lateral to the median nerve before entering the cubital fossa.

of the medial head of the triceps, the radial nerve pierces the lateral intermuscular septum, entering the anterior compartment and lying between the brachioradialis and brachialis muscles as it crosses the elbow joint. There, it supplies the brachioradialis, extensor carpi radialis longus, extensor carpi radialis brevis, and anconeus muscles (see Figs. 2-27, 2-31, 2-35, 2-36, 2-39, and 2-40).

2. The *median nerve* remains in the anterior compartment, anteromedial to the humerus. It runs with the brachial artery, lateral to it in the upper arm and medial to it in the cubital fossa.

3. The *ulnar nerve* lies behind the brachial artery in the anterior compartment of the upper half of the arm. It pierces the medial intermuscular septum about two thirds of the way down the arm to enter the posterior compartment, where it lies with the triceps muscle. It then travels on the back of the medial epicondyle of the humerus, where it is almost subcutaneous in location. Similar to the median nerve, it has no branches in the arm (see Figs. 2-31, 2-37, and 2-39).

## Arteries

The vascular organization of the arm is relatively simple; each nerve takes one artery with it.

1. The brachial artery runs with the median nerve down the medial border of the arm under the biceps brachii muscle and onto the brachialis muscle. The artery can be palpated along its entire length, because the deep fascia of the arm is the only medial covering. The artery lies medial to the humerus in the upper two thirds of the arm. At the elbow, it curves laterally to lie over the anterior surface of the bone, where it may be damaged in supracondylar fractures of the humerus (Figs. 2-28 and 2-29).

2. The *profunda brachii artery* runs with the radial nerve, supplying the triceps brachii muscle (see Figs. 2-35 and 2-36).

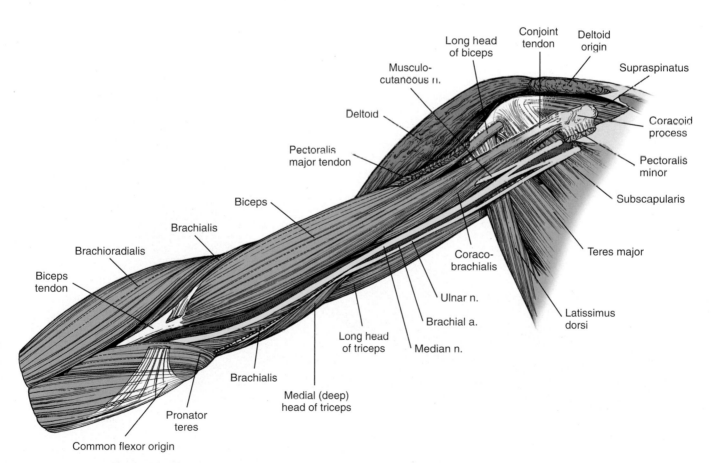

**Figure 2-29** The anterior fibers of the deltoid have been removed. The pectoralis major and minor have been resected at their insertions. Note the relationship of the nerves to the teres major, subscapularis, and latissimus dorsi, as well as the point where the musculocutaneous nerve enters the coracobrachialis muscle. Distally, note the position of the brachial artery and median nerve at the tendinous insertion of the biceps.

3. The *ulnar collateral artery* runs with the ulnar nerve. The three arteries anastomose freely with one another around the elbow joint.

## Landmarks and Incision

### Incisions

A longitudinal incision on the anterior aspect of the arm closely parallels the lines of cleavage of the skin. More proximally, however, the same incision crosses perpendicular to the lines of cleavage. The cosmetic appearance of anterior scars, therefore, is variable and dependent on their location.

A longitudinal incision on the posterior aspect of the humerus crosses the lines of cleavage of the skin at almost 90°. Scars made by posterior incisions are likely to be broad.

## Superficial Surgical Dissection

### Anterolateral Approach to the Humerus

Proximally, the internervous plane lies between the deltoid muscle (which is supplied by the axillary nerve) and the pectoralis major muscle (which is supplied by the lateral and medial pectoral nerves; see Anterior Approach in Chapter 1). Distally, the approach involves the muscles of the flexor compartment of the arm (Figs. 2-30 through 2-32; see Figs. 2-28 and 2-29).

*The coracobrachialis* is a largely vestigial muscle arising from the coracoid process (see Applied Surgical Anatomy of the Anterior Approach in Chapter 1).

The *biceps brachii* is a powerful flexor of the elbow and supinator of the forearm (see Applied Surgical Anatomy of the Anterior Approach in Chapter 1).

The *brachialis* is the main elbow flexor, the workhorse of the upper arm. The biceps only really comes into play when extra strength or speed of flexion is required.

The surgical importance of the brachialis lies in its nerve supply. The lateral part of the muscle is supplied by the radial nerve, and the medial part is supplied by the musculocutaneous nerve. Thus, the muscle can be split longitudinally without either side being denervated. Because the musculocutaneous nerve is the major nerve supply to the brachialis, even cutting the radial nerve supply to the muscle seems to have little clinical effect. That is why the plane between the brachialis and the adjacent lateral muscle, the brachioradialis, is useful in surgery.

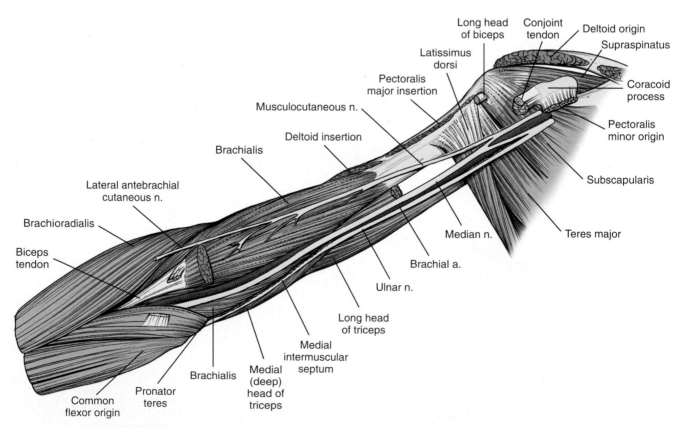

**Figure 2-30** The biceps muscle has been removed at its proximal origins—its conjoined tendon and long head. A portion of the coracobrachialis has been removed to reveal the musculocutaneous nerve running on the brachialis muscle, supplying it. The median nerve and ulnar nerve course through the arm without supplying its muscles.

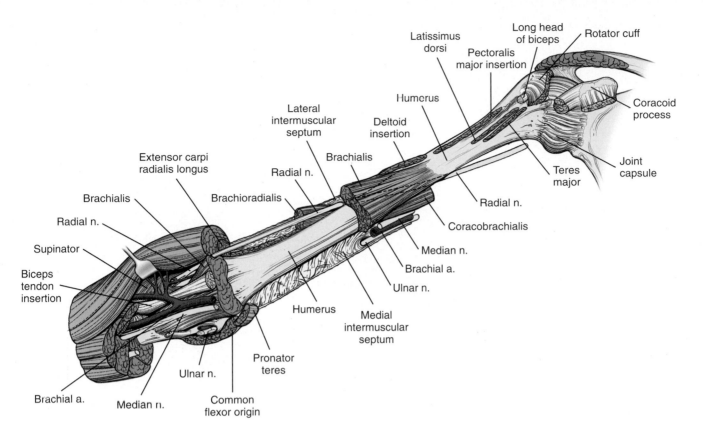

**Figure 2-31** The central portion of the brachialis and the extensor carpi radialis longus have been resected to reveal the distal humerus and the course of the radial nerve as it pierces the lateral intermuscular septum to enter the anterior compartment. The radial nerve continues distally into the elbow before entering the supinator muscle. Medially, the relationships of the median nerve, brachial artery, and ulnar nerve are revealed. The median nerve is anterior to the brachial artery. The ulnar nerve, situated posteriorly, penetrates the medial intermuscular septum to enter the posterior compartment of the arm. The partially resected flexor-pronator group reveals the deeper structures at the level of the elbow.

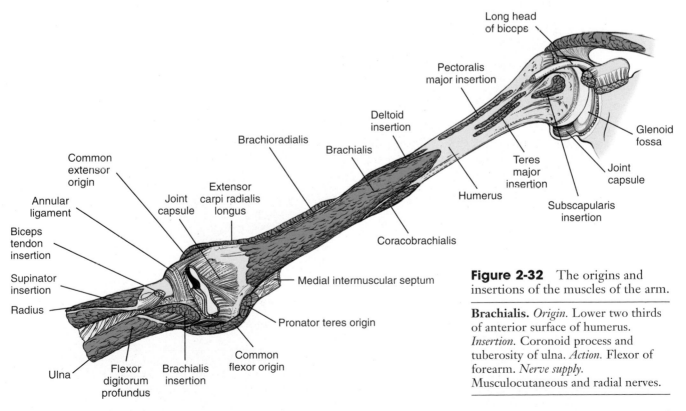

**Figure 2-32** The origins and insertions of the muscles of the arm.

---

**Brachialis.** *Origin.* Lower two thirds of anterior surface of humerus. *Insertion.* Coronoid process and tuberosity of ulna. *Action.* Flexor of forearm. *Nerve supply.* Musculocutaneous and radial nerves.

---

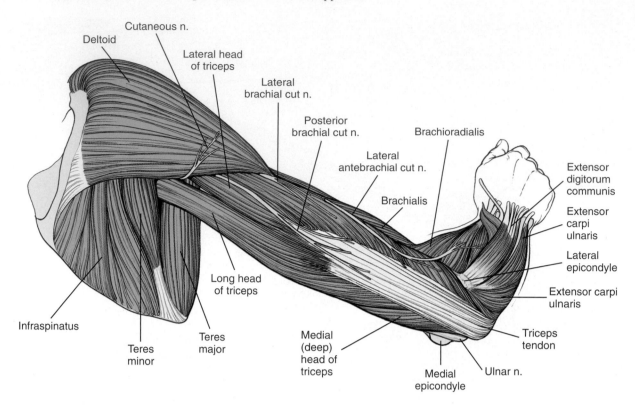

**Figure 2-33**   The anatomy of the posterior aspect of the arm. Note the cleavage plane between the long and lateral heads of the triceps.

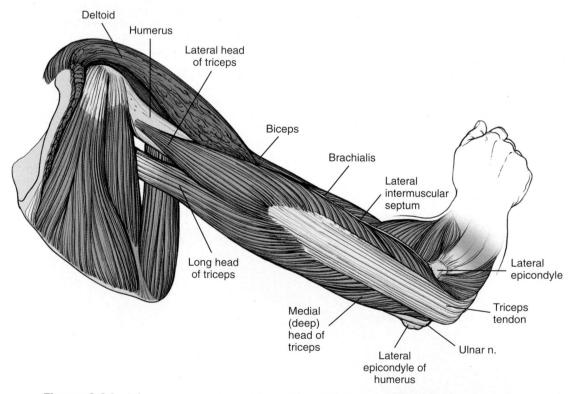

**Figure 2-34**   The most posterior portion of the deltoid muscle has been removed to reveal the origin of the lateral head of the triceps.

**Triceps Brachii.** *Origin.* Long head from infraglenoid tuberosity of scapula. Lateral head from posterior and lateral aspect of humerus. Medial (deep) head from lower posterior surface of humerus. *Insertion.* Upper posterior surface of olecranon. *Action.* Extensor of forearm. Weak adductor of shoulder. *Nerve supply.* Radial nerve.

## Posterior Approach to the Humerus

The posterior approach involves splitting the triceps brachii muscle (Figs. 2-33 through 2-37).

The long head of the triceps brachii receives its radial nerve supply high up in the axilla, close to its origin; the lateral head receives its supply lower, at the upper level of the spiral groove. The two heads can be split up to the level of the spiral groove without compromising the nerve supply of either (Fig. 2-41; see Figs. 2-33 through 2-37).

The medial (deep) head has a dual nerve supply. The medial half receives fibers from the radial nerve. The fibers run alongside the ulnar nerve, so closely bound to it that they once were thought of as branches of the ulnar nerve. They actually are radial fibers that are "hitchhiking" in the ulnar nerve substance.[5]

The lateral half of the medial head receives its nerve supply from the main trunk of the radial nerve as it crosses the back of the humerus in the spiral groove. Because of its dual nerve supply, the medial head may be split longitudinally to expose the posterior surface of the humerus.

## Special Anatomic Points

In some patients, the coracobrachialis muscle has an additional head that attaches to the ligament of Struthers.[6] This ligament connects a supracondylar spur of bone to the medial epicondyle of the humerus. It may trap the median nerve between itself and the underlying bone. Entrapment produces symptoms similar to those of carpal tunnel syndrome.[7] Compression of the median nerve at this level can be differentiated from compression within the carpal tunnel because the flexor muscles of the forearm, as well as the palmar cutaneous branches of the median nerve, are affected. All these branches come off below the ligament and above the carpal tunnel.

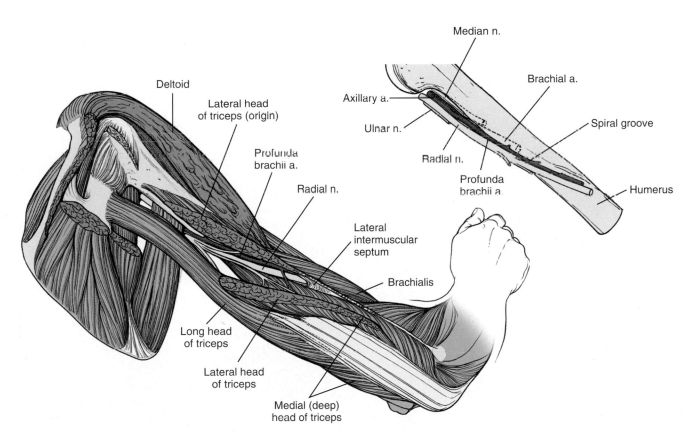

**Figure 2-35** The central portion of the lateral head of the triceps has been removed to reveal the courses of the radial nerve and profunda brachii artery in the spiral groove. The fibers of the medial head of the triceps surround the radial nerve in its groove, protecting it from the bone. Detail of the relationship among the radial nerve, the axillary artery, and the profunda brachii artery (inset). The axillary artery becomes the brachial artery on the anterior surface of the humerus. There it gives off a branch, the profunda brachii artery, which continues posteriorly with the radial nerve through the triangular space and the spiral groove.

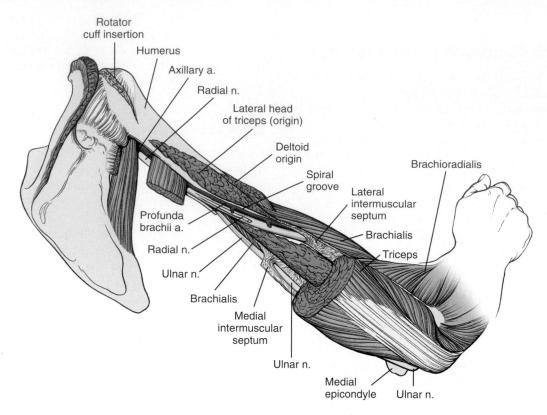

**Figure 2-36** Resection of the proximal half of the triceps. The radial nerve and profunda brachii artery run in the spiral groove between the origins of the lateral and deep heads of the triceps. The nerve and vessel penetrate the lateral intermuscular septum before entering the anterior compartment of the arm. The ulnar nerve pierces the lateral intermuscular septum to gain entrance to the posterior compartment of the arm.

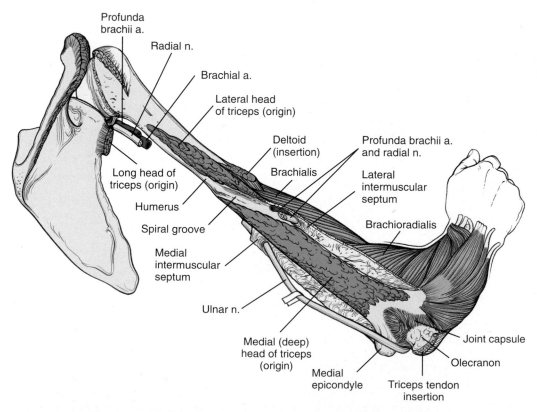

**Figure 2-37** The entire triceps muscle has been removed, uncovering the entire posterior surface of the humerus. The medial and lateral intermuscular septa and the nerves that penetrate them are seen.

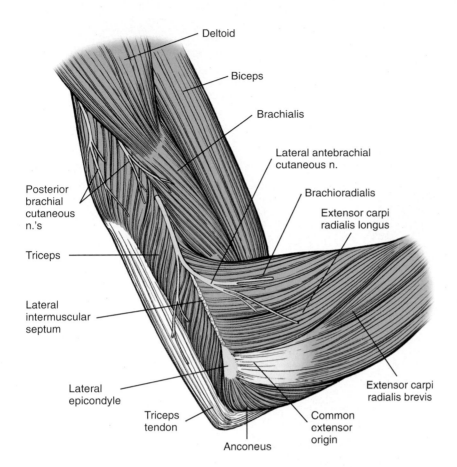

Deltoid

Biceps

Brachialis

Lateral antebrachial
cutaneous n.

Brachioradialis

Extensor carpi
radialis longus

Posterior
brachial
cutaneous
n.'s

Triceps

Lateral
intermuscular
septum

Lateral
epicondyle

Triceps
tendon

Anconeus

Common
extensor
origin

Extensor carpi
radialis brevis

**Figure 2-38**   The lateral aspect of
the humerus, with the overlying
superficial cutaneous nerves.

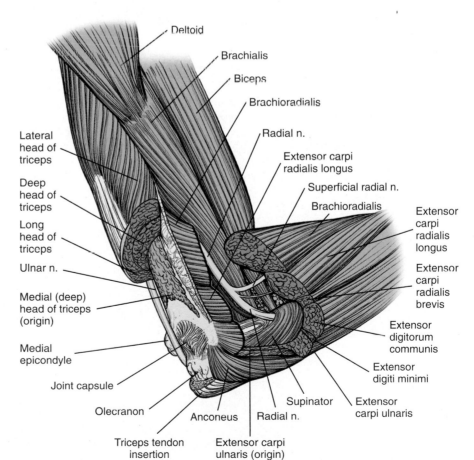

Deltoid

Brachialis

Biceps

Brachioradialis

Radial n.

Extensor carpi
radialis longus

Superficial radial n.

Brachioradialis

Extensor
carpi
radialis
longus

Extensor
carpi
radialis
brevis

Extensor
digitorum
communis

Extensor
digiti minimi

Extensor
carpi ulnaris

Lateral
head of
triceps

Deep
head of
triceps

Long
head of
triceps

Ulnar n.

Medial (deep)
head of triceps
(origin)

Medial
epicondyle

Joint capsule

Olecranon

Triceps tendon
insertion

Anconeus

Extensor carpi
ulnaris (origin)

Radial n.

Supinator

**Figure 2-39**   The posterior
aspect of the humerus and elbow
joint and the course of the ulnar
nerve. The lateral intermuscular
septum runs beneath the
brachioradialis. The main
continuation of the radial nerve is
the posterior interosseous nerve,
which pierces the supinator muscle
through the arcade of Frohse.

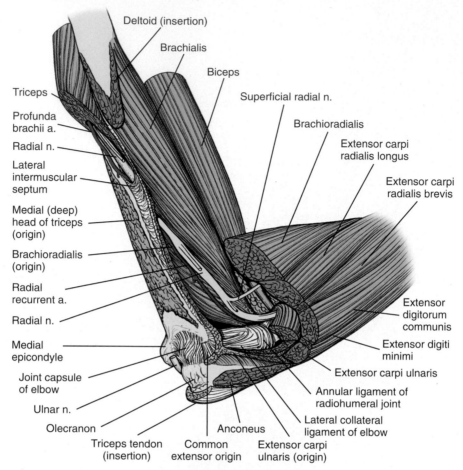

**Figure 2-40**    The lateral intermuscular septum and the course of the radial nerve as it passes from the spiral groove through the intermuscular septum to emerge in the forearm from between the brachialis and the brachioradialis. The muscles covering the posterolateral aspect of the joint have been removed to reveal the joint capsule.

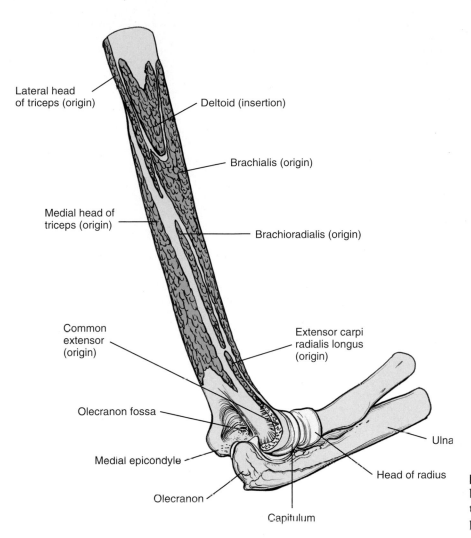

Lateral head
of triceps (origin)

Deltoid (insertion)

Brachialis (origin)

Medial head of
triceps (origin)

Brachioradialis (origin)

Common
extensor
(origin)

Extensor carpi
radialis longus
(origin)

Olecranon fossa

Ulna

Medial epicondyle

Head of radius

Olecranon

Capitulum

**Figure 2-41** The muscles have been removed completely, showing the origins of the musculature of the posterior humerus.

## Minimal Access Approach to the Proximal Humerus

The minimal access approach to the proximal humerus is used for the insertion of intramedullary nails for the treatment of the following:

1. Acute humeral shaft fractures
2. Pathological humeral shaft fractures
3. Delayed union and nonunion of humeral shaft fractures

The presence of the overlying acromion and the fact that the upper end of the humerus is covered entirely with articular cartilage mean that all nails are angled at their upper end and are inserted via the lateral cortex of the humerus. The entry point for an intermedullary nail into the humerus is determined radiographically, with a template of the required nail superimposed over a radiograph of the injured humerus. The entry point depends on the specific design of the nail. The most usual entry point is just lateral to the articular surface of the humeral head and just medial to the greater tuberosity (see Fig. 2-46).

### Position of the Patient

Place the patient in a supine position. Elevate the upper portion of the table approximately 60° (see Fig. 1-65). Position the patient so that the shoulder lies over the edge of the table. Alternatively, use a specialized table that allows radiographic visualization of the shoulder in both anterior-posterior and lateral planes. Ensure that the cervical spine is adequately supported and that lateral flexion of the cervical spine is avoided to prevent a traction lesion of the brachial plexus.

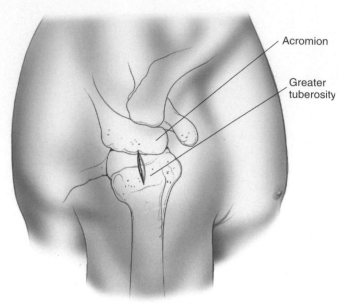

**Figure 2-42**   Palpate the lateral border of the acromion and then make a 2-cm incision from that border down the lateral aspect of the arm.

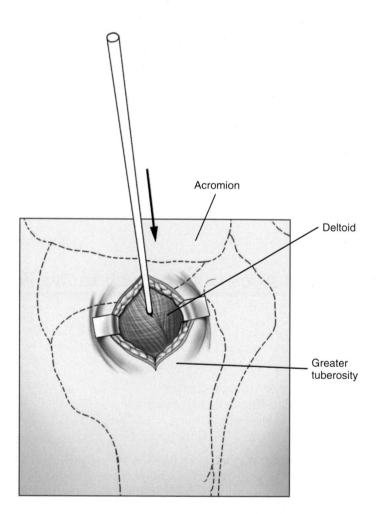

**Figure 2-43**   Insert a guidewire through the substance of the deltoid muscle under image intensifier control.

## Landmarks and Incision

### Landmark

The *acromion* is rectangular. Its bony dorsum and lateral border are easy to palpate on the outer aspect of the shoulder (see Figs. 1-38 and 1-40).

### Incision

Make a 2-cm incision from the outer aspect of the acromion down the lateral aspect of the arm (Fig. 2-42; see Fig. 1-33).

## Internervous Plane

This approach does not exploit an internervous plane. The dissection involves splitting the deltoid muscle.

## Superficial and Deep Surgical Dissections

Insert a wire under image intensifier control through the skin incision, down through the substance of the deltoid muscle and rotator cuff to the correct insertion point on the humerus (Fig. 2-43). This position has been determined on the preoperative x-ray plan. Confirm that the wire is in the correct position by the use of a C-arm image intensifier in both anterior-posterior and lateral planes.

Withdraw the wire and insert a point-ended scalpel blade, following the track of the wire using a C-arm image intensifier to confirm position (Fig. 2-44). Incise a small portion of the deltoid and make a small clean-edged incision through part of the supraspinatus tendon. Withdraw the blade and reinsert the wire. Enter the proximal end of the humerus

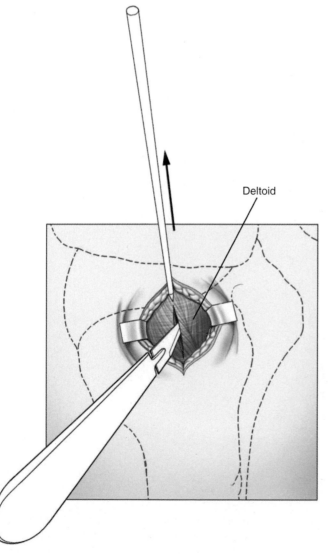

Deltoid

**Figure 2-44** Enlarge the track made by the wire using a point-ended scalpel. You will incise part of the deltoid and part of the supraspinatus tendon.

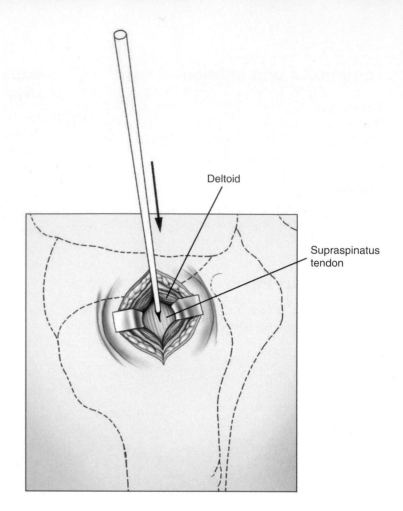

**Figure 2-45** Insert the wire into the proximal end of the humerus under image intensifier control.

Deltoid

Supraspinatus tendon

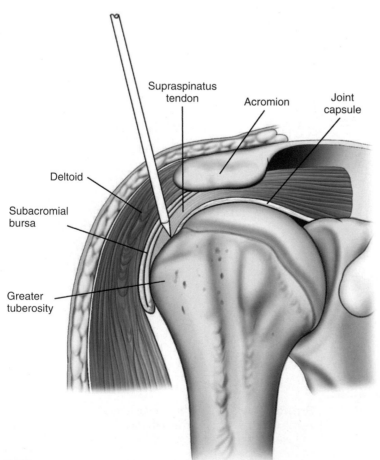

Supraspinatus tendon

Acromion

Joint capsule

Deltoid

Subacromial bursa

Greater tuberosity

**Figure 2-46** Lateral view of the shoulder, revealing insertion of the guidewire. The most common entry point is just lateral to the articular surface of the humeral head and just medial to the greater tuberosity.

using an awl or drill, depending on the nail to be used (Figs. 2-45 and 2-46).

## Dangers

### Nerves

The *axillary nerve* lies approximately 7 cm below the tip of the acromion, running transversely on the deep aspect of the deltoid muscle. This incision should therefore not risk damage to the axillary nerve (see Fig. 1-33).

### Tendons

Part of the *supraspinatus tendon* will be incised by this approach. A degree of damage to the rotator cuff is therefore inevitable in proximal humeral nailing using conventional nails (see Fig. 1-4). Damage to the rotator cuff is minimized by ensuring that any drills used are passed through protection sleeves, but a significant degree of stiffness of the shoulder occurs postoperatively in large numbers of patients following antegrade humeral nailing.

## How to Enlarge the Approach

### Extensile Measures

***Distal Extension.*** The approach can be extended to a formal lateral approach to the proximal humerus. This extension may be needed if closed reduction of proximal humeral fractures cannot be obtained (see Fig. 1-36).

### REFERENCES

1. HENRY AK: Extensile exposure, 2nd ed. Edinburgh, E&S Livingston, 1966
2. HENRY AK: Exposure of the humerus and femoral shaft. Br J Surg 12:84, 1924
3. THOMPSON JE: Anatomical methods of approach in operating on the long bones of the extremities. Ann Surg 68:309, 1918
4. BOYD HB, MCLEOD AC JR: Tennis elbow. J Bone Joint Surg [Am] 55:1183, 1973
5. LAST RJ: Anatomy regional and applied, 6th ed. Edinburgh, Churchill Livingstone, 1978
6. STRUTHERS J: On a peculiarity of the humerus and humeral artery. Monthly J Medical Science 8:264, 1948
7. SUTHERLAND S: Nerves and nerve injuries. Baltimore, Williams & Wilkins, 1968

# Three

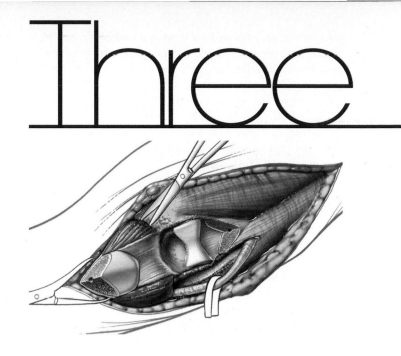

# The Elbow

The elbow is a hinged joint supported by strong collateral ligaments. The key neurovascular structures running down the arm pass anterior and posterior to the joint. The medial and lateral approaches, therefore, avoid the obvious neurovascular dangers, but provide limited access to the elbow because of its bony configuration. Anterior and posterior approaches provide better access to the joint, but may endanger the key neurovascular structures.

Of the five surgical approaches that are described in this chapter, the *posterior approach* provides the best possible exposure to all surfaces of the elbow and is the approach used most often for the internal fixation of complex fractures of this joint. The *medial approach* provides good access to the medial side of the joint, but requires an osteotomy of the medial epicondyle for best exposure. This osteotomy does not involve any part of the articular surface, however. Although the approach is extensile to the distal humerus, it is most useful in dealing with local pathologies of the medial side of the joint. The anterolateral approach exposes the lateral side of the joint; in addition, it can be extended both proximally and distally to expose both the humerus and the radius from the shoulder to the wrist. The *anterior approach* to the cubital fossa is designed primarily for exploration of the critical neurovascular structures that pass in front of the elbow joint. The *posterolateral approach* to the radial head is designed exclusively for surgery on that structure.

The applied anatomy of the elbow is discussed in a single section of this chapter after the various surgical approaches are described, mainly because the keys to the surgical anatomy are the neurovascular bundles that pass across the elbow joint; their positions are important in all the approaches. Separate subsections outline the anatomy that applies to each particular approach.

## Posterior Approach

The posterior approach provides the best possible view of the bones that comprise the elbow joint.[1,2] Although it is basically a safe and reliable operative technique, it does have one major drawback: it usually requires an osteotomy of the olecranon on its articular surface, creating another "fracture" that must be internally fixed. The uses of the posterior approach include the following:

1. Open reduction and internal fixation of fractures of the distal humerus[3,4]
2. Removal of loose bodies within the elbow joint
3. Treatment of nonunions of the distal humerus

Extension contractures of the elbow can be treated by using some portions of this approach to lengthen the triceps muscle, without performing an olecranon osteotomy.

### Position of the Patient

Place the intubated patient prone on the operating table, ensuring adequate padding for the chest and pelvis to allow free movement of the abdomen during respiration. Exsanguinate the limb by elevating it for 3 to 5 minutes and then apply a tourniquet as high up on the arm as possible. Abduct the arm about 90° and place a small sandbag underneath the tourniquet, elevating the upper arm from the operating

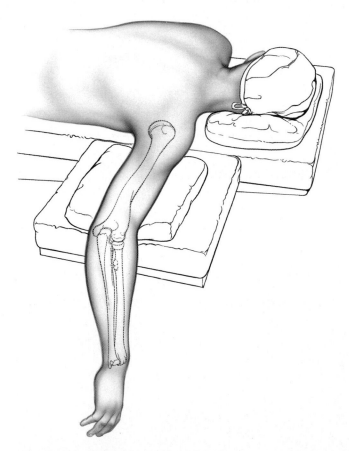

**Figure 3-1**    Position of the patient on the operating table.

table. Allow the elbow to flex and the forearm to hang over the side of the table (Fig. 3-1).

## Landmarks and Incision

### Landmark
Palpate the large, bony *olecranon process* at the upper end of the ulna. It is conical and has a relatively sharp apex.

### Incision
Make a longitudinal incision on the posterior aspect of the elbow. Begin 5 cm above the olecranon in the midline of the posterior aspect of the arm. Just above the tip of the olecranon, curve the incision laterally so that it runs down the lateral side of the process. To complete the incision, curve it medially again so that it overlies the middle of the subcutaneous surface of the ulna. Running the incision around the tip of the olecranon moves the suture line away from devices that are used to fix the olecranon osteotomy and away from the weight-bearing tip of the elbow (Fig. 3-2).

## Internervous Plane

There is no true internervous plane, because the approach involves little more than detaching the extensor mechanism of the elbow. The nerve supply of the triceps muscle (the radial nerve) enters the muscle well proximal to the dissection.

## Superficial Surgical Dissection

Incise the deep fascia in the midline. Palpate the ulnar nerve as it lies in the bony groove on the back of the medial epicondyle and incise the fascia overlying the nerve to expose it. Fully dissect out the ulnar nerve and pass tapes around it so that it can be identified at all times (Fig. 3-3). Do not use these tapes for retraction as this can create a traction lesion to the nerve.

If a screw is going to be used to fix the olecranon osteotomy, drill and tap the olecranon *before* the osteotomy is performed. Score the bone longitudinally with an osteotome so that the pieces can be aligned correctly when the osteotomy is repaired (see Fig. 3-3, *inset*).

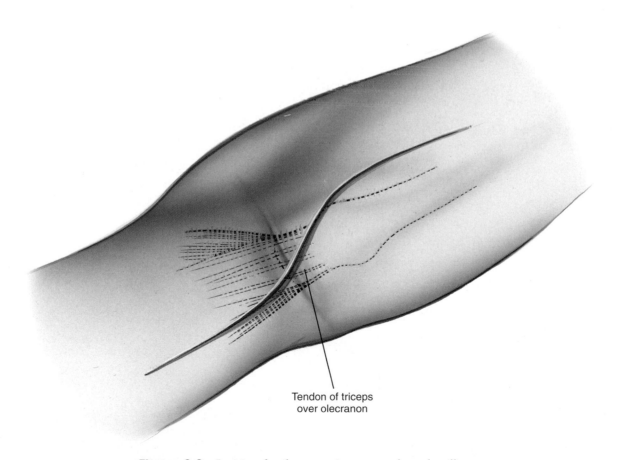

Tendon of triceps
over olecranon

**Figure 3-2**   Incision for the posterior approach to the elbow.

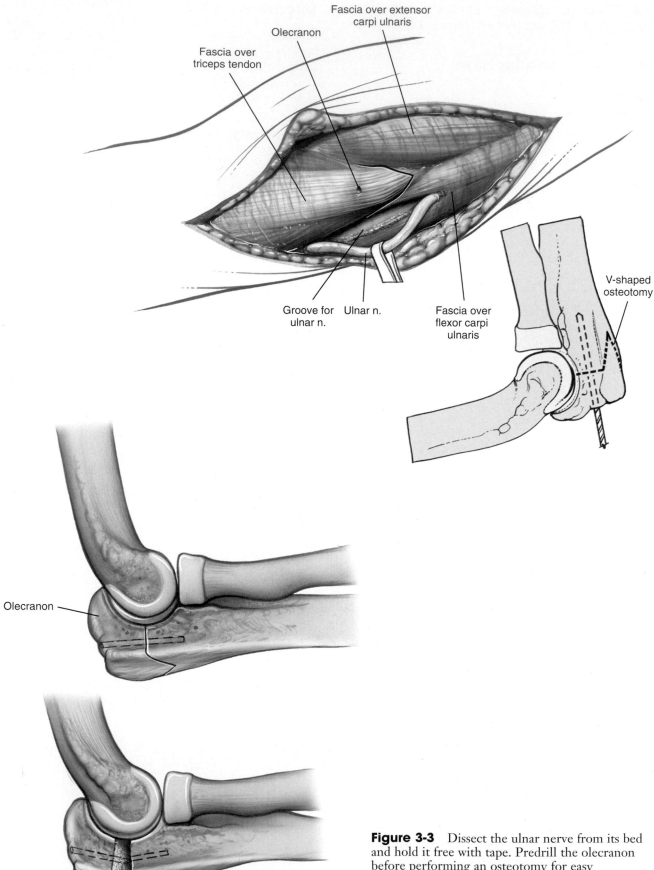

**Figure 3-3**   Dissect the ulnar nerve from its bed and hold it free with tape. Predrill the olecranon before performing an osteotomy for easy reattachment. A V-shaped osteotomy is inherently more stable than a transverse osteotomy.

Make a V-shaped osteotomy of the olecranon about 2 cm from its tip using an oscillating saw. The apex of the V is directed distally. A V-shaped osteotomy gives greater stability than a transverse osteotomy after fixation. Divide the bone until it is cut through almost entirely. Snap the remaining cortex by wedging the two cut surfaces apart with an osteotome. This will cause an irregularity in the osteotomy, allowing it to key together better during repair (see Fig. 3-3, *inset*).

## Deep Surgical Dissection

Strip the soft-tissue attachments off the medial and lateral sides of the portion of the olecranon that has been subjected to osteotomy and retract it proximally, elevating the triceps from the back of the humerus (Fig. 3-4). The posterior aspect of the distal end of the humerus is directly underneath; subperiosteal dissection around the medial and lateral borders of the bone allows exposure of all surfaces of the

distal fourth of the humerus (Fig. 3-5). Note that full exposure seldom will be needed. All the soft-tissue attachments to bone that can be preserved should be, particularly in reductions of fractures. Stripping excessive soft-tissue attachments off the bone leaves the bone fragments without a vascular supply and jeopardizes healing.

Be careful not to extend the dissection proximally above the distal fourth of the humerus, because the radial nerve, which passes from the posterior to the anterior compartment of the arm through the lateral intermuscular septum, may be damaged. Flex the elbow to relax the anterior structures if they need to be elevated off the front of the humerus (see Figs. 2-36 and 2-37).

The ulnar nerve must be kept clear of the operative field during all stages of the dissection. Some surgeons advise routine anterior transposition of the nerve during closure, especially if implant removal is anticipated in the future.

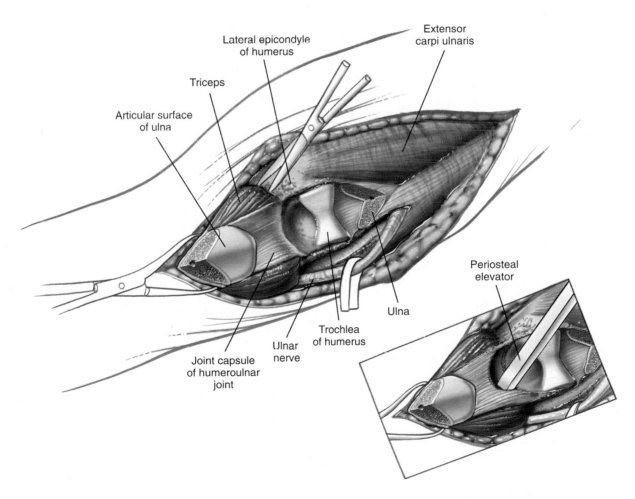

**Figure 3-4**   Perform a V-shaped osteotomy of the olecranon and retract it proximally, with the triceps muscle attached. Strip a portion of the joint capsule with an osteotome.

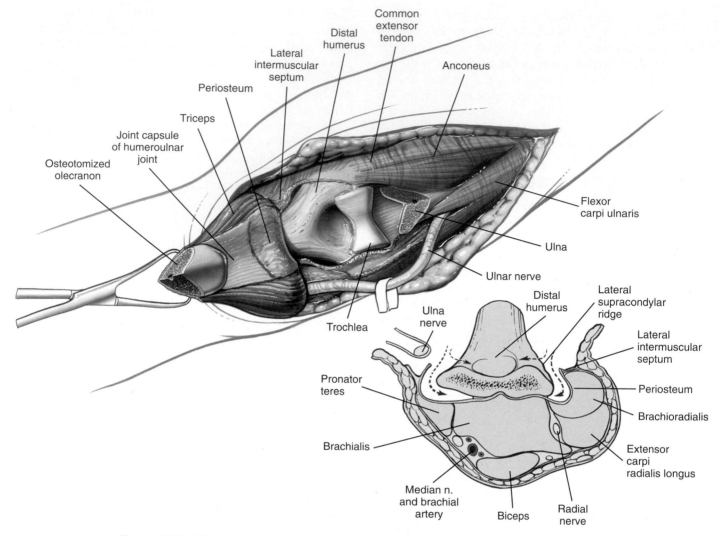

**Figure 3-5**   Dissect around the medial and lateral borders of the bone to expose all the surfaces of the distal fourth of the humerus.

## Dangers

### Nerves

The **ulnar nerve** is in no danger as long as it is identified early and protected, and excessive traction is not placed on it.

The **median nerve** lies anterior to the distal humerus. It may be endangered if the anterior structures are not stripped off the distal humerus. In cases of fracture, this dissection has usually been done for you. In the treatment of nonunions or when the approach is used for osteotomies, a strictly subperiosteal plane must be used to avoid damage to the nerve (see Fig. 3-5, *inset*).

The **radial nerve** is at risk if the dissection ventures farther proximally than the distal third of the humerus, one handbreadth above the lateral epicondyle (see Fig. 2-36).

### Vessels

The **brachial artery** lies with the median nerve in front of the elbow. It should be afforded the same protection as is the nerve (see Fig. 3-5, *inset*).

## Special Points

Great care must be taken to realign the olecranon correctly during closure. Alignment after fractures is easy, because the uneven ends of the bone usually fit snugly, like a jigsaw puzzle. Osteotomies may result in flat surfaces, however, and can make accurate reattachment difficult (see Fig. 3-3).

## How to Enlarge the Approach

### Extensile Measures

*Proximal Extension.* The posterior approach cannot be extended more proximally than the distal third of the humerus because of the danger to the radial nerve (see Fig. 2-36).

*Distal Extension.* The incision can be continued along the subcutaneous border of the ulna, exposing the entire length of that bone (see Applied Surgical Anatomy of the Approach to the Ulna in Chapter 4).

## Medial Approach

The medial approach gives good exposure of the medial compartment of the joint.[5,6] It also can be enlarged to expose the anterior surface of the distal fourth of the humerus. The ulnar nerve (which runs across the operative field), median nerve, and brachial artery may be at risk in this exposure. The uses of the medial approach include the following:

1. Removal of loose bodies
2. Open reduction and internal fixation of fractures of the coronoid process of the ulna
3. Open reduction and internal fixation of fractures of the medial humeral condyle and epicondyle

The medial approach provides poor access to the lateral side of the joint and should not be used for routine exploration of the elbow. The joint may be dislocated during the procedure, however, to gain access to the lateral side of the elbow, if necessary.

### Position of the Patient

Place the patient supine on the operating table, with the arm supported on an arm board or table. Abduct the arm and rotate the shoulder fully externally so that the medial epicondyle of the humerus faces anteriorly. Flex the elbow 90° (Fig. 3-6). Alternatively, flex the patient's shoulder and elbow such that the forearm comes to lie over the front of the face. This allows easier exposure of the medial side of the elbow, but requires an assistant to hold the forearm to provide adequate exposure.

Exsanguinate the limb either by elevating it for 5 minutes or by applying a soft rubber bandage (or exsanguinator). Then, inflate a tourniquet.

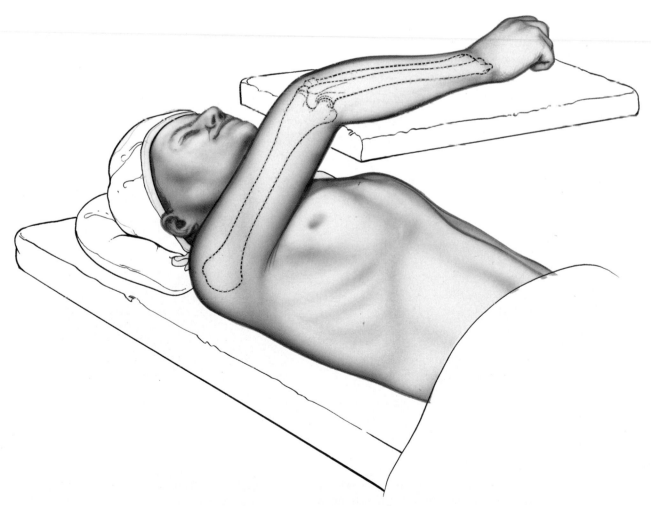

**Figure 3-6**   Position of the patient on the operating table.

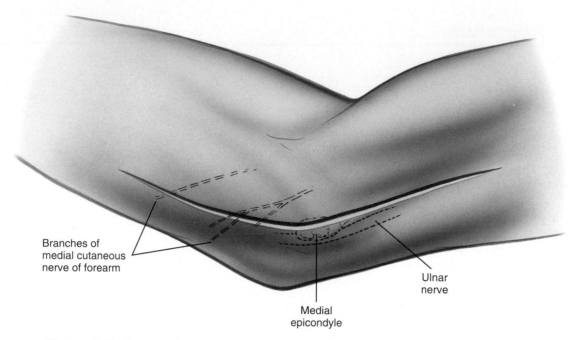

Branches of
medial cutaneous
nerve of forearm

Ulnar
nerve

Medial
epicondyle

**Figure 3-7** Incision for the medial approach to the elbow, centered on the medial epicondyle.

## Landmarks and Incision

### Landmarks

Palpate the *medial epicondyle of the humerus*, the large subcutaneous bony mass that stands out on the medial side of the distal end of the humerus.

### Incision

Make a curved incision 8 to 10 cm long on the medial aspect of the elbow, centering the incision on the medial epicondyle (Fig. 3-7).

## Internervous Plane

*Proximally*, the internervous plane lies between the brachialis muscle (which is supplied by the musculocutaneous nerve) and the triceps muscle (which is supplied by the radial nerve) (Fig. 3-8).

*Distally*, the plane lies between the brachialis muscle (which is supplied by the musculocutaneous nerve) and the pronator teres muscle (which is supplied by the median nerve; see Fig. 3-8).

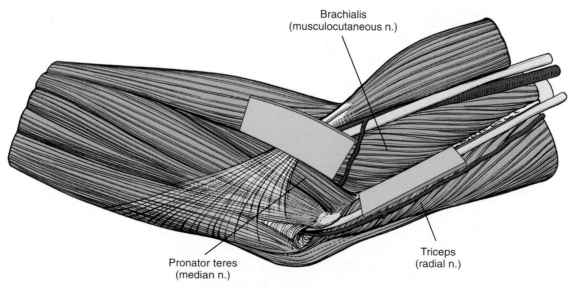

Brachialis
(musculocutaneous n.)

Pronator teres
(median n.)

Triceps
(radial n.)

**Figure 3-8** Internervous plane. Proximally, the plane is between the brachialis (musculocutaneous nerve) and the triceps (radial nerve); distally, it is between the brachialis and the pronator teres (median nerve).

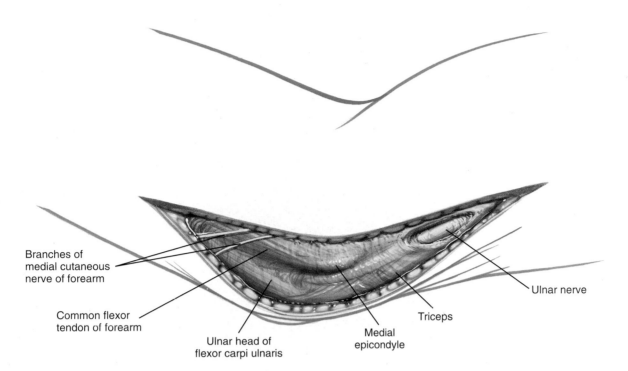

**Figure 3-9**   Superficial surgical dissection. Isolate the ulnar nerve along the length of the incision.

## Superficial Surgical Dissection

Palpate the ulnar nerve as it runs in its groove behind the medial condyle of the humerus. Incise the fascia over the nerve, starting proximal to the medial epicondyle; then, isolate the nerve along the length of the incision (Fig. 3-9).

Retract the anterior skin flap, together with the fascia overlying the pronator teres. The superficial flexor muscles of the forearm now are visible as they pass directly from their common origin on the medial epicondyle of the humerus (Fig. 3-10).

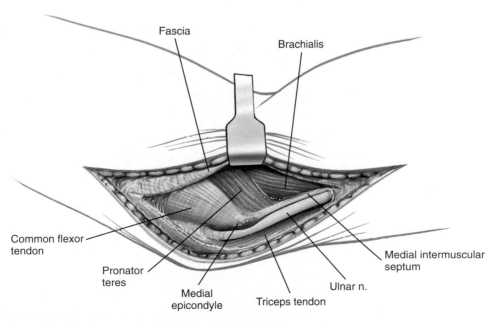

**Figure 3-10**   Retract the skin anteriorly with the fascia to uncover the common origin of the superficial flexor muscles from the medial epicondyle.

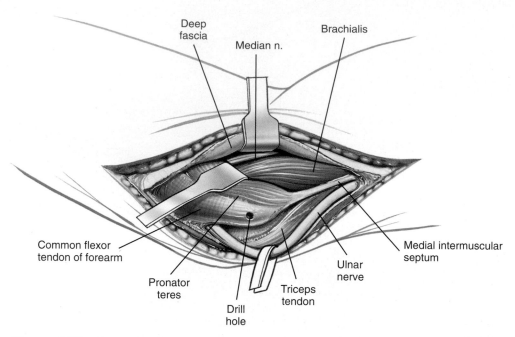

**Figure 3-11**   Enter the interval between the pronator teres and the brachialis. Retract the pronator teres medially.

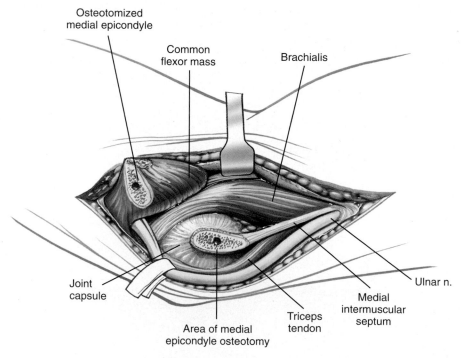

**Figure 3-12**   Subject the medial epicondyle to osteotomy and retract it (gently) with its attached flexors. Vigorous retraction of the epicondyle and its attached muscles may stretch the branch of the median nerve to the flexors.

Define the interval between the pronator teres and brachialis muscles, taking care not to damage the median nerve, which enters the pronator teres near the midline. Gently retract the pronator teres medially, lifting it off the brachialis (Fig. 3-11). Make sure that the ulnar nerve is retracted inferiorly; then, perform osteotomy of the medial epicondyle. Reflect the epicondyle with its attached flexors distally, avoiding traction that might damage the median or anterior interosseous nerves. Superiorly, continue the dissection between the brachialis, retracting it anteriorly, and the triceps, retracting it posteriorly (Fig. 3-12).

## Deep Surgical Dissection

The medial side of the joint now can be seen. Incise the capsule and the medial collateral ligament to expose the joint (Fig. 3-13).

## Dangers

### Nerves

The **ulnar nerve** must be dissected out and isolated before the medial epicondyle undergoes osteotomy (see Fig. 3-11).

The **median nerve** can suffer a traction lesion, with special damage to its multiple branches to the pronator teres muscle, if the medial epicondyle and its superficial flexor muscles are retracted too vigorously in a distal direction. Its major branch, the anterior interosseous nerve, also may suffer a traction lesion (see Fig. 3-12).

## How to Enlarge the Approach

### Local Measures

If a better view of the joint is required, the forearm can be abducted to open its medial side. To dislocate the elbow, the joint capsule and periosteum should be stripped off the distal humerus, working from within the joint. By this means, the mobility of the proximal ulna will be increased significantly. This increased mobility then will allow dislocation of the joint laterally, thereby opening all the surfaces of the joint to inspection.

### Extensile Measures

*Proximal Extension.* Enlarge the exposure proximally by developing the plane between the triceps and brachialis muscles. Subperiosteal dissection and elevation of the brachialis expose the anterior surface of the distal fourth of the humerus (see Figs. 3-13 and 3-39).

*Distal Extension.* The medial epicondyle of the humerus, with its attached flexor muscles, can be retracted only as far as the branches from the median nerve allow. Thus, although the exposure provides an adequate view of the brachialis inserting into the coronoid, it cannot offer a more distal exposure of the ulna.

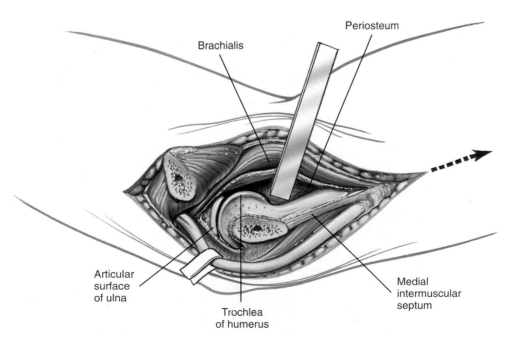

**Figure 3-13**   Incise the joint capsule and the medial collateral ligament to expose the joint.

# Anterolateral Approach

The anterolateral approach exposes the lateral half of the elbow joint, especially the capitulum and the proximal third of the anterior aspect of the radius. Its uses include the following:

1. Open reduction and internal fixation of fractures of the capitulum
2. Excision of tumors of the proximal radius
3. Treatment of aseptic necrosis of the capitulum
4. Drainage of infection from the elbow joint
5. Treatment of neural compression lesions of the proximal half of the posterior interosseous nerve and of the proximal part of the superficial radial nerve—access to the arcade of Frohse, as well as treatment of radial head fractures with paralysis of this nerve
6. Treatment of biceps avulsion from the radial tuberosity
7. Total elbow replacements

This approach is a distal extension of the anterolateral approach to the humerus and a proximal extension of the anterior approach to the radius. Theoretically, the approach can link the two together to expose the entire upper extremity from shoulder to wrist.

## Position of the Patient

Place the patient supine on the operating table, with the arm on an arm board. Exsanguinate the limb either by elevating it for 3 to 5 minutes or by applying a soft rubber bandage or exsanguinator. Then, inflate a tourniquet (Fig. 3-14).

## Landmarks and Incision

### Landmarks
The *brachioradialis* is palpable as part of a thick wad of muscle on the anterolateral aspect of the forearm. This "mobile wad" consists of three muscles; the brachioradialis forms the medial border of the wad.

The *biceps tendon* is a taut band that is palpable on the anterior aspect of the elbow.

### Incision
Make a curved incision along the anterior aspect of the elbow joint. Begin 5 cm above the flexion crease of the elbow, over the lateral border of the biceps muscle. Follow the lateral border of the biceps distally, but curve the incision laterally at the level of the elbow joint to avoid crossing a flexion crease at 90°. Then, continue the incision inferiorly, curving medially and following the medial border of the brachioradialis muscle. The lower limit of the extension depends on the amount of the radius that must be exposed (Fig. 3-15).

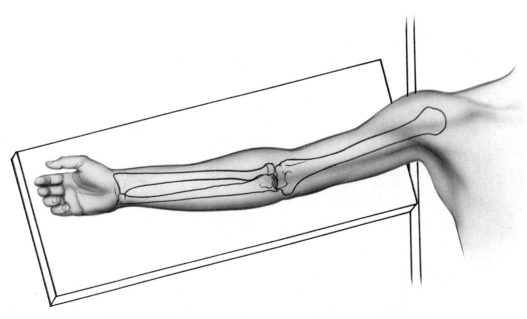

**Figure 3-14**  Position of the patient on the operating table.

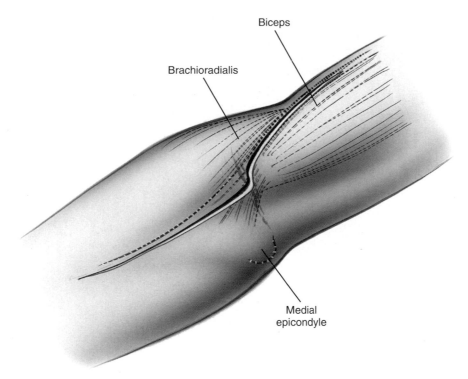

**Figure 3-15** Incision for the anterolateral approach to the elbow. The upper portion of the incision follows the lateral border of the biceps muscle. The lower portion follows the medial border of the brachioradialis muscle.

## Internervous Plane

Proximally, the plane lies between the brachialis muscle (which is supplied by the musculocutaneous nerve) and the brachioradialis muscle (which is supplied by the radial nerve).

Distally, the plane lies between the brachioradialis muscle (which is supplied by the radial nerve) and the pronator teres muscle (which is supplied by the median nerve) (Fig. 3-16).

## Superficial Surgical Dissection

Identify the lateral cutaneous nerve of the forearm (the sensory branch of the musculocutaneous nerve)

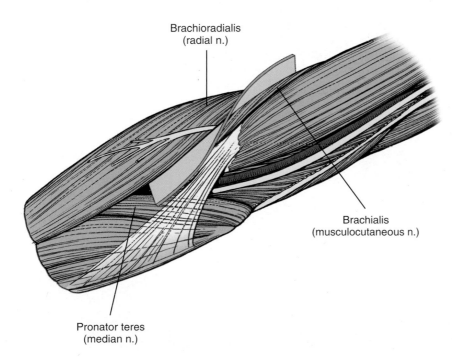

**Figure 3-16** Internervous plane. Proximally, the plane is between the brachialis (musculocutaneous nerve) and the brachioradialis (radial nerve); distally, it is between the brachioradialis and the pronator teres (median nerve).

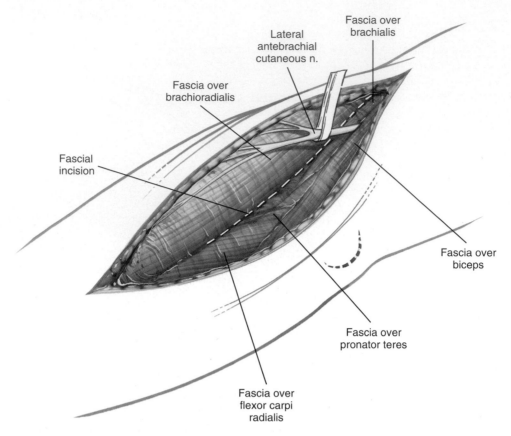

**Figure 3-17**   Superficial surgical dissection. Incise the deep fascia along the medial border of the brachioradialis. Be careful to identify the lateral antebrachial cutaneous nerve and retract it.

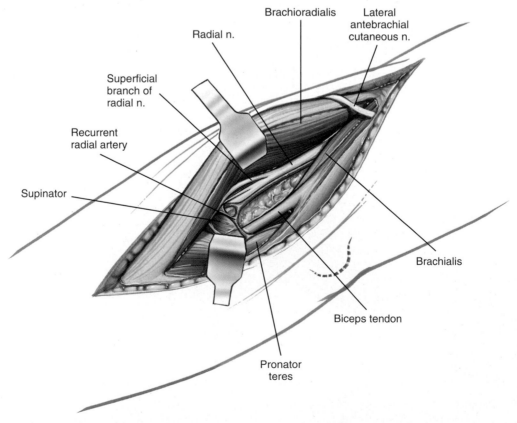

**Figure 3-18**   Identify the interval between the brachioradialis and brachialis muscles. Retract the brachioradialis laterally and the brachialis medially, and identify the radial nerve.

as it becomes superficial to the deep fascia in the distal 2 in. of the arm lateral to the biceps tendon in the interval between it and the brachialis muscle. Retract it with the medial skin flap (Fig. 3-17). It is more superficial than the superficial radial nerve, lying outside the fascial compartment of the brachioradialis; the superficial radial nerve still lies within the compartment at this level.

Incise the deep fascia along the medial border of the brachioradialis (see Fig. 3-17). Identify the radial nerve proximally at the level of the elbow joint between the brachialis and the brachioradialis. It lies deep between the two muscles and cannot be seen fully until they are separated. The intermuscular plane is oblique, with the brachioradialis overlying the brachialis muscle. Develop the plane between the two muscles using your finger, retracting the brachioradialis laterally and the brachialis and the overlying biceps brachii medially (Fig. 3-18).

Follow the radial nerve distally along the intermuscular interval until it divides into its three terminal branches: the posterior interosseous nerve

enters the supinator muscle, the sensory branch passes down the forearm behind the brachioradialis, and the motor branch to the extensor carpi radialis brevis enters that muscle almost immediately. Below the division of the nerve, develop a plane between the brachioradialis on the lateral side and the pronator teres on the medial side. Ligate the recurrent branches of the radial artery and the muscular branches that enter the brachialis just below the elbow so that the muscle can be retracted adequately. Ligation also allows the radial artery, which runs down the proximal third of the forearm on the pronator teres, to be retracted medially (Fig. 3-19).

## Deep Surgical Dissection

To expose the capitulum and the lateral compartment of the elbow, make a longitudinal incision in the anterior capsule of the joint between the radial nerve laterally and the brachialis medially (Fig. 3-20).

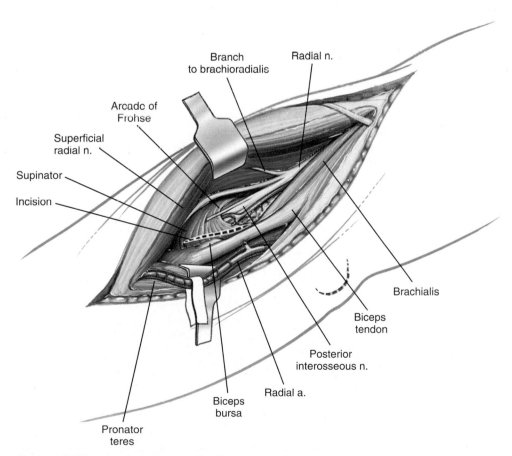

**Figure 3-19** The radial nerve divides into its three terminal branches: the posterior interosseous nerve, the sensory branch (which appears under the brachioradialis), and a motor branch to the extensor carpi radialis brevis. Develop a plane between the brachioradialis and the pronator teres.

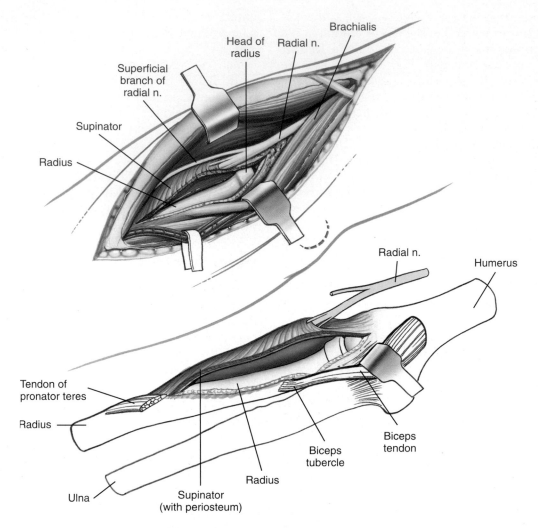

**Figure 3-20**   Deep surgical dissection. Make a longitudinal incision in the anterior capsule of the joint between the radial nerve and the brachialis muscle to expose the radial head and capitulum. To expose the radius further, remove the supinator muscle distally in a subperiosteal manner *(inset)*.

To expose the proximal radius, fully supinate the forearm; note that the origin of the supinator muscle moves anteriorly. Incise the origin of the supinator down the bone, staying just lateral to the insertion of the biceps tendon. Complete the exposure of the proximal radius by circumferential subperiosteal dissection (see Fig. 3-20, *inset*, and Anterior Approach to the Radius in Chapter 4).

## Dangers

### Nerves

The **radial nerve** must be identified in the interval between the brachioradialis and brachialis muscles before this interval is developed fully. Note that the

nerve lies anteromedial to the brachioradialis, within the fascial compartment of that muscle. If it is being sought at the level of the distal humerus or elbow, the intermuscular interval is the best place to find it.

The **posterior interosseous nerve** is vulnerable to injury as it winds around the neck of the radius within the substance of the supinator muscle. To prevent damage to the nerve, ensure that the supinator is detached from its insertion on the radius with the forearm in supination. Do not cut through the muscle body to expose the bone (see Anterior Approach to the Radius in Chapter 4; Fig. 3-21; see Fig. 3-33).

The **lateral cutaneous nerve of the forearm** must be identified and its continuity preserved in the

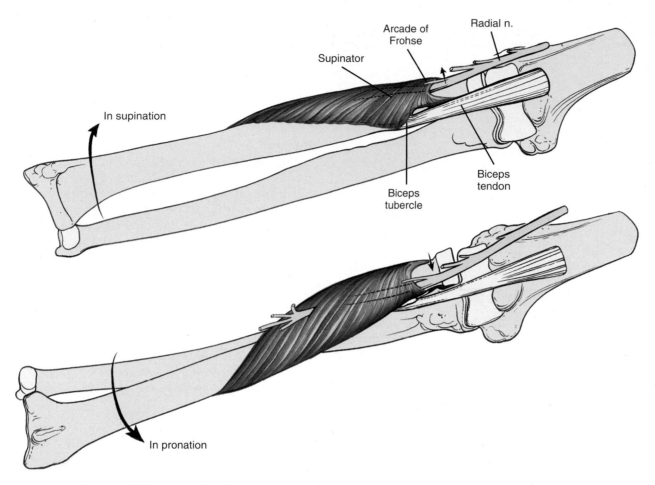

In supination

Arcade of
Frohse

Supinator

Radial n.

Biceps
tubercle

Biceps
tendon

In pronation

**Figure 3-21**    Place the forearm in supination to move the posterior interosseous nerve lateral to the incision into the radiohumeral joint and away from the incision into the origin of the supinator muscle, protecting it.

interval between the brachialis and biceps brachii muscles; retract it with the medial skin flap (see Fig. 3-17).

### Vessels

**Recurrent branches of the radial artery** must be ligated so that the brachioradialis can be mobilized fully. Ligation also reduces postoperative bleeding and avoids the risk of an ischemic contracture developing postoperatively as a result of the pressure caused by a postoperative bleed (see Fig. 3-19).

## How to Enlarge the Approach

### Extensile Measures

*Proximal Extension.* The anterolateral approach can be extended easily into an anterolateral approach

to the distal humerus by developing the plane between the brachialis and triceps muscles. Remember that the radial nerve crosses the lateral border of the humerus about one handbreadth above the lateral epicondyle. (For details, see Anterolateral Approach to the Distal Humerus.)

*Distal Extension.* The anterolateral approach can be extended easily to expose the entire anterior surface of the radius by developing the plane proximally between the brachioradialis muscle (which is supplied by the radial nerve) and the pronator teres muscle (which is supplied by the median nerve), and distally between the brachioradialis muscle (which is supplied by the radial nerve) and the flexor carpi radialis muscle (which is supplied by the median nerve). (For details, see Anterior Approach to the Radius in Chapter 4.)

# Anterior Approach to the Cubital Fossa

The anterior approach may be the least commonly used surgical approach to the elbow and provides access to the neurovascular structures that are found in the cubital fossa. Its uses include the following:

1. Repair of lacerations to the median nerve
2. Repair of lacerations to the brachial artery
3. Repair of lacerations to the radial nerve
4. Reinsertion of the biceps tendon
5. Repair of lacerations to the biceps tendon
6. Release of posttraumatic anterior capsular contractions
7. Excision of tumor

## Position of the Patient

Place the patient supine on the operating table with the arm in the anatomic position. Exsanguinate the limb either by elevating it for 3 to 5 minutes or by applying a soft rubber bandage or exsanguinator. Then, apply a tourniquet (see Fig. 3-14).

## Landmarks and Incision

### Landmarks

The *brachioradialis* is a fleshy muscle that forms the lateral border of the supinated forearm.

The *tendon of the biceps* is a taut, easily palpable, band-like structure that runs downward across the anterior aspect of the cubital fossa.

### Incision

Make a curved, "boat-race" incision* over the anterior aspect of the elbow. Begin 5 cm above the flexion crease on the medial side of the biceps. Curve the incision across the front of the elbow, then complete it by incising the skin along the medial border of the brachioradialis muscle. Curving the incision avoids crossing the flexion crease at 90° (Figs. 3-22 and 3-23).

## Internervous Plane

*Distally,* the internervous plane lies between the brachioradialis muscle (which is supplied by the radial nerve) and the pronator teres muscle (which is supplied by the median nerve) (Fig. 3-24).

---

*The term boat-race refers to the annual Oxford and Cambridge boat race held in London, England. Because the course from Putney to Mortlake contains three large bends, the term can be used for any incision that involves multiple curves.

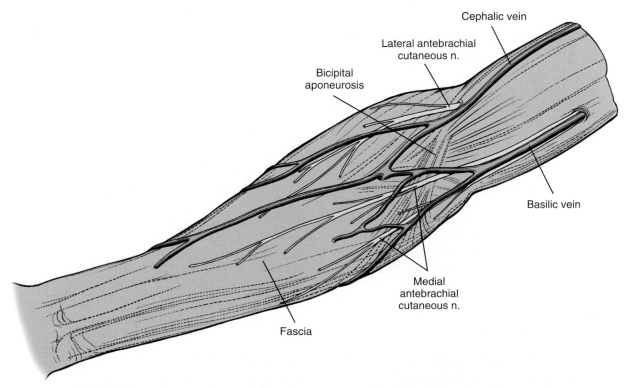

**Figure 3-22** Superficial view of the elbow and forearm, showing superficial veins and nerves.

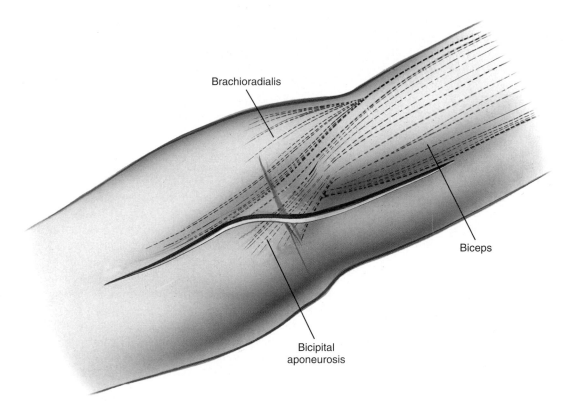

**Figure 3-23** Incision for the anterior approach to the cubital fossa.

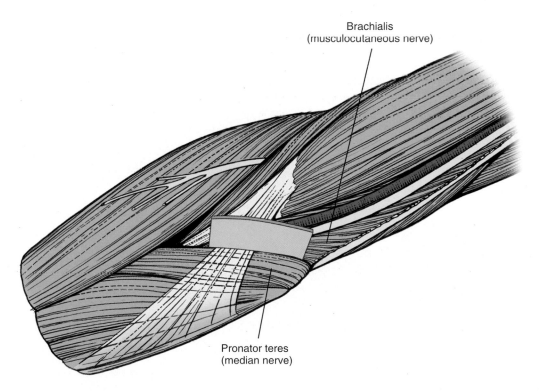

**Figure 3-24** Internervous plane. Distally, the plane is between the brachioradialis (radial nerve) and the pronator teres (median nerve); proximally, it is between the brachioradialis (radial nerve) and brachialis (musculocutaneous nerve).

*Proximally*, the plane lies between the brachioradialis muscle (which is supplied by the radial nerve) and the brachialis muscle (which is supplied by the musculocutaneous nerve).

## Superficial Surgical Dissection

Mobilize the skin flaps widely. Incise the deep fascia in line with the skin incision and ligate the numerous veins that cross the elbow in this area.

The lateral cutaneous nerve of the forearm (the sensory branch of the musculocutaneous nerve) must be preserved. To find it, locate the interval between the biceps tendon and the brachialis muscle. The nerve emerges there to run down the lateral side of the forearm subcutaneously (Fig. 3-25).

Next, identify the bicipital aponeurosis (lacertus fibrosus), which is a band of fibrous tissue coming from the biceps tendon and swinging medially across the forearm, running superficial to the proximal part of the superficial flexor muscles (see Fig. 3-25). Cut the aponeurosis close to its origin at the biceps tendon and reflect it laterally. Be careful not to injure the brachial artery, which runs immediately under the aponeurosis (Fig. 3-26).

Identify the radial artery as it passes the biceps tendon and trace it proximally to its origin from the brachial artery. Note that both the brachial vein and the median nerve lie medial to the artery. To identify the radial nerve, look between the brachialis and the brachioradialis; the nerve crosses in front of the elbow joint.

Identifying these structures and understanding their relationship are the keys to operating successfully in the cubital fossa (see Fig. 3-26).

## Deep Surgical Dissection

If the anterolateral approach is to be used only for exploration of the neurovascular structures, deep dissection is not required. If you require access to the anterior capsule of the elbow joint, retract the biceps and brachialis muscle medially and the brachioradialis muscle laterally. Fully supinate the forearm and identify the origin of the supinator muscle from the anterior aspect of the radius. Incise the origin of this muscle and dissect it off the bone in a subperiosteal plane, carefully reflecting it laterally. Take care not to insert a retractor on the lateral aspect of the proximal radius as this may compress the posterior interosseous nerve. The anterior capsule of the elbow joint is now exposed and may be incised to expose the anterior aspect of the elbow joint (Fig. 3-28).

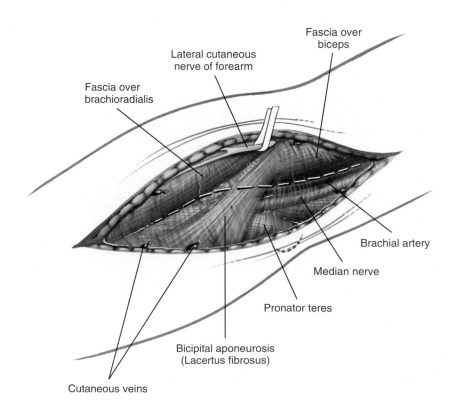

Fascia over biceps

Lateral cutaneous nerve of forearm

Fascia over brachioradialis

Brachial artery

Median nerve

Pronator teres

Bicipital aponeurosis (Lacertus fibrosus)

Cutaneous veins

**Figure 3-25** Superficial surgical dissection. Locate the lateral cutaneous nerve of the forearm in the interval between the biceps tendon and the brachialis, and preserve it.

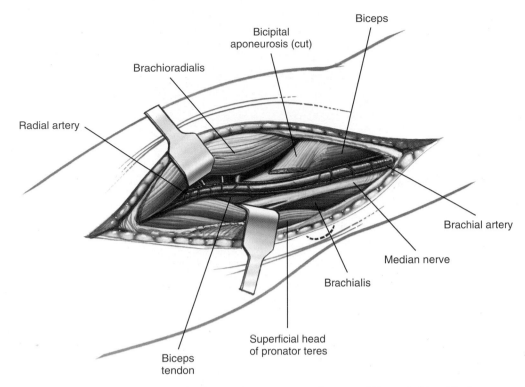

**Figure 3-26** After cutting the bicipital aponeurosis (lacertus fibrosus), identify the brachial artery. Note that the median nerve lies medial to the artery. The brachial vein, which accompanies the artery, consists of a series of small, fine vessels, the venae comitantes.

## Dangers

Because this approach exposes the neurovascular structures of the fossa so quickly, they may be damaged if care is not taken.

Three points are crucial, as follows:

1. The lateral cutaneous nerve of the forearm (the sensory branch of the musculocutaneous nerve) is vulnerable to injury in the distal fourth of the arm during incision of the deep fascia. Pick it up in the interval between the biceps and brachialis muscles in the arm, trace it downward, and preserve it (see Fig. 3-25).
2. The radial artery lies immediately deep to the bicipital aponeurosis; the aponeurosis must be incised carefully to avoid damage to the artery (see Fig. 3-26).
3. The posterior interosseous nerve is vulnerable to injury as it winds round the neck of the radius within the substance of the supinator muscle. To prevent damage to the nerve, ensure that the supinator is detached from its insertion on the radius with the forearm in supination (see Fig. 3-20).

## How to Enlarge the Approach

### Extensile Measures

The approach may be extended for more extensive exposure of the neurovascular structures (see Figs. 4-16 through 4-22).

### *Median Nerve*

*Proximal Extension.* Extend the incision superiorly along the medial border of the biceps, and incise the deep fascia in line with the incision. The brachial artery lies immediately under the fascia, between the biceps muscle and the underlying brachialis muscle. The medial nerve runs with the artery.

*Distal Extension.* Trace the median nerve as it disappears into the pronator teres muscle. Simple retraction of the muscle may provide adequate exposure. Take care not to cut any branches of the median nerve going to the flexor-pronator group of muscles that pass from the medial side of the median nerve at the level of the elbow joint. This incision lies

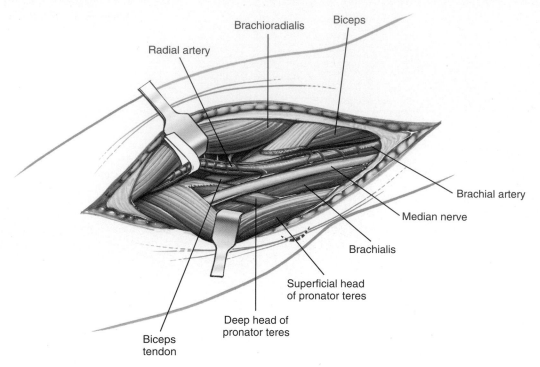

**Figure 3-27** Trace the median nerve distally into the pronator teres. Incise a portion of the muscle superficial to the nerve, if necessary, to expose the nerve. The incision lies between the humeral and ulnar heads of the pronator teres.

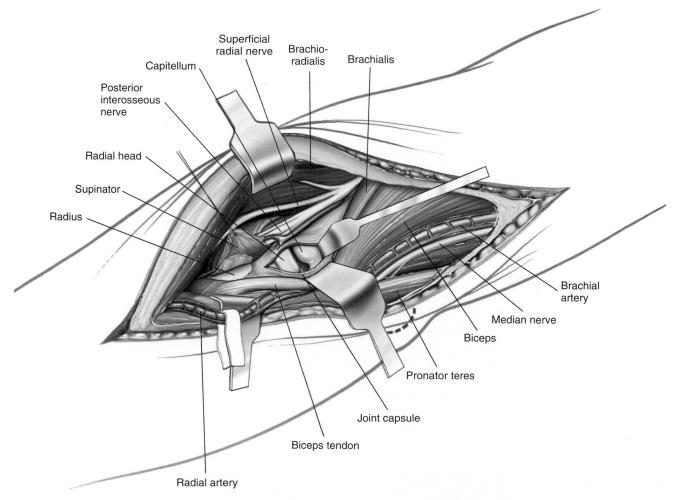

**Figure 3-28** Retract the biceps tendon and carefully detach and retract the proximal supinator muscle to gain access to the anterior joint capsule, which may be incised to expose the elbow joint.

between the humeral and ulnar heads of the pronator teres and allows the plane between the two heads to be developed for the distal exposure of the nerve (Fig. 3-27).

### Brachial Artery
The brachial artery runs with the median nerve and is exposed in the same way.

### Radial Artery
To expose the radial artery, trace it distally as it crosses the surface of the pronator teres, running toward the lateral side of the forearm. Developing the plane proximally between the pronator teres and brachioradialis muscles, and distally between the flexor carpi radialis and brachioradialis muscles allows the artery to be followed to the wrist.

# Posterolateral Approach to the Radial Head

The posterolateral approach to the radial head[7] is useful for all surgeries to the radial head, including excision of the radial head and insertion of a prosthetic replacement.[8,9]

Because the incision cannot be extended below the annular ligament without risking damage to the posterior interosseous nerve, avoid extending the incision to the upper part of the radial shaft.

## Position of the Patient

Place the patient supine on the operating table, with the affected arm positioned over the chest. Pronate the forearm.[10] Exsanguinate the limb either by applying a soft rubber bandage or an exsanguinator or by elevating it for 3 to 5 minutes. Then, inflate a tourniquet (Fig. 3-29).

## Landmarks and Incision

### Landmarks
One of the landmarks is the *lateral humeral epicondyle.*

To identify the *radial head*, palpate the lateral epicondyle of the humerus, moving the fingers 2.5 cm distally until a depression is detected. The

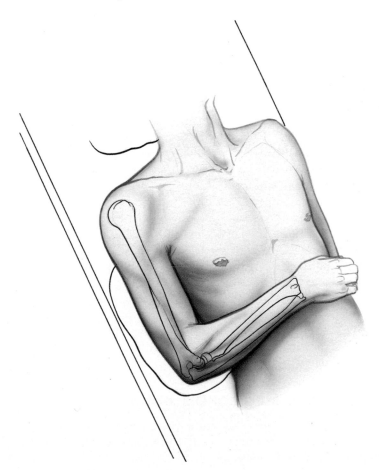

**Figure 3-29** Position of the patient on the operating table.

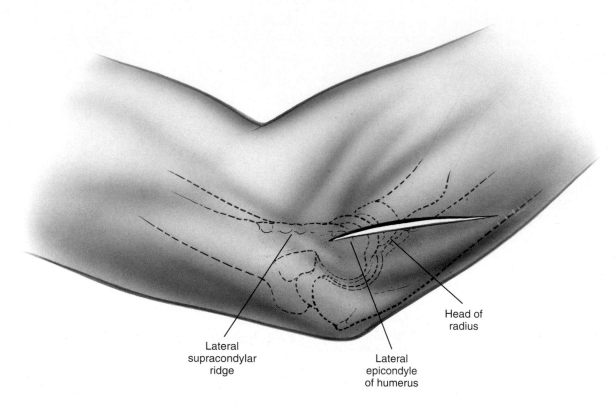

**Figure 3-30** Make a longitudinal incision based proximally on the lateral humeral epicondyle.

radial head lies deep within this depression. It is palpable through the muscle mass of the wrist extensors. As the forearm is pronated and supinated, movement of the radial head can be felt beneath the surgeon's fingers. In cases of fracture of the radial head, the normal landmarks are lost because of hemorrhage and swelling. Crepitus at the fracture site often is quite obvious and helpful in placing the incision.

The *olecranon* is the proximal subcutaneous end of the ulna.

### Incision

Make a gently curved incision, beginning over the posterior surface of the lateral humeral epicondyle and continuing downward and medially to a point over the posterior border of the ulna, about 6 cm distal to the tip of the olecranon.

Alternatively, make a 5-cm longitudinal incision based proximally on the lateral humeral epicondyle. This incision follows the skin fold and lies directly over the radial head (Fig. 3-30).

### Internervous Plane

The internervous plane lies between the anconeus, which is supplied by the radial nerve, and the exten-

sor carpi ulnaris, which is supplied by the posterior interosseous nerve (Fig. 3-31).

### Superficial Surgical Dissection

Incise the deep fascia in line with the skin incision. To find the interval between the extensor carpi ulnaris and the anconeus, look distally where the plane is easy to identify; proximally, the two muscles share a common aponeurosis (Fig. 3-32). Detach part of the superior origin of the anconeus as it arises from the lateral epicondyle of the humerus. Then, separate the anconeus and extensor carpi ulnaris muscles, using retractors (Fig. 3-33).

In cases of trauma, there often has been bleeding and contusion in this area, and it is difficult to identify the interval between the extensor carpi ulnaris and anconeus muscles. In this case, it is safe to dissect straight down onto the lateral epicondyle of the humerus, because this structure always can be palpated easily.

### Deep Surgical Dissection

Fully pronate the forearm to move the posterior interosseous nerve away from the operative field (see Fig. 3-33, *inset*).

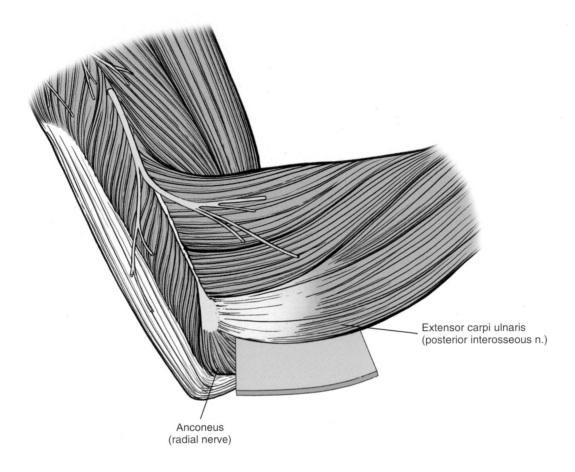

Extensor carpi ulnaris
(posterior interosseous n.)

Anconeus
(radial nerve)

**Figure 3-31**   The internervous plane lies between the anconeus (radial nerve) and the extensor carpi ulnaris (posterior interosseous nerve).

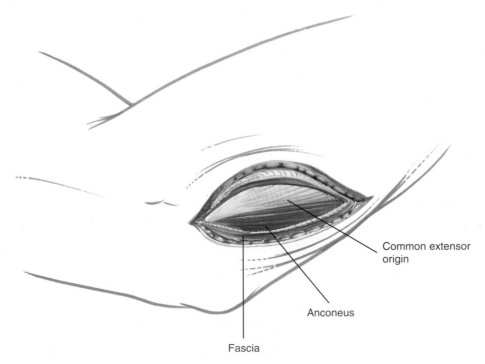

Common extensor
origin

Anconeus

Fascia

**Figure 3-32**   Find the interval between the extensor carpi ulnaris and the anconeus distally. Proximally, the two muscles merge.

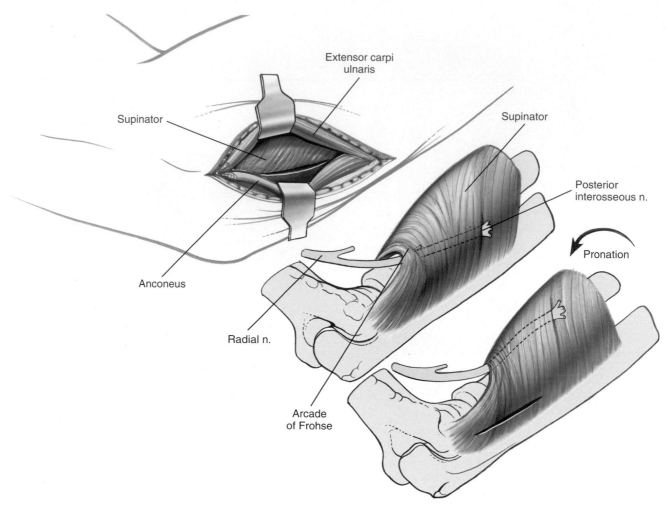

**Figure 3-33**    Detach the superior origin of the anconeus from the lateral epicondyle, and separate the anconeus and the extensor carpi ulnaris. Pronation of the forearm moves the posterior interosseous nerve medially away from the operative field *(insets)*.

Incise the capsule of the elbow joint longitudinally to reveal the underlying capitulum, the radial head, and the annular ligament. Do not incise the capsule too far anteriorly; the radial nerve runs over the front of the anterolateral portion of the elbow capsule. Do not continue the dissection below the annular ligament or retract vigorously, distally, or anteriorly, because the posterior interosseous nerve lies within the substance of the supinator muscle and is vulnerable to injury (Fig. 3-34).

ligament. Pronation of the forearm keeps the nerve as far from the operative field as it possibly can be (see Fig. 3-33, *inset*). To ensure the safety of the nerve, take great care to place the retractors directly on bone and be careful in their placement. Because the posterior interosseous nerve actually may touch the bone of the radial neck, directly opposite the bicipital tuberosity, placing retractors behind it poses a risk.[11]

The **radial nerve** is safe as long as the elbow joint is opened laterally and not anteriorly.

## Dangers

### Nerves

The **posterior interosseous nerve** is in no danger as long as the dissection remains proximal to the annular

## How to Enlarge the Approach

### Local Measures

For more complete exposure of the lateral half of the distal humerus, extend the superficial dissection by

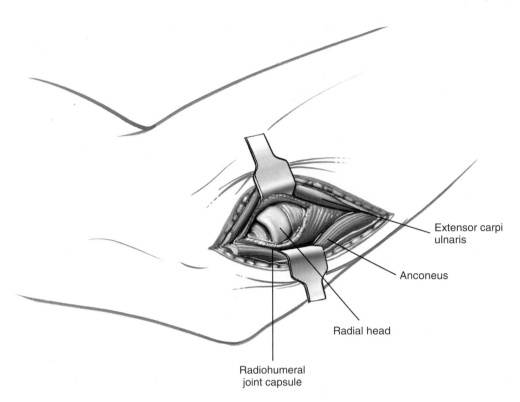

**Figure 3-34** Incise the joint capsule longitudinally to expose the capitulum and radial head.

cutting down on the lateral supracondylar ridge. Strip the tissues off subperiosteally both anteriorly and posteriorly to gain access to the distal humerus and to expose the capitellum. The extension is most useful for fixing fractures internally and for removing loose bodies in the lateral compartment of the elbow

(see Anterolateral Approach to the Distal Humerus in Chapter 2).

### Extensile Measures

There is no way to extend this approach profitably in any direction.

# Applied Surgical Anatomy

## Overview

The elbow is the hinge (ginglymus) joint between the lower end of the humerus and the upper end of the radius and ulna. It communicates with the superior radioulnar joint.

The lower end of the humerus articulates in two areas:

1. The lateral *capitulum* articulates with the radial head. Its shape is reminiscent of a hemisphere.
2. The medial *trochlea* articulates with the ulna. Its shape resembles a spool of thread. It extends further distally than the capitulum, resulting in a configuration that gives a tilt to the lower end of the humerus and produces the "carrying angle" of

the joint. The trochlea is grooved; the groove's boundaries are marked medially by a prominent, sharp ridge and laterally by a lower, more blunted ridge.

The two articulations are separated by a ridge of bone.

The elbow is supported by strong medial and lateral collateral ligaments. The anterior and posterior ligaments are mainly thickened sections in the capsule, which is exactly what would be expected from a hinge joint. The shape of the bones that comprise the elbow joint and the presence of the strong collateral ligaments make it difficult to explore the joint completely without extensive dissection. Medial and lateral approaches to the joint provide limited access unless they are extended. Complete exposure is obtained most easily through a posterior approach, and then only if an olecranon osteotomy is performed. Four groups of muscles cross the elbow joint:

1. Anteriorly, the flexors of the elbow, which are supplied by the musculocutaneous nerve
2. Posteriorly, the extensor of the elbow, which is supplied by the radial nerve
3. Medially, the flexor-pronator group of muscles (the flexors of the wrist and fingers, and the pronators of the forearm), which are supplied by the median and ulnar nerves. They arise from the medial epicondyle of the humerus.
4. Laterally, the extensors of the wrist and fingers, and the supinators of the forearm, which are supplied by the radial and posterior interosseous nerves. They arise from the lateral epicondyle of the humerus.

Between each pair of muscle groups is an intermuscular plane; two are internervous planes and can be explored. A third internervous plane lies within the lateral group, as follows:

1. Between the *anterior* and *lateral* muscle groups, which are supplied by the musculocutaneous and radial nerves, respectively. The anterolateral approach uses the interval between the brachialis and brachioradialis muscles (see Fig. 3-16).
2. Between the *anterior* and *medial* muscle groups, which are supplied by the musculocutaneous and median nerves, respectively. The medial approach uses the interval between the brachialis and pronator teres muscles (see Figs. 3-8 and 3-24).
3. Between two members of the lateral group: the anconeus muscle (which is supplied by the radial nerve) and the extensor carpi ulnaris muscle (which is supplied by the posterior interosseous nerve, a major branch of the radial nerve; see Fig. 3-31). The posterolateral approach to the radial head uses this plane.

The intermuscular plane between the lateral and posterior groups of muscles is not an internervous plane, because both groups are supplied by the radial nerve. The plane is useful, though, because the radial nerve gives off its branches well proximal to the elbow. This pseudo-internervous plane, which is used in the lateral approach, falls in the interval between the brachioradialis and triceps muscles (see Fig. 2-24*A*).

The medial and lateral groups of muscles converge in the forearm, forming a triangular fossa known as the cubital fossa, which is bordered by the pronator teres medially and the brachioradialis later-

ally. The superior border of the triangle consists of an imaginary line joining the medial and lateral epicondyle of the humerus.

## Neurovascular Structures

### Nerves

The *median nerve* crosses the front of the joint on its medial side and is covered by the bicipital aponeurosis (lacertus fibrosus) in the cubital fossa. It disappears between the two heads of the pronator teres muscle as it leaves the fossa and runs down the forearm, adhering to the deep surface of the flexor digitorum superficialis muscle (see Fig. 4-12).

The *radial nerve* crosses the front of the elbow joint in the interval between the brachialis and brachioradialis muscles. It divides in the cubital fossa at the radiohumeral joint line into the posterior interosseous nerve (which enters the substance of the supinator muscle) and the superficial radial nerve (which descends the lateral side of the forearm under cover of the brachioradialis muscle; see Fig. 3-19).

The *ulnar nerve* crosses the joint in the groove on the back of the medial epicondyle, where it is easy to palpate. The nerve enters the anterior compartment of the forearm by passing between the two heads of the flexor carpi ulnaris muscle, which it supplies and where it may be entrapped. It then runs down the forearm on the anterior surface of the flexor digitorum profundus (see Figs. 3-40 and 3-43). In the proximal third of the forearm, it supplies the ring and little fingers.

### Vessels

The *brachial artery* enters the cubital fossa, running on the lateral side of the median nerve and lying on the brachialis muscle. The median nerve passes under the bicipital aponeurosis, which separates it from the median basilic vein, a frequent site of venous puncture (see Fig. 3-35). In the days when bleeding was a recognized form of treatment and venesection was done with lancets rather than with needles, this site was a frequent one used by barber surgeons. The reason this site was preferred is because the bicipital aponeurosis protects the vital structures of the artery and nerve, which provided these early practitioners with a margin of safety, because their patients often moved on insertion of the lancet. Halfway down the cubital fossa, the artery divides into two terminal branches: the radial and ulnar arteries. Similar to the median nerve, the artery may be damaged in supracondylar fractures of the humerus (see Fig. 3-26).

The *radial artery* passes medial to the biceps tendon before turning anteriorly, lying on the supinator muscle and the insertion of the pronator teres muscle. In the upper forearm, it lies under the brachioradialis muscle (see Fig. 4-11).

The *ulnar artery* usually disappears from the cubital fossa by passing deep to the deep head of the pronator teres, the muscle that separates it from the median nerve (see Fig. 4-13).

## Applied Surgical Anatomy *of* the Medial Approach

Five flexor muscles of the forearm fan out from the common flexor origin on the medial epicondyle of the humerus:

1. The pronator teres
2. The flexor carpi radialis
3. The flexor digitorum superficialis
4. The palmaris longus
5. The flexor carpi ulnaris (Fig. 3-36)

The first four muscles are supplied by the median nerve; the flexor carpi ulnaris is supplied by the ulnar nerve. The pronator teres, the most proximal muscle, forms the medial border of the cubital fossa.

All five muscles are retracted distally after osteotomy of the medial epicondyle. They can be retracted only a short distance because the median nerve, passing through the pronator teres muscle, "anchors" the group and prevents distal retraction (Figs. 3-35 through 3-39).

## Applied Surgical Anatomy of the Anterolateral Approach

Two groups of muscles arise from the lateral epicondyle and the supracondylar ridge of the humerus (see Applied Surgical Anatomy of the Posterior Approach to the Radius in Chapter 4):

1. The mobile wad of three muscles, consisting of the brachioradialis, the extensor carpi radialis longus, and the extensor carpi radialis brevis
2. Four muscles arising from the common extensor origin: the extensor digitorum communis, the extensor digiti minimi, the extensor carpi ulnaris, and the anconeus

The *anconeus* is purely a muscle of the elbow; its function is unclear. Its more distal fibers run almost vertically and act as a weak extensor of the elbow, whereas its proximal fibers are almost horizontal and adduct and rotate the ulna. This unlikely movement occurs to a slight degree at the elbow. Electromyographic studies suggest that the muscle is most active during extension,[12] but it probably functions more as a stabilizer while other muscles act on the elbow as prime movers, functioning in much the same way as does the rotator cuff in the shoulder.

Its major surgical importance lies in the fact that it forms one boundary of the internervous plane that is used in the posterolateral approach to the radial head.

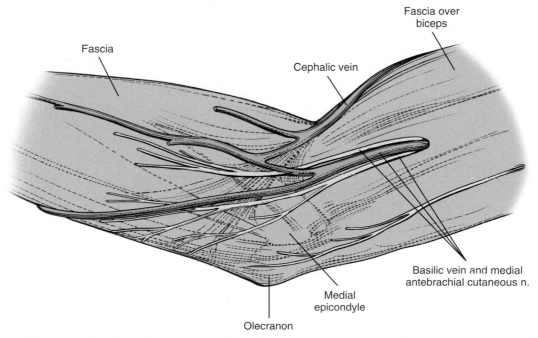

**Figure 3-35**   Medial view of the elbow. Note the sensory nerves and veins on the medial side of the elbow joint.

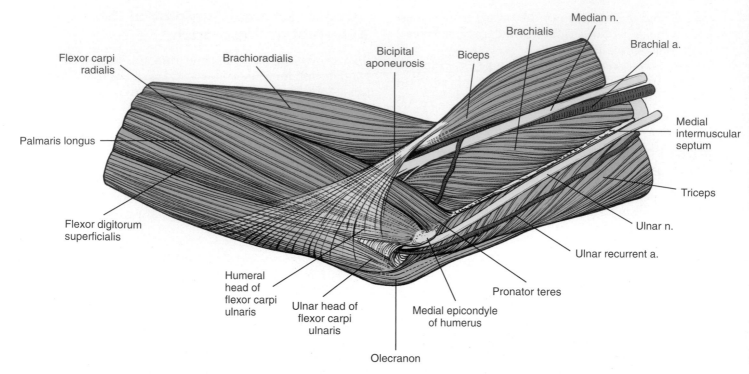

**Figure 3-36**    The five muscles of the forearm have a common flexor origin on the medial epicondyle. All five are supplied by the median nerve. The ulnar nerve passes between the two heads of the flexor carpi ulnaris. The median nerve runs beneath the bicipital aponeurosis.

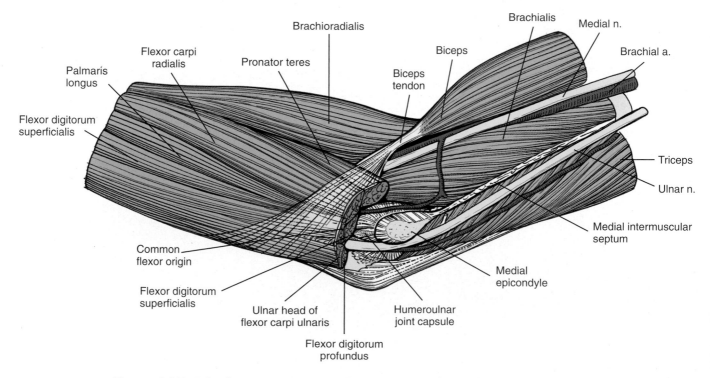

**Figure 3-37**    The flexor-pronator group has been resected, revealing the course of the ulnar nerve as it runs around the medial epicondyle, passing distally before entering the plane between the flexor carpi ulnaris and the flexor digitorum profundus.

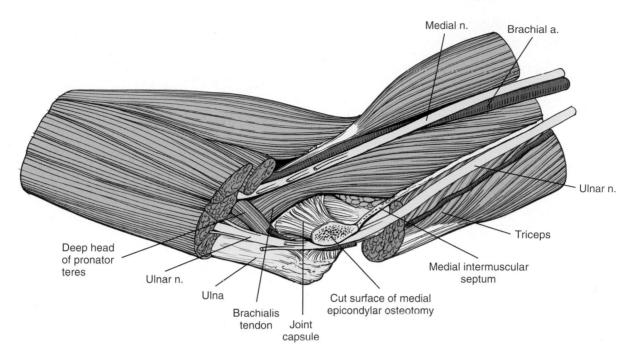

**Figure 3-38** The flexor muscles have been resected further. The medial epicondyle has been subjected to osteotomy. Distally, the ulnar nerve crosses the forearm between the flexor carpi ulnaris and the profundus. The median nerve enters the forearm between the two heads of the pronator teres, lying on the tendon of the brachialis.

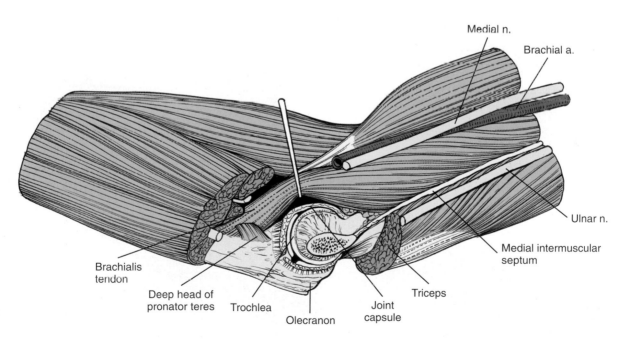

**Figure 3-39** The joint capsule has been opened. The brachialis is elevated from the capsule.

## Applied Surgical Anatomy of the Anterior Approach

Two flexors, the brachialis and biceps brachii muscles, cross the anterior aspect of the elbow joint. Both are supplied by the musculocutaneous nerve, which runs between the biceps and the brachialis in the upper arm. In front of the elbow, they diverge; the biceps runs laterally to the bicipital tuberosity of the radius, and the brachialis runs medially to the coronoid process of the ulna.

(For a discussion of the brachialis, see Applied Surgical Anatomy of the Anterior Compartment of the Forearm in Chapter 4. For a discussion of the biceps brachii, see Applied Surgical Anatomy of the Anterior Approach in Chapter 1.)

In front of the elbow, the biceps brachii develops a flat tendon, which also overlies the brachialis. The tendon rotates so that its anterior surface faces laterally as it passes between the two bones of the forearm before inserting into the back of the radius at the bicipital tuberosity. A bursa separates the tendon from the anterior part of the tuberosity.

As the biceps tendon crosses the front of the elbow, it gives off fibrous tissue from its medial side.

This *bicipital aponeurosis*, or *lacertus fibrosus*, sweeps across the forearm by way of the deep fascia to insert into the subcutaneous border of the upper end of the ulna.

The bicipital aponeurosis forms part of the roof of the cubital fossa. It separates superficial nerves and vessels from deep ones. Lying superficial are the median cephalic vein, the median basilic vein, and the medial cutaneous nerve of the forearm. Lying deep are the median nerve and the brachial artery.

The relationship of the median nerve, brachial artery, and brachial vein can be remembered easily through the mnemonic "VAN" (vein, artery, nerve), which labels the structures from the lateral to the medial aspect. They all pass medial to the biceps tendon under the lacertus fibrosus (see Fig. 3-27).

## Applied Surgical Anatomy of the Posterior Approach

See Figures 3-40 through 3-43.

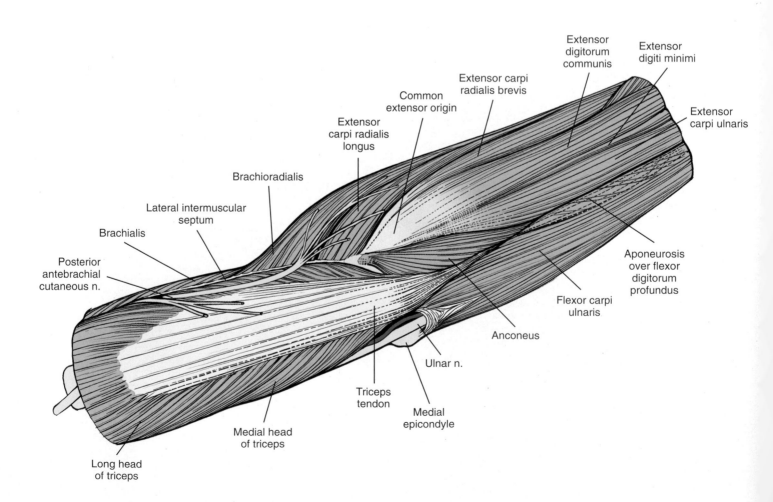

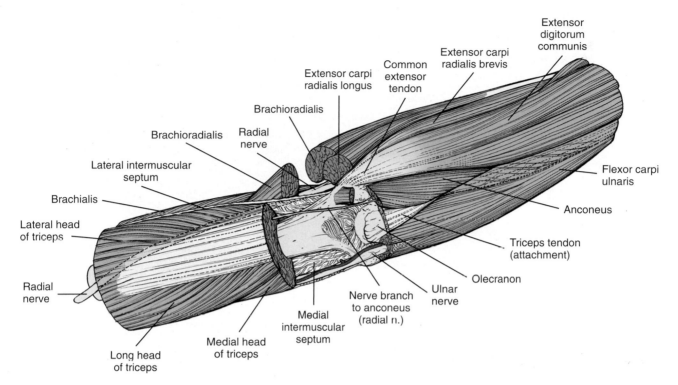

**Figure 3-41**    The distal part of the triceps, the origins of the flexors and flexor carpi ulnaris, and the extensor tendons have been resected. The ulnar nerve enters the plane between the two heads of the flexor carpi ulnaris. On the radial side, the radial nerve lies anterior to the intermuscular septum, between the brachioradialis and brachialis muscles.

**Figure 3-40**    Superficial view of the posterior aspect of the elbow. The triangular aponeurosis of the triceps runs down to its triangular insertion into the ulna. The ulnar nerve lies in its groove on the posterior aspect of the elbow. The brachial cutaneous nerve crosses the intermuscular septum on the posterior aspect of the elbow.

**Anconeus.** *Origin.* Lateral epicondyle of humerus and posterior joint capsule of elbow. *Insertion.* Lateral side of olecranon and posterior surface of ulna. *Action.* Extensor of elbow. *Nerve supply.* Radial nerve.

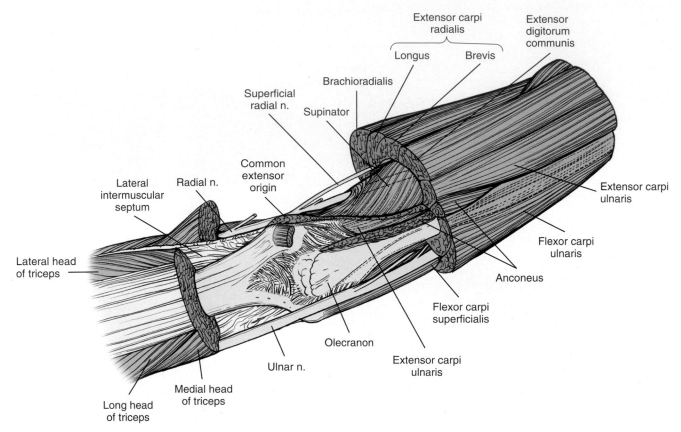

**Figure 3-42**   The insertion of the anconeus, the origin of the extensor carpi ulnaris, and the common extensor origin are revealed. The radial nerve divides into its main continuation, the posterior interosseous nerve, as it enters the supinator muscle through the arcade of Frohse. The superficial branch (sensory branch) of the radial nerve enters the undersurface of the brachioradialis. The ulnar nerve gives off its branches to the flexor carpi ulnaris immediately after it passes around the groove between the olecranon and the medial epicondyle.

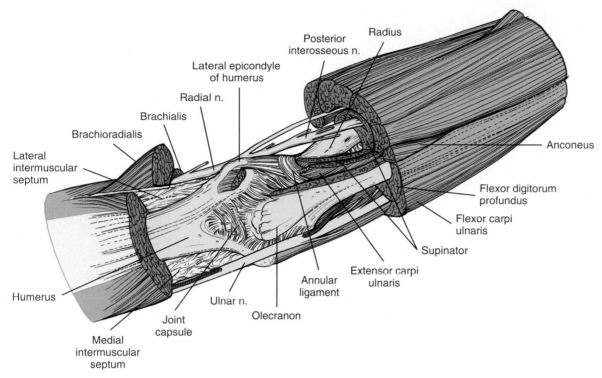

**Figure 3-43** The supinator muscle has been resected, revealing the distal course of the posterior interosseous nerve through its distal portion. The annular portion of the radiohumeral ligament is defined clearly.

## REFERENCES

1. CASSEBAUM WH: Operative treatment of T and Y fractures of the lower end of the humerus. Am J Surg 83:265, 1952
2. DE BOER P, STANLEY D: Surgical approaches to the elbow. In: Stanley D, Kay N. Surgery of the elbow: practical and scientific aspects. London, Arnold, 1998
3. MULLER ME, ALLGOWER M, WILLENEGGER H: Manual of internal fixation. New York, Springer-Verlag, 1970
4. JOHANSSON H, OLLERUD S: Operative treatment of intercondylar fractures of the humerus. J Trauma 11:836, 1971
5. CAMPBELL WC: Incision for exposure of the elbow joint. Am J Surg 15:65, 1932
6. MOLKSWORTH WHL: Operation for complete exposure of the elbow joint. Br J Surg 18:303, 1930
7. KOCHER T: Textbook of operative surgery, 3rd ed. London, Adam and Charles Black, 1911. Stiled HL, Paul CB, translators
8. MACKAY S: Silastic replacement of the head of the radius in trauma. J Bone Joint Surg [Br] 61:494, 1979
9. SWANSON AB, JAEGER SH, LAROCHELLE D: Comminuted fractures of the radial head: the role of silicone implant replacement arthroplasty. J Bone Joint Surg [Am] 63:1039, 1981
10. STRACHAN JCH, ELLIS BW: Vulnerability of the posterior interosseous nerve during radial head excision. J Bone Joint Surg [Br] 53:320, 1971
11. SPINNER M: Injuries to the major peripheral nerves of the forearm, 2nd ed, Section VII. Philadelphia, WB Saunders, 1978
12. TRAVEILLE AA: Electromyographic study of the extensor apparatus of the forearm. Anat Rec 144:373, 1962

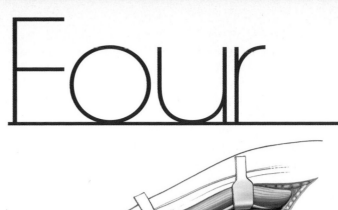

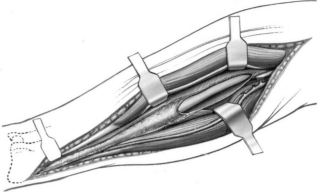

# The Forearm

The surgical anatomies of the two bones of the forearm differ significantly. The ulna has a subcutaneous border that extends for its entire length; the bone can be reached simply and directly without endangering other structures. In contrast, the upper two thirds of the radius are enclosed by a sheath of muscles. All surgery in the upper third of the radius is complicated further by the posterior interosseous nerve, which winds spirally around the bone close to, if not in contact with, its periosteum.

Three surgical approaches to the forearm are described in this chapter, all of which allow for the complete exposure of bone. In nearly every case, only part of the approach is required. The *anterior approach to the radius* is one of the classic extensile approaches, relying on subperiosteal dissection for protection of the posterior interosseous nerve. The *posterior approach to the radius* also makes use of an internervous plane, but still requires identification and preservation of the posterior interosseous nerve. The *approach to the ulna* cuts directly onto its subcutaneous border. The anatomy of the anterior approach to the radius, the approach to the ulna, and the anatomy of the posterior compartment of the forearm are considered separately. Because of the critical importance of the posterior interosseous nerve, its course is described in both anatomic sections.

# Anterior Approach to the Radius

The anterior approach offers an excellent, safe exposure of the radius, uncovering the entire length of the bone. Exposing the proximal third of the radius endangers the posterior interosseous nerve. By stripping the supinator muscle off the radius subperiosteally and using it to protect the nerve, however, the anterior approach avoids this danger. Still, great care must be taken in positioning retractors, because the nerve actually may touch the bone at the level of the distal portion of the neck of the radius, opposite the bicipital tuberosity, and posteriorly placed retractors can compress it against the bone. The approach first was described by Henry, and his name usually is associated with it.[1]

The uses of the anterior approach include the following:

1. Open reduction and internal fixation of fractures[2]
2. Bone grafting and fixation of fracture nonunions
3. Radial osteotomy
4. Biopsy and treatment of bone tumors
5. Excision of sequestra in chronic osteomyelitis
6. Anterior exposure of the bicipital tuberosity

This section describes an approach that exposes the entire length of the bone. Ordinarily, only a portion of the approach is required.

## Position of the Patient

Place the patient supine on the operating table, with the arm on an arm board. Place a tourniquet on the arm, but do not exsanguinate it fully before inflating the tourniquet. Venous blood left in the arm makes the vascular structures easier to identify. Finally, supinate the forearm (Fig. 4-1).

## Landmarks and Incision

### Landmarks

Palpate the *biceps tendon*, which is a long, taut structure that crosses the front of the elbow joint just medial to the brachioradialis muscle.

Palpate the *brachioradialis*, which is a fleshy muscle that arises with the extensor carpi radialis longus and brevis muscles from the lateral epicondyle of the elbow. The three muscles form a "mobile wad" of muscle that runs down the lateral aspect of the supinated forearm.

Palpate the *styloid process of the radius*. Note that this bony process is truly lateral when the hand is in the anatomic (supinated) position. The styloid process is the most distal part of the lateral side of the radius.

### Incision

Make a straight incision from the anterior flexor crease of the elbow just lateral to the biceps tendon down to the styloid process of the radius. The length of the incision depends on the amount of bone that needs to be exposed (Fig. 4-2).

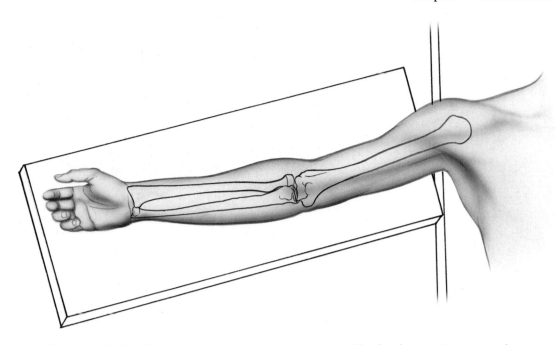

**Figure 4-1** Position of the patient on the operating table, for the anterior approach to the radius.

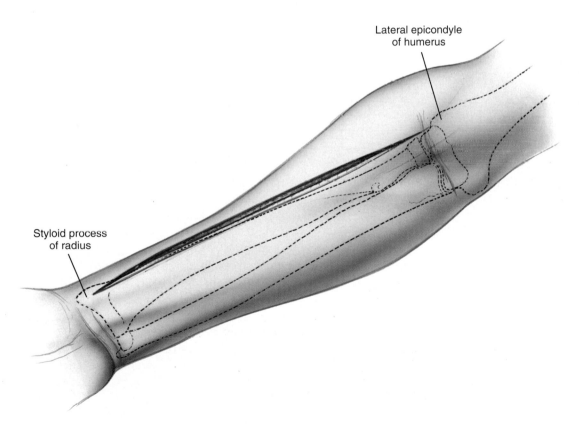

Lateral epicondyle
of humerus

Styloid process
of radius

**Figure 4-2** Make a straight incision on the anterior part of the forearm, from the flexor crease on the lateral side of the biceps down to the styloid process of the radius.

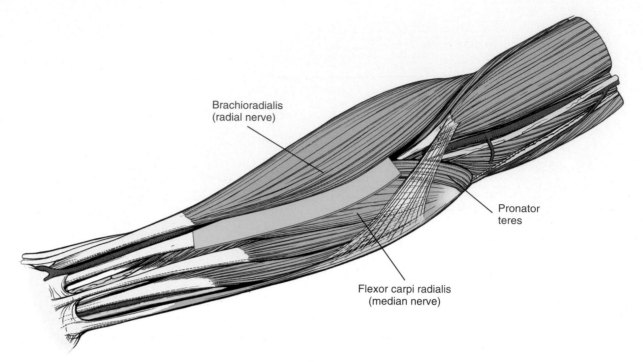

**Figure 4-3**   Internervous plane. The plane lies between the brachioradialis (radial nerve) and the flexor carpi radialis (median nerve).

## Internervous Plane

Distally, the internervous plane lies between the *brachioradialis* muscle, which is innervated by the radial nerve, just proximal to the elbow joint, and the *flexor carpi radialis* muscle, which is innervated by the median nerve (Fig. 4-3). Proximally, the internervous plane lies between the brachioradialis muscle, which is innervated by the radial nerve, and the pronator teres muscle, which is innervated by the median nerve.

## Superficial Surgical Dissection

Incise the deep fascia of the forearm in line with the skin incision. Identify the medial border of the brachioradialis as it runs down the forearm, and develop a plane between it and the flexor carpi radialis distally. More proximally, the plane lies between the pronator teres and brachioradialis muscles (Fig. 4-4). Note that the medial border of the brachioradialis is surprisingly far across the forearm. At the level of the elbow the brachioradialis extends almost halfway across the forearm.

Begin dissection distally and work proximally. Identify the superficial radial nerve running on the undersurface of the brachioradialis and moving with it. The brachioradialis receives a number of arterial branches from the radial artery (called the recurrent radial artery) just below the elbow joint. Ligate this recurrent leash of vessels to make it easier to move the brachioradialis laterally (Fig. 4-5). Take care to ligate these vessels and not avulse them, as avulsion is a potent cause of postoperative hematoma formation.

The radial artery lies beneath the brachioradialis in the middle part of the forearm; therefore, it is quite close to the medial edge of the wound. It runs with its two venae comitantes, which remain prominent if the limb is not exsanguinated before the tourniquet is applied. Often, the artery may have to be mobilized and retracted medially to achieve adequate exposure of the deeper muscular layer, particularly at the upper and lower ends of the approach (see Fig. 4-5).

The superficial radial nerve, which is a sensory nerve in the forearm, also runs under cover of the brachioradialis muscle. Preserve the nerve, because damage to it may create a painful neuroma at the operative site (see Fig. 4-5). It is retracted laterally with the brachioradialis muscle.

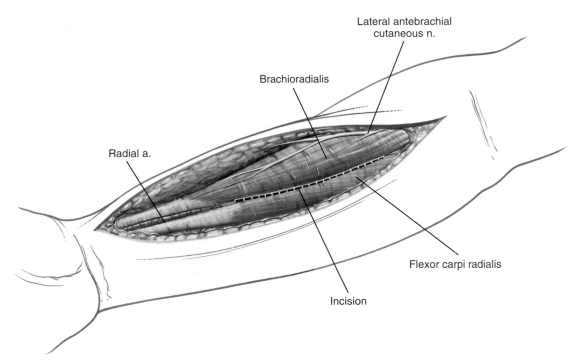

**Figure 4-4**   Incise the fascia and develop the plane between the brachioradialis and the flexor carpi radialis.

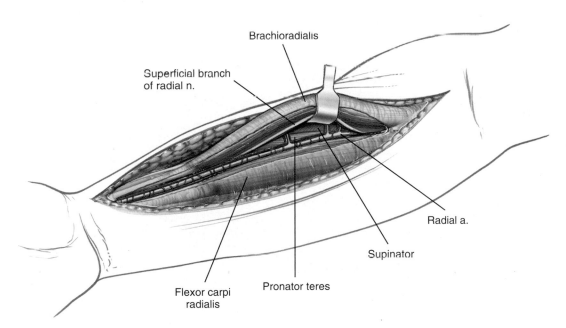

**Figure 4-5**   A leash of vessels from the radial artery supplies the brachioradialis. The vessels must be ligated to mobilize the brachioradialis laterally. Retract the superficial branch of the radial nerve with the brachioradialis muscle.

## Deep Surgical Dissection

### Proximal Third

Follow the biceps tendon to its insertion into the bicipital tuberosity of the radius. Just lateral to the tendon is a small bursa; incise the bursa to gain access to the proximal part of the shaft of the radius. Because the radial artery lies superficial and just *medial* to the tendon at this point, deepen the wound on the *lateral* side of the biceps tendon (Fig. 4-6).

The proximal third of the radius is covered by the supinator muscle, through which the posterior interosseous nerve passes on its way to the posterior compartment of the forearm.

The posterior interosseous nerve is the single most important structure left vulnerable by this approach. To displace the nerve laterally and posteriorly (away from the surgical area), fully supinate the forearm, exposing, at the same time, the insertion of the supinator muscle into the anterior aspect of the radius (Fig. 4-7).

Next, incise the supinator muscle along the line of its broad insertion. Continue subperiosteal dissection laterally, stripping the muscle off the bone (see Fig. 4-7). Lateral retraction of the muscle lifts the posterior interosseous nerve clear of the operative field, but be careful! Excessive traction may cause a neurapraxia of the nerve, and it recovers very slowly, tak-

ing up to 6 to 9 months. Finally, do not place retractors on the posterior surface of the radial neck, because they may compress the posterior interosseous nerve against the bone in patients whose nerve comes into direct contact with the posterior aspect of the radial neck (about 25% of all patients).[3]

### Middle Third

The anterior aspect of the middle third of the radius is covered by the pronator teres and flexor digitorum superficialis muscles. To reach the anterior surface of the bone, pronate the arm so that the insertion of the pronator teres onto the lateral aspect of the radius is exposed (Fig. 4-8; see Fig. 4-6). Detach this insertion from the bone and strip the muscle off medially. Preserve as much soft tissue as you can compatible with accurate reduction and fixation of the fracture. This maneuver detaches the origin of the flexor digitorum superficialis from the anterior aspect of the radius as well (Fig. 4-9).

### Distal Third

Two muscles, the flexor pollicis longus and the pronator quadratus, arise from the anterior aspect of the distal third of the radius. To reach bone, partially supinate the forearm and incise the periosteum of the lateral aspect of the radius lateral to the pronator quadratus and the flexor pollicis longus. Then, con-

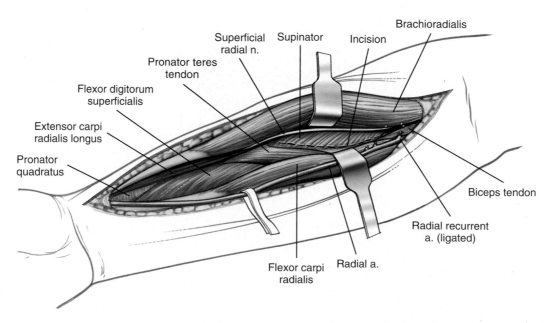

**Figure 4-6**    Deep to the brachioradialis and the flexor carpi radialis are the supinator muscle, the pronator teres, the flexor digitorum superficialis, and, most distally, the pronator quadrants.

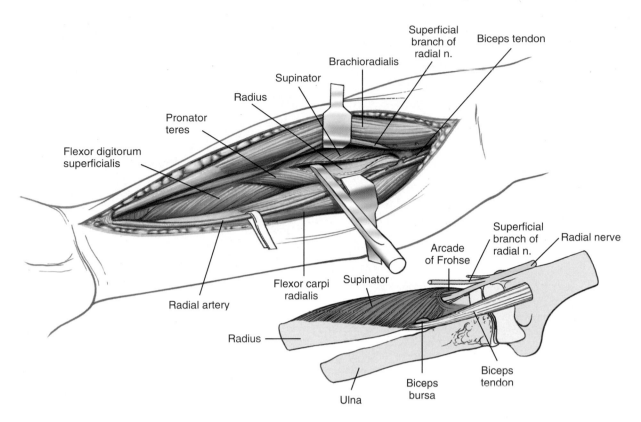

**Figure 4-7** With the patient's arm in the supinated position, resect the origin of the supinator. Reflect the muscle laterally. Leave the posterior interosseous nerve in the muscle's substance. The radial nerve enters the supinator through the arcade of Frohse *(inset)*. Turning the forearm upward moves the nerve laterally, away from the operative field. The origin of the supinator muscle is easier to identify if the surgeon stays lateral to the biceps tendon and locates the bursa between it and the supinator.

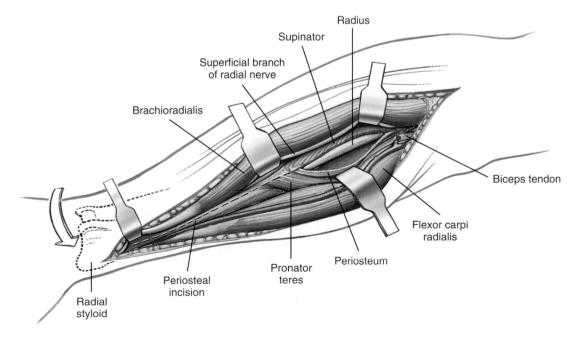

**Figure 4-8** Turn the arm downward to identify the pronator teres muscle. Resect it along its insertion on the lateral aspect of the radius.

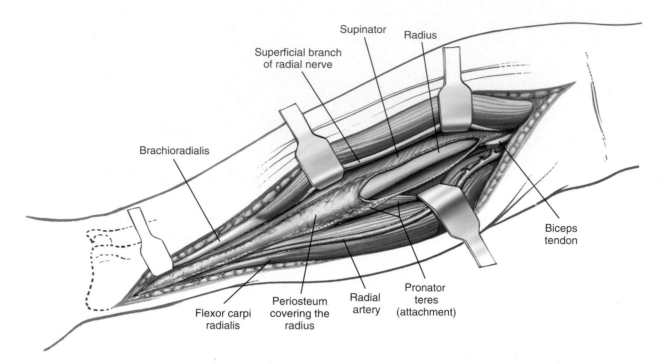

**Figure 4-9** Continue dissection distally to uncover the distal part of the radius. Leave the periosteum intact.

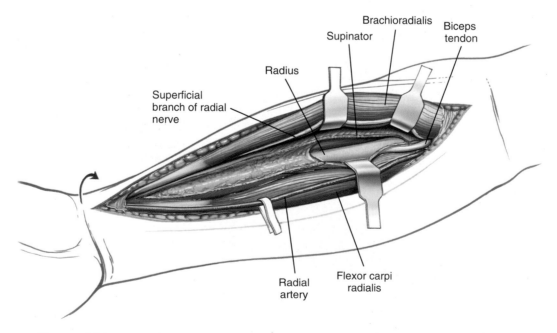

**Figure 4-10** With the arm in partial supination, remove the flexor pollicis longus and the pronator quadratus from the bone to expose the entire radius from its proximal to distal end.

tinue the dissection distally, retracting the two muscles medially and lifting them off the radius (Fig. 4-10).

## Dangers

### Nerves

The **posterior interosseous nerve** is vulnerable as it winds around the neck of the radius within the substance of the supinator muscle. The key to ensuring its safety is to detach correctly the insertion of the supinator muscle from the radius. The insertion of the muscle is exposed completely only when the arm is supinated fully. Once the subperiosteal dissection is begun, the nerve is comparatively safe, but overzealous retraction still can lead to a neurapraxia (see Figs. 4-7, *inset*, and 4-13).

The **superficial radial nerve** runs down the forearm under the brachioradialis muscle. It becomes vulnerable when the "mobile wad" of three muscles is mobilized and retracted laterally (see Fig. 4-5). The superficial radial nerve is vulnerable to neurapraxia if it is retracted vigorously. Take great care, therefore, when retracting the nerve and warn your patients preoperatively that temporary paresthesia in the distribution of the superficial branch of the radial nerve may occur in the early postoperative phase.

### Vessels

The **radial artery** runs down the middle of the forearm under the brachioradialis muscle. It is vul-nerable twice during the anterior approach to the radius:

1. During mobilization of the brachioradialis. Protection depends on recognizing the artery. Its two accompanying venae comitantes are the best surgical guide, because the artery is surprisingly small after a tourniquet has been used (see Fig. 4-5).
2. In the proximal end of the wound, as the artery passes to the medial side of the biceps tendon. Damage to the artery at that level can be avoided by remaining lateral to the tendon (see Fig. 4-13).

The **recurrent radial arteries** are a leash of vessels that arise from the radial artery just below the elbow joint. They consist of two groups, anterior and posterior, which pass in front of and behind the superficial radial nerve, respectively, before entering the brachioradialis muscle. They must be ligated to allow mobilization of both the artery and the nerve (see Figs. 4-9 and 4-12).

## How to Enlarge the Approach

The anterior approach provides complete access to the entire length of the radius. The approach can be extended distally to expose the wrist joint.[4] Although it can be extended into an anterolateral approach to the elbow and humerus, such extension rarely is required.

# Applied Surgical Anatomy of the Anterior Compartment of the Forearm

## Overview

### Muscles

Two muscle groups form the musculature of the anterior aspect of the forearm: the *mobile wad of three* (the brachioradialis, extensor carpi radialis longus, and extensor carpi radialis brevis), which is supplied by the radial nerve, forms the lateral border of the supinated forearm; and the flexor-pronator muscles, which are supplied by the median and ulnar nerves, comprise the rest.

The flexor-pronator group is arranged in three layers. In the *superficial layer*, four muscles arise from the common flexor origin on the medial humeral epicondyle and fan out across the forearm. They are easy to remember by the following simple maneuver. Place the butt of the opposite hand over the medial epicondyle, with the palm on the anterior surface of the forearm: the thumb points in the direction of the pronator teres, the index finger represents the flexor carpi radialis, the middle finger represents the palmaris longus, and the ring finger represents the flexor carpi ulnaris (Fig. 4-11).

The *middle layer* consists of the flexor digitorum superficialis (Fig. 4-13).

The *deep layer* is comprised of three muscles: the flexor digitorum profundus, the flexor pollicis longus, and the pronator quadratus. (A fourth deep muscle, the supinator, is critical to the surgical anatomy of the area, but is not strictly a flexor muscle [Fig. 4-14].)

The keys to the surgical anatomy of the anterior aspect of the forearm are the following three practi-

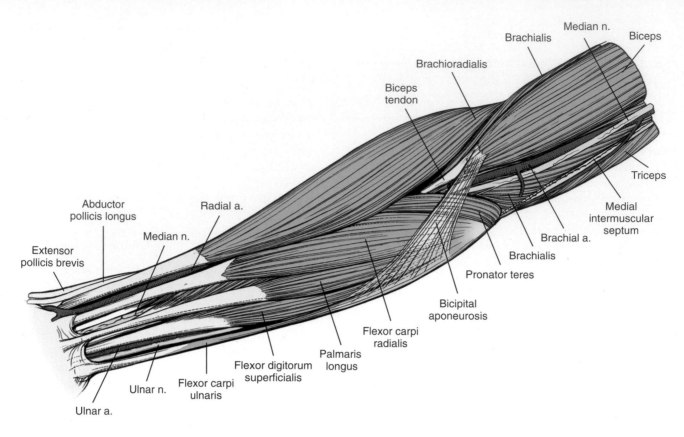

**Figure 4-11** Superficial layer of the forearm muscles and vessels.

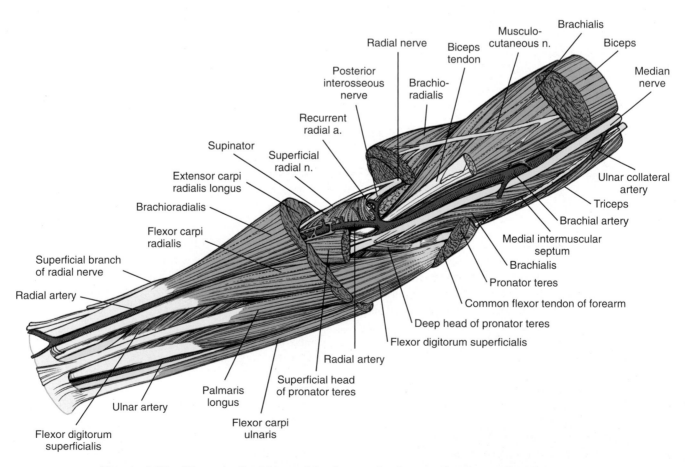

**Figure 4-12** The superficial layer of the forearm has been resected, revealing the vessels and nerves. The median nerve pierces the gap between the two heads of the pronator teres. Note the leash of vessels of the radial artery and the recurrent radial artery.

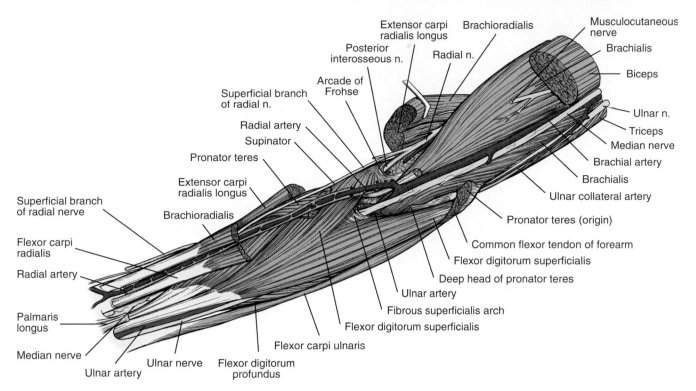

**Figure 4-13**    The middle layer of the forearm, with the superficial branch of the radial nerve. In the proximal part of the wound, the median nerve enters the undersurface of the superficialis.

---

**Flexor Carpi Radialis** *Origin.* Common flexor origin on medial epicondyle of humerus. *Insertion.* Bases of second and third metacarpals. *Action.* Flexor and radial deviator of wrist. *Nerve supply.* Median nerve.

---

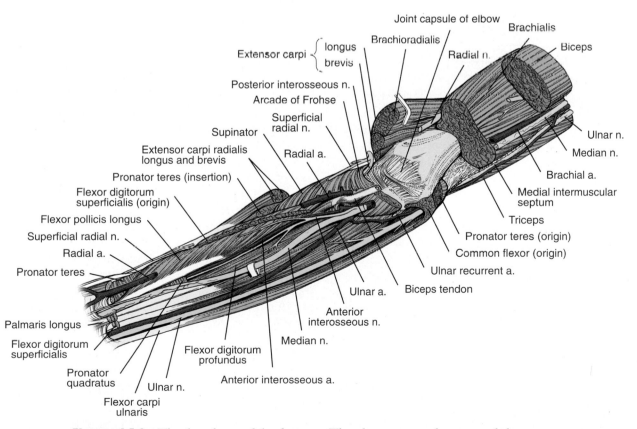

**Figure 4-14**    The deep layer of the forearm. The ulnar nerve and artery and the median nerve lie on the flexor digitorum profundus. Note the position of the anterior interosseous nerve and artery.

cal internervous planes that are used in operative approaches:

1. Between the radial and median nerves: a dissection between the brachioradialis muscle, the most medial of the three muscles (which is supplied by the radial nerve), and the flexor carpi radialis and pronator teres muscles, the most lateral of the flexor-pronator group (which are supplied by the median nerve; see Fig. 4-3)
2. Between the median and ulnar nerves: a dissection between the flexor carpi ulnaris muscle (which is supplied by the ulnar nerve) and the flexor digitorum superficialis muscle, the most medial of the flexor muscles (which is supplied by the median nerve; see Fig. 5-29)
3. Between the ulnar and posterior interosseous nerves: a dissection between the flexor carpi ulnaris muscle (which is supplied by the ulnar nerve) and the extensor carpi ulnaris muscle (which is supplied by the posterior interosseous nerve; see Fig. 4-19)

The first of these planes is used in the anterior approach to the radius, the second exposes the ulnar nerve in the forearm, and the third is used for exposure of the ulna.

### Nerves and Vessels

The neurovascular architecture of the anterior aspect of the forearm is relatively simple: the forearm is "framed" by its nerves. The superficial *radial nerve* runs down the radial aspect of the forearm, with the radial artery lying on its medial side in the distal half of the forearm (see Fig. 4-13). The *ulnar nerve* runs down the ulnar side of the forearm, with the ulnar artery lying on its lateral side in the distal half of the forearm. The *median nerve* runs down the middle of the forearm (see Fig. 4-14).

Both the *radial and the ulnar arteries* are arteries of transit in the forearm; they both are branches of the brachial artery. Because the brachial artery lies in the middle of the anterior aspect of the elbow, with the median nerve lying on its medial side, the ulnar artery and median nerve must cross in the upper forearm, with the nerve superficial to the artery; this crossing occurs at the level of the musculotendinous region of the pronator teres muscle (see Fig. 4-13). The anterior interosseous nerve (which is a branch of the median nerve) and the anterior interosseous artery (which is a branch of the common interosseous artery, which itself is a branch of the ulnar artery) also run down the middle of the forearm, but deeper than the median nerve (see Fig. 4-14).

## Incision

Because the incision runs transversely across the lines of cleavage in the forearm, the resultant scar may be broad. Making the incision as a series of gentle curves brings the skin incision closer to the lines of cleavage in the forearm. Such an incision has the effect of reducing tension on the subsequent skin repair.

## Superficial Surgical Dissection and its Dangers

### Muscles

Superficial surgical dissection opens the plane between the mobile wad of three muscles (the brachioradialis, extensor carpi radialis longus, and extensor carpi radialis brevis) and the pronator teres muscle proximally and flexor carpi radialis muscle distally (see Fig. 4-11).

The mobile wad of three muscles, on the radial side of the forearm, is supplied by the radial nerve. All three muscles take some of their origin from the common extensor origin on the lateral epicondyle of the humerus (see Fig. 4-13).

The *brachioradialis* pronates the forearm when it is supinated and supinates it when it is pronated. Therefore, it may act as a deforming force in distal radial fractures if the forearm is immobilized in either full pronation or full supination after reduction of the fracture. Its action is one reason for immobilizing distal radial fractures with the forearm in the neutral position.

The brachioradialis is the only muscle in the body to take origin from the distal end of one bone and insert onto the distal end of another (Fig. 4-15; see Fig. 4-11).

During recovery from high radial nerve palsy, the *extensor carpi radialis longus* is one of the first muscles to be reinnervated. If the patient recovering from a high radial nerve palsy is asked to extend the wrist, the muscle extends with radial deviation, because the balancing muscle, the extensor carpi ulnaris, is supplied farther distally by a branch from the posterior interosseous nerve. Reinnervation of the brachioradialis, however, probably is the best way to diagnose both clinically and electrically (by electromyographic studies) a recovering high radial nerve palsy (see Figs. 4-12 and 4-22).

The *extensor carpi radialis brevis* muscle is a wrist extensor that deviates the wrist neither toward the radius nor toward the ulna. It may be involved in tennis elbow.

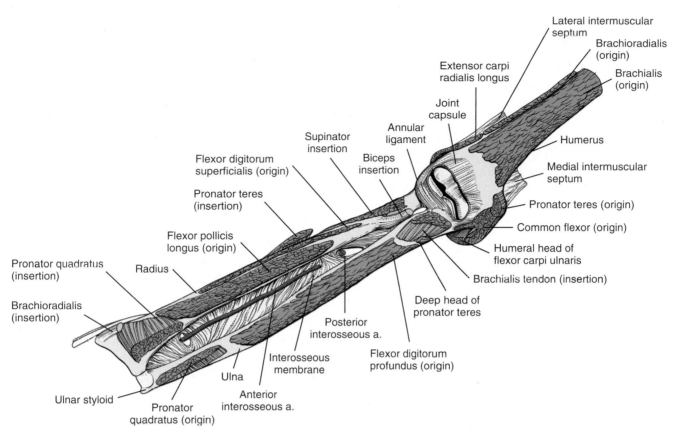

**Figure 4-15** The origins and insertions of the muscles of the forearm. Note the anterior interosseous artery lying on the interosseous membrane.

**Brachioradialis.** *Origin.* Upper two thirds of lateral supracondylar ridge of humerus. *Insertion.* Styloid process of radius. *Action.* Flexor of elbow. Pronator and supinator of forearm. *Nerve supply.* Radial nerve.

**Flexor Digitorum Superficialis.** *Origin.* Medial epicondyle of humerus, medial ligament of elbow, medial border of coronoid process of ulna, fibrous arch connecting coronoid process of ulna with anterior oblique line of radius. *Insertion.* Volar aspect of middle phalanges of fingers. *Action.* Flexor of proximal interphalangeal joints, metacarpophalangeal joints, and wrist joint. *Nerve supply.* Median nerve.

**Flexor Pollicis Longus.** *Origin.* Middle part of anterior surface of radius. *Insertion.* Distal phalanx of thumb. *Action.* Main flexor of thumb. *Nerve supply.* Anterior interosseous nerve.

**Pronator Quadratus.** *Origin.* Lower fourth of volar surface of ulna. *Insertion.* Lower fourth of lateral aspect of radius. *Action.* Weak pronator of forearm. *Nerve supply.* Anterior interosseous nerve.

**Palmaris Longus.** *Origin.* Common flexor origin on humerus. *Insertion.* Palmar aponeurosis. *Action.* Weak flexor of wrist. *Nerve supply.* Median nerve.

**Flexor Digitorum Profundus.** *Origin.* Upper three fourths of anterior surface of ulna. *Insertion.* Distal phalanges of fingers. *Action.* Flexor of distal interphalangeal joints, proximal interphalangeal joints, metacarpophalangeal joints, and wrist joint. *Nerve supply.* Median and ulnar nerves.

**Flexor Carpi Ulnaris.** *Origin.* From two heads. Humeral head: from common flexor origin on medial epicondyle of humerus. Ulnar head: from medial border of olecranon and upper three fourths of subcutaneous border of ulna. *Insertion.* Hamate and fifth metacarpal. *Action.* Flexor and ulnar deviator of wrist. Also weak flexor of elbow. *Nerve supply.* Ulnar nerve.

### Nerves and Vessels

Palsies of the posterior interosseous nerve caused by compression of the nerve by the tendinous origin of the extensor carpi radialis brevis muscle have been described.

Two structures that lie under the brachioradialis muscle must be preserved during superficial surgical dissection:

1. The *radial artery* originates from the brachial artery in the cubital fossa. Proximally, it lies just medial to the biceps tendon in a somewhat superficial position. The radial artery angles across the arm as it descends, lying on the supinator, the pronator teres, the origin of the flexor pollicis longus, and the lower part of the anterior surface of the radius, where it can be palpated easily (see Fig. 4-13).
2. The *superficial radial nerve* is purely sensory in the forearm. It runs along the lateral side, crossing the supinator, the pronator teres, and the flexor digitorum superficialis. Damage to the nerve in the forearm produces an area of diminished sensation on the dorsoradial aspect of the hand. The most important problem associated with such damage is not the sensory loss, however, but the painful neuroma that may result. The nerve runs lateral to the radial artery when the two are together (see Figs. 4-13 and 4-32).

## Deep Surgical Dissection and its Dangers

Five muscles must be detached from the radius to expose fully the anterior aspect of the bone. From the proximal to the distal aspect, they are as follows:

1. The supinator
2. The pronator teres
3. The flexor digitorum superficialis
4. The flexor pollicis longus
5. The pronator quadratus

The nerve supply of the *supinator* muscle, the posterior interosseous nerve, passes through a fibrous arch known as the arcade of Frohse as it enters the muscle (see Figs. 4-12 and 4-13).[5] The arch is formed by the thickened edge of the superficial head of the supinator. Compression of the nerve at that point produces paralysis or dysfunction of all the extensor muscles of the forearm, fingers, and thumb, a lesion that may be incomplete. Compression at the arcade of Frohse is one of the causes of a posterior interosseous nerve entrapment syndrome and can be relieved by incising the fibrous arch.[6–9] It also is a cause of pain restricted to this area, which may present as a resistant "tennis elbow" (see Fig. 4-13).[10]

The nerve supply of the pronator teres, the median nerve, enters the forearm between the muscle's two heads of origin (see Fig. 4-12). The great variations that occur in the site, size, and quality of the ulnar head of the muscle sometimes cause the nerve to become trapped as it traverses the muscle, producing the pronator syndrome, which mimics the carpal tunnel syndrome, but includes pain and paresthesia to the proximal end of the volar aspect of the forearm.[11,12] Understandably, the syndrome occurs when the muscle contracts and further compresses the nerve. In this syndrome, the intrinsic muscles of the thumb become weak, but the muscles that are innervated by the anterior interosseous nerve (the flexor pollicis longus, the flexor profundus to the index and middle fingers, and the pronator quadratus) are spared (see Fig. 4-12).

The median nerve passes under the fibrous arch of origin of the *flexor digitorum superficialis*. It may be compressed by a thickened arch, producing pain or a median nerve palsy (see Fig. 4-13).[13] The tendons of the muscle form well above the wrist. Functionally, it is four separate muscles; it can flex each finger independently, in contrast to the mass action of the flexor digitorum profundus.

Part of the origin of the flexor digitorum superficialis may have to be detached to expose the anterior part of the shaft of the radius (see Figs. 4-13 and 4-15).

The origin of the *flexor pollicis longus*, which is the sole long flexor of the thumb, must be stripped off the radius for the bone to be accessible (see Figs. 4-14 and 4-15).

The insertion of the *pronator quadratus* must be stripped off to expose the distal fourth of the radius (see Fig. 4-15). Because the muscle is relaxed totally when the forearm is pronated fully, some authors suggest that distal radial fractures should be immobilized in pronation. Clearly, however, the pronator quadratus is not the only possible deforming force on the distal radius; the best position for immobilizing reduced fractures of the distal radius still is a matter of debate.

## Dangers

### Nerves

The **posterior interosseous nerve** is the motor nerve of the extensor compartment of the forearm. A branch of the radial nerve, it passes between the two heads of origin of the supinator muscle and actually may come in direct contact with the periosteum of the neck of the radius. At that point, it may be trapped beneath incorrectly positioned plates or retractors. After emerging from the supinator muscle, the nerve passes down over the origin of the abductor pollicis longus muscle to reach the interosseous membrane. It continues distally on the interosseous membrane to the wrist joint, which it supplies with some sensory branches. The nerve supplies the muscles that arise from the common extensor origin and the deep muscles of the extensor compartment of the forearm.

The posterior interosseous nerve is vulnerable during all approaches to the upper third of the radial shaft. Although the nerve can be protected if the insertion of the supinator is detached and the muscle is stripped off the bone subperiosteally, it can be argued that the only certain protection as the upper third of the radius is plated comes from identifying and preserving the nerve via a posterior approach (see Figs. 4-32 and 4-33).

Proximally, the **median nerve** usually passes between the heads of the pronator teres muscle, whereas the ulnar artery passes deep to both the heads. Distal to the pronator teres, the median nerve joins the ulnar artery and passes beneath the fibrous arch of origin of the flexor digitorum superficialis muscle. Then, it runs down the flexor aspect of the forearm, roughly in the midline (see Figs. 4-13 and 4-14).

Because of its proximity to the flexor digitorum superficialis muscle, the median nerve sometimes is mistaken for the superficial tendon to the index finger. To differentiate nerve from tendon, try to find an artery on the structure in question: the median nerve has the median artery running along its surface. The artery, derived from the anterior interosseous artery, is the original fetal axial artery (see Fig. 4-14).

## Special Anatomic Points

The main surgical use of the palmaris longus muscle is as a graft for tendon repairs. Because it is absent in 10% of the population, it must be identified in the conscious patient before surgery is undertaken. To find it, instruct the patient to touch the thumb and little fingers together while flexing the wrist against resistance. Then, palpate the tendon, which stands out prominently in the forearm (see Fig. 4-11).

Note that the median nerve is immediately below the palmaris longus at the wrist. In the patient with an absent palmaris longus, the nerve actually may be mistaken for the tendon (see Fig. 4-11).

The tendons of the *flexor digitorum profundus* arise at or below the level of the wrist joint. Therefore, contraction of the muscle produces movement in all

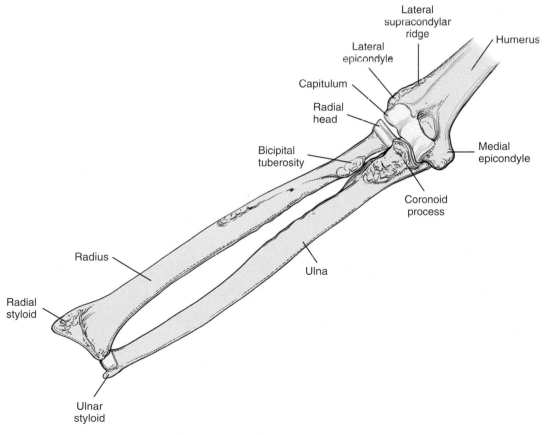

**Figure 4-16**   The bones of the forearm.

four tendons, making it a mass action muscle that is used mainly for power grip.

The *anterior interosseous* nerve arises from the median nerve shortly after the median nerve enters the forearm; the two lie under the tendinous origin of the deep head of the pronator teres (see Figs. 4-11 and 4-13). The anterior interosseous nerve may be compressed at this point, producing the anterior interosseous nerve syndrome: paralysis of the flexor pollicis longus and flexor profundus tendons to the index and middle fingers, as well as of the pronator quadratus muscle.[14–16]

## Exposure of the Shaft of the Ulna

Exposing the shaft of the ulna is the simplest of all forearm approaches, uncovering the entire length of bone. The exposure uses the internervous plane between the extensor carpi ulnaris and flexor carpi ulnaris muscles. Both muscles attach by a shared aponeurosis into the subcutaneous border of the ulna, the border of bone that is exposed initially during the approach.

Because the two muscles that form the boundaries of the internervous plane share a common aponeurosis, they cannot be separated at their origin, and the plane is difficult to define. Fibers of the extensor carpi ulnaris usually have to be detached from the aponeurosis.

The uses of the approach include the following:

1. Open reduction and internal fixation of ulnar fractures
2. Treatment of delayed union or nonunion of ulnar fractures
3. Osteotomy of the ulna
4. Treatment of chronic osteomyelitis
5. Treatment of the fibrous anlage of the ulna in cases of ulnar clubhand[2]
6. Ulnar lengthening (in Kienböck's disease)[17]
7. Ulnar shortening (in cases of distal radial malunion)

### Position of the Patient

Place the patient supine on the operating table with the arm placed across the chest to expose the subcutaneous border of the ulna. Exsanguinate the limb either by elevating it for 3 to 5 minutes or by applying a soft rubber bandage and then a tourniquet (Fig. 4-17).

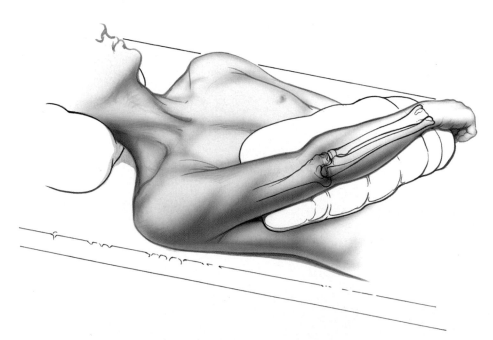

**Figure 4-17**   Position of the patient on the operating table, for exposure of the shaft of the ulna.

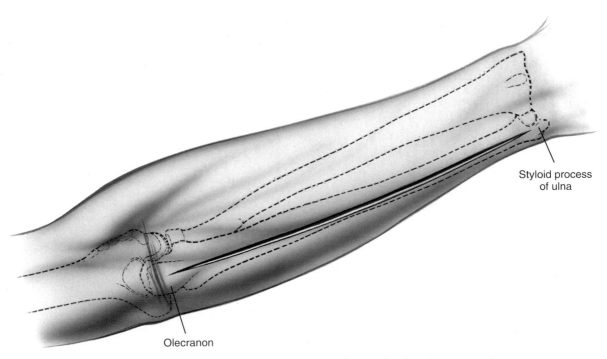

Styloid process
of ulna

Olecranon

**Figure 4-18**   Incision for ulnar exposure. Make a longitudinal incision over the subcutaneous border of the ulna.

## Landmarks and Incision

### Landmarks
The *subcutaneous border of the ulna* can be palpated along its entire length. It is felt most easily in the proximal and distal thirds of the bone.

### Incision
Make a linear, longitudinal incision over the subcutaneous border of the ulna. The length of the incision depends on the amount of bone that is to be exposed. In cases of fracture, center the incision over the fracture site (Fig. 4-18).

## Internervous Plane

The internervous plane lies between the *extensor carpi ulnaris* muscle, which is supplied by the posterior interosseous nerve, and the *flexor carpi ulnaris* muscle, which is supplied by the ulnar nerve (Fig. 4-19).

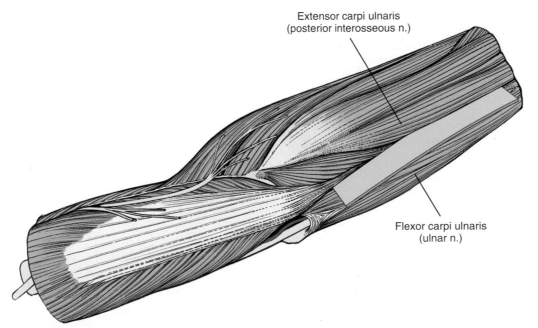

Extensor carpi ulnaris
(posterior interosseous n.)

Flexor carpi ulnaris
(ulnar n.)

**Figure 4-19**   The internervous plane lies between the extensor carpi ulnaris (posterior interosseous nerve) and the flexor carpi ulnaris (ulnar nerve).

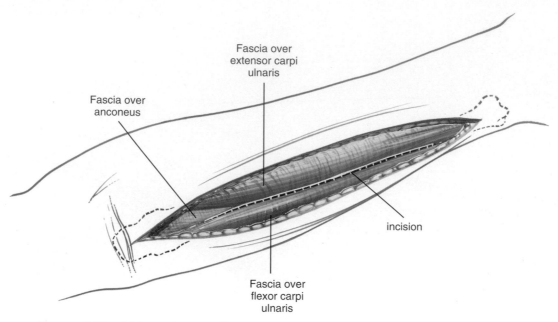

Fascia over
extensor carpi
ulnaris

Fascia over
anconeus

incision

Fascia over
flexor carpi
ulnaris

**Figure 4-20**  Make an incision through the fascia onto the subcutaneous border of the ulna.

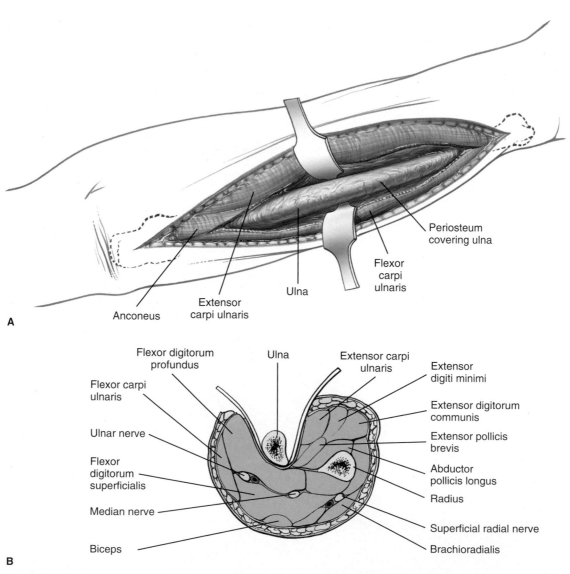

Periosteum
covering ulna

Flexor
carpi
ulnaris

Ulna

Extensor
carpi ulnaris

Anconeus

**A**

Flexor digitorum
profundus

Ulna

Extensor carpi
ulnaris

Flexor carpi
ulnaris

Extensor
digiti minimi

Ulnar nerve

Extensor digitorum
communis

Flexor
digitorum
superficialis

Extensor pollicis
brevis

Median nerve

Abductor
pollicis longus

Radius

Biceps

Superficial radial nerve

**B**

Brachioradialis

**Figure 4-21**  **(A)** Lift the periosteum longitudinally on the posterior aspect of the ulna, both radially and medially, to expose the entire posterior length of the ulna. **(B)** Subperiosteal dissection around the ulna is safe; the muscle masses on each side protect the vital structures.

## Superficial Surgical Dissection

Beginning in the distal half of the incision, incise the deep fascia along the same line as the skin incision; continue the dissection down to the subcutaneous border of the ulna (Fig. 4-20). Even though the bone feels subcutaneous in its middle third, the fibers of the extensor carpi ulnaris muscle nearly always have to be divided to reach the bone.

In the region of the olecranon, the flexor carpi ulnaris and anconeus muscles run along the plane of dissection. The plane still is an internervous plane, because the anconeus is supplied by the radial nerve and the flexor carpi ulnaris is supplied by the ulnar nerve.

## Deep Surgical Dissection

Incise the periosteum over the ulna longitudinally. Continue the dissection around the bone in a subperiosteal plane to reveal either the flexor or the extensor aspects of the bone, as needed (Fig. 4-21).

In the proximal fifth of the ulna, part of the insertion of the triceps tendon will need to be detached to gain access to the bone. This insertion is very broad and long, and it blends in with the periosteum of the subcutaneous surface of the olecranon.

## Dangers

### Nerves

The **ulnar nerve,** which travels down the forearm under the flexor carpi ulnaris, lies on the flexor digi-torum profundus. The nerve is safe as long as the flexor carpi ulnaris is stripped off the ulna subperiosteally. If the dissection strays into the substance of the muscle, however, the nerve may be damaged. Because the nerve is most vulnerable during very proximal dissections, it should be identified as it passes through the two heads of the flexor carpi ulnaris *before* the muscle is stripped off the proximal fifth of the bone (Fig. 4-22).

### Vessels

The **ulnar artery** travels down the forearm with the ulnar nerve, lying on its radial side. Therefore, it also is vulnerable when dissection of the flexor carpi ulnaris is not carried out subperiosteally (see Fig. 4-21B).

## How to Enlarge the Approach

### Local Measures

The approach described provides excellent exposure of the entire bone and cannot be enlarged usefully by local measures.

### Extensile Measures

The approach cannot be extended usefully distally. It can be extended over the olecranon and up the back of the arm, however, either to expose the elbow joint through an olecranon osteotomy or to approach the posterior aspect of the distal two thirds of the humerus.

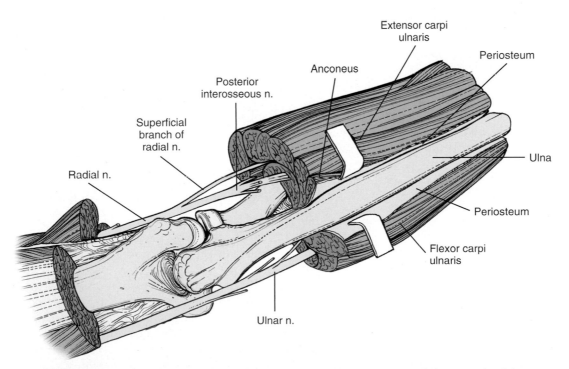

**Figure 4-22**   The ulnar nerve is vulnerable during the most proximal dissections of the ulna. It must be identified before muscle is stripped from bone in the proximal fifth.

# Applied Surgical Anatomy of the Approach to the Ulna

## Anatomy of the Surgical Dissection and its Dangers

Two muscles are separated in the approach to the ulna: the flexor carpi ulnaris (which is supplied by the ulnar nerve) and the extensor carpi ulnaris (which is supplied by the posterior interosseous nerve; see Fig. 4-22).

The muscular branch of the ulnar nerve, which innervates the flexor carpi ulnaris, effectively tethers the nerve, preventing further distal mobilization during decompression at the elbow. Compression lesions of the nerve have been described (see Fig. 3-40).[18,19]

The *extensor carpi ulnaris* is the most medial of the muscles that are innervated by the posterior interosseous nerve. Thus, it forms one border of the internervous plane between the muscles that are innervated by the posterior interosseous nerve and those that are innervated by the ulnar nerve, the most medial of which is the flexor carpi ulnaris (see Fig. 4-19).

The *ulnar nerve* runs down the medial side of the forearm between the flexor digitorum profundus and the flexor digitorum superficialis, and under the flexor carpi ulnaris. In the forearm, it supplies the flexor carpi ulnaris and the ulnar half of the flexor digitorum profundus (see Figs. 3-40 and 4-14).

The *ulnar artery* is a terminal branch of the brachial artery. It usually enters the forearm deep to the deep head of the pronator teres before angling medially across the forearm and passing under the fibrous arch of the flexor digitorum superficialis, where it runs just deep to the median nerve (see Figs. 4-12 through 4-14). In the distal two thirds of the forearm, the artery runs on the lateral side of the ulnar nerve, lying on the flexor digitorum profundus and under the flexor carpi ulnaris. The artery has one major branch in the forearm, the common interosseous artery, which divides almost immediately into two tributaries, the anterior interosseous artery (which runs down the forearm in the midline, lying on the interosseous membrane) and the posterior interosseous artery (which pierces the interosseous membrane, running down the forearm in its posterior compartment; see Fig. 4-14).

The ulnar nerve and ulnar artery may be endangered during superficial dissection if the dissection strays to the flexor side of the bone.

# Posterior Approach to the Radius

The posterior approach to the radius provides good access to the entire dorsal aspect of the radial shaft.[20] The principal aim of the approach is to isolate and retract the posterior interosseous nerve before exposing the highest parts of the radial shaft, keeping the nerve under direct observation during all stages of the subsequent procedure and protecting it from damage. The uses of the posterior approach include the following:

1. Open reduction and internal fixation of radial fractures (the approach provides access to the extensor side of the bone; this is the tensile side of the bone, where plates should be placed, if possible)
2. Treatment of delayed union or nonunion of fractures of the radius
3. Access to the posterior interosseous nerve; decompression of the nerve as it passes through the arcade of Frohse for nerve paralysis or resistant tennis elbow[9]
4. Radial osteotomy
5. Treatment of chronic osteomyelitis of the radius
6. Biopsy and treatment of bone tumors

## Position of the Patient

Situate the patient in one of two positions:

1. Place the patient supine on the operating table, with the arm on an arm board. Pronate the patient's arm to expose the extensor compartment of the forearm.
2. Place the patient's arm across the chest. Supinate the forearm to expose its extensor compartment (Fig. 4-23). If the ulna must be approached as well as the radius, this position will allow easier access to the ulna through a separate incision.

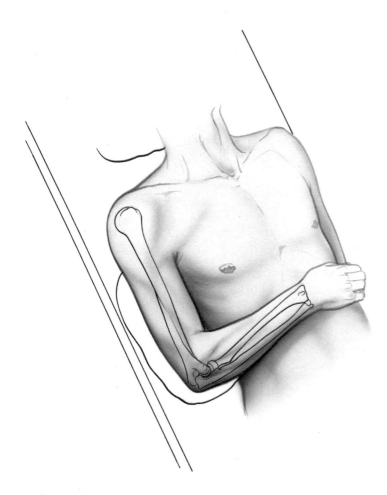

**Figure 4-23** Position of the patient's arm on the operating table, for the posterior approach to the radius.

In both positions, exsanguinate the limb by elevating the arm for 3 to 5 minutes or by applying a soft rubber bandage or exsanguinator. Then, apply a tourniquet.

## Landmarks and Incision

### Landmarks
Palpate the *lateral epicondyle of the humerus* just lateral to the olecranon process on the distal humerus. It is a prominent bony landmark, but is somewhat smaller and less defined than the medial epicondyle of the humerus.

*Lister's tubercle* (the dorsoradial tubercle) lies about a third of the way across the dorsum of the wrist from the styloid process of the radius. It feels like a small, longitudinal bony prominence or nodule.

### Incision
Make either a straight or a gently curved incision, extending from a point anterior to the lateral epi-condyle of the humerus (along the dorsal aspect of the forearm) to a point just distal to the ulnar side of Lister's tubercle at the wrist (Fig. 4-24).

Normally, only part of this incision is required for any given operation. In cases of fracture, the incision should be centered over the fracture site.

## Internervous Plane

*Proximally*, the internervous plane lies between the extensor carpi radialis brevis muscle (which is supplied by the radial nerve) and the extensor digitorum communis muscle (which is supplied by the posterior interosseous nerve; Fig. 4-25). The common aponeurosis of these muscles is the cleavage plane.

*Distally*, the internervous plane lies between the extensor carpi radialis brevis muscle (which is supplied by the radial nerve) and the extensor pollicis longus muscle (which is supplied by the posterior interosseous nerve).

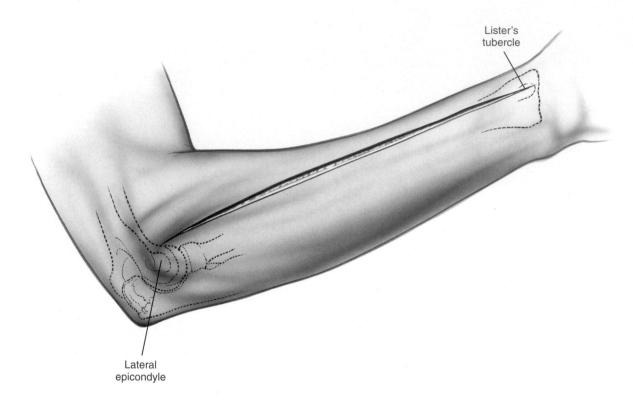

**Figure 4-24**    The long incision extends from just anterior to the lateral epicondyle of the humerus to just distal to the ulnar side of Lister's tubercle at the wrist.

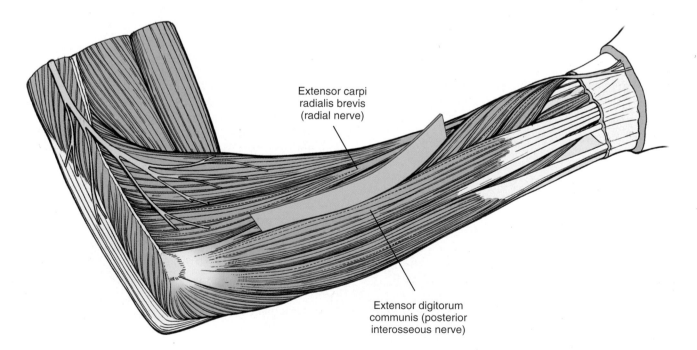

**Figure 4-25**    The internervous plane lies between the extensor carpi radialis brevis (radial nerve) and the extensor digitorum communis (posterior interosseous nerve).

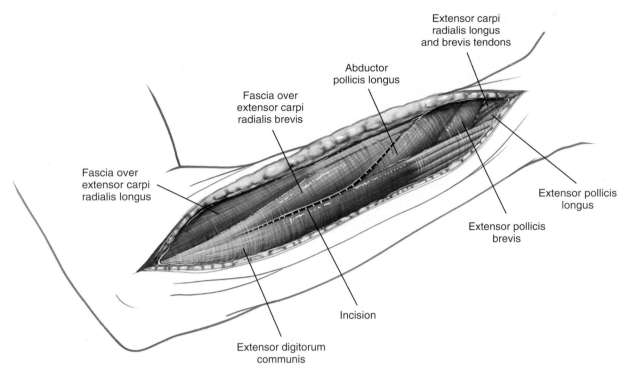

**Figure 4-26**  Incise the deep fascia and identify the space between the extensor carpi radialis brevis and the extensor digitorum communis. The identification is easier distally.

## Superficial Surgical Dissection

Incise the deep fascia in line with the skin incision and identify the space between the extensor carpi radialis brevis and the extensor digitorum communis.

This gap is more obvious distally, where the abductor pollicis longus and the extensor pollicis brevis emerge from between the two muscles. Proximally, the extensor carpi radialis brevis and the extensor digitorum communis share a common aponeurosis (Figs. 4-26 and 4-27).

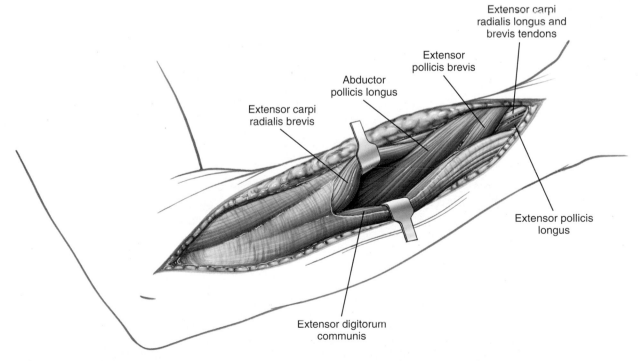

**Figure 4-27**  The interval between the extensor carpi radialis brevis and the extensor digitorum communis.

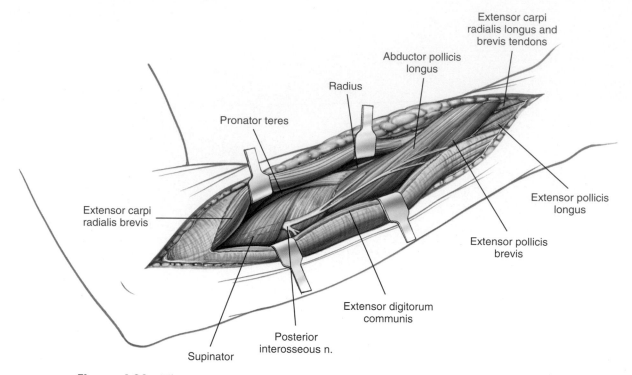

**Figure 4-28** The supinator muscle, beneath the extensor carpi radialis brevis and the extensor pollicis longus.

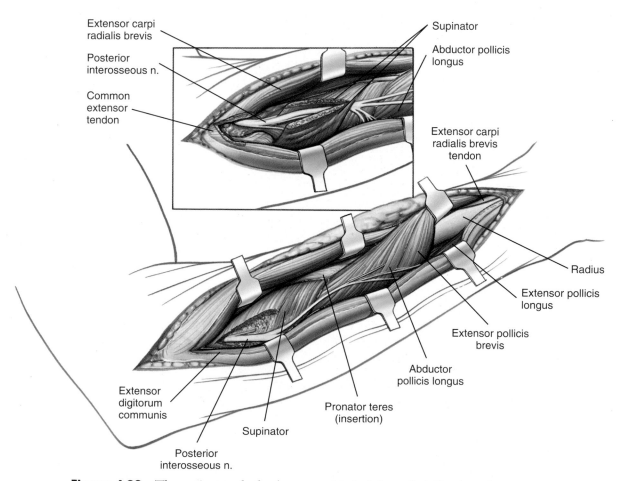

**Figure 4-29** The supinator cloaks the upper third of the radius; the posterior interosseous nerve runs through its substance. The nerve must be protected and identified as it traverses the muscle. The interosseous nerve is seen in the substance of the supinator *(inset).*

Continue the dissection proximally, separating the two muscles to reveal the upper third of the shaft of the radius, which is covered by the enveloping supinator muscle.

Below the abductor pollicis longus and the extensor pollicis brevis, identify the intermuscular plane between the extensor carpi radialis brevis and the extensor pollicis longus. Separating the two muscles exposes the lateral aspect of the shaft of the radius (Figs. 4-28 and 4-29).

## Deep Surgical Dissection

### Proximal Third

The supinator muscle cloaks the dorsal aspect of the upper third of the radius; the posterior interosseous nerve runs within its substance between the superficial and deep heads. The nerve emerges from between the superficial and deep heads of the supinator muscle about 1 cm proximal to the distal edge of the muscle. At this point, it divides into branches that supply the extensors of the wrist, fingers, and thumb (see Fig. 4-29).

Two methods exist for successfully identifying and preserving this nerve as it traverses the muscle.

1. Proximal to distal (see Fig. 4-29, *inset*). Detach the origin of the extensor carpi radialis brevis and part of the origin of the extensor carpi radialis longus from the lateral epicondyle and retract these two muscles laterally. Next, identify the posterior interosseous nerve proximal to the proximal end of the supinator muscle by palpating the nerve. Now, carefully dissect the nerve out through the substance of the supinator, in a proximal to distal direction, taking great care to preserve the multiple motor branches to the muscle itself.

2. Distal to proximal (see Fig. 4-29). Identify the nerve as it emerges from the supinator. Note that it emerges about 1 cm proximal to the distal end of the muscle. Now, follow the nerve proximally through the substance of the muscle, taking care to preserve all muscular branches.

When the nerve has been identified and preserved successfully, fully supinate the arm to bring the anterior surface of the radius into view. Detach the insertion of the supinator muscle from the anterior aspect of the radius. Strip the supinator off the bone subperiosteally to expose the proximal third of the shaft of the radius (Fig. 4-30).

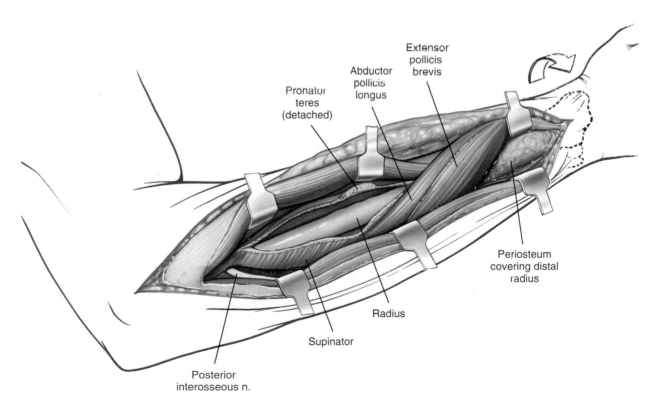

**Figure 4-30** Detach the insertion of the supinator from the anterior aspect of the radius, with the arm in full supination to bring the origin of the supinator into view and to move the posterior interosseous nerve away from the area of incision. Along the distal third of the bone, the extensor carpi radialis brevis has been separated from the extensor pollicis longus, uncovering the lateral border of the radius.

### Middle Third

Two muscles, the abductor pollicis longus and the extensor pollicis brevis, blanket this approach as they cross the dorsal aspect of the radius before heading distally and radially across the middle third of the radius. To retract them off the bone, make an incision along their superior and inferior borders. Then, they can be separated easily from the underlying radius and retracted either distally or proximally, depending on the exposure that is required (see Fig. 4-30). Plates can be slid underneath these muscles if required for fixation.

### Distal Third

Separating the extensor carpi radialis brevis from the extensor pollicis longus already has led directly onto the lateral border of the radius (see Fig. 4-30).

## Dangers

There are two ways in which to preserve the critical posterior interosseous nerve, which is the key to this dissection:

1. *Identification of the nerve.* In 25% of patients, the posterior interosseous nerve actually touches the dorsal aspect of the radius opposite the bicipital tuberosity; plates placed high on the dorsal surface of the radius may trap the nerve underneath.[21] Identifying and preserving the nerve in the supinator muscle is the only means of ensuring that it will not be trapped beneath any plate that is applied for a radial fracture (see Fig. 4-29).

2. *Protecting the nerve with the supinator muscle.* Strip the supinator off the anterior aspect of the radius and retract it radially, with the nerve still enclosed in its substance. This technique often is used in the anterior approach to the radius, exposing the anterior surface of the bone. The dorsal aspect of the radius can be exposed in the same way, but because the posterior interosseous nerve actually touches the periosteum in one of four patients, the safest procedure is to dissect the nerve out fully before stripping the muscle from the bone (see Fig. 4-30).

## How to Enlarge the Approach

### Local Measures

To widen the plane between the extensor carpi radialis brevis and extensor digitorum communis muscles, detach the origin of the extensor carpi radialis brevis from the common extensor origin on the lateral epicondyle of the humerus.

### Extensile Measures

The approach can be extended to the dorsal side of the wrist (see Dorsal Approach to the Wrist in Chapter 5). It can be extended proximally to expose the lateral epicondyle of the humerus (see Lateral Approach to the Distal Humerus in Chapter 2). These extensions, however, rarely are required.

---

# Applied Surgical Anatomy of the Posterior Approach to the Radius

## Overview

Twelve muscles appear on the dorsal aspect of the forearm. They are divided into three groups, as follows:

1. The *mobile wad of three* (the brachioradialis, extensor carpi radialis longus, and extensor carpi radialis brevis) runs along the lateral side of the forearm. These three muscles arise from a continuous line on the lateral supracondylar ridge and lateral epicondyle of the humerus.
2. The *four superficial extensor muscles* fan out from the lateral epicondyle of the humerus. From the ulnar to the radial side of the forearm, they consist of the anconeus, the extensor carpi ulnaris, the extensor digiti minimi, and the extensor digitorum communis (Fig. 4-31). Two internervous planes exist in this layer of musculature: between the extensor carpi ulnaris muscle (which is supplied by the posterior interosseous nerve) and the flexor carpi ulnaris muscle (which is supplied by the ulnar nerve) on the ulnar side (see Fig. 4-19), and between the extensor carpi radialis brevis muscle[22] (which is supplied by the radial nerve) and the extensor digitorum communis muscle (which is supplied by the posterior interosseous nerve) on the radial side (see Fig. 4-25).
3. Of the *five deep muscles*, three (the abductor pollicis longus, the extensor pollicis brevis, and the

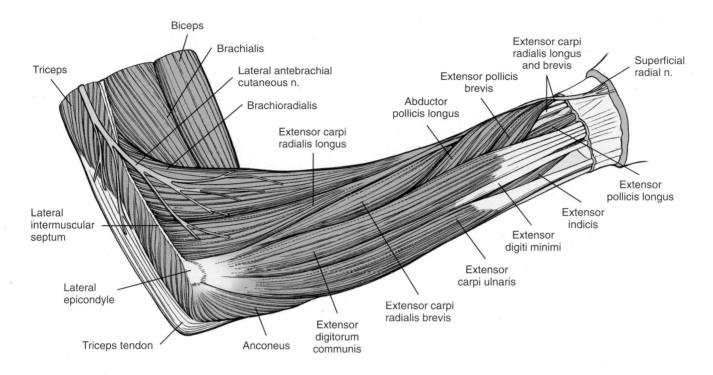

**Figure 4-31** Superficial muscles of the posterior aspect of the forearm.

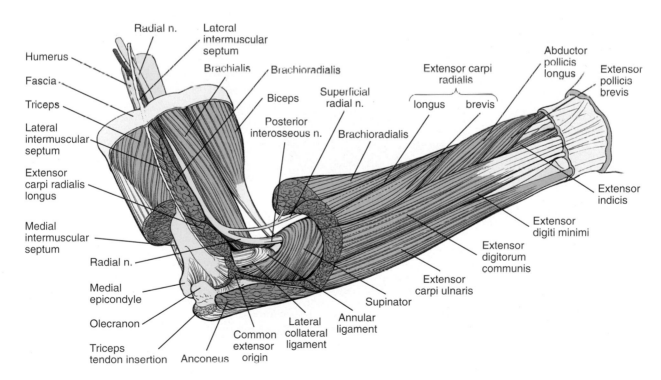

**Figure 4-32** The superficial muscles have been removed to reveal the course of the posterior interosseous nerve as it enters the supinator muscle through the arcade of Frohse and the course of the superficial radial nerve, which is sensory and supplies no muscles of the forearm.

extensor pollicis longus) supply the thumb. The three cross the forearm obliquely from the ulnar to the radial side, and two of them (the abductor pollicis longus and the extensor pollicis brevis) wind around the dorsal and lateral aspects of the radius. The remaining two muscles of the deep group are the supinator and the extensor indicis (Fig. 4-33).

The critical nerve in the area, the posterior interosseous nerve, innervates the muscles of the extensor compartment; it is the key anatomic structure from an operative point of view. The only major arterial supply of the compartment is the posterior interosseous artery.

## Landmarks and Incision

### Landmarks

The lateral epicondyle of the humerus, located just lateral to the olecranon process, is smaller than the medial epicondyle, but its lateral supracondylar line, which runs superiorly, is longer than the medial supracondylar line, extending almost to the deltoid tuberosity. The lateral epicondyle is the site of the common origin of the superficial muscles of the extensor compartment of the forearm. The extensor carpi radialis brevis, extensor digitorum communis, extensor digiti minimi, and extensor carpi ulnaris all originate from fused tendons that attach just anterior

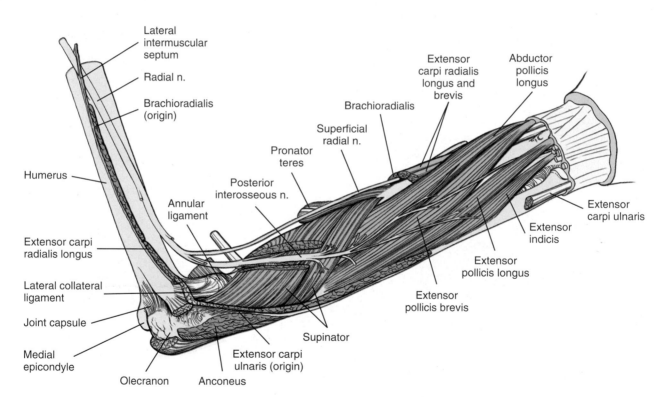

**Figure 4-33**   The course of the posterior interosseous nerve through the supinator muscle, as it runs to supply muscles in the forearm.

**Extensor Carpi Ulnaris.** *Origin.* Common extensor origin on lateral epicondyle of humerus and subcutaneous border of ulna. (Shared origin with flexor carpi ulnaris.) *Insertion.* Base of fifth metacarpal. *Action.* Extensor and ulnar deviator of wrist. *Nerve supply.* Posterior interosseous nerve.
**Extensor Digitorum Communis.** *Origin.* Common extensor origin on lateral epicondyle of humerus. *Insertion.* Into extensor apparatus of fingers. *Action.* Extensor of wrist and fingers. *Nerve supply.* Posterior interosseous nerve.

to the epicondyle. The brachioradialis and extensor carpi radialis longus arise from the lateral supracondylar ridge.

Tenderness over the common extensor origin occurs in lateral epicondylitis; the pain that is characteristic of this condition can be reproduced by providing resistance to extension of the wrist.

Compression of the posterior interosseous nerve at the arcade of Frohse may produce a syndrome similar to lateral epicondylitis. In these cases, the tenderness usually is elicited more distally in the course of the posterior interosseous nerve or anteriorly over the arcade of Frohse. Both conditions can exist in a single patient.[23]

## Incision

A longitudinal incision on the posterior aspect of the forearm crosses the lines of cleavage of the skin at right angles and often leaves a broad scar.

## Superficial Surgical Dissection

In the proximal half of the wound, dissection opens the plane between the extensor carpi radialis brevis and the extensor communis. In the distal third of the wound, the internervous plane lies between the extensor carpi radialis brevis and the extensor pollicis longus (see Fig. 4-31).

## Deep Surgical Dissection

For the proximal third of the radius, dissection consists of detaching the insertion of the supinator muscle from the radius while preserving the posterior interosseous nerve (see Fig. 4-30).

For the middle third of the bone, dissection involves mobilizing and retracting two muscles, the abductor pollicis longus and the extensor pollicis brevis (see Fig. 4-30).

In the distal third of the radius, dissection opens the internervous plane between the extensor pollicis longus and the extensor carpi radialis brevis.

The proximal third of the radius is covered by the supinator muscle, through which the posterior interosseous nerve passes on its way to the posterior compartment of the forearm (see Figs. 4-32 and 4-33). For additional information on the supinator muscle, see the section regarding the anterior approach to the radius.

## Dangers

### Nerves

The **posterior interosseous nerve** is the motor nerve of the posterior compartment of the forearm. A branch of the radial nerve, it passes between the two heads of the supinator muscle and actually may come in direct contact with the neck of the radius. At that point, it may be trapped beneath incorrectly positioned plates. After emerging from the supinator muscle, the nerve passes distally over the origin of the abductor pollicis longus muscle to reach the interosseous membrane. It continues distally on the interosseous membrane to the level of the wrist joint, which it supplies with some sensory branches. The nerve supplies those muscles that arise from the common extensor origin and the deep muscles of the extensor compartment of the forearm (see Fig. 4-33).

When performing deep surgical dissection, it is important to remember that the posterior interosseous nerve is vulnerable during all approaches to the proximal third of the radial shaft. Although the nerve can be protected by detaching the insertion of the supinator and stripping the muscle off the bone subperiosteally, the only certain protection of the posterior interosseous nerve during plating of the upper third of the radius may come with full dissection via a posterior approach.

### Vessels

The **posterior interosseous artery** accompanies the posterior interosseous nerve as it runs along the interosseous membrane in the proximal two thirds of the forearm. The posterior interosseous artery enters the extensor compartment of the forearm by passing between the radius and the ulna through the interosseous membrane (Fig. 4-34). The artery then joins the posterior interosseous nerve distal to the distal edge of the deep head of the supinator muscle.

The posterior interosseous artery is too small to be dissected easily down to the level of the wrist. Most of the blood supply for the posterior area comes from an anterior interosseous artery via branches that perforate the interosseous membrane. The tendons running in this area may have a marginal blood supply.

Although the artery may be damaged during the posterior approach to the radius, good collateral circulation appears to protect the extremity from any functional deficits.

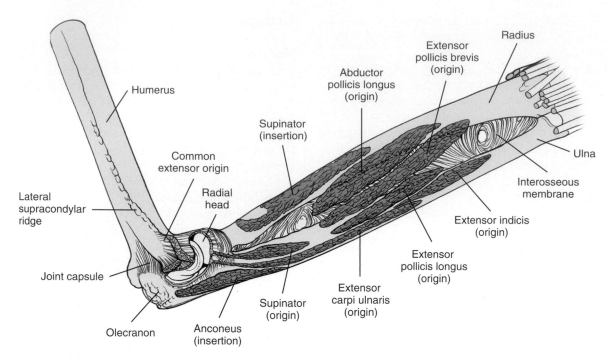

**Figure 4-34**   The origins and insertions of the muscles of the posterior aspect of the forearm.

---

**Extensor Carpi Radialis Longus.** *Origin.* Lower third of lateral supracondylar ridge of humerus, lateral intermuscular septum of arm. *Insertion.* Base of second metacarpal. *Action.* Extensor and radial deviator of wrist. *Nerve supply.* Radial nerve.

**Extensor Carpi Radialis Brevis.** *Origin.* Common extensor origin on lateral epicondyle of humerus and radial collateral ligament of elbow. *Insertion.* Base of third metacarpal. *Action.* Extensor and radial deviator of wrist. *Nerve supply.* Radial nerve.

**Supinator.** *Origin.* From two heads. Superficial head: from lateral epicondyle of humerus, lateral collateral ligament of elbow, and supinator crest of ulna. Deep head: from supinator crest and fossa of ulna. *Insertion.* Anterior aspect of radius. *Action.* Supinator of forearm. Weak flexor of elbow. *Nerve supply.* Posterior interosseous nerve.

**Extensor Pollicis Longus.** *Origin.* Posterior surface of ulna in its middle third and from interosseous membrane. *Insertion.* Distal phalanx of thumb. *Action.* Extensor of thumb and wrist. *Nerve supply.* Posterior interosseous nerve.

**Abductor Pollicis Longus.** *Origin.* Posterior surface of ulna, posterior interosseous membrane, and middle third of posterior surface of radius. *Insertion.* Base of thumb metacarpal. *Action.* Abductor and extensor of thumb. *Nerve supply.* Posterior interosseous nerve.

**Extensor Pollicis Brevis.** *Origin.* Posterior surface of radius and interosseous membrane. *Insertion.* Base of proximal phalanx of thumb. *Action.* Extensor of proximal phalanx of thumb. *Nerve supply.* Posterior interosseous nerve.

**Extensor Indicis.** *Origin.* Posterior surface of ulnar shaft and interosseous membrane. *Insertion.* Extensor apparatus of index finger via ulnar side of tendon of extensor digitorum that runs to index finger. *Action.* Extensor of index finger. *Nerve supply.* Posterior interosseous nerve.

**Extensor Digiti Minimi.** *Origin.* Common extensor origin on lateral epicondyle of humerus. *Insertion.* Extensor apparatus of little finger. *Action.* Extensor of little finger. *Nerve supply.* Posterior interosseous nerve.

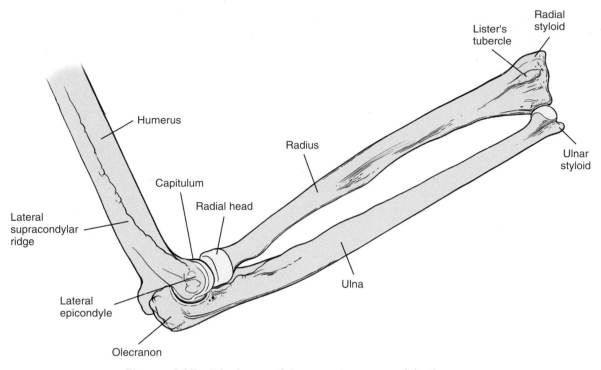

**Figure 4-35**  The bones of the posterior aspect of the forearm.

## REFERENCES

1. HENRY AK: Extensile exposure, 2nd ed. Baltimore, Williams & Wilkins, 1970:100
2. STRAUB LB: Congenital absence of the ulna. Am J Surg 109: 300, 1965
3. SPINNER M: Injuries to the major branches of peripheral nerves of the forearm, 2nd ed. Philadelphia, WB Saunders, 1978
4. MULLER ME, ALLGONER M, WILLENGER H: Manual of internal fixation. New York, Springer-Verlag, 1970
5. FROHSE F, FRANKEL M: Die Muskeln des Menschlichen Armes. In: Bardelehen's Handbuch der Anatomie des Menschlichen. Jena, Germany, Fisher, 1980
6. CAPENER N: Posterior interosseous nerve lesions: proceedings of the second hand club. J Bone Joint Surg [Br] 46:361, 1964
7. SHARRARD WJW: Posterior interosseous neuritis. J Bone Joint Surg [Br] 48:777, 1966
8. WEINBERGER LM: Non-traumatic paralysis of the dorsal interosseous nerve. Surg Gynecol Obstet 69:358, 1939
9. SPINNER M: The arcade of Prohse and its relationship to posterior interosseous nerve paralysis. J Bone Joint Surg [Br] 50:809, 1968
10. ROLES NC, MAUDSLET RH: Radial tunnel syndrome: resistant tennis elbow as a nerve entrapment. J Bone Joint Surg [Br] 54: 499, 1972
11. SOLNITZKY O: Pronator syndrome: compression neuropathy of the median nerve at level of pronator teres muscle. Georgetown Med Bull 13:232, 1960
12. KOPELL HP, THOMPSON WAL: Pronator syndrome. N Engl J Med 239:713, 1958
13. SPINNER M: Injuries to the major branches of peripheral nerves of the forearm, 2nd ed. Philadelphia, WB Saunders, 1978: 195
14. KILOH LG, NEKN S: Isolated neuritis of the anterior interosseous nerve. BMJ 1:850, 1952
15. SPINNER M: The anterior interosseous nerve syndrome, with special attention to its variations. J Bone Joint Surg [Am] 54A:84, 1970
16. FEARN CB, GOODFELLOW JW: Anterior interosseous nerve palsy. J Bone Joint Surg [Br] 47:91, 1965
17. ARMISTEAD RB, LINSCHEID RL, DOBYNS JH ET AL: Ulnar lengthening in the treatment of Kienböck's disease. J Bone Joint Surg [Am] 64:170, 1982
18. OSBORNE G: Compression neuritis at the elbow. Hand 10, 1970
19. VANDERPOOL DW, CHALMERS J, LAMB DW ET AL: Peripheral compression lesions of the ulnar nerve. J Bone Joint Surg [Br] 50:792, 1968
20. THOMPSON JE: Anatomical methods of approach in operations on the long bones of the extremities. Ann Surg 68:309, 1918
21. DAVIES F, LAIRD M: The supinator muscle and the deep radial (posterior interosseous) nerve. Anat Rec 101:243, 1948
22. SALSBURY CR: The nerve to extensor carpi radialis brevis. Br J Surg 26:9597, 1938
23. SPINNER O: Management of peripheral nerve problems. In: Management of nerve compression lesions of the upper extremity. Philadelphia, WB Saunders, 1980:569

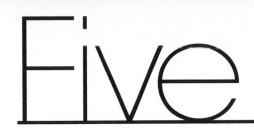

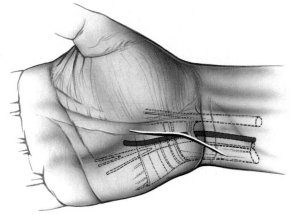

# The Wrist and Hand

Seven approaches to the wrist and hand are described in this chapter: three to the wrist and two each to the flexor tendons and scaphoid.

The *dorsal approach to the wrist joint* is used mainly for treating rheumatoid arthritis and working on the bones of the carpus; the *volar approach* is used primarily for exploring the carpal tunnel and its enclosed structures. The applied anatomy of each approach is considered separately in this chapter.

The *volar approach to the flexor tendons* is used most often. It also provides excellent exposure of the digital nerves and vessels. The *midlateral approach* is useful in the treatment of phalangeal fractures. A discussion of the applied anatomy of the finger flexor tendons follows the description of these two approaches in this chapter.

*Dorsal and volar approaches to the scaphoid* are outlined together, with a brief description of the blood supply of that bone.

Infection within the hand is a common clinical problem. The methods of drainage used for these conditions are described together, with an introduction to the general principles of drainage in the hand. Of all the infections of the hand that require surgery, paronychia and felons are by far the most common.

Throughout this book, we have related anatomy to surgical approaches. In the hand, however, the majority of wounds encountered arise from trauma, not from planned incisions. A brief review of the overall anatomy of the hand is vital to explain the damage that may be caused by a particular injury. Although clinical findings are the key to the accurate diagnosis of tissue trauma, knowledge of the underlying anatomy is crucial in bringing to light all possibilities and minimizing the risk that a significant injury will be overlooked. For example, arterial hemorrhage from a digital artery in a finger nearly always is associated with damage to a digital nerve, because the nerve lies volar to the severed artery. Arterial hemorrhage in a finger should alert the surgeon to the possibility of nerve injury, which often appears clinically as a change in the quality of sensation rather than as complete anesthesia, and can be overlooked in a brief examination.

Therefore, this chapter ends with a section on the topographic anatomy of the hand. This information is presented in one section rather than on an approach-by-approach basis to provide a clear and integrated picture of hand anatomy.

# Dorsal Approach to the Wrist

The dorsal approach provides excellent exposure of all the extensor tendons that pass over the dorsal surface of the wrist. It also allows access to the dorsal aspect of the wrist itself, the dorsal aspect of the carpus, and the dorsal surface of the proximal ends of the middle metacarpals. Its uses include the following:

1. Synovectomy and repair of the extensor tendons in cases of rheumatoid arthritis; dorsal stabilization of the wrist[1,2]
2. Wrist fusion[3]
3. Excision of the lower end of the radius for benign or malignant tumors
4. Open reduction and internal fixation of certain distal radial and carpal fractures and dislocations, including dorsal metacarpal dislocations, displaced intraarticular dorsal lip fractures of the radius, and transscaphoid perilunate dislocations
5. Proximal row carpectomy[4,5]

## Position of the Patient

Place the patient supine on the operating table. Pronate the forearm and put the arm on an arm board. Exsanguinate the limb by applying a soft rubber bandage, and then inflate a tourniquet (Fig. 5-1).

## Landmarks and Incision

### Landmarks

Palpate the *radial styloid*, the most common distal extension of the lateral side of the radius.

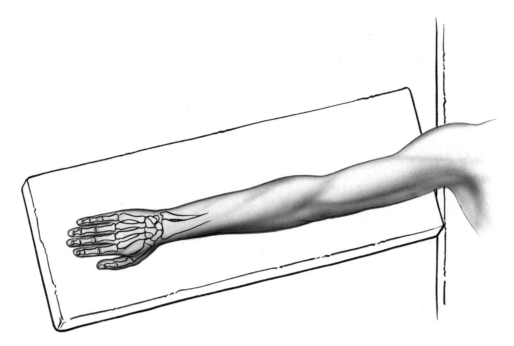

**Figure 5-1**    Place the patient supine on the operating table. Turn the forearm downward and place the arm on a board, for the dorsal approach to the wrist joint.

Palpate the *ulnar styloid* on the dorsal aspect of the distal end of the ulna.

### Incision

Make an 8-cm longitudinal incision on the dorsal aspect of the wrist, crossing the wrist joint midway between the radial and ulnar styloids. The incision begins 3 cm proximal to the wrist joint and ends about 5 cm distal to it. It can be lengthened if necessary (Fig. 5-2).

Because the skin on the dorsum of the wrist is pliable and redundant, the incision does not cause a contracture of the wrist joint, even though it crosses a major skin crease at right angles.

## Internervous Plane

There is no true internervous plane, because both the extensor carpi radialis longus muscle and the extensor carpi radialis brevis muscle are supplied by the radial nerve. Because both muscles receive their nerve supply well proximal to the incision, however, the intermuscular plane between them can be used safely.

## Superficial Surgical Dissection

Incise the subcutaneous fat in line with the skin incision to expose the extensor retinaculum that covers the tendons in the six compartments on the dorsal aspect of the wrist (Fig. 5-3).

## Deep Surgical Dissection

The deep dissection depends on the procedure to be performed.

### Synovectomy

Incise the extensor retinaculum over the extensor carpi radialis longus and brevis muscles in the second compartment of the wrist. The compartment is on the radial side of Lister's tubercle. To expose the other compartments, incise the ulnar edge of the cut retinaculum by sharp dissection in an ulnar direction to deroof sequentially the four compartments on the ulnar side. Then, dissect the radial edge of the cut extensor retinaculum radially to deroof the first compartment. The extensor retinac-

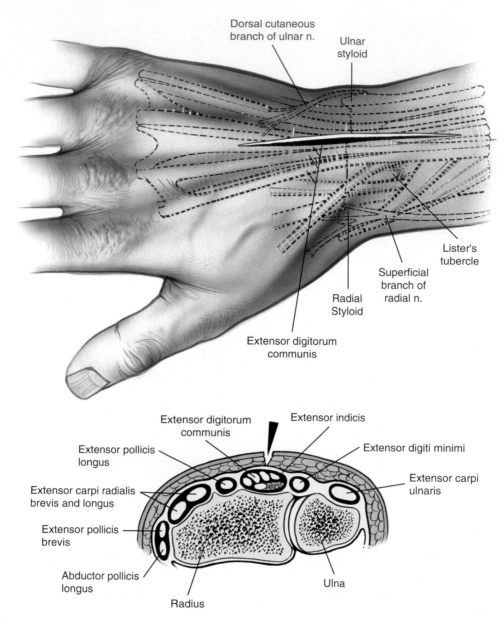

**Figure 5-2**   Skin incision for the dorsal approach to the wrist joint. A cross section at the distal portion of the radius is seen.

ulum should be preserved; during closure, it can be sutured underneath the extensor tendons to prevent them from being abraded by the bones, which can be deformed grossly by rheumatoid arthritis (see Fig. 5-8).

## Full Exposure of the Wrist Joint

Incise the extensor retinaculum over the extensor digitorum communis and extensor indicis proprius muscles in the fourth compartment of the wrist. Mobilize the tendons of the compartment, lifting them from their bed in an ulnar and radial direction to expose the underlying radius and joint capsule (Fig. 5-4). Incise the joint capsule longitudinally on the dorsal aspect of the radius and carpus (Fig. 5-5). Continue the dissection below the capsule (the dorsal radiocarpal ligament) toward the radial and ulnar sides of the radius to expose the entire distal end of the radius and carpal bones (Figs. 5-6 and 5-7).

The tendons of the extensor carpi radialis longus and brevis muscles, which attach to the bases of the second and third metacarpals and lie in a tunnel on the radial side of Lister's tubercle, must be retracted radially to expose fully the dorsal aspect of the carpus.

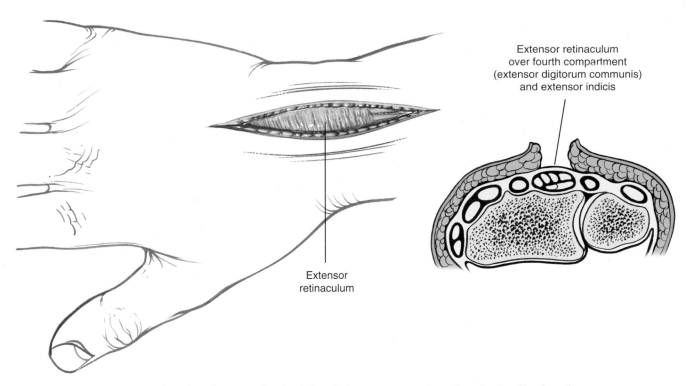

Extensor retinaculum over fourth compartment (extensor digitorum communis) and extensor indicis

Extensor retinaculum

**Figure 5-3** Skin flaps are developed, and the extensor retinaculum is visualized in the deeper portion of the wound. Cross section reveals the approach to the fourth tunnel, which contains the extensor digitorum communis and the extensor indicis proprius.

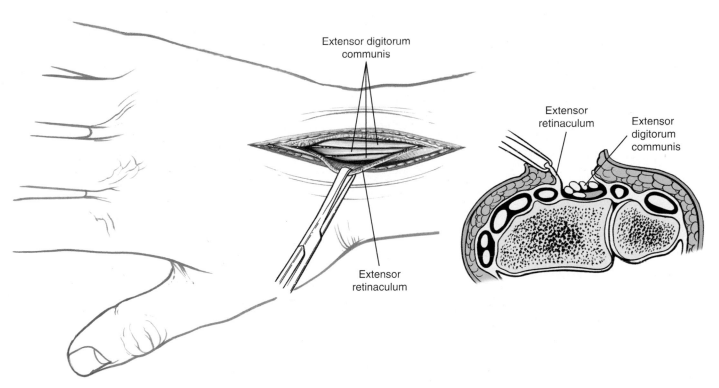

Extensor digitorum communis

Extensor retinaculum

Extensor digitorum communis

Extensor retinaculum

**Figure 5-4** The retinaculum over the fourth compartment has been opened, revealing the communis tendons.

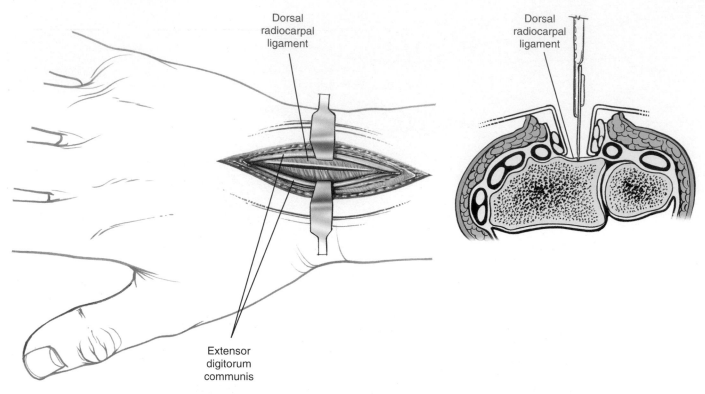

**Figure 5-5**   The extensor communis tendons and extensor indicis proprius have been retracted, revealing the dorsal radiocarpal ligament and the joint capsule, which then is incised.

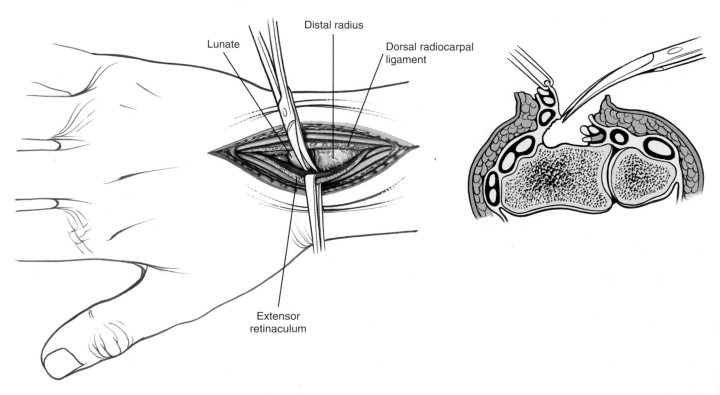

**Figure 5-6**   The dorsal radiocarpal ligament and the extensor tendons are elevated from the posterior aspect of the radius to expose the entire dorsal end of the bone.

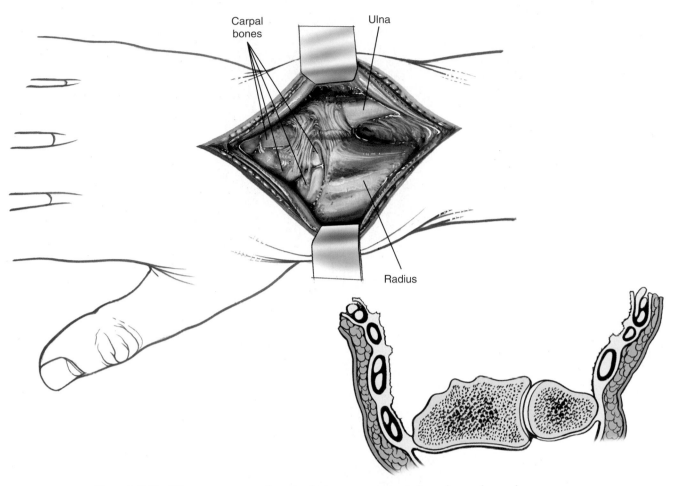

**Figure 5-7** The extensor tendons in their compartments have been elevated to expose the distal end of the radius and ulna.

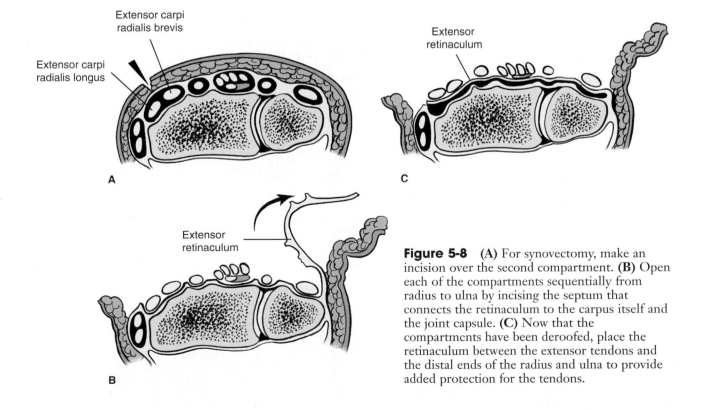

**Figure 5-8** **(A)** For synovectomy, make an incision over the second compartment. **(B)** Open each of the compartments sequentially from radius to ulna by incising the septum that connects the retinaculum to the carpus itself and the joint capsule. **(C)** Now that the compartments have been deroofed, place the retinaculum between the extensor tendons and the distal ends of the radius and ulna to provide added protection for the tendons.

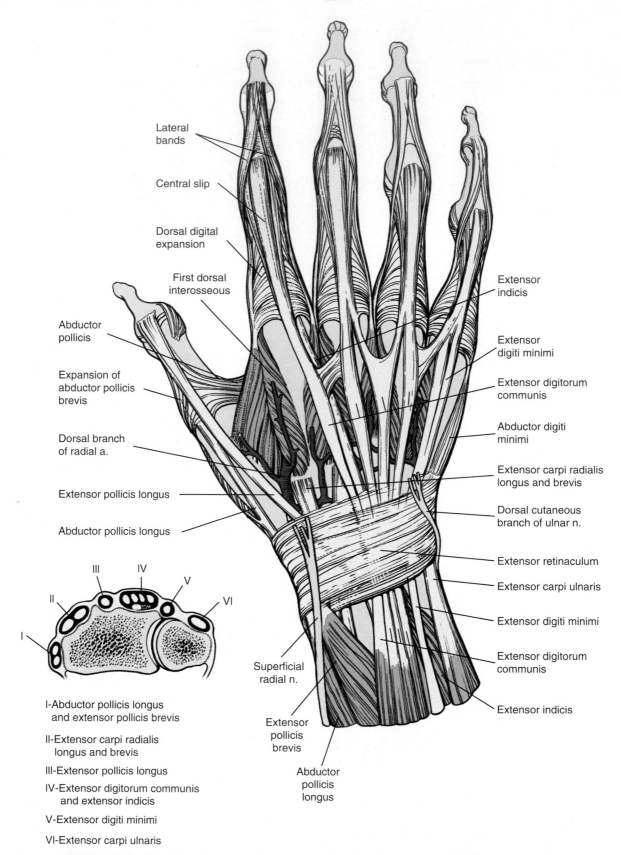

Lateral bands

Central slip

Dorsal digital expansion

First dorsal interosseous

Abductor pollicis

Expansion of abductor pollicis brevis

Dorsal branch of radial a.

Extensor pollicis longus

Abductor pollicis longus

Extensor indicis

Extensor digiti minimi

Extensor digitorum communis

Abductor digiti minimi

Extensor carpi radialis longus and brevis

Dorsal cutaneous branch of ulnar n.

Extensor retinaculum

Extensor carpi ulnaris

Extensor digiti minimi

Extensor digitorum communis

Extensor indicis

Superficial radial n.

Extensor pollicis brevis

Abductor pollicis longus

III  IV  V  VI  II  I

I-Abductor pollicis longus and extensor pollicis brevis

II-Extensor carpi radialis longus and brevis

III-Extensor pollicis longus

IV-Extensor digitorum communis and extensor indicis

V-Extensor digiti minimi

VI-Extensor carpi ulnaris

**Figure 5-9**    The dorsal aspect of the wrist and hand. Cross section of the distal forearm *(inset)*. Note the compartmentalization of tendons into six distinct tunnels at the dorsal aspect of the distal forearm.

## Dangers

### Nerves

The **radial nerve** (superficial radial nerve) emerges from beneath the tendon of the brachioradialis muscle just above the wrist joint before traveling to the dorsum of the hand. The skin incision lies between skin that is supplied by cutaneous branches of the ulnar nerve and skin that is supplied by cutaneous branches of the radial nerve. Damage to cutaneous nerves occurs only if the dissection is begun within the fat. If the incision is taken down to the extensor retinaculum before the ulnar and radial flaps are elevated, the nerves are protected by the full thickness of the fat (Fig. 5-9).

Cutting a cutaneous nerve may result in a painful neuroma, but the resultant sensory defect rarely is significant.

### Vessels

The **radial artery** crosses the wrist joint on its lateral aspect. As long as the dissection at the level of the wrist joint remains below the periosteum, the artery is difficult to damage.

## How to Enlarge the Approach

Because it does not make use of an internervous plane, the incision cannot be extended proximally to expose the rest of the radius. It can be extended to expose the distal half of the dorsal aspect of the radius, however, by retracting the abductor pollicis longus and extensor pollicis brevis muscles, which cross the operative field obliquely.

To expose the entire dorsal surface of the metacarpals, extend the incision distally and retract the extensor tendons. (This type of extension seldom is required in practice.) The approach provides excellent exposure of the wrist joint and allows easy access to all six compartments of the extensor tunnel.

---

# Applied Surgical Anatomy of the Dorsal Approach to the Wrist

## Overview

Twelve tendons cross the dorsal aspect of the wrist joint and pass beneath the extensor retinaculum, which is a thickening of the deep fascia of the forearm. The extensor retinaculum prevents the tendons from "bowstringing." Fibrous septa pass from the deep surface of the retinaculum to the bones of the forearm, dividing the extensor tunnel into six compartments. These septa must be separated from the retinaculum so that each compartment can be opened in surgery (see Fig. 5-9).

## Landmarks and Incision

### Landmarks

Two bony landmarks lie on the dorsal aspect of the wrist. The *styloid process* is the distal end of the lateral side of the radius. It also is the site of attachment of the tendon of the brachioradialis muscle. Its medial part articulates with the scaphoid bone (see Fig. 5-12A). Strong and sudden radial deviation of the wrist may cause the radial styloid process to slam into the scaphoid and fracture it (see Fig. 5-12B).

The styloid process often is excised when the scaphoid fails to reunite or after arthritic changes in the wrist joint have affected the radial margin of the radioscaphoid joint.

*Lister's tubercle* (the dorsoradial tubercle) is a small bony prominence on the dorsum of the radius. The tendon of the extensor pollicis longus muscle angles around its distal end, changing direction about 45° as it does so. When the wrist is hyperextended, the base of the third metacarpal comes very close to Lister's tubercle, and the two bones can crush the trapped tendon of the extensor pollicis longus. This probably is the reason the tendon suffers delayed rupture in some cases of minimal or undisplaced fractures of the distal radius; the tendon sustains a vascular insult at the time of the original injury, even though it remains intact (see Fig. 5-12C).[4]

### Incision

Longitudinal incisions crossing the lines of cleavage of the skin almost perpendicularly on the dorsum of the wrist can cause broad scarring. Nevertheless, because the skin on the wrist is so loose, this is one of those rare occasions when a skin incision *can* cross a major skin crease at right angles without causing a joint contracture.

## Superficial and Deep Surgical Dissection

The extensor retinaculum is a narrow (2-cm) fibrous band that lies obliquely across the dorsal aspect of the wrist. Its radial side is attached to the anterolateral border of the radius; its ulnar border is attached to the pisiform and triquetral bones. (Were it attached to both bones of the forearm instead, pronation and supination would be impossible, because its fibrous tissue is incapable of stretching the necessary 30%.)

Fibrous septa pass from the deep surface of the extensor retinaculum to the bones of the carpus, dividing the extensor tunnel into six compartments (Fig. 5-10). From the radial (lateral) to the ulnar (medial) aspect, the compartments contain the following:

1. *Abductor pollicis longus and extensor pollicis brevis.* These tendons lie over the lateral aspect of the radius. They may become trapped or inflamed beneath the extensor retinaculum in their fibro-osseous canal, producing de Quervain's disease (tenosynovitis stenosans).
2. *Extensor carpi radialis longus and extensor carpi radialis brevis.* These muscles run on the radial side of Lister's tubercle before reaching the dorsum of the hand. The tendon of the extensor carpi radialis longus is used frequently in tendon transfers. The tendons run in separate synovial sheaths.
3. *Extensor pollicis longus.* This tendon passes into the dorsum of the hand on the ulnar side of Lister's tubercle. It may rupture in association with fractures or rheumatoid arthritis. The oblique passage of this tendon on the dorsal aspect of the wrist creates significant problems for plate fixation of fractures of the distal radius. Tendon irritation and even rupture may occur due to abrasion of the tendon on the surface of the plate. Similar problems apply to a lesser degree with all the other extensor tendons.[6]
4. *Extensor digitorum communis and extensor indicis.* The indicis tendon is used commonly in tendon transfers.
5. *Extensor digiti minimi.* This tendon overlies the distal radioulnar joint.
6. *Extensor carpi ulnaris.* This tendon passes near the base of the ulnar styloid process. It is used sometimes in tendon transfers (Fig. 5-11; see Fig. 5-10).

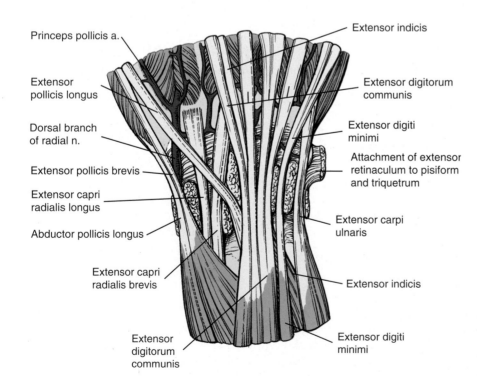

Princeps pollicis a.

Extensor pollicis longus

Dorsal branch of radial n.

Extensor pollicis brevis

Extensor capri radialis longus

Abductor pollicis longus

Extensor capri radialis brevis

Extensor digitorum communis

Extensor indicis

Extensor digitorum communis

Extensor digiti minimi

Attachment of extensor retinaculum to pisiform and triquetrum

Extensor carpi ulnaris

Extensor indicis

Extensor digiti minimi

**Figure 5-10** Anatomy of the distal forearm, with the extensor retinaculum excised and the septa remaining. The retinaculum on the ulnar side inserts into the triquetrum and pisiform bones.

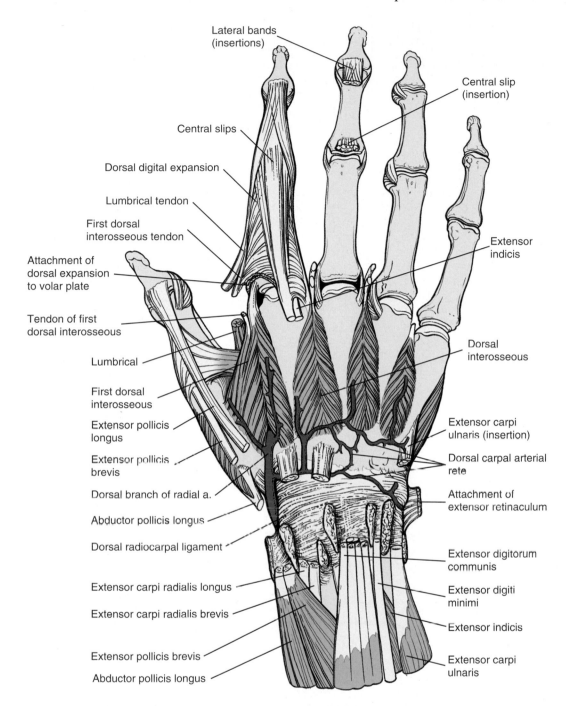

Lateral bands
(insertions)

Central slip
(insertion)

Central slips

Dorsal digital expansion

Lumbrical tendon

First dorsal
interosseous tendon

Extensor
indicis

Attachment of
dorsal expansion
to volar plate

Tendon of first
dorsal interosseous

Lumbrical

First dorsal
interosseous

Dorsal
interosseous

Extensor pollicis
longus

Extensor pollicis
brevis

Extensor carpi
ulnaris (insertion)

Dorsal carpal arterial
rete

Dorsal branch of radial a.

Abductor pollicis longus

Attachment of
extensor retinaculum

Dorsal radiocarpal ligament

Extensor carpi radialis longus

Extensor digitorum
communis

Extensor carpi radialis brevis

Extensor digiti
minimi

Extensor pollicis brevis

Extensor indicis

Abductor pollicis longus

Extensor carpi
ulnaris

**Figure 5-11**   The extensor tendons have been removed, revealing the dorsal
radiocarpal ligament. The radial artery is seen piercing the first dorsal interosseous
muscle and contributing to the dorsal carpal rete. Note the hood mechanism for the
index finger; contributions are made to it by the first dorsal interosseous and the first
lumbrical muscles.

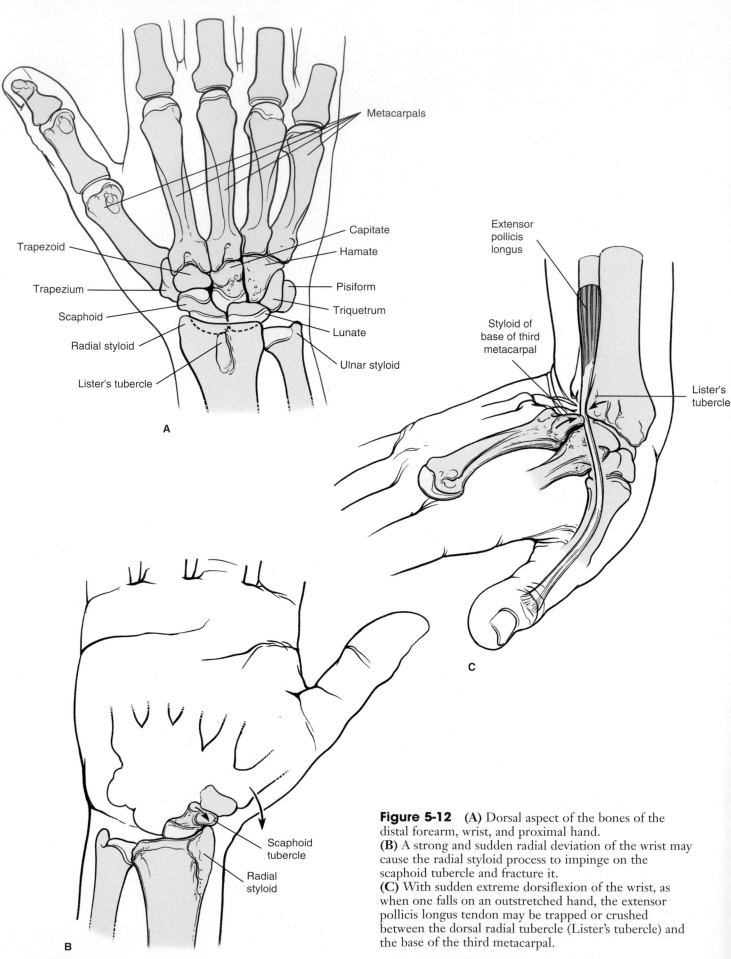

Trapezoid

Trapezium

Scaphoid

Radial styloid

Lister's tubercle

Metacarpals

Capitate

Hamate

Pisiform

Triquetrum

Lunate

Ulnar styloid

**A**

Extensor
pollicis
longus

Styloid of
base of third
metacarpal

Lister's
tubercle

**C**

Scaphoid
tubercle

Radial
styloid

**B**

**Figure 5-12** **(A)** Dorsal aspect of the bones of the distal forearm, wrist, and proximal hand.
**(B)** A strong and sudden radial deviation of the wrist may cause the radial styloid process to impinge on the scaphoid tubercle and fracture it.
**(C)** With sudden extreme dorsiflexion of the wrist, as when one falls on an outstretched hand, the extensor pollicis longus tendon may be trapped or crushed between the dorsal radial tubercle (Lister's tubercle) and the base of the third metacarpal.

## Volar Approach to the Wrist

Decompression of the median nerve within the carpal tunnel is one of the most common operations of the hand. Two anatomic structures, the motor and palmar cutaneous branches of the median nerve, determine how the tunnel is approached. Both structures vary considerably in the paths they take; they are so unpredictable that "blind" procedures, which are acceptable elsewhere, must be avoided. The tunnel must be decompressed through a full incision and under direct vision. The uses of the incision include the following:

1. Decompression of the median nerve[7,8]
2. Synovectomy of the flexor tendons of the wrist
3. Excision of tumors within the carpal tunnel
4. Repair of lacerations of nerves or tendons within the tunnel
5. Drainage of sepsis tracking up from the mid-palmar space
6. Open reduction and internal fixation of certain fractures and dislocations of the distal radius and carpus, including volar lip fractures of the radius

### Position of the Patient

Place the patient supine on an operating table. Rest the forearm on a hand table in the supinated position so that the palm faces upward. Use an exsanguinating bandage (Fig. 5-13).

### Landmarks and Incision

#### Landmarks
The *thenar crease* runs around the base of the thenar eminence. The *transverse skin* crease of the wrist overlies the wrist joint. The *tendon of the palmaris longus* muscle bisects the anterior aspect of the wrist. Its distal end bisects the anterior surface of the carpal tunnel. It is easy to palpate in the distal forearm if the patient is instructed to pinch the fingers together and flex the wrist.

#### Incision
Begin the incision just to the ulnar side of the thenar crease, about one third of the way into the hand. Curve it proximally, remaining just to the ulnar side of the thenar crease, until the flexion crease of the wrist is almost reached: to avoid problems in skin healing, do not wander into the thenar crease itself. Then, curve the incision toward the ulnar side of the forearm so that the flexion crease is not crossed transversely (Fig. 5-14).

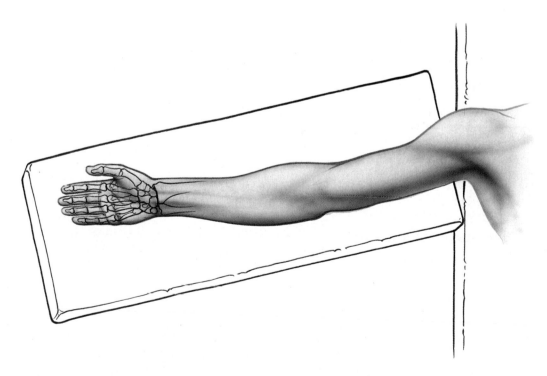

**Figure 5-13**   Position of the patient for volar approaches to the wrist and hand.

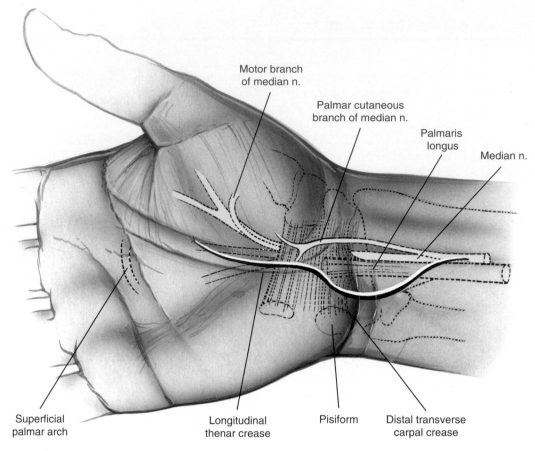

**Figure 5-14** The incision for the volar approach to the wrist. The incision should be made on the ulnar side of the palmaris longus tendon to protect the palmar cutaneous branch of the median nerve.

## Internervous Plane

There is no internervous plane. The approach is a true anatomic dissection in which the major nerves are identified, dissected out, and preserved. No muscles are transected except, on occasion, some fibers of the abductor pollicis brevis and palmaris brevis that cross the midline.

## Superficial Surgical Dissection

Carefully incise the skin flaps. Remember that the palmar cutaneous branch of the median nerve, which usually presents on the ulnar side of the flexor carpi radialis, has a variable course. Dissection should be carried out meticulously, with particular attention paid to the location of the nerve (see Fig. 5-14). After the fat is incised, the fibers of the superficial palmar

fascia come into view; section them in line with the incision.

Retract the curved flaps medially, exposing the insertion of the palmaris longus muscle into the flexor retinaculum (the transverse carpal ligament; Fig. 5-15). Retract the tendon toward the ulna and identify the median nerve between the tendons of the palmaris longus muscle and the flexor carpi radialis muscle. The nerve lies closer to the palmaris longus than to the flexor carpi radialis (Fig. 5-16).

Pass a blunt, flat instrument (such as a McDonald dissector) down the carpal tunnel between the flexor retinaculum and the median nerve (Fig. 5-17). Carefully incise the retinaculum, cutting down on the dissector to protect the nerve. Make the incision on the ulnar side of the nerve to avoid possible damage to its motor branch to the thenar muscle. Divide the entire length of the retinaculum (Fig. 5-18).

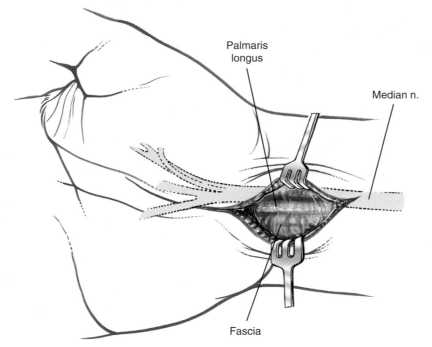

Palmaris
longus

Median n.

Fascia

**Figure 5-15** The skin is retracted, and the deep fascia and tendon of the palmaris longus are inspected.

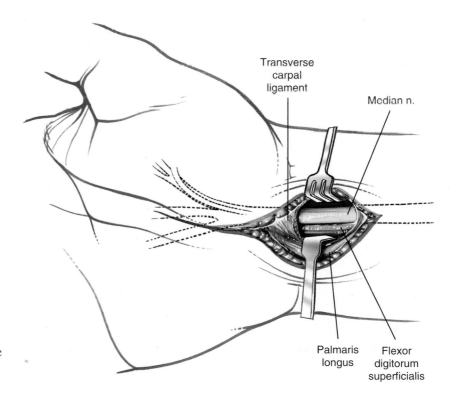

Transverse
carpal
ligament

Median n.

Palmaris
longus

Flexor
digitorum
superficialis

**Figure 5-16** The deep fascia is incised. The palmaris longus is retracted toward the ulna, revealing the median nerve as it enters the carpal tunnel.

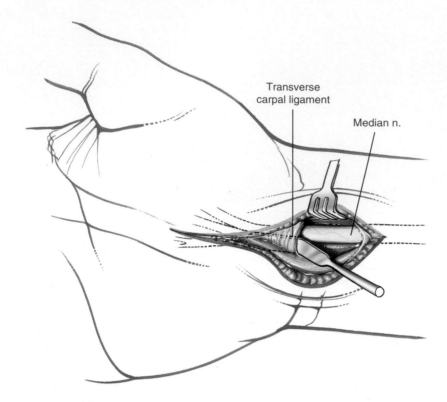

**Figure 5-17**   A spatula is placed under the transverse carpal ligament to protect the median nerve as the ligament is incised.

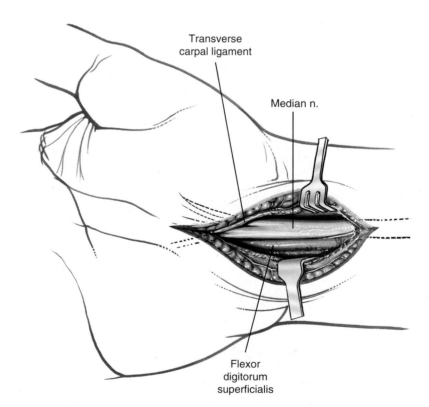

**Figure 5-18**   The transverse carpal ligament is released on the ulnar side of the nerve to avoid damage to the motor branch of the thenar muscle.

## Deep Surgical Dissection

Identify the motor branch of the median nerve. It usually arises from the anterolateral side of the median nerve just as the nerve emerges from the carpal tunnel. The motor branch then curves radially and upward to enter the thenar musculature between the abductor pollicis brevis and flexor pollicis brevis muscles. Sometimes, however, the motor branch arises within the tunnel and pierces the flexor retinaculum to reach the thenar musculature. In these rare cases, the motor nerve itself may have to be decompressed before the patient's symptoms will be relieved fully (see Fig. 5-18).

It rarely is necessary to gain access to the volar aspect of the wrist joint. If this is required, mobilize the median nerve in the carpal tunnel and retract it radially to avoid stretching its motor branch. Next, mobilize and retract the flexor tendons in the carpal tunnel (Fig. 5-19). Incising the base of the tunnel longitudinally exposes the volar aspect of the carpus. Extending the incision proximally provides access to the volar aspect of the wrist joint and the distal radius (Fig. 5-20). The most convenient approach for access to the volar aspect of the distal radius is the distal portion of the anterior approach to the radius (see Chapter 4).

## Dangers

### Nerves

The **palmar cutaneous branch of the median nerve** arises 5 cm proximal to the wrist joint and runs down along the ulnar side of the tendon of the flexor carpi radialis muscle before crossing the flexor retinaculum. The greatest threat to this nerve occurs if the skin incision is not angled to the ulnar side of the forearm (see Fig. 5-14).

The **motor branch of the median nerve** to the thenar muscles exhibits considerable anatomic variation. The risk to the nerve is minimized if the incision is made into the carpal tunnel on the ulnar side of the median nerve (see Applied Surgical Anatomy of the Volar Aspect of the Wrist and Fig. 5-32).

### Vessels

The **superficial palmar arch** crosses the palm at the level of the distal end of the outstretched thumb. Blind slitting of the flexor retinaculum may damage this arterial arcade if the instrument passes too far distally. The arch is in no danger if the flexor retinaculum is cut carefully under direct observation for its entire length (see Figs. 5-14 and 5-32).

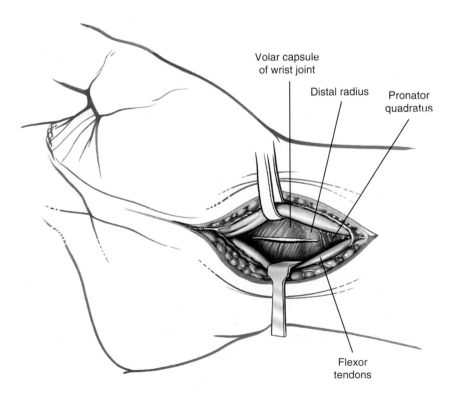

Volar capsule
of wrist joint

Distal radius

Pronator
quadratus

Flexor
tendons

**Figure 5-19** The median nerve is retracted radially and the flexor tendons are retracted toward the ulna, revealing the distal radius and joint capsule. An incision then is made into the capsule to expose the carpus.

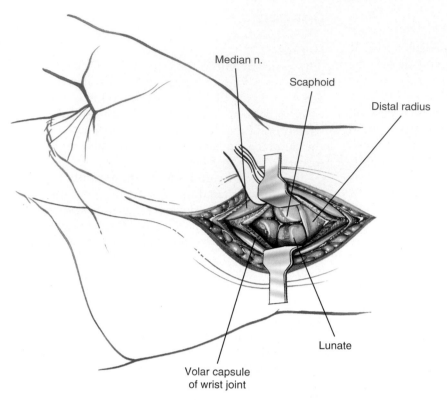

Median n.

Scaphoid

Distal radius

Lunate

Volar capsule
of wrist joint

**Figure 5-20**   Incise the joint capsule to expose the carpus.

## How to Enlarge the Approach

### Extensile Measures

***Proximal Extension.***   The approach can be extended to expose the median nerve. To accomplish this, extend the skin incision proximally, running it up the middle of the anterior surface of the forearm (Fig. 5-21). Incise the deep fascia of the forearm between the palmaris longus and flexor carpi radialis muscles. Retract the flexor carpi radialis in a radial direction and the palmaris longus in an ulnar direction, exposing the muscle belly of the flexor digitorum superfi-

**Figure 5-21**   Extend the wrist incision proximally to expose the distal forearm and median nerve.

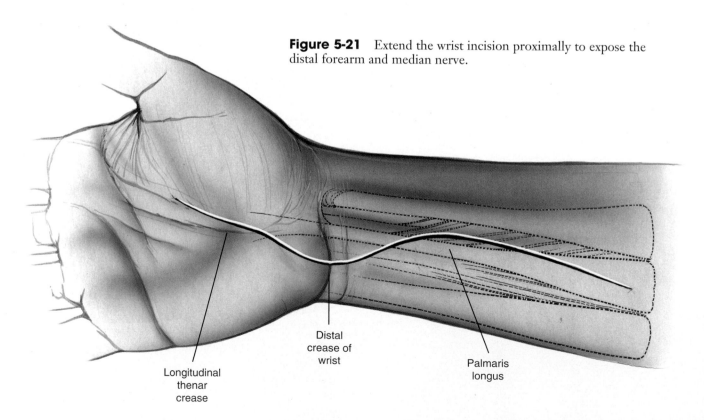

Longitudinal
thenar
crease

Distal
crease of
wrist

Palmaris
longus

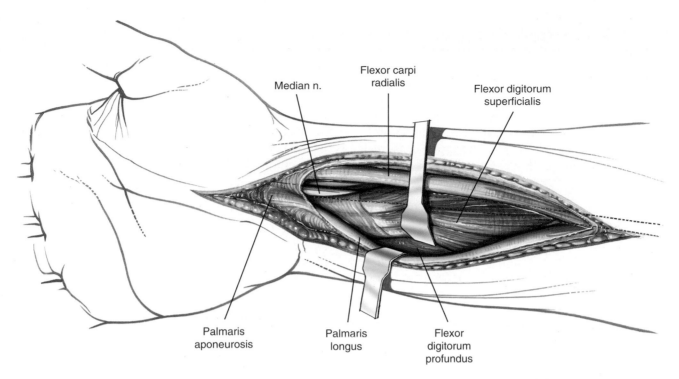

**Figure 5-22**   Incise the fascia on the forearm between the palmaris longus and the flexor carpi radialis to expose the tendons and muscles on the flexor digitorum superficialis.

cialis muscle in the distal two thirds of the forearm (Fig. 5-22). The median nerve adheres to the deep surface of the flexor digitorum superficialis, held there by fascia. Thus, if the flexor digitorum superficialis is reflected, the nerve goes with it (Fig. 5-23).

***Distal Extension.***   The skin incision can be extended into a volar zigzag approach for any of the fingers, providing complete exposure of all the palmar structures (see Volar Approach to the Flexor Tendons and Fig. 5-38).

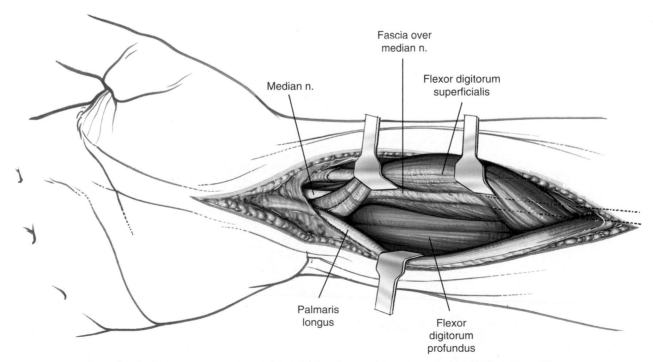

**Figure 5-23**   Reflect the flexor digitorum superficialis and note that the median nerve moves with it, because it is attached to the muscle via the posterior fascia of the muscle.

# Volar Approach to the Ulnar Nerve

The volar approach is used for exploration of the ulnar nerve at the wrist. It is used primarily to decompress the canal of Guyon in cases of ulnar nerve compression. It also permits exploration of the ulnar nerve in cases of trauma. The approach is freely extensile proximally, allowing exposure of the nerve all the way up the forearm.

## Position of the Patient

Place the patient supine on the operating table. Rest the hand on a hand table in the supinated position, so that the palm faces upward. Use an exsanguinating soft bandage, then inflate a tourniquet (see Fig. 5-13).

## Landmarks and Incision

### Landmarks

The *hypothenar eminence* is a readily palpable group of muscles on the ulnar border of the hand. The *transverse skin crease* of the wrist overlies the wrist joint.

### Incision

Make a curved incision, following the radial border of the hypothenar eminence and crossing the wrist joint obliquely at about 60°. Extend the incision onto the volar aspect of the distal forearm. The incision should be about 5 to 6 cm long (Fig. 5-24).

## Internervous Plane

There is no internervous plane. The approach is a true anatomic dissection in which the nerve and vessels are dissected out and preserved.

## Superficial Surgical Dissection

Deepen the incision in the line of the skin incision and identify the tendon of the flexor carpi ulnaris in the proximal end of the wound (Fig. 5-25). Mobilize the tendon by incising the fascia on its radial border, and retract the muscle and tendon in an ulnar direction to reveal the ulnar nerve and artery (Fig. 5-26).

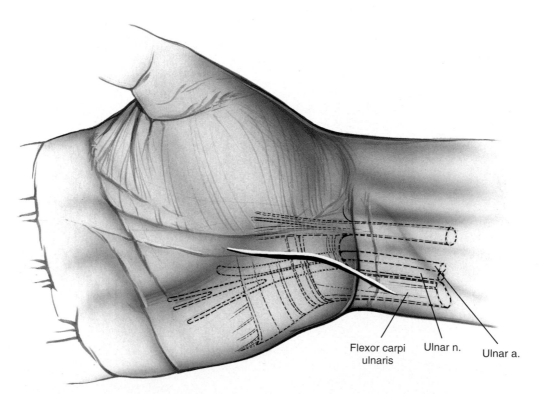

Flexor carpi ulnaris   Ulnar n.   Ulnar a.

**Figure 5-24**   Incision for the exposure of the ulnar nerve in the canal of Guyon.

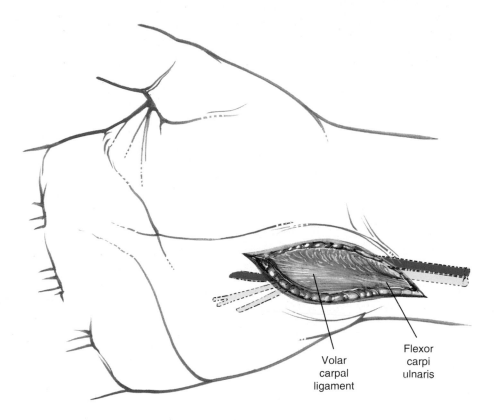

**Figure 5-25**   The volar carpal ligament is seen as a continuation of the deep palmar fascia and fibers of the flexor carpi ulnaris.

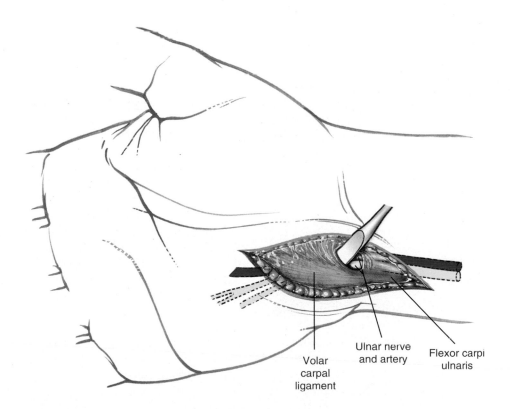

**Figure 5-26**   The volar carpal ligament is isolated and the nerve is protected in preparation for sectioning of the volar carpal ligament.

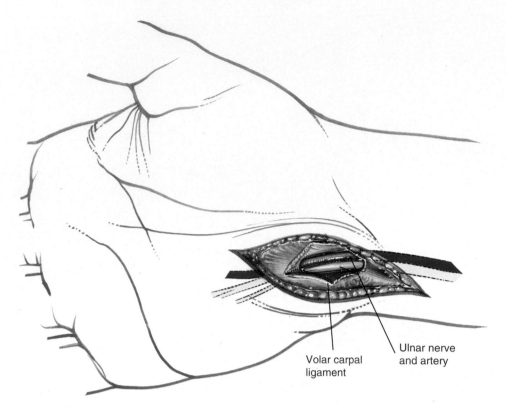

**Figure 5-27**    The roof of the canal has been incised, revealing the ulnar nerve and artery.

Volar carpal
ligament

Ulnar nerve
and artery

## Deep Surgical Dissection

Trace the nerve and artery distally, incising overlying fibrous tissue, the volar carpal ligament. During this procedure, take great care to protect the nerve and vessel. The ulnar nerve now is exposed across the wrist joint; the canal of Guyon is decompressed (Fig. 5-27).

## Dangers

### Nerves

The **ulnar nerve** is vulnerable during two phases of the dissection:

1. When the fascia on the radial side of the flexor carpi ulnaris is incised to allow retraction of the muscle, during superficial surgical dissection
2. When the volar carpal ligament is incised, during deep surgical dissection

If care is taken during these two phases of the procedure, the nerve should be safe.

## How to Enlarge the Approach

### Extensile Measures

*Proximal Extension.* Extend the skin incision proximally on the anterior aspect of the forearm, running it longitudinally up the middle of the forearm (Fig. 5-28). Incise the deep fascia in line with the incision and identify the radial border of the flexor carpi ulnaris. Develop a plane between the flexor carpi ulnaris muscle (which is supplied by the ulnar nerve) and the flexor digitorum superficialis muscle (which is supplied by the median nerve), retracting the flexor carpi ulnaris toward the ulna to reveal the ulnar nerve. This incision can expose the ulnar nerve almost to the level of the elbow joint (Fig. 5-29), where it passes between the two heads of the flexor carpi ulnaris muscle.

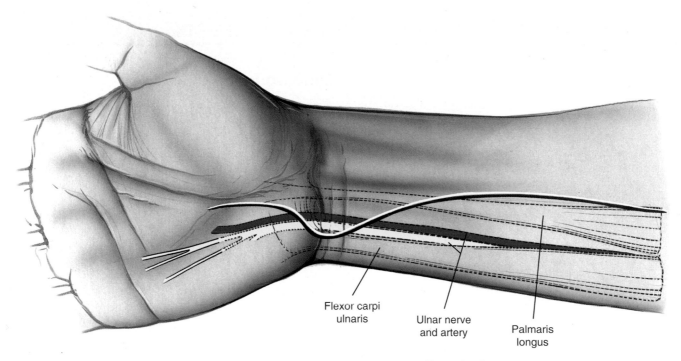

Flexor carpi
ulnaris

Ulnar nerve
and artery

Palmaris
longus

**Figure 5-28** Explore the ulnar nerve proximally in the forearm.

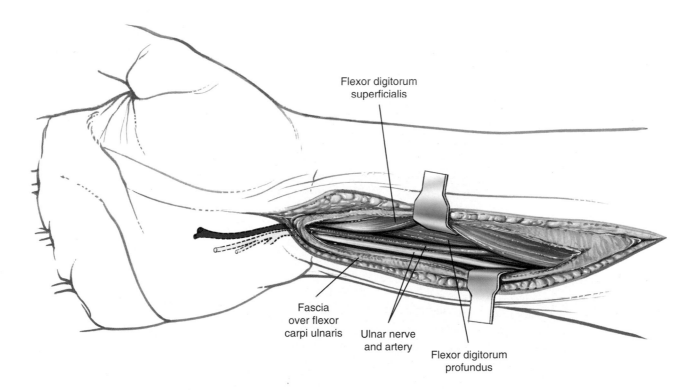

Flexor digitorum
superficialis

Fascia
over flexor
carpi ulnaris

Ulnar nerve
and artery

Flexor digitorum
profundus

**Figure 5-29** Develop the plane between the flexor carpi ulnaris and the flexor digitorum superficialis. In the depth of the wound, the ulnar nerve is visualized running under the reflected head of the flexor carpi ulnaris.

# Applied Surgical Anatomy of the Volar Aspect of the Wrist

## Overview

The carpal tunnel is a fibro-osseous canal on the volar surface of the carpus. Its base is formed by the deeply concave surface of the volar aspect of the carpal bones, and its roof is formed by the flexor retinaculum (Fig. 5-30). The ulnar nerve runs over the surface of the flexor retinaculum; it is enclosed in its own fibro-osseous canal, the canal of Guyon (Fig. 5-31).

## Landmarks and Incision

The four attachments of the flexor retinaculum all are palpable (Figs. 5-35 and 5-36*A*):

1. The *pisiform*. This is located on the ulnar border of the wrist. The pisiform is a mobile sesamoid bone lying within the tendon of the flexor carpi ulnaris muscle. The bone sometimes is used by artisans to tap nails into soft wood or leather.

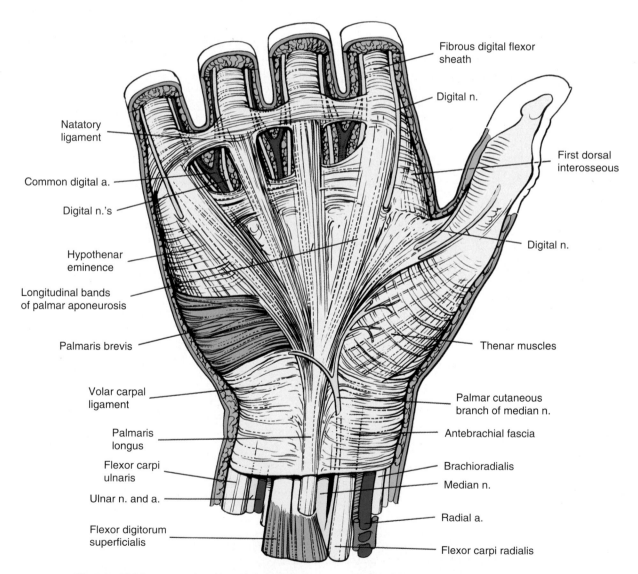

**Figure 5-30** Superficial anatomy of the wrist and palm. Note the course of the cutaneous branch of the median nerve. The longitudinal bands of the palmar aponeurosis are continuations of the palmaris longus tendon.

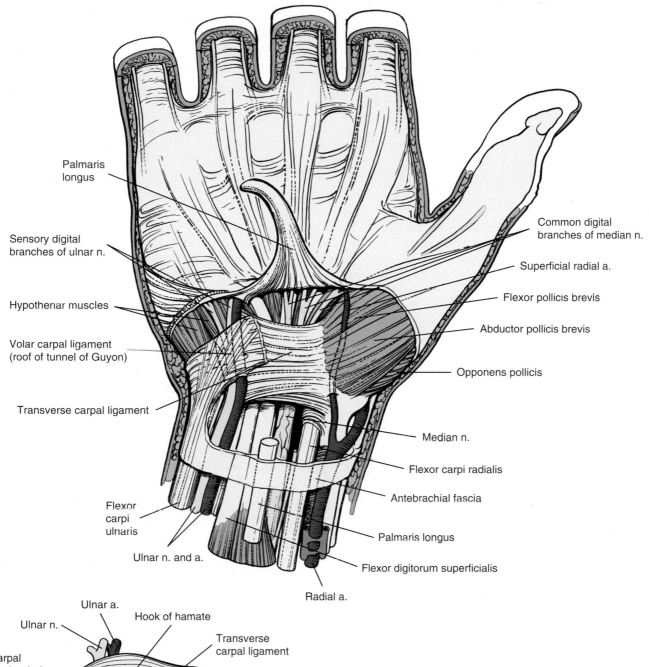

Palmaris longus

Sensory digital branches of ulnar n.

Hypothenar muscles

Volar carpal ligament (roof of tunnel of Guyon)

Transverse carpal ligament

Flexor carpi ulnaris

Ulnar n. and a.

Common digital branches of median n.

Superficial radial a.

Flexor pollicis brevis

Abductor pollicis brevis

Opponens pollicis

Median n.

Flexor carpi radialis

Antebrachial fascia

Palmaris longus

Flexor digitorum superficialis

Radial a.

Ulnar a.

Ulnar n.

Volar carpal ligament (roof of tunnel of Guyon)

Pisiform

Pisohamate ligament

Flexor carpi ulnaris

Triquetrum

Lunate

Hook of hamate

Transverse carpal ligament

Scaphoid

**Figure 5-31**   The palmar aponeurosis and fascia have been elevated to reveal the transverse carpal ligament. The fascia of the forearm and the expansions of the flexor carpi ulnaris (volar carpal ligament) are left intact where they form the roof of the tunnel of Guyon. The canal of Guyon looking from proximal to distal *(inset)*. The transverse carpal ligament forms the floor of the tunnel of Guyon; the roof is formed by the volar carpal ligament, which is a condensation of the fascia of the forearm and expansions of the flexor carpi ulnaris tendon. The canal is formed medially by the pisiform bone and laterally by the hook of the hamate bone.

Stress fractures have been noted in cobblers who use the pisiform for this purpose.

2. The *hook of the hamate*. This is slightly distal and radial to the pisiform. To locate it, place the interphalangeal joint of the thumb on the pisiform, pointing the tip toward the web space between the thumb and index finger, and rest the tip of the thumb on the palm. The hook of the hamate lies directly under the thumb. Because it is buried under layers of soft tissue, one must press firmly to find its rather shallow contours. The deep branch of the ulnar nerve lies on the hook, and neurapraxia of the nerve has been described in cases of fracture.

3. The *ridge of the trapezium*. The trapezium lies on the radial side of the carpus, where it articulates with the first metacarpal. To palpate the ridge, identify the joint between the trapezium and the thumb's metacarpal bone by moving the joint passively. The ridge feels like a prominent lump on the volar aspect of the trapezium (see Fig. 5-36*A*).

4. The *tubercle of the scaphoid*. This small protuberance is barely palpable just distal to the distal end of the radius on the volar aspect of the wrist joint (see Figs. 5-35 and 5-36*A*).

On its radial side, the retinaculum also attaches across the groove on the trapezium, converting the groove into a tunnel through which the tendon of the flexor carpi radialis muscle runs before it attaches to the base of the second and third metacarpals (see Figs. 5-35 and 5-36*A*).

## Superficial Surgical Dissection and its Dangers

Three structures run across the surface of the flexor retinaculum (see Fig. 5-30):

I. *Tendon of the palmaris longus.* The palmaris longus is a vestigial muscle of no functional importance. Its tendon is used frequently for tendon grafting. It is important to test for the presence of this tendon before surgery, because it is absent in about 10% of the population. The tendon also is used as an anatomic landmark for the injection of steroid into the carpal tunnel. If the patient is asked to flex the wrist against resistance, the tendon of the palmaris longus (if it is present) is easily palpable together with the thicker and more radially located tendon of the flexor carpi radialis. The easily defined gap between the two tendons is the site where the needle should be inserted for injection of the carpal tunnel. The needle should be inserted here dorsally and distally at an angle of almost 45°. Note also that because the carpal tunnel is a distensible space, if problems are encountered in injecting it, then the tip of the needle either still is in the flexor retinaculum or is imbedded in one of the tendons in the tunnel. Correctly positioned syringes should enter the space without encountering much resistance to pressure.

II. *Palmar cutaneous branch of the median nerve.* The course of the palmar cutaneous branch of the median nerve may vary in four important ways (see Fig. 5-30):

A. Normally, the nerve branches off 5 cm proximal to the wrist. It runs along the ulnar side of the tendon of the flexor carpi radialis before crossing the flexor retinaculum. On rare occasions, the nerve actually may be enclosed by parts of the flexor retinaculum and, thus, may run in a tunnel of its own on the wrist.

   The nerve divides into two major branches, medial and lateral, while crossing the flexor retinaculum. The lateral is the larger branch. Both supply the skin of the thenar eminence.

B. Less often, the nerve arises from the median nerve in two distinct branches, which travel separately across the wrist.[9]

C. The palmar cutaneous branch may arise *within* the carpal tunnel and penetrate the flexor retinaculum to supply the skin of the thenar eminence.

D. The palmar cutaneous branch may be absent, replaced by a branch derived from the radial nerve, the musculocutaneous nerve, or the ulnar nerve.[9]

   The skin incision described above avoids cutting the nerve by angling across the distal forearm in an ulnar direction. One must be aware, however, that considerable variability exists in the course of the nerve. Because damage can result in the formation of a painful neuroma, transverse incisions on the volar aspect of the distal forearm must be avoided. (Compression lesions of the nerve have been reported, but these are rare.)[10,11]

III. *Ulnar nerve.* The ulnar nerve runs down the volar surface of the distal forearm under cover of the flexor carpi ulnaris muscle (see Fig. 5-31). The ulnar artery lies on its radial side. The tendon of the flexor carpi ulnaris inserts into the pisiform, which then joins with the hamate and fifth metacarpal via ligaments. Just proximal to the wrist, the artery and nerve emerge from under the muscle to pass over the flexor retinaculum (the transverse carpal ligament) of the wrist (see Fig. 5-31).

At this level, the anatomic arrangement of these structures can be remembered by the mnemonic "ANT": the *a*rtery is the most lateral structure, then the *n*erve, and, finally, the *t*endon of the flexor carpi ulnaris (see Fig. 5-31).

At the wrist, the nerve is particularly vulnerable to damage by lacerations. The grim triad of lacerations of the tendon of the flexor carpi ulnaris, the ulnar artery, and the ulnar nerve is a common sequela of falling through a window with the ulnar border of the wrist flung forward to protect the face.

As the nerve crosses the flexor retinaculum, it is covered with a tough fibrous tissue that is continuous with the deep fascia of the forearm, the volar carpal ligament. The tunnel thus formed, the canal of Guyon, has four boundaries: a floor, the flexor retinaculum (transverse carpal ligament); a medial wall, the pisiform; a lateral wall, the hamate; and a roof, the volar carpal ligament (distal fascia of the forearm; see Fig. 5-31).

Around the pisiform, the ulnar nerve divides into two branches. The superficial branch supplies the palmaris brevis muscle and the skin of the small finger and ulnar half of the ring finger. The deep branch supplies all the small intrinsic muscles of the hand, except those of the thenar eminence and the radial two lumbricals (see Figs. 5-32 through 5-35).

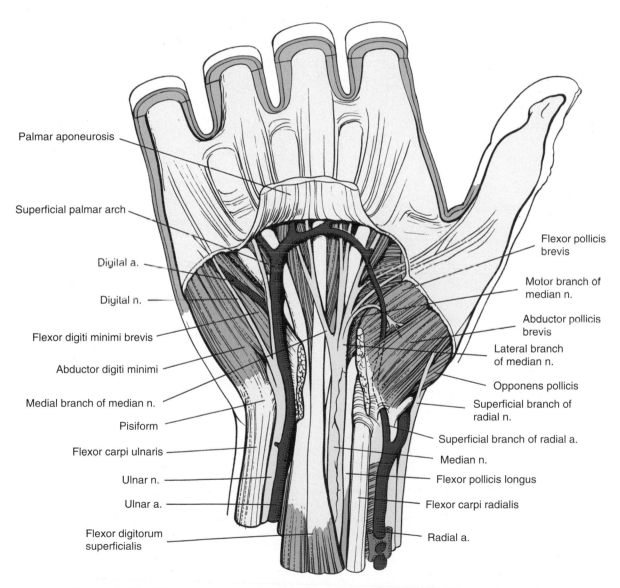

**Figure 5-32**  The palmar aponeurosis has been resected further distally to expose the superficial palmar arterial arch. The transverse carpal ligament also has been resected. The median nerve lies superficial to the tendons of the profundus, but at the same level with the superficialis muscle tendons. Note the motor branch of the median nerve to the thenar muscles. The location of its division from the median nerve is quite variable.

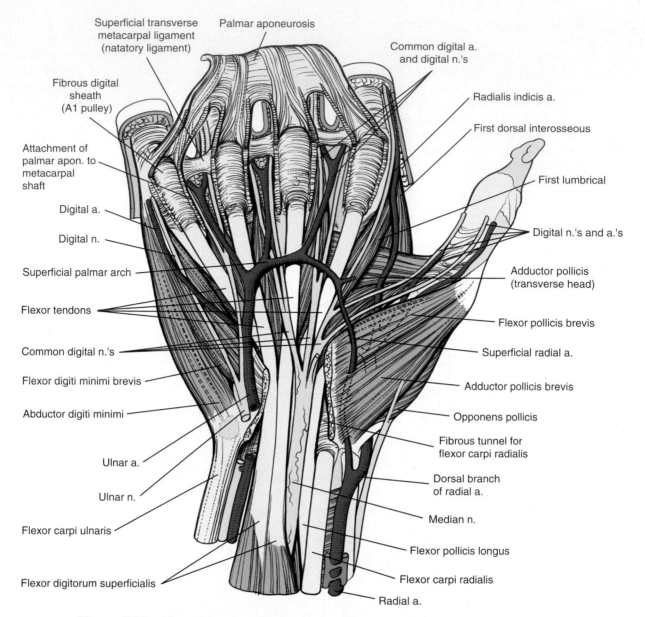

**Figure 5-33** The palmar aponeurosis has been elevated up to its attachment to the digital flexor sheaths. Its deeper attachments to the carpal plate and bone have been cut. The flexor tendons and digital nerves are shown in continuity, as are the superficial palmar arch and the thenar and hyperthenar muscles. Note that the digital nerves and vessels go deep or dorsal to the natatory ligaments.

**Flexor Pollicis Brevis.** *Origin.* Flexor retinaculum. *Insertion.* Radial border of proximal phalanx of thumb. *Action.* Flexor of metacarpophalangeal joint of thumb. *Nerve supply.* Median nerve (motor or recurrent branch).

**Abductor Pollicis Brevis.** *Origin.* Flexor retinaculum and tubercle of scaphoid. *Insertion.* Radial side of base of proximal phalanx of thumb. *Action.* Abduction of thumb at metacarpophalangeal joint and rotation of proximal phalanx of thumb. *Nerve supply.* Median nerve (motor or recurrent branch).

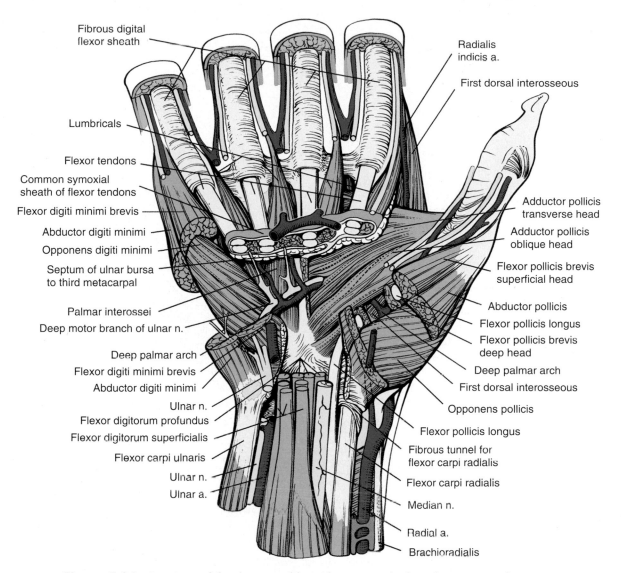

Fibrous digital flexor sheath
Lumbricals
Flexor tendons
Common symoxial sheath of flexor tendons
Flexor digiti minimi brevis
Abductor digiti minimi
Opponens digiti minimi
Septum of ulnar bursa to third metacarpal
Palmar interossei
Deep motor branch of ulnar n.
Deep palmar arch
Flexor digiti minimi brevis
Abductor digiti minimi
Ulnar n.
Flexor digitorum profundus
Flexor digitorum superficialis
Flexor carpi ulnaris
Ulnar n.
Ulnar a.

Radialis indicis a.
First dorsal interosseous
Adductor pollicis transverse head
Adductor pollicis oblique head
Flexor pollicis brevis superficial head
Abductor pollicis
Flexor pollicis longus
Flexor pollicis brevis deep head
Deep palmar arch
First dorsal interosseous
Opponens pollicis
Flexor pollicis longus
Fibrous tunnel for flexor carpi radialis
Flexor carpi radialis
Median n.
Radial a.
Brachioradialis

**Figure 5-34** Portions of the thenar and hypothenar muscles have been resected to reveal their layering. The ulnar nerve passes between the origin of the abductor digiti minimi and the flexor digiti minimi. In the thenar region, the course of the flexor pollicis longus is seen as it crosses between the two heads of the flexor pollicis brevis. Portions of the long flexors of the fingers have been resected to show their layering. The superficial palmar arch runs superficial to the tendons, whereas the deep palmar arch is immediately deep to the tendons. Note that potential spaces develop on the undersurface of the flexor tendons and their sheaths, and on the deep intrinsic muscles of the hand, the interosseous on the hyperthenar side and the adductor pollicis on the thenar side. A septum that runs from the undersurface of the flexor tendons to the third metacarpal divides the two spaces. More distally, the superficial transverse ligament has been resected, revealing the course of the lumbricals and the digital vessels that run superficial or palmar to the deep transverse metacarpal ligaments.

**Adductor Pollicis.** *Origin.* Oblique head from bases of second and third metacarpals, trapezoid, and capitate. Transverse head from palmar border of third metacarpal. *Insertion.* Ulnar side of base of proximal phalanx of thumb via ulnar sesamoid. *Action.* Adduction of thumb. Opposition of thumb. *Nerve supply.* Deep branch of ulnar nerve.
**Opponens Pollicis.** *Origin.* Flexor retinaculum. *Insertion.* Radial border of thumb metacarpal. *Action.* Opposition of metacarpal bone of thumb. *Nerve supply.* Median nerve (motor or recurrent branch).

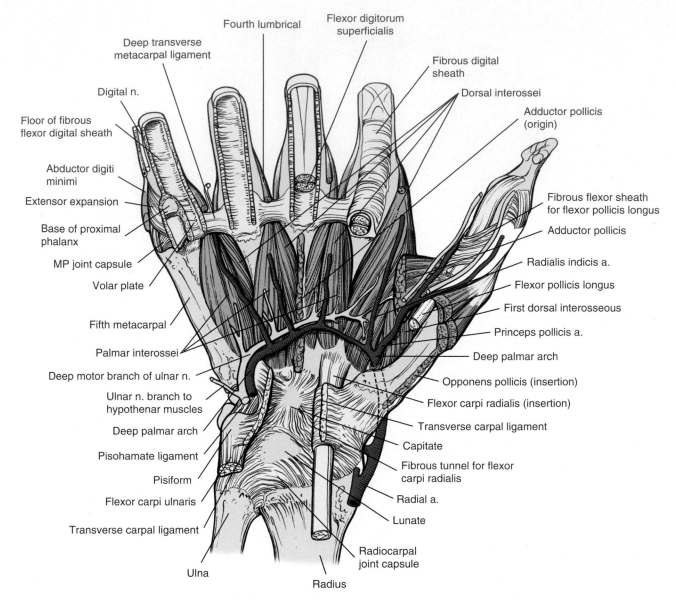

**Figure 5-35** The deepest layer of the palm is revealed. The deep palmar arterial arch lies deep to the long flexor tendon and superficial to the interosseous muscles. It crosses the palm with the deep branch (motor branch) of the ulnar nerve. The nerve supplies all the interosseous muscles. More distal, the interosseous muscles are seen running deep (dorsal) to the deep transverse ligament. The deep transverse metacarpal ligaments attach to the palmar plate, which is seen on the fifth metacarpal. The pulleys of the thumb are seen in relationship to the digital nerves.

## Deep Surgical Dissection and its Dangers

### Median Nerve

The median nerve crosses the volar aspect of the distal forearm deep to the flexor digitorum superficialis muscle. Just above the wrist, it becomes superficial and lies between the tendons of the palmaris longus and flexor carpi radialis muscles. It enters the palm by traversing the carpal tunnel (see Fig. 5-31).

Within the tunnel, the nerve lies superficial to the tendons of the flexor digitorum profundus and flexor pollicis longus muscles. The superficialis tendons lie toward the ulnar side of the nerve. At the distal border of the flexor retinaculum, the nerve divides into two branches (see Figs. 5-32 and 5-33).

1. The *medial branch* sends cutaneous branches to the adjacent sides of the ring and middle fingers, and to the adjacent sides of the middle and index fingers.
2. The *lateral branch* sends cutaneous branches to the radial side of the index finger and to both sides of the thumb. The lateral branch usually also sends off the motor, or recurrent, nerve (see Fig. 5-32), which is the key surgical landmark and major surgical danger in carpal tunnel decompression.

The motor nerve supplies the muscles of the thenar eminence. Its course may take any one of seven significant variations[10]:

1. The classic course (seen in 50% of patients). The branch arises from the volar radial aspect of the median nerve distal to the radial end of the carpal tunnel. The nerve hooks radially and upward to enter the thenar muscle group between the flexor pollicis brevis and abductor pollicis brevis muscles.

    The position of the motor branch can be estimated by drawing one vertical line from the web space between the middle and index fingers, drawing another from the radial origin of the first web space, then connecting to the hook of the hamate (Kaplan's cardinal line). The intersection of these two lines marks the origin of the motor branch (see Fig. 5-36B).[12]
2. A variation that occurs in about 30% of patients. The branch arises from the anterior surface of the nerve within the carpal tunnel. It passes through the tunnel with its parent nerve and hooks around the distal end of the flexor retinaculum to enter the thenar group between the flexor pollicis brevis and abductor pollicis brevis muscles.
3. A variation that occurs in about 20% of patients. The branch arises from the anterior surface of the nerve within the carpal tunnel. It travels radially to pierce the flexor retinaculum and enter the thenar group of muscles between the abductor pollicis brevis and flexor pollicis brevis muscles.[13]
4. A rare variation. The branch arises from the ulnar side of the median nerve.[14] It crosses the median nerve within the tunnel, then hooks around the distal end of the flexor retinaculum to enter the thenar muscle group. It also may pass through the flexor retinaculum and lie anterior to it.[15]

5. Another rare variation. The nerve arises from the anterior surface of the median nerve within the carpal tunnel. At the distal end of the flexor retinaculum, the branch hooks radially over the top of the retinaculum. The nerve crosses the distal part of the retinaculum almost transversely before entering the thenar group of muscles.
6. A very rare variation (multiple motor branches).[16] Double nerves may follow any of the courses described above.
7. A third rare variation (high division of the median nerve).[17] The nerve may divide into medial and lateral branches high up in the forearm. The thenar branch, originating from the lateral branch, may leave the carpal tunnel either in the conventional manner or by piercing the flexor retinaculum on its radial side.

All these variations should be considered when the nerve is exposed. If the tunnel is opened on the ulnar side of the nerve, the motor branch will be preserved unless it lies on the same side. Patients with exceptionally rare variations usually have large palmaris brevis muscles, which should alert the surgeon to the possibility during the approach.[10]

### Flexor Digitorum Superficialis
Within the carpal tunnel, the tendons to the middle and ring fingers are superficial to the tendons of the index and little fingers. This arrangement dictates correct repair in cases of multiple tendon laceration (see Fig. 5-31).

### Flexor Digitorum Profundus
The tendons of the flexor digitorum profundus lie deep to the tendons of the flexor digitorum superficialis. The tendon to the index finger is separate; the other three still may be attached partially to each other as they pass through the carpal tunnel (see Fig. 5-31).

### Flexor Pollicis Longus
The tendon of the flexor pollicis longus lies deep to that of the flexor carpi radialis and is found on the most radial aspect of the canal at the same depth as the profundus tendons (see Figs. 5-31 and 5-34).

### Flexor Carpi Radialis
The flexor carpi radialis muscle perforates the flexor retinaculum to lie in the groove of the trapezium before it inserts into the bases of the second and third metacarpals. It does not pass through the carpal tunnel (see Fig. 5-35).

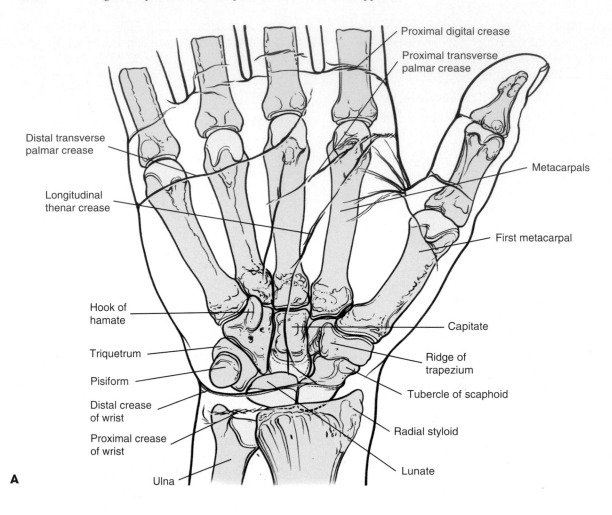

Proximal digital crease

Proximal transverse palmar crease

Distal transverse palmar crease

Longitudinal thenar crease

Metacarpals

First metacarpal

Hook of hamate

Capitate

Triquetrum

Ridge of trapezium

Pisiform

Tubercle of scaphoid

Distal crease of wrist

Radial styloid

Proximal crease of wrist

Lunate

Ulna

**A**

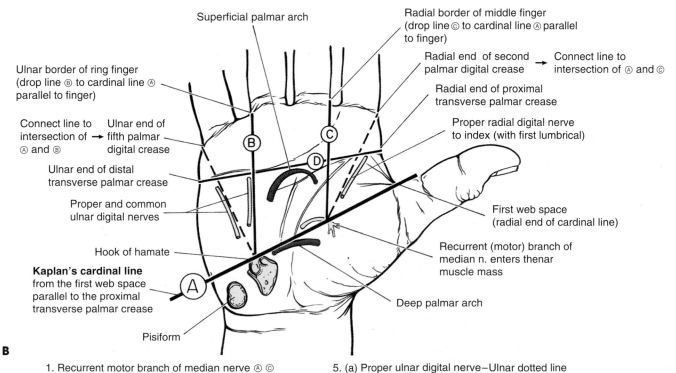

Superficial palmar arch

Radial border of middle finger (drop line ⓒ to cardinal line Ⓐ parallel to finger)

Radial end of second palmar digital crease → Connect line to intersection of Ⓐ and ⓒ

Ulnar border of ring finger (drop line Ⓑ to cardinal line Ⓐ parallel to finger)

Radial end of proximal transverse palmar crease

Proper radial digital nerve to index (with first lumbrical)

Connect line to intersection of → Ⓐ and Ⓑ

Ulnar end of fifth palmar digital crease

Ulnar end of distal transverse palmar crease

First web space (radial end of cardinal line)

Proper and common ulnar digital nerves

Recurrent (motor) branch of median n. enters thenar muscle mass

Hook of hamate

**Kaplan's cardinal line** from the first web space parallel to the proximal transverse palmar crease

Deep palmar arch

Pisiform

**B**

1. Recurrent motor branch of median nerve Ⓐ ⓒ
2. Superficial palmar arch ⓓ
3. Deep palmar arch Ⓐ
4. Proper radial digital nerve to index—Radial dotted line
5. (a) Proper ulnar digital nerve–Ulnar dotted line
   (b) Common ulnar digital nerve Ⓑ
6. Hook of hamate Ⓐ + Ⓑ
7. Pisiform Ⓐ

# Volar Approach to the Flexor Tendons

The volar approach provides the best possible exposure of the flexor tendons within their fibrous sheaths.[18] It also provides excellent exposure of both neurovascular bundles in the finger. The skin incision can be extended into the palm, the volar surface of the wrist, and the anterior surface of the forearm, making it a suitable approach in cases of trauma, where many levels may have to be exposed. Its other major advantage is that many skin lacerations can be incorporated into the skin incision. Its uses include the following:

1. Exploration and repair of flexor tendons
2. Exploration and repair of digital nerves and vessels
3. Exposure of the fibrous flexor sheath for drainage of pus
4. Excision of tumors within the fibrous flexor sheath
5. Excision of palmar fascia in Dupuytren's contracture

## Position of the Patient

Place the patient supine on the operating table with the arm abducted and lying on an arm board. Adjust the height of the table to make sitting comfortable. Most right-handed surgeons prefer to sit on the ulnar side of the affected arm. An exsanguinating bandage and tourniquet, as well as good lighting, are essential (see Fig. 5-13).

## Landmarks and Incision

### Landmarks

Three major skin creases traverse the fingers: the *distal phalangeal crease*, just proximal to the distal interphalangeal joint; the *proximal phalangeal crease*, just proximal to the proximal interphalangeal joint; and the *palmar digital crease*, well distal to the metacarpophalangeal joint. The course of the volar zigzag incision takes these creases into account, running diagonally across the finger between creases (Fig. 5-37).

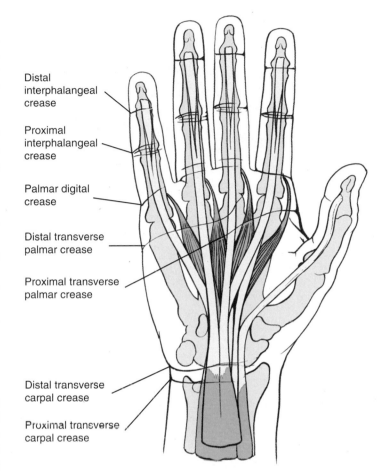

Distal interphalangeal crease

Proximal interphalangeal crease

Palmar digital crease

Distal transverse palmar crease

Proximal transverse palmar crease

Distal transverse carpal crease

Proximal transverse carpal crease

**Figure 5-37**   The relationship of the skin creases to the tendons and joints of the wrist and hand is seen.

### Incision

Before the fingers are incised, mark the skin with methylene blue to outline the proposed site. The angles of the zigzag should be about 90° to each other (or to the transverse skin crease); angles considerably less than 90° to each other may lead to necrosis of the corners (Fig. 5-38*A*). The angles should not be placed too far in a dorsal direction; otherwise, the neuromuscular bundle may be damaged when the skin flaps are mobilized (see Fig. 5-38*B*). Of course, the basic zigzag pattern should be

**Figure 5-36**   **(A)** The bones of the wrist and palm and the proximal metacarpals are seen in relationship to the creases of the wrist. The necks of the metacarpals are at the level of the distal palmar crease. The distal wrist crease runs from the proximal portion of the pisiform to the proximal portion of the tubercle of the scaphoid and marks the proximal level of volar carpal ligament. The proximal transverse palmar crease is at the radiocarpal joint. **(B)** Kaplan's cardinal line. Used to locate the motor branch of the median nerve to the thenar muscles.

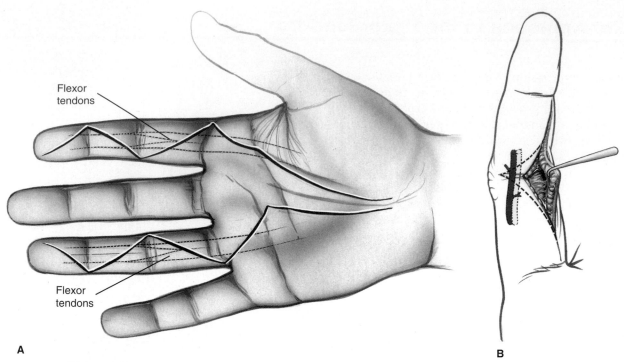

**A**

**B**

**Figure 5-38**   **(A)** Basic zigzag incision for exposure of the flexor tendons of the palm and fingers. **(B)** If an incision is placed too far laterally or medially, the neurovascular bundle may be damaged.

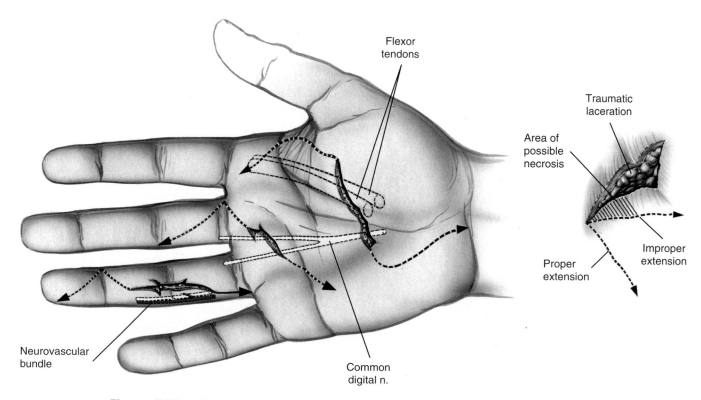

**Figure 5-39**   The basic zigzag pattern should be adapted to preexisting lacerations for exploration of the underlying structures. When adapting the skin incisions to previously existing lacerations, attempt to maintain an angle of about 90° to prevent necrosis of the corners of the incision *(inset)*.

modified to accommodate any preexisting lacerations (Fig. 5-39).

## Internervous Plane

There is no true internervous plane. The skin at the site of the incision is innervated by nerves coming from either side of the incision, so no areas of anesthesia are created.

## Superficial Surgical Dissection

Reflect the skin flaps carefully with a skin hook, starting at the apex. Elevate the flaps along with some underlying fat. Do not mobilize the flaps widely until the level of the flexor sheath is reached, to ensure thick flaps and reduce the risk of skin flap necrosis (Fig. 5-40).

## Deep Surgical Dissection

To expose the flexor tendons, carefully incise the subcutaneous tissues along the midline in a longitudinal fashion (Fig. 5-41). The flexor tendons lie directly underneath, within their fibrous flexor sheaths.

To expose the digital nerve and vessel, gently separate the subcutaneous tissues at the lateral border of the fibrous flexor sheath. The neurovascular bundle is separated from the volar subcutaneous flap by a thin layer of fibrous tissue known as Grayson's ligament. This layer must be opened for full exposure of the neurovascular bundle. The easiest way to pry the tissues apart is to open gently a small pair of closed scissors so that the blades separate the tissues in a longitudinal plane. The blades actually are working along the line of the digital nerve, maximizing expo-

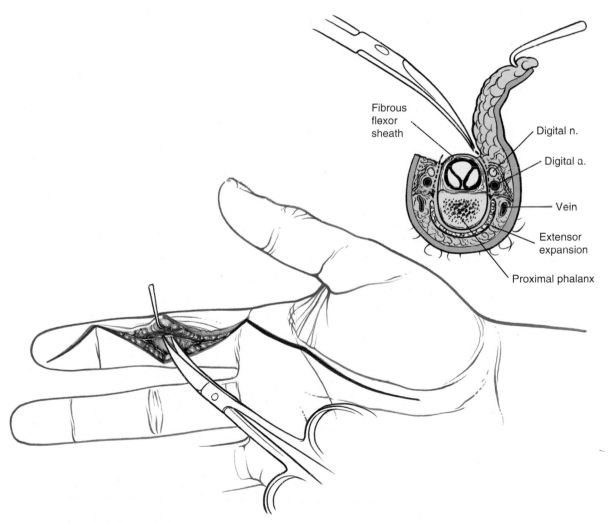

**Figure 5-40** Elevate thick skin flaps. Stay as close to the sheath as possible to prevent damage to the laterally placed neurovascular structures.

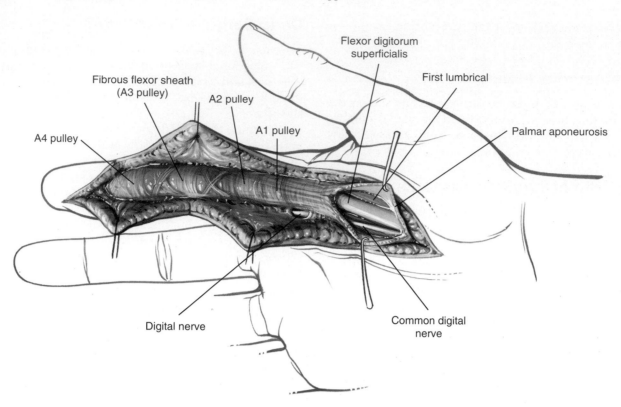

**Figure 5-41** Expose the flexor tendons in a longitudinal fashion. The digital nerves lie lateral to the tendons. Maintain the A2 and A4 pulleys.

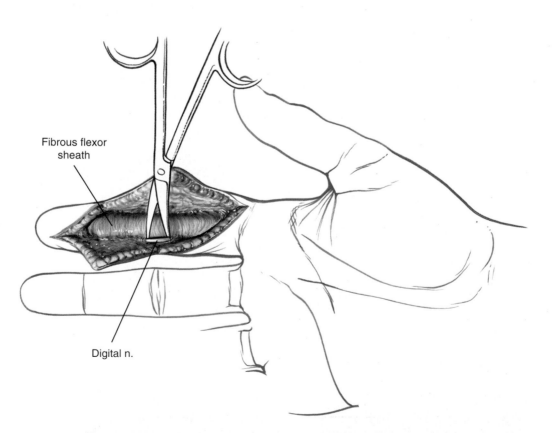

**Figure 5-42** Identify the neurovascular bundles and preserve them.

sure of the nerve while minimizing the chance of accidental laceration (Fig. 5-42; see Fig. 5-40).

To expose the bone, create a plane between the edge of the fibrous flexor sheath and the digital nerves and vessels. (In practice, it seldom is necessary to go this deep; surgery on the osseous structures usually is safer through a midlateral or dorsal incision [Fig. 5-43].)

Incising the fibrous flexor sheath, retracting the tendons, and incising the periosteum from the volar surface of the bone lead to adhesions within the fibrous flexor sheath. It is very important to note that

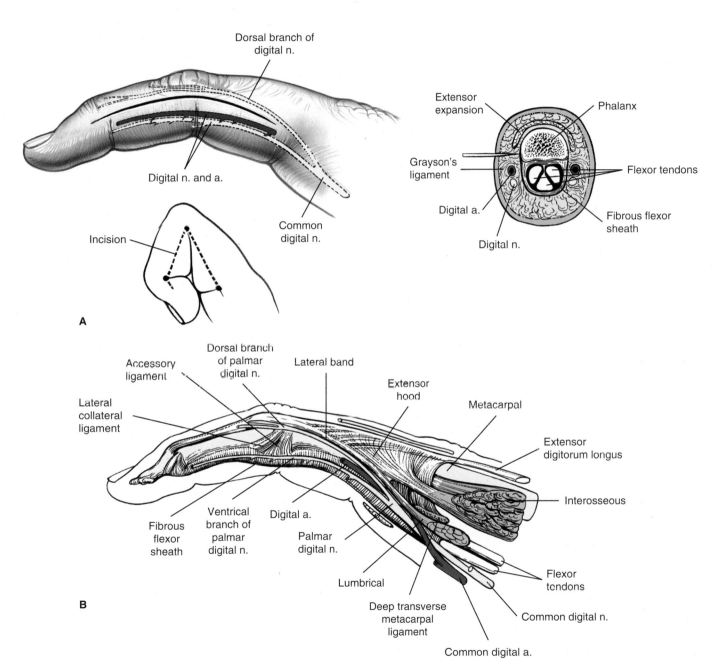

**Figure 5-43** **(A)** Incision for the midlateral approach to the finger. The incision lies between the proper digital nerve, which runs toward the palm, and its dorsal branch. The incision also can be made with the finger flexed; connect the dorsal portions of the interphalangeal creases *(inset)*. **(B)** Lateral view of the anatomy of the finger. Note the division of the proper (common) digital nerve into dorsal and palmar branches, the relationship of the palmar division of the nerve to the flexor tendon sheath, and the insertion of the lumbrical and interossei muscles into the hood mechanism.

the consequences of this will be the loss of full function of the finger. Therefore, every effort should be made to avoid this at all costs.

## Dangers

**Digital nerves and vessels** can be damaged if the skin mobilization extends too far in a dorsal direction.

**Skin flaps** should not be cut at too acute an angle, and skin sutures should be meticulous to ensure closure. Skin flaps should be thick enough to avoid skin necrosis (see Fig. 5-39). The tourniquet should be removed and hemostasis secured before closure is undertaken.

## How to Enlarge the Approach

### Proximal Extension

The zigzag skin incision can be extended onto the palm, eventually joining the curved incision parallel to the thenar crease that is used for exposure of the structures of the palm, volar surface of the wrist, and anterior surface of the forearm. The key to making these incisions is to avoid crossing flexion creases at 90°, thus preventing the development of flexion contractures, and to leave skin flaps with substantial corners (see Fig. 5-39).

## Midlateral Approach to the Flexor Sheaths

The midlateral approach is a popular way of reaching the flexor tendons and digital nerves in the fingers. It affords access to the neurovascular bundle on the incised side of the finger; at the same time, it is difficult to extend into the palm. Its uses include the following:

1. Open reduction and stabilization of phalangeal fractures
2. Exposure of the fibrous flexor sheath and its contents
3. Exposure of the neurovascular bundle

## Position of the Patient

Place the patient supine on the operating table, with the arm stretched out on an arm board. Good lighting and a good exsanguinating bandage and tourniquet are essential (see Fig. 5-13).

## Landmarks and Incision

### Landmarks

The *proximal and distal interphalangeal creases* are the key to this skin incision. They extend around the medial and lateral surfaces of the fingers and end slightly nearer the dorsal than the volar surface of the finger.

The creases may disappear if the finger is very swollen or if it is struck in full extension. If so, the surgical landmark for the skin incision is the junction between the wrinkled dorsal and the smooth volar skin on the side of the finger (see Fig. 5-43).

### Incision

Make a longitudinal incision on the lateral aspect of the finger, starting at the most dorsal point of the proximal finger crease. Continue cutting distally to the distal interphalangeal joint, passing just dorsal to the dorsal end of the flexor skin crease. Extend the incision farther distally toward the lateral end of the fingernail. The incision actually is dorsolateral rather than truly lateral (see Fig. 5-43). Alternatively, flex the finger and make an incision connecting dorsal end points of the interphalangeal crease.

## Internervous Plane

There is no true internervous plane, because no intermuscular interval is developed. The nerve supply to the finger comes mainly from two sources, the dorsal digital nerves and the volar, or palmar, digital nerves. Because the skin incision marks the division between these two supplies, it causes no significant areas of hypoesthesia.

## Superficial Surgical Dissection

Develop a volar skin flap by incising the subcutaneous flap in line with the skin incision. The fat over the proximal interphalangeal joint is quite thin; take care not to incise the joint itself. Continue the dissection toward the midline of the finger, angling slightly in a volar direction. The main neuromuscular bundles lie in the volar flap (Fig. 5-44).

## Deep Surgical Dissection

Incise the fibrous flexor sheath longitudinally to expose the underlying tendon (Fig. 5-45). The neuromuscular bundles also can be dissected out from within the volar flap (Fig. 5-46).

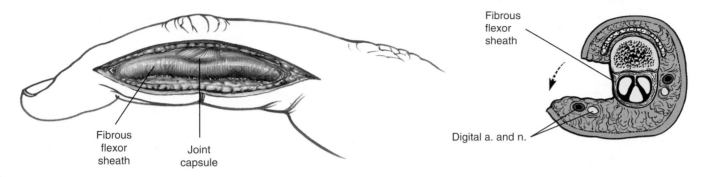

**Figure 5-44** Develop the skin flap down to the flexor sheath, maintaining the neurovascular bundle in the volar flap.

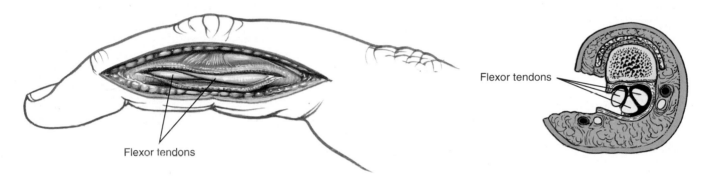

**Figure 5-45** Incise the flexor sheath longitudinally to reveal the tendons.

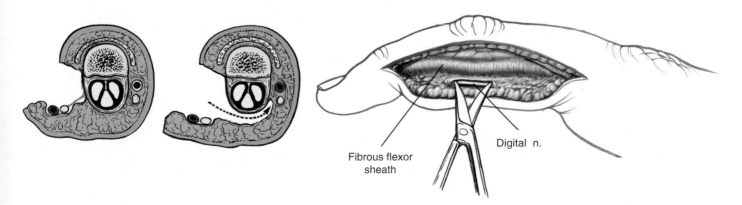

**Figure 5-46** By longitudinal dissection, the neurovascular structures are revealed within the volar flap. Careful dissection of the flexor sheath can expose the entire palmar aspect of the bundle.

## Dangers

### Nerves

The **palmar digital nerve** is in danger if the skin incision and approach drift too far in a volar direction. This approach always should begin just dorsal to the end of the interphalangeal creases. If the approach does begin at this site, the danger to the palmar digital nerve will be diminished (see Fig. 5-43*A*).

### Vessels

The **volar digital artery** runs with the digital nerve on its inner side. It also may be damaged if the approach moves too far in a volar direction (see Fig. 5-43).

## How to Enlarge the Exposure

Continue the dissection around the fibrous sheath to expose the neurovascular bundle on the opposite side. Note that the exposure gained is not as good as that offered by a zigzag volar approach.

# Applied Surgical Anatomy of the Finger Flexor Tendons

This section describes only the anatomy of the finger flexor tendons. For a general description of the palmar anatomy, see Applied Surgical Anatomy of the Volar Aspect of the Wrist.

## Overview

The anatomy of the finger flexor tendons provides the key to the treatment and prognosis of flexor tendon injuries. Nowhere else in the body are the links between anatomy, pathology, and treatment illustrated so clearly. The structure of the tendons, their blood supply, and their special relationship to other structures all relate to the pathogenesis of injury and repair.

The anatomy of the finger flexor tendons encompasses five zones, each of which is separated from the others by anatomic landmarks. The zones all must be treated differently in cases of tendon laceration. We shall consider the anatomy from the proximal to the distal aspect, from zone 5 to zone 1, as devised by Milford (Fig. 5-47).[19]

## Zone 5

Zone 5 is in the anterior compartment of the forearm, proximal to the flexor retinaculum and the carpal tunnel (see Fig. 5-42). At that point, nine distinct tendons run into the hand toward the digits. Each finger has two tendons, one each from the flexor digitorum superficialis muscle and the flexor digitorum profundus muscle. The thumb has one long flexor, the flexor pollicis longus.

The tendons in zone 5 are not enclosed in a tight canal, but are surrounded by a synovial sheath in the distal part of the forearm. Tendon repairs carried out in this area generally are successful, and independent finger flexion usually returns.

## Zone 4

Zone 4 encompasses the tendons as they run through the carpal tunnel. All the tendons remain in a common synovial sheath throughout the carpal tunnel.

Tendon repairs carried out in zone 4 have a good prognosis, but not as good as the prognosis of those carried out in zone 5, because the tendons are enclosed in a fibro-osseous tunnel. The tunnel must be opened for repairs, and adhesions may form after surgery.

## Zone 3

Zone 3 is the zone of the lumbrical origin. As the flexor digitorum profundus tendons traverse the palm, a lumbrical muscle arises from each tendon. The radial two lumbricals arise from a single head, from the radial side of the profundus tendons to the index and middle fingers. The ulnar two lumbricals arise from two heads, from the adjacent sides of the profundus tendons between which they lie. The tendons of the lumbricals pass along the radial sides of the metacarpophalangeal joints before they insert into the dorsal expansion. They pass volar to the axes of the metacarpophalangeal joints; thus, they act as flexors of those joints, even as they extend the interphalangeal joints (see Fig. 5-34).

Lacerations in zone 3 almost invariably involve damage to the lumbrical muscles. Most surgeons do not recommend repairing the lumbricals; the increased tension on the muscles caused by the repair produces fixed flexion at the metacarpophalangeal joints and limited flexion at the interphalangeal joints, resulting in an intrinsic plus hand.

## Zone 2

Zone 2 stretches from the distal palmar crease to the middle of the middle phalanx. In this area, the two

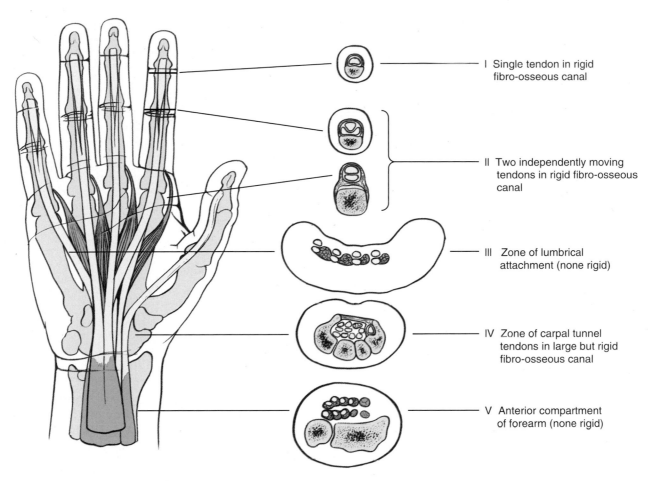

I   Single tendon in rigid fibro-osseous canal

II   Two independently moving tendons in rigid fibro-osseous canal

III   Zone of lumbrical attachment (none rigid)

IV   Zone of carpal tunnel tendons in large but rigid fibro-osseous canal

V   Anterior compartment of forearm (none rigid)

**Figure 5-47**   The five zones of the wrist and hand (according to Milford).

tendons for each finger run together in a common fibro-osseous sheath.

The sheaths run from the level of the metacarpal heads (the distal palmar crease) to the distal phalanges. They are attached to the underlying bone and prevent the tendons from bowstringing.

Thickenings in the fibrous flexor sheath are constant (Fig. 5-48). They act as pulleys, directing the sliding movement of the tendons. There are two types: annular and cruciate. Annular pulleys are composed of a single fibrous band (ring); cruciate pulleys have two crossing fibrous strands (cross). Annular pulleys act much like the rings on a fishing rod. Without the ring, the fishing line would pull away from the rod as it bends. This effect is known as bowstringing; in human terms, it results in the loss of range of movement and power in the affected finger. Annular pulleys include the following:

1. The A1 pulley, which overlies the metacarpophalangeal joint. It is incised during trigger finger release.

2. The A2 pulley, which overlies the proximal end of the proximal phalanx. It must be preserved (if at all possible) to prevent bowstringing.
3. The A3 pulley, which lies over the proximal interphalangeal joint.
4. The A4 pulley, which is located about the middle of the middle phalanx. It must be preserved to prevent bowstringing.

Cruciate pulleys, none of which are critical for flexor function, include the following:

1. The C1 pulley, which is located over the middle of the proximal phalanx
2. The C2 pulley, which is located over the proximal end of the middle phalanx
3. The C3 pulley, which is located over the distal end of the middle phalanx

The two tendons enter each fibro-osseous canal with the superficialis tendon on top of the profundus tendon. Over the proximal phalanx, the superficialis

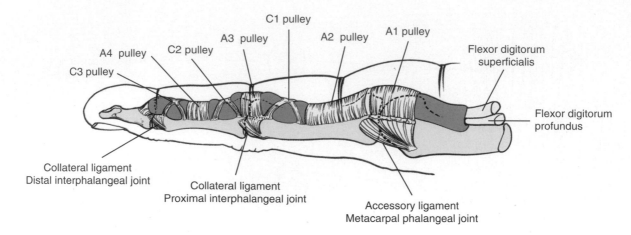

**Figure 5-48**    The annular and cruciate ligaments of the flexor tendon sheath, lateral view. Note the relationship of the pulleys to the skin creases and joint lines.

tendon divides into halves, which spiral around the profundus tendon, meeting on its deep surface and forming a partial decussation (chiasma). The two then run as one tendon underneath the profundus tendon before attaching to the base of the middle phalanx. Thus, the superficialis tendon actually provides part of the bed on which the profundus tendon runs. Distal to the attachment of the superficialis tendon, the profundus tendon inserts into the base of the terminal phalanx (see Fig. 5-64). Within the fibro-osseous sheath, the nutrition of the flexor tendons is provided for by blood vessels that enter the tendons from synovial folds called vincula (Fig. 5-49).

Extremely difficult conditions for full recovery exist after lacerations in zone 2, mainly because the flexor tendons are enclosed within a nondistensible fibro-osseous canal, and also because, for full function, the tendons must run over each other. It is important to remember that any adhesion between the two can cause malfunction of the involved finger.

Repairs in this zone have the worst prognosis of all the zones.[20] It has been nicknamed "no-man's land" by Bunnell.[21]

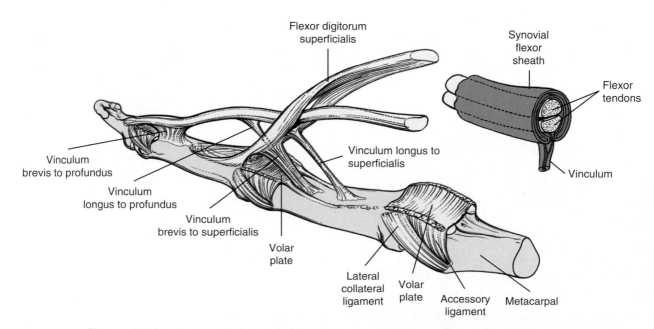

**Figure 5-49**    The vincula longa and brevia are main blood supplies to the flexor tendons. Note the relationship of the vincula to the flexor tendon synovial sheath (inset).

### Zone 1

Zone 1 is the area distal to the insertion of the superficialis tendon. Although the profundus tendon still is enclosed tightly within a fibro-osseous sheath here, it runs alone. Therefore, the prognosis for the repair of lacerations in this zone is better than that for zone 2, although not as good as that for zones 3, 4, and 5.

### Vascular Supply of the Tendons

Within the fibrous sheath, the flexor tendons are enveloped in a double layer of synovium (see Fig. 5-49, *inset*). Each tendon receives its blood supply from arteries that arise from the palmar surface of the phalanges. These vessels are encased in the vinculum (mesotenon). Two vincula supply each tendon, as follows:

I. Profundus tendon.
   A. The short vinculum runs to the tendon close to its insertion onto the distal phalanx.
   B. The long vinculum passes to the tendon from between the halves of the superficialis tendon at the level of the proximal phalanx.
II. Superficialis tendon.
   A. The short vinculum runs to the tendon near its attachment onto the middle phalanx.
   B. The long vinculum is a double vinculum, passing to each half of the tendon from the palmar surface of the proximal phalanx.

Injection studies on fresh cadaveric material have found that this classic arrangement does not always hold true. The long vincula to both tendons may be absent in the long or ring fingers. When they are present, the long vinculum to the superficialis tendon may attach to either or both of its slips, and the long vinculum to the profundus tendon may arise at the level of the insertion of the superficialis tendon.[22]

These variations should be borne in mind as the flexor tendons are explored within their sheaths. The vincula should be preserved, if possible, to preserve the blood supply to the tendon.

Other injection studies have found that the volar aspects of the flexor tendons are largely avascular; their nutrition may be derived from synovial fluid. Therefore, sutures placed in the volar aspects of the tendons do not interfere materially with the blood supply to the tendons themselves.[23]

### Landmarks and Incision

The critical landmarks of hand surgery are the skin creases, all of which are situated where the fascia attaches to the skin. There are four major creases: the distal palmar crease corresponds roughly to the palmar location of the metacarpophalangeal joints and the location of the proximal (A1) pulley, the palmar digital crease marks the palmar location of the A2 pulley, the proximal interphalangeal crease marks the proximal interphalangeal joint, and the thenar crease outlines the thenar eminence (see Figs. 5-37, 5-47, and 5-48).

The nerve supply to the skin of the fingers comes from two sources: the volar aspect is supplied by the volar digital nerves, and the dorsal aspect is innervated by the dorsal nerves of the radial and ulnar nerves, as well as by the dorsal contribution from the volar digital nerves for the distal 1½ phalanges of the index, long, and ring fingers. The dorsa of the thumb and small finger are served exclusively by the radial and ulnar nerves, respectively. Because of this anatomic arrangement, the midlateral approach to the flexor sheath does not cause skin denervation (see Fig. 5-43).

## Volar Approach to the Scaphoid

The volar approach provides good exposure of the scaphoid bone.[24] It also avoids damaging the dorsal blood supply to the bone's proximal half, as well as the superficial branch of the radial nerve. It does pose a threat to the radial artery, however, which is close to the operative field. It leaves a more cosmetic scar than does the dorsal approach, and its uses include the following:

1. Bone grafting for nonunion of the scaphoid
2. Excision of the proximal third of the scaphoid

3. Excision of the radial styloid, either alone or combined with one of the above procedures
4. Open reduction and internal fixation of fractures of the scaphoid. In such cases this approach frequently is combined with the dorsolateral approach to the scaphoid.

### Position of the Patient

Place the patient supine on the operating table, with the arm lying on an arm board. Supinate the forearm to expose the volar aspect of the wrist, and apply an exsanguinating bandage and tourniquet (see Fig. 5-13).

## Landmarks and Incision

### Landmarks
Palpate the *tuberosity of the scaphoid* on the volar aspect of the wrist, just distal to the skin crease of the wrist joint.

The *flexor carpi radialis* muscle lies radial to the palmaris longus muscle at the level of the wrist. It crosses the scaphoid before inserting into the base of the second and third metacarpal just on the ulnar side of the radial pulse.

### Incision
Make a vertical or curvilinear incision on the volar aspect of the wrist, about 2 to 3 cm long. Base it on the tuberosity of the scaphoid and extend it proximally between the tendon of the flexor carpi radialis muscle and the radial artery (Fig. 5-50).

## Internervous Plane

There is no true internervous plane; the only muscle mobilized is the flexor carpi radialis (which is supplied by the median nerve).

## Superficial Surgical Dissection

Incise the deep fascia in line with the skin incision and identify the radial artery on the lateral (radial) side of the wound (Fig. 5-51). Retract the radial artery and lateral skin flap to the lateral side. Identify the tendon of the flexor carpi radialis muscle and trace it distally, incising that portion of the flexor retinaculum that lies superficial to it. After the tendon has been freed from its tunnel in the flexor retinaculum, retract it medially to expose the volar aspect of the radial side of the wrist joint (Fig. 5-52).

## Deep Surgical Dissection

Incise the capsule of the wrist joint over the scaphoid to expose the distal two thirds of the scaphoid. This

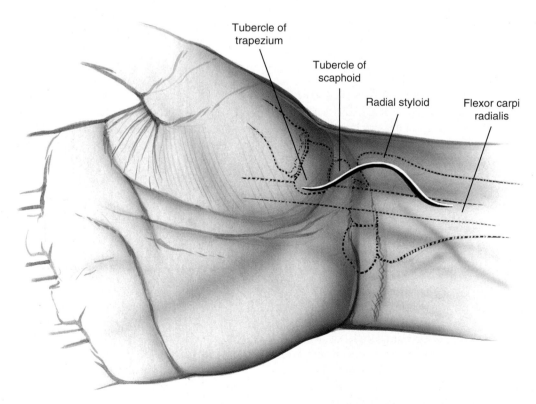

**Figure 5-50**   Incision for the volar approach to the scaphoid. Base the incision on the tuberosity of the scaphoid and extend it proximally and distally. The proximal extension is between the tendon of the flexor carpi radialis and the radial artery.

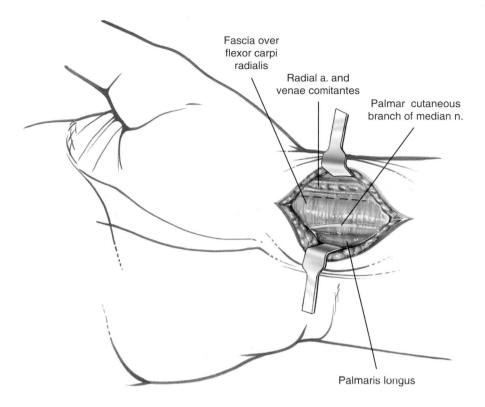

Fascia over
flexor carpi
radialis

Radial a. and
venae comitantes

Palmar cutaneous
branch of median n.

Palmaris longus

**Figure 5-51** Incise the deep fascia between the radial artery and the flexor carpi radialis.

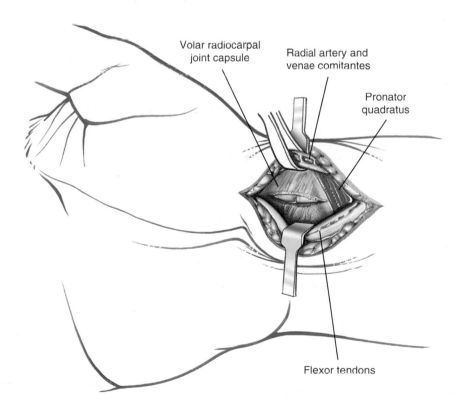

Volar radiocarpal
joint capsule

Radial artery and
venae comitantes

Pronator
quadratus

Flexor tendons

**Figure 5-52** Retract the radial artery and skin flap laterally and the flexor carpi radialis medially to expose the volar aspect of the radial side of the wrist joint capsule.

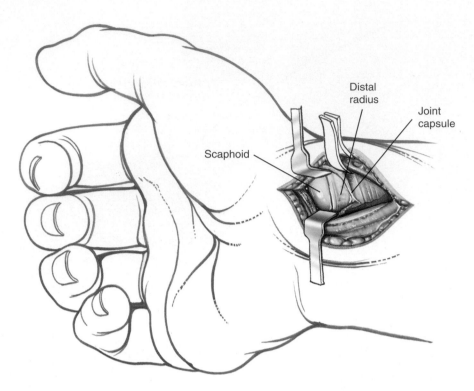

**Figure 5-53**   Incise the joint capsule. Dorsiflex the wrist to gain exposure of the proximal articular third of the bone.

anterior area of bone is nonarticular. To gain the best view of the proximal third of the bone, place the wrist in marked dorsiflexion (Fig. 5-53).

## Dangers

### Vessels

The **radial artery** lies close to the lateral border of the wound and can be incised accidentally at any time during the dissection. Therefore, it must be identified early in the procedure.

Note that this approach exposes the distal two thirds of the scaphoid.

## How to Enlarge the Approach

The incision can be extended usefully to a limited extent. Proximally, extend the skin incision along the line of the flexor carpi radialis muscle. Identify the distal border of the pronator quadratus muscle and elevate it gently from the underlying bone. This will create adequate exposure of the distal end of the radius, allowing a bone graft to be taken from this site. Adequate exposure also will be obtained to allow excision of the radial styloid, if this is indicated.

The key to exposing the scaphoid lies in forceful dorsiflexion of the wrist. This will expose the proximal pole of the scaphoid, which is the site of most cases of nonunion. If the location of the fracture is not completely clear, place a small, radiopaque mark at the operative site and carry out a radiographic examination on the operating table. Bone grafting can be carried out adequately with this exposure, but the insertion of a screw may require a combined dorsal and volar approach to the scaphoid.[25]

# Dorsolateral Approach to the Scaphoid

The dorsolateral approach offers an excellent and safe exposure of the scaphoid bone. Its major drawback is that it endangers the superficial branch of the radial nerve, and it also may interfere with the dorsal blood supply of the scaphoid.[26] Its uses include the following:

1. Bone grafting for nonunion
2. Excision of the proximal fragment of a nonunited scaphoid
3. Excision of the radial styloid in combination with either of the two above procedures
4. Open reduction and internal fixation of fractures of the scaphoid. When this approach is used for this indication, it is frequently combined with a volar approach to the scaphoid.[25]

## Position of the Patient

Place the patient supine on the operating table, with the arm extended on an arm board. Pronate the forearm to expose the dorsoradial aspect of the wrist, and apply an exsanguinating bandage and tourniquet (see Fig. 5-1).

## Landmarks and Incision

### Landmarks

The *radial styloid process* is truly lateral when the hand is in the anatomic position. Palpate it in this position and then pronate the arm, keeping a finger on the styloid process.

The *anatomic snuff-box* is a small depression that is located immediately distal and slightly dorsal to the radial styloid process. The scaphoid lies in the floor of the snuff-box. Ulnar deviation of the wrist causes the scaphoid to slide out from under the radial styloid process, and it becomes palpable. The radial pulse is palpable in the floor of the snuffbox, just on top of the scaphoid.

The *first metacarpal* can be palpated between the snuff-box and the metacarpophalangeal joint.

### Incision

Make a gently curved, S-shaped incision centered over the snuff-box. The cut should extend from the base of the first metacarpal to a point about 3 cm above the snuff-box (Fig. 5-54).

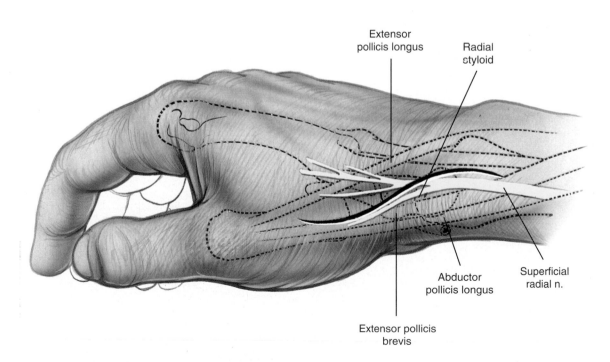

**Figure 5-54**    Incision for dorsolateral exposure of the scaphoid. Make a gently curved S-shaped incision centered over the snuff-box. The superficial branch of the radial nerve crosses directly beneath the incision.

## Internervous Plane

There is no true internervous plane, because the plane of dissection falls between the tendons of the extensor pollicis longus and extensor pollicis brevis muscles, both of which are supplied by the posterior interosseous nerve. Because both muscles receive their nerve supply well proximal to this dissection, using this plane does not cause denervation.

## Superficial Surgical Dissection

Identify the tendons of the extensor pollicis longus muscle dorsally and the extensor pollicis brevis muscle ventrally (Fig. 5-55). To confirm their identity, pull on the tendons and observe their action on the thumb. Open the fascia between the two tendons, taking care not to cut the sensory branch of the superficial radial nerve, which lies superficial to the tendon of the extensor pollicis longus muscle. The radial nerve usually has divided into two or more branches at this level. Both branches cross the interval between the tendons of the extensor pollicis brevis and the extensor pollicis longus, lying superficial to the tendons. Their course is variable, and they must be sought during superficial dissection (see Figs. 5-54 and 5-55).

Now, separate the tendons, retracting the extensor pollicis longus dorsally and toward the ulna, and the extensor pollicis brevis ventrally. Identify the radial artery as it traverses the inferior margin of the wound, lying on the bone (Fig. 5-56). Find the tendon of the extensor carpi radialis longus muscle as it lies on the dorsal aspect of the wrist joint. Mobilize it and retract it in a dorsal and ulnar direction, together with the tendon of the extensor pollicis longus muscle, to expose the dorsoradial aspect of the wrist joint.

## Deep Surgical Dissection

Incise the capsule of the wrist joint longitudinally (Fig. 5-57). Reflect the capsule dorsally and in a volar direction to expose the articulation between the distal end of the radius and the proximal end of the scaphoid. The radial artery retracts radially and in a volar direction with the joint capsule.

Place the wrist in ulnar deviation and continue stripping the capsule off the scaphoid to expose the joint completely (Fig. 5-58).

## Dangers

### Nerves

The **superficial radial nerve** is at risk during this exposure. Because it lies directly over the tendon of the extensor pollicis longus muscle, it is extremely easy to cut as the tendon is mobilized. Incising the nerve may produce a troublesome neuroma, as well as an awkward (although not handicapping) area of hypoesthesia on the dorsal aspect of the hand.

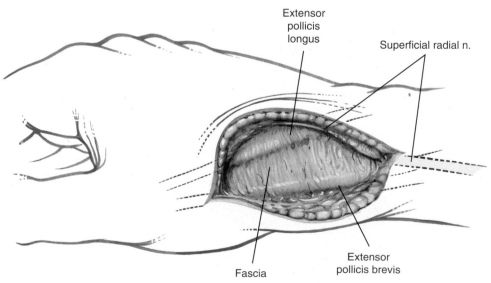

**Figure 5-55**    Identify the superficial branch of the radial nerve and retract it with the dorsal skin flap. Identify the tendons of the extensor pollicis longus dorsally and the extensor pollicis brevis ventrally. Incise the fascia between the tendons.

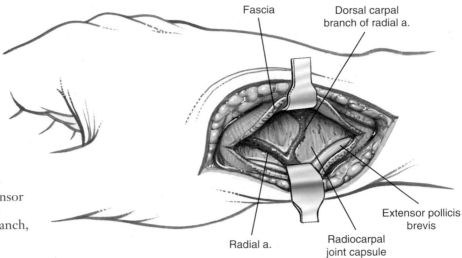

**Figure 5-56** Retract the extensor pollicis longus dorsally and the extensor pollicis brevis ventrally. Identify the radial artery and its dorsal carpal branch, taking care to preserve the arterial branch.

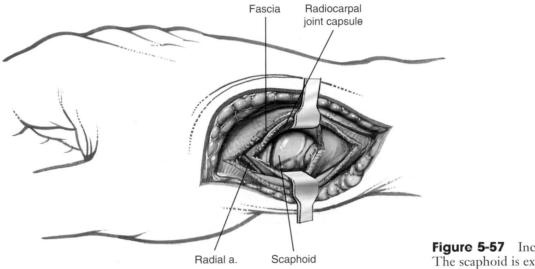

**Figure 5-57** Incise the joint capsule. The scaphoid is exposed.

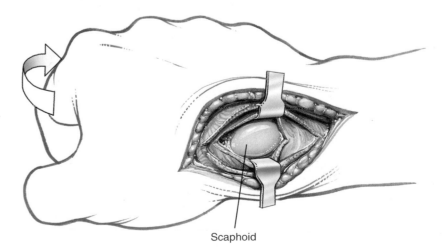

**Figure 5-58** Place the wrist in ulnar deviation to expose the proximal third of the scaphoid in its entirety.

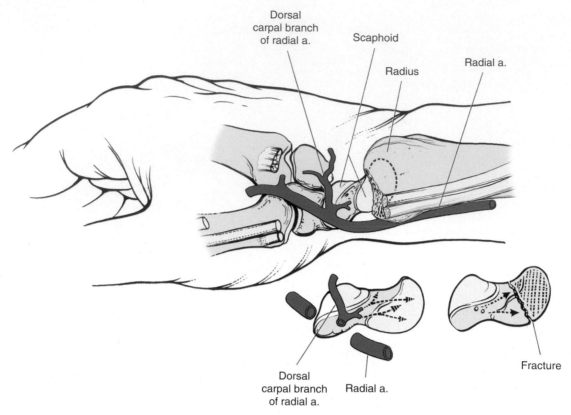

**Figure 5-59** Blood supply to the scaphoid. Most branches enter the scaphoid from the dorsal aspect. These branches must be preserved to prevent necrosis of its proximal fragment.

# Drainage of Pus in the Hand

Hand infections are an important source of patient morbidity. They cause an enormous loss of time from work and can produce permanent deficits in hand function. Until recently, the availability of more prompt medical care and the administration of antibiotics had caused a dramatic decrease in the incidence of major hand infections; however, the intravenous and subcutaneous use of narcotics among drug addicts has increased, reintroducing serious hand infections to the field of surgery.

The keys to the surgical treatment of hand infections are as follows:

1. *Accurate localization of the infection.* Each particular infection has characteristic physical signs, according to the anatomy of the particular compartment that is infected.
2. Timing of the operation. The timing of surgical drainage is critical to the outcome of surgical treatment. If an infection is incised too early, the surgeon may incise an area of cellulitis and actually cause the infection to spread. In contrast, if pus is left in the hand too long, particularly

around the tendon, it may induce irreversible changes in the structures it surrounds.

The correct timing for a given surgical procedure is difficult to determine. In the body, the cardinal physical sign of an abscess is the presence of a fluctuant mass within an area of inflammation; however, because there often is only a small amount of pus present in the hand, an abscess there can be hard to find. In addition, pus frequently is found in tissues that contain fat. At body temperature, fat itself is fluctuant, further complicating the physical diagnosis of an abscess. Nevertheless, some guidelines for the detection of pus do exist:

1. Pus may be seen subcutaneously.
2. The longer an infection has been present, the more likely it is that pus will be present. Infections of less than 24 hours' duration are unlikely to have developed pus.
3. Classically, if the patient cannot sleep at night because of pain in the hand, pus probably has formed.

4. If slight passive extension of the finger produces pain along the finger and in the palm, the tendon sheath is likely to be infected; it should be explored to drain the pus.

The last guideline, signs of tendon sheath infection, is one of the four cardinal signs of acute suppurative tenosynovitis described by Kanavel.[27] The other three follow below:

1. Swelling around the tendon sheath
2. Tenderness to palpation
3. Flexion deformity of the affected finger

Despite these guidelines, it still may be difficult to determine whether there is pus in the hand. If doubt exists, elevate the arm and treat the patient with intravenous antibiotics and warm soaks, reexamining him or her at frequent intervals. If signs of inflammation diminish rapidly, avoid surgery.

## Optimum Operative Conditions

1. Use a general anesthetic or a distal nerve block. Injecting a local anesthetic at the site of infection is ineffective and actually may spread the infection within fascial planes.
2. Use a tourniquet. The arm should not be exsanguinated with a bandage, to avoid spreading the infection by mechanical compression. The arm should be elevated for 3 minutes before the tourniquet is applied.
3. Perfect lighting is critical for all explorations of pus in the hand. All relevant neurovascular bundles must be identified to ensure their preservation.
4. Draining abscesses of the hand is not like draining abscesses anywhere else in the body. Boldly incising an abscess space without approaching it carefully is to be condemned.
5. Leave all wounds open after incision.
6. Immobilize the hand in the functional position after surgery by applying a dorsal or volar splint, or both, with the metacarpophalangeal joints at 80° of flexion and the proximal and distal interphalangeal joints at 10° of flexion. At this position, the collateral ligaments of the metacarpophalangeal, proximal interphalangeal, and distal interphalangeal joints are at their maximum length and will not develop contractures during immobilization.
7. Elevate the arm postoperatively. Continue administering intravenous antibiotics until signs of inflammation begin to diminish. Mobilize the affected part as soon as signs of inflammation subside. Begin extensive rehabilitation, which may last several months.

Of the eight major infection sites listed below, the first three are seen most often:

I. Paronychia
II. Pulp space (felon)
III. Web space
IV. Tendon sheath
V. Deep palmar area
   A. Lateral space (thenar space)
   B. Medial space (midpalmar space)
VI. Radial bursa
VII. Ulnar bursa

Surgical approaches to each of these areas are discussed below.

# Drainage of Paronychia

Paronychia is infection of a nail fold. Perhaps the most common hand infection, it is caused most often by *Staphylococcus aureus*. It occurs in individuals from all walks of life.[1] Hairdressers often are affected because hair from their clients may become embedded between the cuticle and the bony nail. Tearing the cuticle to remove a "hangnail" probably is the most common cause of this infection.

It usually is easy to see where the pus distends the cuticle. The paronychia may occur on either side or it may lift the whole of the cuticle upward. It even may extend underneath the nail.

## Position of the Patient

Place the patient supine on the operating table, with the arm extended on an arm board (see Fig. 5-13).

## Incision

Make a short, longitudinal incision at one or both corners of the nail fold (Fig. 5-60A).

## Internervous Plane

There is no internervous plane involved. The nerve supply of the skin in this region is derived from cutaneous nerves that overlap one another considerably. No area of skin becomes denervated.

## Superficial Surgical Dissection

Raise the skin flap outlined by the skin incision at the base of the nail, evacuating the pus between the

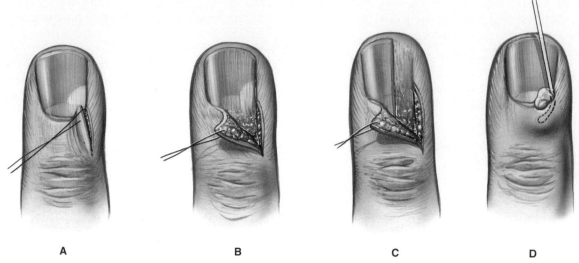

A          B          C          D

**Figure 5-60** (**A** through **D**) Incisions for the evacuation of pus at the base of the nail (paronychia).

cuticle and the nail. If pus extends under the nail, excise either one corner of the base of the nail or half of the nail itself, depending on how it has been undermined and lifted off the nail bed (see Fig. 5-60*B,C*). Occasionally, a nick into the soft-tissue cuticle parallel with the nail will release the pus (see Fig. 5-60*D*).

## Dangers

If the nail bed is damaged, the new nail will develop a ridge, which is a minor cosmetic deformity.

## How to Enlarge the Approach

The approach cannot be extended usefully by either local or extensile measures.

# Drainage of a Pulp Space Infection (Felon)

Distal finger pulp space infections are the hand infections that most often require surgical drainage. Infection usually is caused by a penetrating injury to the pulp, an injury that may be quite trivial in itself. Superficial infections cause skin necrosis and point early, usually on the volar aspect of the pulp. Deeper infections are more likely to cause osteomyelitis of the underlying distal phalanx, a condition that is known as a felon or whitlow.

Depending on the depth of the infection, two different techniques exist for draining pus in this site:

1. If the abscess is pointing in a volar direction in the distal pulp of the finger, as it commonly is, make a small incision on the lateral side of the volar surface and enter the abscess cavity obliquely. Midline incisions may produce painful scars.
2. If the abscess is deep, the surgery described below may be necessary.

## Position of the Patient

Place the patient on the operating table, with the arm lying on an arm board.

## Incision

Make a straight incision on the lateral aspect of the terminal phalanx of the finger, extending to the tip of the finger close to the nail. The incision should not extend proximally to the distal interphalangeal joint; more proximal incisions may damage the digital nerve, causing a painful neuroma, or they may contaminate the joint with purulent material.

The incision should be dorsal and distal to the distal end of the distal interphalangeal crease (Fig. 5-61). It should not extend distally beyond the distal corner of the nail. Avoid the ulnar aspect of the thumb and the radial aspect of the index and long fingers to avoid creating a scar that interferes with pinch.

## Internervous Plane

There is no internervous plane in this incision. The skin incision lies between skin that is supplied by the dorsal cutaneous nerve and skin that is supplied by branches of the volar digital nerves.

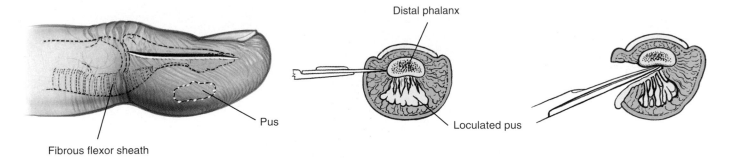

Distal phalanx

Pus

Loculated pus

Fibrous flexor sheath

**Figure 5-61**   Incision for drainage of pulp space infection (felon). The septa must be cut to ensure appropriate drainage.

## Superficial Surgical Dissection

The pulp of the terminal phalanx contains numerous fibrous septa that connect the distal phalanx with the volar skin, creating loculi. The infection easily can invade several of these loculi. To ensure that all pockets of infection are drained, deepen the skin incision transversely across the pulp of the finger, remaining on the volar aspect of the terminal phalanx, until the skin of the opposite side of the finger is reached. Do not penetrate this skin (see Fig. 5-61). Now, bring the scalpel blade distally, detaching the origins of the fibrous septa from the bone. Proximally, take care not to extend the dissection beyond a point 1 cm distal to the distal interphalangeal crease; otherwise, the flexor tendon sheath may be damaged and infection introduced into it.

## Dangers

### Nerves
The **digital nerves** may be damaged if the skin incision drifts too far proximally. Painful neuromas can result without an appreciable area of hyperesthesia on the finger.

### Muscles and Ligaments
The fibrous flexor sheath of the profundus tendon may be incised accidentally if the incision is carried too far proximally.

## Special Points

The fibrous septa that connect the distal phalanx to the skin make this an ideal site for loculation of pus. Take care to open all the loculi so that adequate drainage takes place. Unsuccessful treatment of a deep abscess may result in osteomyelitis of the distal phalanx.

## How to Enlarge the Approach

The approach cannot be enlarged usefully by either local or extensile measures.

# Web Space Infection

Web space infections, which involve pus in one of the four webs of the palm, are quite common. The abscess usually points dorsally, because the skin on the dorsal surface of the web is thinner than the skin on the palmar surface. Characteristically, a large amount of edema appears on the dorsum of the hand, and the two fingers of the affected web are spread farther apart than normal (Fig. 5-62).

The web spaces all communicate via the canal of the lumbrical muscles into the palm; therefore, a neglected web space infection can cause a more extensive infection by spreading up the lumbrical canal and into the palm.

## Position of the Patient

Place the patient supine on the operating table, with the arm on an arm board. Use a general anesthetic or an axillary or brachial block, then raise the arm for 3 minutes before inflating an arm tourniquet (see Fig. 5-13).

## Incision

Make a curved transverse incision in the volar skin of the palm, following the contour of the web space about 5 mm proximal to it (Fig. 5-63).

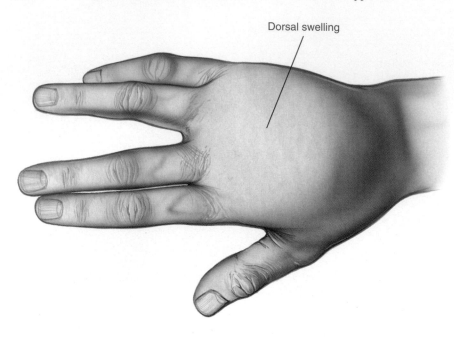

Dorsal swelling

**Figure 5-62**   Web space infection. A large amount of edema usually appears on the dorsum of the hand, and the two fingers of the affected web space are spread farther apart than normal.

## Internervous Plane

There is no true internervous plane in this approach.

## Superficial Surgical Dissection

Carefully deepen the skin incision by blunt dissection. The digital nerves and vessels lie immediately under the incision and may be damaged if the cut is too deep, mainly because the dissection is being carried out in a transverse rather than a longitudinal plane. The abscess cavity usually is located just below the skin; it can be entered with very little additional dissection.

## Dangers

### Nerves

Both digital nerves of the web space are vulnerable with this transverse skin incision. Make sure that an effective tourniquet, proper lighting, and fine instruments are used in the operation. As long as the skin

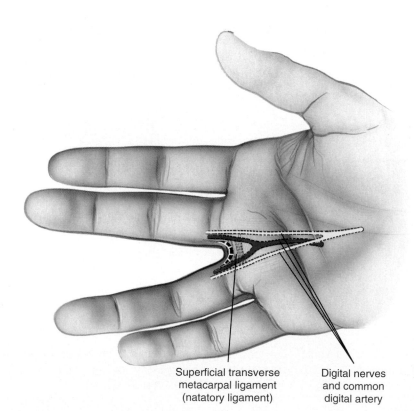

Superficial transverse metacarpal ligament (natatory ligament)

Digital nerves and common digital artery

**Figure 5-63**   Make a curved transverse incision in the volar skin of the palm, following the contour of the web space.

is incised with care, the nerves should not be damaged.

Longitudinal incisions in the web space avoid the threat to the neurovascular bundle, but scarring during the healing process may reduce significantly the ability of the two fingers of the web space to separate. That is why a transverse skin incision is recommended.

## How to Enlarge the Approach

The approach cannot be extended usefully. Some surgeons recommend a second, dorsal, skin incision over the pointing area to improve drainage without appreciably increasing the morbidity of the procedure.

## Anatomy of the Web Space of the Fingers

There are three webs between the four fingers. The spaces are surprisingly long (about 2 cm), extending from the edge of the skin to the metacarpophalangeal joints. They contain both the superficial and the deep transverse ligaments of the palm, the digital nerves and vessels, and the tendons of the interossei and lumbricals. Between these various structures lies loose, fibrous, fatty tissue, tissue that can be displaced easily by infection and the formation of abscesses (Fig. 5-64; see Fig. 5-33).

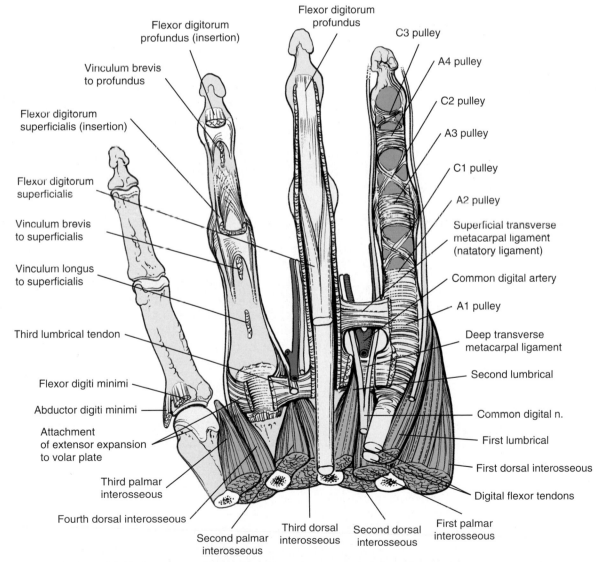

**Figure 5-64**   Anatomy of the web space. The neurovascular bundle runs deep to or dorsal to the superficial transverse ligament (natatory ligament) and palmar to the deep transverse metacarpal ligament. The lumbrical muscle runs along with the neurovascular bundle palmar to the deep transverse ligament, whereas the interossei pass dorsal to the deep transverse metacarpal ligament.

The important structures in the web space are listed below:

1. *Superficial transverse ligament of the palm (natatory ligament).* This ligament lies immediately beneath the palmar skin and supports the free margins of the webs. The ligament runs superficial (palmar) to the digital nerves and vessels, and attaches to the palmar aponeurosis.
2. *Digital nerves and vessels.* These structures lie immediately deep to the superficial transverse ligament of the palm, with the nerves on the palmar side of the arteries.
3. *Tendons of the lumbricals.* These muscles arise from the four tendons of the flexor digitorum profundus muscle in the middle of the palm. Each lumbrical tendon passes along the radial side of its metacarpophalangeal joint before inserting into the extensor expansion on the dorsum of the proximal phalanx. Infection in the web space can spread proximally along the lumbrical tendon and enter the palm (see Fig. 5-66).
4. *Deep transverse ligament of the palm.* This strong ligament connects the volar plates (palmar ligaments) of the metacarpophalangeal joints. It is 3 to 4 cm proximal to the superficial transverse ligaments. The lumbrical tendons are volar or palmar to it, as is the neurovascular bundle (see Fig. 5-64).
5. *Interosseous tendons.* These muscles, which arise from the metacarpals, insert into the dorsal expansion over the proximal phalanges. Their tendons pass dorsal to the deep transverse ligament, in contrast to the lumbrical tendons, which pass on the ligament's volar side (see Fig. 5-64).

## Anatomy of the Web Space of the Thumb

The thumb is far more mobile than are any of the fingers. Its increased mobility is reflected in the unique anatomy of its web space: both the superficial and the deep transverse ligaments are absent and the bulk of the web is filled with two muscles, the transverse head of the adductor pollicis and the first dorsal interosseous (see Figs. 5-33 through 5-35).

### Adductor Pollicis Muscle

See the section regarding the anatomy of the palm.

### First Dorsal Interosseous Muscle

The dorsal interosseous muscle is the largest of all the interossei. It arises from the adjacent borders of the first and second metacarpals, runs deep to the adductor pollicis, and inserts into the fibrous extensor expansion on the dorsum of the index finger. The muscle bulk provides most of the substance of the thumb's web space; wasting is easy to detect clinically by gently pinching the web while the patient pinch-grips. The pinch also forms the basis for one test of an ulnar nerve lesion, because the muscle is supplied by the ulnar nerve (see Fig. 5-9).

### Arteries

Two branches of the radial artery, the radialis indicis and the princeps pollicis, emerge from between the two muscles of the thumb web. The radialis indicis artery runs to the radial border of the index finger, and the princeps pollicis goes to the thumb, where it divides into two palmar digital arteries. Approaches made in the center of the web space avoid damage to either artery (see Fig. 5-35).

## Tendon Sheath Infection

An infection within the synovial sheath of the flexor tendons is one of the most serious of all hand infections. Prompt surgical drainage is critical, for a long-standing infection almost always results in fibrosis within the tendon sheath and subsequent tethering of the tendon itself. Sheath infections are caused by spread from a pulp infection or by puncture wounds, particularly at the flexor creases.

The diagnosis is made clinically. The finger held in a flexed position is grossly swollen and tender. The slightest active or passive extension of the digit produces severe pain, which is the cardinal physical symptom on which the diagnosis is based.

These infections are not as common as they used to be as a result of earlier diagnosis and treatment of superficial finger infections. Nevertheless, they still occur and offer a true orthopaedic emergency.

## Position of the Patient

Place the patient supine on the operating table, with the arm extended on an arm board. A tourniquet is essential, but the arm should not be exsanguinated as it is with general anesthesia or a proximal local block (either brachial or axillary). Good lighting and fine instruments minimize the risk of damaging the vital structures within the hand (see Fig. 5-13).

## Landmarks and Incision

### Landmarks

The *distal palmar crease* roughly marks the palmar site of the metacarpophalangeal joints and the proximal border of the fibrous flexor sheath of the flexor tendons.

The *distal interphalangeal crease* is the surface marking of the distal interphalangeal joint and lies just proximal to the distal end of the fibrous flexor sheath.

### Incision

Make a small transverse incision just proximal to the distal palmar crease and over the infected flexor tendon. The incision should be 1.5 to 2.0 cm long (Fig. 5-65).

A second incision usually is necessary if there is turbid fluid within the sheath. Make a *midlateral* cut

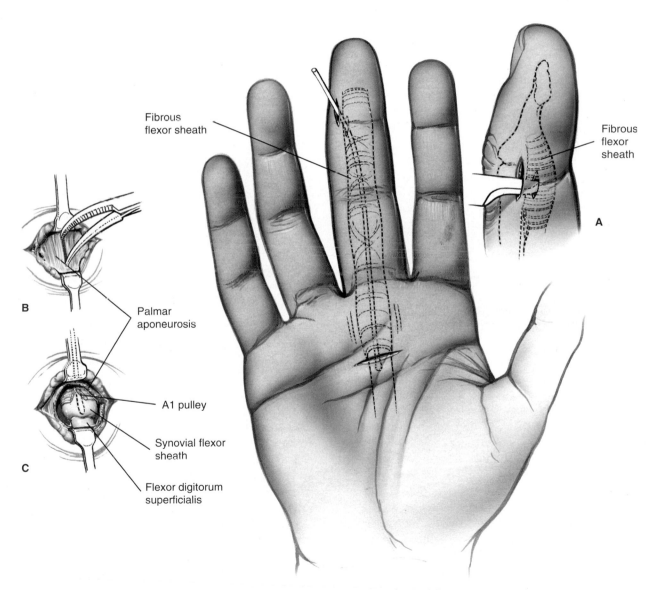

Fibrous flexor sheath

Fibrous flexor sheath

A

B

Palmar aponeurosis

A1 pulley

Synovial flexor sheath

C

Flexor digitorum superficialis

**Figure 5-65**  Incision for infection of the flexor digital sheath. Make a small transverse incision just proximal to the distal palmar crease, over the infected flexor tendon. **(A)** A second incision may be necessary, and this should be made over the distal end of the middle phalanx in the midlateral position. **(B)** Separate the longitudinally running fibers of the palmar aponeurosis. **(C)** Incise the A1 pulley to reveal the underlying synovial sheath, which then should be opened.

over the distal end of the middle phalanx in the line connecting the dorsal ends of the proximal and distal interphalangeal creases (see Fig. 5-65*A*).

## Internervous Plane

There is no internervous plane in this approach. The midlateral approach is roughly in the line of demarcation between skin that is supplied by the digital nerves and skin that is supplied by the dorsal cutaneous nerves.

## Superficial Surgical Dissection

Separate the longitudinally running fibers of the palmar aponeurosis by blunt dissection, by opening a closed hemostat so that the dissection is carried out parallel to, rather than across, the main neurovascular bundles of the palm (see Fig. 5-65*B*). Proceed deeper onto the proximal end of the fibrous flexor sheath. At this level, the proximal (A1) pulley is visible. Incise the pulley longitudinally to reveal turbid fluid or, more rarely, frank pus (see Fig. 5-65*C*). If turbid fluid is found, make the second skin incision and deepen it, coming down dorsal to the digital nerves and vessels. Incise the fibrous flexor sheath at the distal end of the middle phalanx.

This second incision allows through-and-through irrigation to be carried out, if it is required (see Fig. 5-65*A*).

## Dangers

### Nerves

The digital nerves and vessels are at risk in both incisions. If the skin incision in the finger is made too far in a volar direction, it may threaten the neurovascular bundle. The bundle is safe as long as the skin incision remains just dorsal to the dorsal end of the proximal and distal interphalangeal creases (see Fig. 5-65 and Midlateral Approach to the Flexor Sheaths).

Because the skin palmar incision crosses the neurovascular bundles at right angles, and because the bundles lie immediately deep to the palmar aponeurosis, the bundles may be damaged by overzealous incision of the skin. Separating the fibers of the palmar aponeurosis by blunt dissection in the line of the fibers avoids damage to the nerves.

## How to Enlarge the Approach

The approach cannot be enlarged effectively. Infections in the radial or ulnar bursae require a separate incision.

# Deep Palmar Space Infection

Deep palmar infections are extremely serious; they often lead to diminished hand function. The infected area usually lies deep to the flexor tendons and lumbricals, but superficial to the metacarpals and their muscles, the adductor pollicis and the interossei.

The central compartment of the palm is subdivided by a septum of fascia that arises from the fascia surrounding the flexor tendons of the middle finger and attaches to the third metacarpal. The area on the lateral side of the septum sometimes is called the thenar space, and the area on the medial side is called the midpalmar space. In this text, the terms *lateral space* and *medial space* are used, because the term *thenar space* can be confusing, as this area has nothing to do with the space that is occupied by the thenar muscles of the thenar eminence (Fig. 5-66; see Fig. 5-34).

Infections of the medial space cause local pain, tenderness, and swelling of the palm. The middle and ring fingers lose their ability to move actively, and moving them passively produces severe pain. The hand is grossly swollen, resembling an inflated rubber glove.

Infections of the lateral space produce symptoms and signs similar to those of infections of the medial space, but the index finger and thumb are the digits that lose the ability to move.

Deep palmar infections are among the rarest encountered in hand surgery. These deep infections are being seen more frequently now, however, primarily because of the increase in drug addiction. More than any other infection in the hand, they can cause systemic illness associated with high fevers.

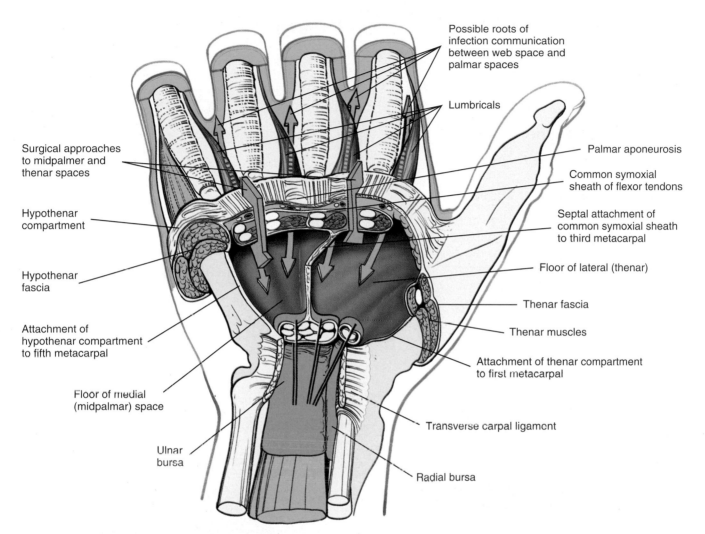

Possible roots of infection communication between web space and palmar spaces

Lumbricals

Surgical approaches to midpalmer and thenar spaces

Hypothenar compartment

Hypothenar fascia

Attachment of hypothenar compartment to fifth metacarpal

Floor of medial (midpalmar) space

Ulnar bursa

Palmar aponeurosis

Common symoxial sheath of flexor tendons

Septal attachment of common symoxial sheath to third metacarpal

Floor of lateral (thenar)

Thenar fascia

Thenar muscles

Attachment of thenar compartment to first metacarpal

Transverse carpal ligament

Radial bursa

**Figure 5-66** Within the central compartment of the palm, a potential deep space exists between the undersurface of the flexor tendons and the upper surfaces of the interossei and adductor pollicis muscles. This deep palmar space is subdivided into medial midpalmar and lateral thenar spaces by the oblique septum that arises from the connective tissue surrounding the middle finger flexor tendons and runs to the palmar surface of the middle metacarpal. Infections involving the web space may travel along the lumbrical muscle to enter these two potential spaces.

# Drainage of the Medial (Midpalmar) Space

## Incision

Make a curved transverse incision on the palm just proximal to the distal palmar crease and over the swelling. The length of the incision should be determined by the size of the abscess to be drained (Fig. 5-67).

## Internervous Plane

There is no internervous plane in this approach.

## Superficial Surgical Dissection

Incise the skin carefully; the line of the skin incision crosses the paths of the digital nerves. Open the palmar fascia by blunt dissection at the distal end of the wound and identify the long flexor tendon to the ring finger. Enter the medial midpalmar space by blunt dissection on the radial border of this tendon (Figs. 5-68 through 5-70).

## Dangers

### Nerves

The **digital nerves** to the little and ring fingers run immediately under the palmar aponeurosis and cross the line of the skin incision. No part of the palmar aponeurosis should be incised transversely until these nerves have been dissected out fully (see Fig. 5-69).

### Vessels

The **digital arteries** run with the digital nerves and also may be in danger. For this reason, the digital arteries should be identified before the palmar aponeurosis is incised.

## How to Enlarge the Approach

The incision, which is a drainage procedure, cannot be extended usefully.

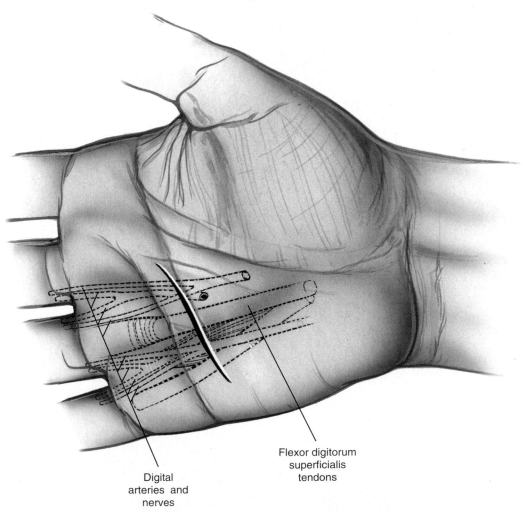

Digital
arteries and
nerves

Flexor digitorum
superficialis
tendons

**Figure 5-67**   Incision for drainage of the medial space (midpalmar space).

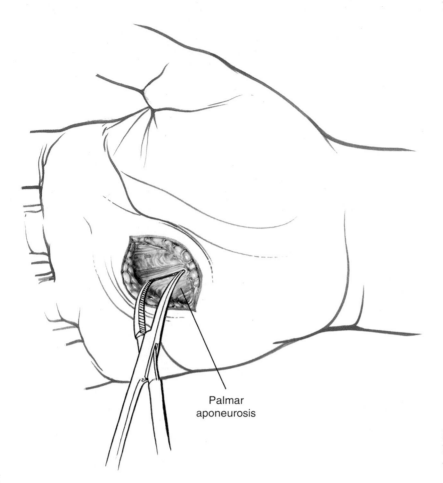

Palmar
aponeurosis

**Figure 5-68**   Open the palmar fascia
by blunt dissection at the distal end of
the wound.

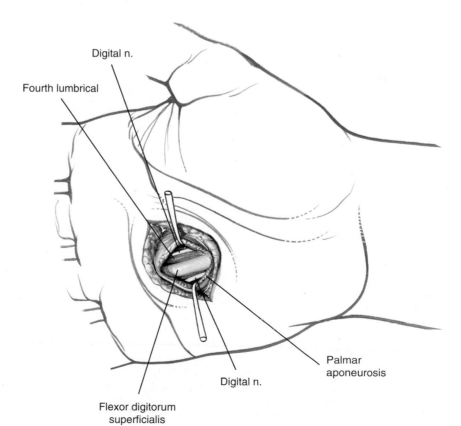

Digital n.

Fourth lumbrical

Palmar
aponeurosis

Digital n.

Flexor digitorum
superficialis

**Figure 5-69**   The long flexor
tendon to the ring finger is
identified. The neurovascular
structures run parallel to it on each
side, and the lumbrical is visible on
its radial side.

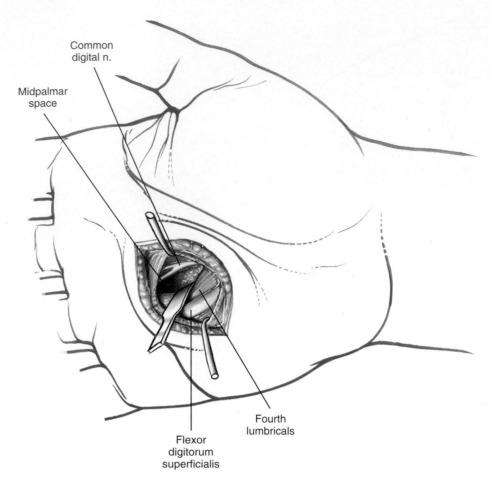

Common
digital n.

Midpalmar
space

Fourth
lumbricals

Flexor
digitorum
superficialis

**Figure 5-70**   The deep palmar space is entered by retracting the lumbrical and its tendon medially.

# Drainage of the Lateral (Thenar) Space

## Incision

Make a curved incision about 4 cm long, just on the ulnar side of the thenar crease (Fig. 5-71).

## Internervous Plane

There is no internervous plane in this approach.

## Superficial Surgical Dissection

Deepen the dissection in line with the skin incision, taking care to identify and preserve the digital nerves to the index finger. Identify the long flexor tendon to the index finger (Figs. 5-72 and 5-73). Deep to these tendons is the lateral space; enter it by blunt dissection (Fig. 5-74).

## Dangers

### Nerves

The **digital nerves** to the index finger are directly in line with the skin incision. Take care not to damage them during incision of the palmar aponeurosis.

The **motor branch to the thenar muscles** emerges from the deep surface of the median nerve as the median nerve leaves the carpal tunnel. Note, however, that the location of its division from the median nerve is quite variable. This nerve hooks around the distal end of the flexor retinaculum to supply the muscles. Make sure to identify the branch at the proximal end of the incision so as to avoid damaging it (see Fig. 5-32).

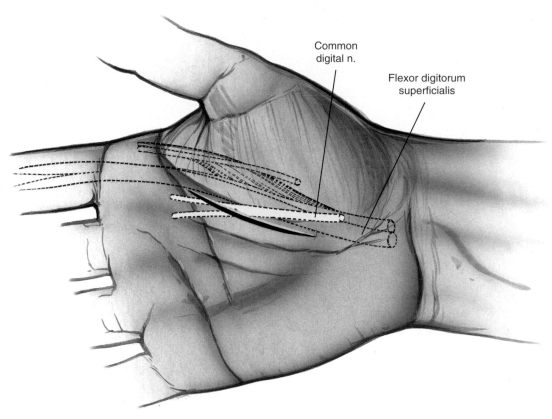

Common
digital n.

Flexor digitorum
superficialis

**Figure 5-71** Incision for drainage of the lateral space (thenar space). The incision is made just to the ulnar side of the thenar crease.

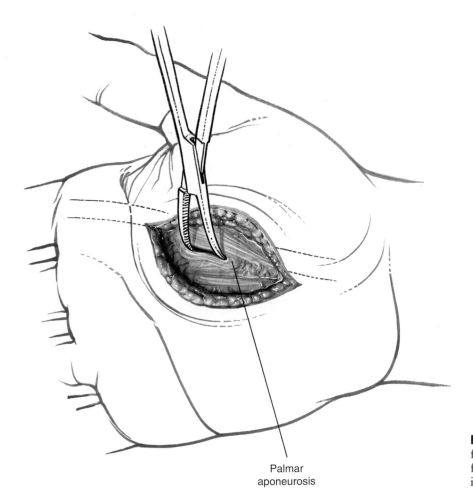

Palmar
aponeurosis

**Figure 5-72** Identify the palmar fascia and spread it in line with its fibers over the flexor tendon to the index finger.

**235**

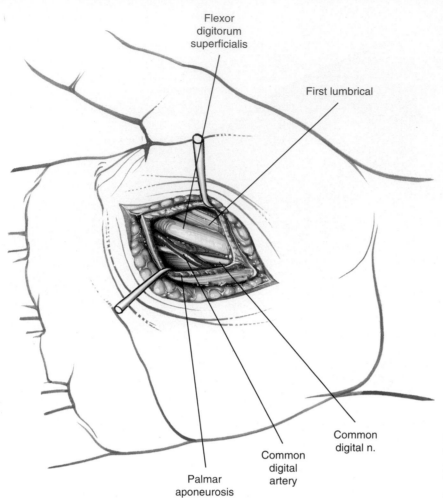

Flexor
digitorum
superficialis

First lumbrical

Common
digital n.

Common
digital
artery

Palmar
aponeurosis

**Figure 5-73**  Identify the flexor tendon to the index finger. The neurovascular bundles lie to each side. The lumbrical is seen on the radial side.

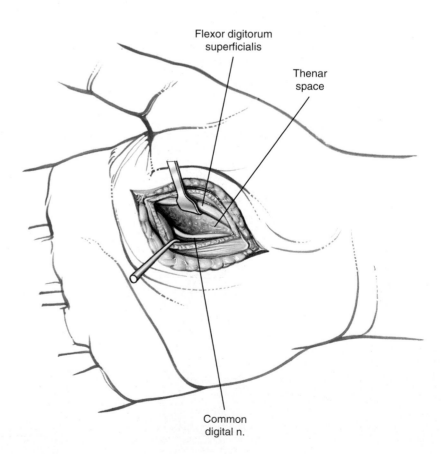

Flexor digitorum
superficialis

Thenar
space

Common
digital n.

**Figure 5-74**  Retract the tendon and lumbrical radially, and enter the space beneath them by blunt dissection.

# Applied Surgical Anatomy of the Deep Palmar Space

The palm is divided into spaces by fibrous septa that pass through it before attaching to the metacarpals. There are two major septa: the *thenar septum* originates from the palmar aponeurosis and inserts into the first metacarpal, separating the three muscles of the thenar eminence from the central palmar structures; and the *hypothenar septum* originates on the ulnar side of the palmar aponeurosis and inserts into the fifth metacarpal, separating the three muscles of the hypothenar eminence from the central palmar structures (see Figs. 5-34 and 5-66).

Thus, the palm is divided into three compartments: a thenar compartment, a hypothenar compartment, and a central compartment.

The central compartment contains the long flexor tendons to the fingers and the adductor pollicis muscle, as well as the digital nerves and vessels and the superficial and deep palmar arches.

Within the central compartment, a *potential deep space* exists between the undersurface of the flexor tendons and the upper surface of the interosseous and adductor pollicis muscles. This deep palmar space is divided into medial (midpalmar) and lateral (thenar) spaces by the *oblique septum* that arises from the connective tissue surrounding the middle finger flexor tendons and runs to the palmar surface of the middle metacarpal.[28] This septum is the anatomic basis for the clinical division of deep palmar infection into two distinct, separate spaces.[27]

## Lateral Space (Thenar Space)

The lateral space usually contains the first lumbrical muscle, which runs with the long flexor tendon to the index finger. Infections in the first web space may track down into the lateral space along the lumbrical muscle, although this is rare. Although lateral space infections may be drained through the first web space, such an incision drains less thoroughly than does the procedure described in the previous section (see Figs. 5-71 through 5-74).

The space lies anterior to the adductor pollicis muscle. A second potential space exists behind that muscle and in front of the interossei. Infection of this "posterior adductor space" is very rare.[29]

## Medial Space (Midpalmar Space)

The medial space contains the lumbrical muscles for the middle, ring, and little fingers, which run from the long flexor tendons of the middle, ring, and little fingers (the volar boundary of the space). The deep boundary is formed by the interossei and metacarpals of the third and fourth spaces. Thus, infection in the web spaces between the middle and ring fingers, and between the ring and little fingers, in theory, may spread to the medial space (see Fig. 5-66). The medial space may be drained through an incision in these webs, but the result is not as good as that obtained with direct drainage (see Figs. 5-67 through 5-70).

# Drainage of the Radial Bursa

The long flexor tendon of the thumb is surrounded by a synovial sheath that extends from the tendon's insertion into the distal phalanx through the palm and carpal tunnel to the forearm just proximal to the proximal end of the flexor retinaculum. The proximal end of this sheath is known as the radial bursa (Fig. 5-75).

Infection of this space is diagnosed on the same clinical grounds as are infections of the synovial sheaths of the other fingers: fusiform swelling of the thumb, with extreme pain on active or passive extension of the digit.

## Position of the Patient

Place the patient supine on the operating table, with the arm on an arm board. A general anesthetic or an axillary or brachial block is essential. Use a nonexsanguinating tourniquet and have an excellent light source available (see Fig. 5-12).

## Landmark and Incision

### Landmark

The *interphalangeal crease of the thumb* is the surface marking for the interphalangeal joint of the thumb. It lies just proximal to the distal end of the fibrous flexor sheath of the thumb.

### Incision

Two incisions are required for complete drainage. First, make a small longitudinal incision on the lateral side of the proximal phalanx of the thumb, just

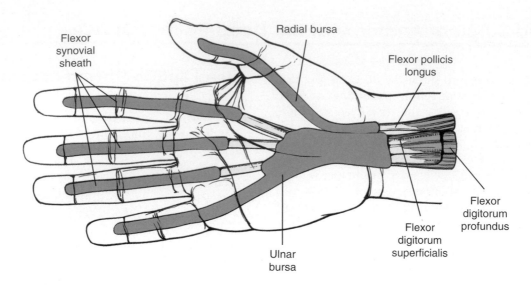

**Figure 5-75** Anatomy of the synovial sheaths of the fingers and the radial and ulnar bursae.

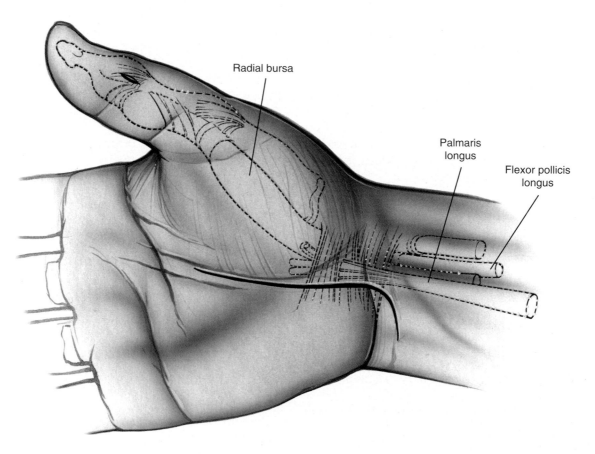

**Figure 5-76** Incision for drainage of the radial bursa. Two incisions are required for complete drainage. Distally, make a small longitudinal incision on the lateral side of the proximal phalanx of the thumb, just dorsal to the interphalangeal crease. Make a second incision over the medial aspect of the thenar eminence on the volar aspect of the wrist, and carry the incision proximally to the end of the radial bursa. Care must be taken to protect the median nerve and its motor branch to the thenar muscles.

dorsal to the dorsal termination of the interphalangeal crease (Fig. 5-76). Then, make a second incision over the medial aspect of the thenar eminence (beware of the motor branch) or on the volar aspect of the wrist (the proximal end of the radial bursa).

## Internervous Plane

There is no internervous plane in this approach. The skin incision in the finger lies between skin that is supplied by the dorsal digital nerves and skin that is supplied by the volar digital nerves.

## Superficial Surgical Dissection

Deepen the wound in line with the first skin incision, remaining dorsal to the radial neurovascular bundle of the thumb. Identify the fibrous flexor sheath covering the flexor pollicis longus tendon and incise it longitudinally, just proximal to the tendon's insertion into the distal phalanx. Incise the synovium within the sheath to drain the pus.

Now, pass a probe proximally along the flexor sheath until the point of the probe can be felt on the volar aspect of the wrist. Make a small longitudinal skin incision over this point and dissect carefully down to the probe. The tip of the probe may be proximal to the proximal end of the flexor retinaculum, or it may be actually in the carpal tunnel itself. If it is in the carpal tunnel, then formally incise the flexor retinaculum, taking great care not to damage the underlying median nerve with its motor branch to the thenar eminence. This is the only situation in which the median nerve is approached necessarily from its radial aspect in the carpal tunnel.

As is the case in the treatment of tendon sheath infections, a small catheter may be left in the distal end of the flexor sheath to irrigate the flexor tendon (Fig. 5-77).

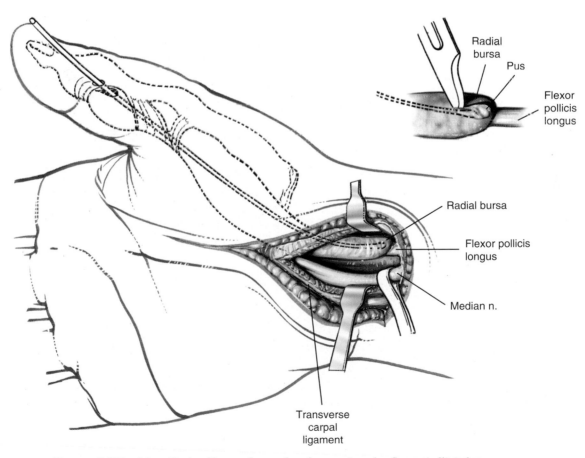

**Figure 5-77**   Identify the fibrous flexor sheath covering the flexor pollicis longus tendon and incise it longitudinally just proximal to the tendon's insertion into the distal phalanx. Incise the synovium in the sheath to drain the pus and then pass a probe proximally along the flexor sheath. Make a small longitudinal incision over the probe at the level of the wrist to ensure complete drainage.

## Dangers

If the midlateral approach to the thumb is made too far in a volar direction, its radial neurovascular bundle may be incised accidentally.

## Special Points

Do not cut blindly down on the tip of the probe at the wrist; the median nerve, the motor branch of the median nerve, or the palmar cutaneous branch of the median nerve may be cut (see Applied Surgical Anatomy of the Volar Aspect of the Wrist).

## How to Enlarge the Approach

This approach cannot be enlarged effectively by either local or extensile measures.

# Drainage of the Ulnar Bursa

The synovial sheath surrounding the flexor tendons to the little finger extends from the insertion of the profundus tendon on the distal phalanx of the little finger to the volar aspect of the wrist, just proximal to the proximal end of the flexor retinaculum. The flexor tendons to the index, middle, and ring fingers also are invested by this layer of synovium as they pass through the carpal tunnel. The distal extension of the synovial compartment ends at the origin of the lumbrical muscle from the tendons to the ring, middle, and index fingers. It is known as the ulnar bursa (see Fig. 5-75).

Infection of the synovial sheath of the little finger may lead to infection of the ulnar bursa. The physical signs include a tenosynovitis affecting the little finger, with active or passive extension producing extreme pain. In addition, pain may be referred to the palm when the other fingers are extended.

## Position of the Patient

Place the patient supine on the operating table, with the arm extended on an arm board. Use a nonexsanguinating tourniquet and either a general anesthetic or a proximal local block (an axillary or brachial block).

## Landmark and Incision

### Landmark

The *distal interphalangeal crease of the little finger* is the surface marking for the distal interphalangeal joint. It lies just proximal to the distal end of the fibrous sheath of the little finger.

### Incision

Make a short midline incision on the ulnar side of the little finger over the distal end of the middle phalanx (Fig. 5-78, *inset*). The incision should be just dorsal to the line connecting the dorsal termination of the proximal and distal interphalangeal creases. Make a second longitudinal incision on the lateral aspect of the hypothenar eminence at the level of the wrist.

## Internervous Plane

There is no internervous plane. The finger skin incision lies between skin that is supplied by the dorsal digital nerves and skin that is supplied by the volar digital nerves.

## Superficial Surgical Dissection

Deepen the approach in line with the incision, staying to the dorsal side of the neurovascular bundle. Identify the fibrous flexor sheath and incise it longitudinally. Next, incise the synovium to allow drainage of the pus. Pass a probe gently along the tendon until it can be felt on the volar aspect of the wrist, just proximal to the proximal end of the flexor retinaculum.

Carefully incise the skin longitudinally over the probe and dissect down to it layer by layer. The probe should be just proximal to the proximal end of the flexor retinaculum. It may be in the carpal tunnel, however, in which case, the flexor retinaculum will have to be incised meticulously, taking care to avoid damage to the underlying median nerve. If the probe is lying in the forearm, then take great care not to damage the ulnar nerve and artery, which are very close to the flexor digitorum superficialis tendon to the little finger (see Fig. 5-78).

As is true in the case of other tendon sheath infections, a small catheter may be inserted in the distal wound to allow continuous or intermittent irrigation of the tendon sheath.

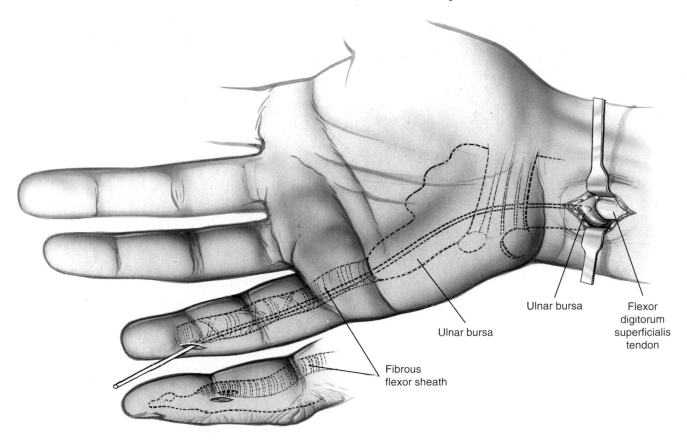

**Figure 5-78**   Drainage of the ulnar bursa. Make a short midline incision on the ulnar side of the little finger over the distal end of the middle phalanx. Make a second longitudinal incision over the lateral aspect of the hyperthenar eminence at the level of the wrist. Pass a probe from the distal aspect to the proximal aspect, and cut down onto the probe at its proximal end, a point that marks the proximal end of the ulnar bursa.

## Dangers

The digital nerve to the ulnar side of the little finger is in danger if the skin incision on the finger is made too far in a volar direction. The distal vessels run with the nerves.

## How to Enlarge the Approach

The approach cannot be enlarged effectively by either local or extensile measures.

## Anatomy of the Hand

Two characteristics of the normal hand reveal what happens when it is damaged:

1. The hand has a *natural resting position*. At rest, both the metacarpophalangeal and the interphalangeal joints normally hold a position of slight flexion. The fingers all adopt a slightly different degree of rotation, such that the volar surfaces of the terminal phalanges face progressively more toward the thumb as one moves from the index finger to the little finger. It is critical to appreciate the different degrees of rotation in the finger when assessing displacement in phalangeal or metacarpal fractures. The degree of flexion increases as one passes from the index finger to the little finger. This configuration is a result of muscle balance; if one element is deficient or absent, the resting position of the hand changes.

In cases of acute trauma, a cut flexor tendon may leave a finger extended. An abnormal resting position often is indicative of tendon damage.

2. The concept of *muscle balance* also can be applied to chronic conditions of the hand. In patients with long-standing ulnar nerve lesions, in which the intrinsic muscles of the hand are paralyzed, the hand develops an abnormal attitude because of muscle imbalance. The intrinsic muscles normally flex the fingers at the metacarpophalangeal joints and extend them at the proximal and distal interphalangeal joints. The absence of intrinsic function leads to extension of the metacarpophalangeal joints and flexion of the proximal and distal interphalangeal joints of the affected fingers, resulting in an ulnar clawhand.

## Palm

### Skin

The skin of the palm and the palmar aspect of the fingers is a tough structure, characterized by flexure creases in the palm and fingerprints in the fingers. The skin has very little laxity because of the series of tough fibrous bands that tie it to the palmar aponeurosis. These bands divide the subcutaneous fat into small loculi, which are capable of withstanding considerable pressure. The skin's lack of mobility means that it is difficult to close even small defects in it without resorting to plastic procedures such as *V-Y advancement flaps* or skin grafting.

The blood supply of the palmar skin is extremely good, and even long, distally based flaps may survive. In an elective incision, however, the angle at the apex of a triangular flap should be more than 60°, and distally based flaps should be avoided, if possible.

To avoid flexion contractures, the flexure creases should not be crossed at 90°. Cutting within a flexure crease itself avoids this problem, but the wound created is difficult to close without inverting the skin edges. That is the reason that many incisions parallel natural flexure creases.

### Palmar Aponeurosis

The palmar aponeurosis is a tough fibrous sheath that lies under the skin of the palm (see Fig. 5-30). It is continuous with the tendon of the palmaris longus muscle, spreading distally from the distal border of the flexor retinaculum to cover the central area of the palm between the thenar and hypothenar eminences. At the bases of the fingers, it divides into four bands, one for each finger. At the level of the distal palmar crease, these bands divide into two and run into the fingers to insert into the bases of the proximal phalanges and the fibrous flexor sheaths (see Fig. 5-30).

The nerves and vessels to the palm lie immediately deep to the palmar aponeurosis and actually are in contact with its deep surface. In patients with Dupuytren's contracture, the palmar fascia thickens; contracted and fibrous tissue grows all around the digital nerves and vessels to enclose them.[30]

The fascia over the thenar and hypothenar muscles is thinner than that over the central palm because of the greater mobility required from the first and fifth digits.

The palmar aponeurosis has deep connections to the first and fifth metacarpals at its lateral and medial borders, dividing the hand into three major compartments: the thenar, hypothenar, and palmar spaces. There also are deep connections between the palmar aponeurosis and the metacarpals in the distal part of the hand (see Fig. 5-33).

### Thenar Muscles

The thenar eminence consists of three short muscles: the abductor pollicis brevis, the flexor pollicis brevis, and the opponens pollicis (see Figs. 5-33 and 5-34). All three are supplied by the median nerve via its motor branch, which enters the eminence between the short abductor and the flexor.

The flexor pollicis brevis also receives a nerve supply from the ulnar nerve to its deep head. This dual nerve supply explains the clinical observation that a complete median nerve palsy does not necessarily produce complete flattening of the thenar eminence, because the bulky deep head of the flexor pollicis brevis does not atrophy.

The three short muscles of the thumb lie in two layers. The superficial layer consists of the short abductor and the short flexor, with the abductor lying on the radial side of the flexor. The deep layer consists of the opponens pollicis, which produces rotation of the thumb metacarpal at its saddle-shaped joint with the trapezium. The ability to oppose the thumb and the other fingers is one of the major structural advantages that the human hand has over the ape hand. It is a complex movement requiring several muscles. The abductor pollicis brevis abducts the thumb, rotation is achieved by the opponens pollicis, and the movement is completed by the thumb flexors. The abductor pollicis brevis is the most important muscle in this group. Median nerve paralysis destroys opposition; the resultant hand often is known as a simian (apelike) hand.

### Hypothenar Muscles

The hypothenar eminence consists of three muscles: the abductor digiti minimi, the flexor digiti minimi, and the opponens digiti minimi. These muscles (all of which are supplied by the ulnar nerve) are arranged in the same layering as are those of the thenar eminence. The superficial layer consists of the abductor and flexor, with the abductor lying on the ulnar side; the deep layer consists of the opponens digiti minimi. Together, these muscles help deepen the cup of the palm of the hand. Very little genuine opposition of the fifth finger is possible compared with that of the thumb (see Figs. 5-33 and 5-34).

Lying superficial to the muscles of the hypothenar eminence is the palmaris brevis muscle, the only muscle that is supplied by the superficial branch of the ulnar nerve.

## Nerves and Vessels

The second layer of the palm consists of the superficial nerves and vessels (see Figs. 5-32 and 5-33).

The *superficial palmar arch* is an arterial arcade that is formed largely by the ulnar artery. The arcade is completed by the superficial palmar branch of the radial artery, but this branch often is missing. When it is, the arch remains incomplete. Four *palmar digital arteries* arise from the arcade and pass distally. The most ulnar of the arteries supplies the ulnar border of the little fingers; the other three common digital arteries divide in the web space into two vessels that supply adjacent fingers.

Note that this arterial arcade is superficial to the nerves in the palm, an arrangement that is opposite of that of the finger, and that the thumb and the radial side of the index finger are not supplied by its branches.

The *digital nerves* lie immediately deep to the superficial palmar arch. The ulnar nerve divides into a superficial and a deep branch at the distal border of the flexor retinaculum. The superficial branch supplies the ulnar 1½ fingers with sensation. The median nerve divides into two sensory branches after giving off its motor branch to the thenar muscles. The medial branch supplies the radial side of the ring finger, the middle finger, and the ulnar side of the index finger. The lateral branch supplies the radial side of the index finger and the whole of the thumb.

## Long Flexor Tendons

The third layer of structures in the palm is composed of the long flexor tendons. The tendons of the flexor digitorum superficialis muscle overlie those of the flexor digitorum profundus muscle. Each flexor profundus tendon gives rise to a lumbrical muscle, which passes along the radial side of the metacarpophalangeal joint before inserting into the extensor expansion from the dorsum of the proximal phalanx. Lumbricals that arise by two heads from adjacent profundus tendons (usually the ulnar two) are supplied by the ulnar nerve; lumbricals that arise from one tendon (usually the radial two) are supplied by the median nerve.

## Deep Palmar Arch

The deep palmar arch, which is an arterial arcade, lies deep to the long flexor tendons and forms a fourth layer in the palm (see Figs. 5-34 and 5-35). The arterial arch consists of the terminal branch of the radial artery, which enters the palm by passing between the oblique and transverse heads of the adductor pollicis muscle, and the deep branch of the ulnar artery. Running with the ulnar artery is the deep branch of the ulnar nerve, which supplies all the interossei with muscular branches at this level.

## Deep Muscles of the Palm

The adductor pollicis muscle and the interossei are the deepest muscles in the palm (see Fig. 5-35).

The interossei can be divided into two groups, dorsal and palmar. The dorsal interossei arise by two heads from adjacent sides of the metacarpals and insert into the proximal phalanges so that they abduct the fingers away from the line drawn through the center of the third finger.

The three palmar interossei are much smaller. Each arises from only one metacarpal and inserts into the base of the proximal phalanx, adducting the finger toward the middle finger.

All interossei are supplied by the deep branch of the ulnar nerve. (The function of the interossei can be remembered by the mnemonics "PAD" and "DAB": the *p*almar interossei *ad*duct, and the *d*orsal interossei *ab*duct.)[31]

## Other Structures

Two structures in the palm, the deep branch of the ulnar nerve and the radial artery, have courses that do not follow the layering concept. The way in which they run through the wrist and hand ties the rest of the anatomy together.

The *radial artery* lies on the volar aspect of the distal radius. It reaches the dorsum of the hand under the tendons of the abductor pollicis longus muscle and the extensor pollicis brevis muscle, lying on the scaphoid bone in the anatomic snuffbox. To return to the volar aspect of the palm, it pierces the deepest layer of the palmar structures, passing between the two heads of the first dorsal interosseous muscle. At that point, it gives off two branches, the radialis indicis artery and the princeps pollicis artery, which supply the index finger and thumb, respectively. The main arterial trunk then passes between the two heads of the adductor pollicis and lies superficial to the deepest muscles as it forms the deep palmar arch.

The *ulnar nerve* enters the hand superficial to the flexor retinaculum within the canal of Guyon. There, it divides into superficial and deep branches (see Fig. 5-31). The superficial branch gives off digital nerves and lies in the same plane as the superficial arterial arcade. The deep branch descends through the layers of the palm, passing between the heads of origin of the opponens digiti minimi to lie on the interossei in the same plane as the radial artery. There, it supplies all the interossei, the two ulnar lumbrical muscles, both heads of the adductor pollicis muscle, the three hypothenar muscles, and the deep head of the flexor pollicis brevis muscle (see Figs. 5-34 and 5-35).

## Dorsum of the Hand

The anatomy of the dorsum of the hand is far simpler than that of the palm. The *skin* is thinner than the palmar skin and is more mobile to allow for finger flexion. The subcutaneous tissue contains very little fat, but a large number of veins. Venous return runs via the dorsum of the hand because the pressure of gripping otherwise would impede it. The blood supply of the dorsal skin is not as good as that of the palmar skin, and distally based skin flaps are less likely to survive.

The backs of the radial 3½ digits are supplied by the terminal branches of the superficial radial nerve as far as the middle of the middle phalanx. The ends of these fingers are supplied by branches of the median nerve that are derived from the volar digital nerves.

The dorsal aspects of the ulnar 1½ digits are supplied by the ulnar nerve, the proximal 1½ phalanges are supplied by dorsal branches of the ulnar nerve, and the distal 1½ phalanges are supplied by branches of the ulnar nerve (the volar digital nerves).

The clinical importance of this arrangement is that the terminal phalanx, including the nail bed, can be anesthetized by an injection of local anesthetic around the volar digital nerves.

The only tendons of the dorsum of the hand are those of the long extensors. Just proximal to the metacarpophalangeal joint, these tendons are united by three oblique bands, which limit retraction of the tendon if it is cut. As each long extensor tendon passes over its metacarpophalangeal joint, its deepest part becomes continuous with the dorsal capsule of that joint. The tendon becomes much broader before dividing into three slips over the dorsal surface of the proximal phalanx. The central slip inserts into the base of the middle phalanx and the two marginal slips receive attachments from interossei and lumbrical tendons to form a broad extensor expansion, or hood, which overlies the metacarpal head and the proximal part of the proximal phalanx. The hood is anchored firmly on each side to the volar plate of the metacarpophalangeal joint. Each hood receives some of the insertion of each of two interossei, with the rest going to the proximal phalanx itself. The amount varies considerably from finger to finger. The entire insertion of the lumbrical tendon attaches to the extensor hood (see Fig. 5-9).

Over the dorsum of the middle phalanx, the intrinsic tendons are joined to each other by transversely running fibers (the triangular ligament). Initially, the two marginal slips of the long extensor tendon pass outward from the midline to insert into the base of the distal phalanx. By inserting into this extensor expansion from the palmar side, the lumbrical and interosseous muscles not only can abduct and adduct the fingers at the metacarpophalangeal joint, but also can flex the metacarpophalangeal joint while extending the distal and proximal interphalangeal joints. In this way, each extended finger can be flexed independently.

Disruption of the central slip of the extensor tendon and the triangular ligament may produce a flexion deformity at the proximal interphalangeal joint. The two marginal slips then pass volar to the joint and act as flexors of that joint, and the joint "buttonholes" between these two slips. This deformity is known as a boutonniere deformity or, as the French put it, "le buttonhole."

## REFERENCES

1. KESSLER I, VAINIK K: Posterior (dorsal) synovectomy for rheumatoid involvement of the hand and wrist: a follow up study of sixty six procedures. J Bone Joint Surg [Am] 48: 1035, 1966
2. KULICK RG, DEFIORE JC, STRAUB LR ET AL: Long term results of dorsal stabilization in the rheumatoid wrist. J Hand Surg [Am] 6:272, 1981
3. MACKENZIE IG: Arthrodesis of the wrist in reconstructive surgery. J Bone Joint Surg [Br] 42:60, 1960
4. JORGENSEN EC: Proximal row carpectomy. J Bone Joint Surg [Am] 51:1104, 1969
5. CRABBE NA: Excision of the proximal row of the carpus. J Bone Joint Surg [Br] 46:708, 1964
6. RING D, JUPITER JB, BRENNWALD J ET AL: Prospective multicenter trial of a plate for dorsal fixation of distal radius fractures. J Hand Surg [Am] 22(5):777, 1997
7. PHALEN GS, GARDNER WJ, LALONDE AA: Neuropathy of the median nerve due to compression beneath the transverse carpal ligament. J Bone Joint Surg [Am] 32:109, 1950
8. DOYLE JR, CARROLL RE: The carpal tunnel syndrome: a review of 100 patients treated surgically. Calif Med J 108:263, 1968
9. SONDERLAND S: Nerves and nerve injuries. Baltimore, Williams & Wilkins, 1968
10. SPINNER M: Injuries to the major branches of peripheral nerves in the forearm. Philadelphia, WB Saunders, 1978:215
11. STELLBRINK G: Compression of the palmar branch of the median nerve by atypical palmaris longus muscle. Handchirurgie 4:155, 1972
12. KAPLAN EB: Functional and surgical anatomy of the hand. Philadelphia, JB Lippincott, 1953
13. JOHNSON EK, SHREWSBURY MM: Anatomical course of the thenar branch of the median nerve—usually in a separate tunnel through the transverse carpal ligament. J Bone Joint Surg [Am] 52:269, 1970
14. ENTIN MA: Carpal tunnel syndrome and its variants. Surg Clin North Am 48:1097, 1968
15. MANNERFELT L, HYBRINETTE CH: Important anomaly of the thenar branch of the median nerve. Bull Hosp Jt Dis 33:15, 1972

16. GRAHAM WP III: Variations of the motor branch of the median nerve at the wrist. Plast Reconstr Surg 51:90, 1973
17. LANZ V: Anatomical variations of the median nerve in the carpal tunnel. J Hand Surg [Am] 2:44, 1977
18. BRUNER JM: The flexor tendons in the hand. J Bone Joint Surg [Am] 53:84, 1973
19. MILFORD L: The hand. In: Edmonson AS, Crenshaw AH, eds. Campbell's operative orthopaedics. St Louis, CV Mosby, 1980
20. FURLONG R: Injuries of the hand. Boston, Little, Brown & Co, 1957
21. BUNNELL S: The early treatment of hand injuries. J Bone Joint Surg [Am] 33:807, 1951
22. OCHIAAI N, MATSUI T, MIYAJI ET AL: Vascular anatomy of flexor tendon, I: vincular system and blood supply of the profundus tendon in the digital sheath. J Hand Surg [Am] 4:321, 1979
23. LUNDBORG G, MYRHAGE R, RYDEVIK B: The vascularization of human flexor tendons within the digital synovial sheath region: Structural and functional aspects. J Hand Surg [Am] 2:417, 1977
24. RUSSE O: Fracture of the carpal navicular. J Bone Joint Surg [Am] 42:759, 1960
25. HERBERT TJ, FISHER WE: Management of the fractured scaphoid using a new bone screw. J Bone Joint Surg [Br] 66B:114, 1984
26. TALEISNIK J, KELLY PJ: The extraosseous and interosseous blood supply of the scaphoid bone. J Bone Joint Surg [Am] 48:1125, 1966
27. KANAVEL AB: Infections of the hand: a guide to the surgical treatment of acute and chronic suppurative processes in the fingers, hands, and forearm, 7th ed. Philadelphia, Lea & Febiger, 1939
28. FLYNN JE: Clinical and anatomical investigations of deep fascial space infections of the hand. Am J Surg 55:467, 1942
29. LANNON J: The posterior adductor and posterior interosseous spaces of the hand. S Afr Med J 22:283, 1948
30. DUPUYTREN G: Permanent retraction of the fingers produced by an affection of the palmar fascia. Lancet 2:222, 1834
31. LAST RJ: Anatomy regional and applied, 6th ed. Edinburgh, Churchill Livingstone, 1978

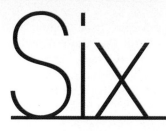

# Six

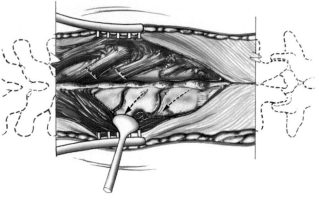

# The Spine

The anatomy of the spine varies from region to region. The cervical spine is light, small, and flexible; the thoracic spine is larger and relatively immobile because of its associated ribs. The lumbar spine, especially the lower part, has more mobility than the thoracic spine, but less than the cervical spine. Pathology is seen most commonly in the cervical and lumbar spines, which are the most mobile portions of the axial skeleton; they require surgery most frequently.

It is important to be able to reach the spine surgically through either an anterior or a posterior approach to treat pathology of its anterior and posterior elements. Pathologies such as vertebral body infection, fracture, and tumor often require anterior approaches. There are many anterior approaches to the spinal column; we present the basic ones that allow access to all the anterior parts of the spine.

Posterior approaches are used more often. The midline posterior approaches are the most common, permitting access to all the posterior spinal elements, as well as to the spinal cord and intervertebral discs.

Frequently, portions of the spine must be fused. Because the ilium is the best site from which to obtain bone graft material, this chapter concludes with the anterior and posterior approaches to the ilium that are used in conjunction with spinal approaches.

# Posterior Approach to the Lumbar Spine

The posterior approach is the most common approach to the lumbar spine. Besides providing access to the cauda equina and the intervertebral discs, it can expose the posterior elements of the spine: the spinous processes, laminae, facet joints, and pedicles. The approach is through the midline, and it may be extended proximally and distally.

The uses of the posterior approach include the following:

1. Excision of herniated discs[1]
2. Exploration of nerve roots[2]
3. Spinal fusion[3,4]
4. Removal of tumors[5]

## Position of the Patient

The posterior approach can be undertaken with the patient in either of two positions:

1. Place the patient in a prone position. Be sure that bolsters are placed longitudinally under the patient's sides to allow the abdomen to be entirely free, reducing venous plexus filling around the spinal cord by permitting the venous plexus to drain directly into the inferior vena cava (Fig. 6-1A).
2. Place the patient on his or her side, with the affected side upward. Flex the patient's hips and knees to flex the lumbar spine and open up the interspinous spaces. Make sure that the patient is positioned with the involved spinal level over the table break. Jackknifing the table can open further the intervertebral space on the upper side of the patient by putting the lumbar spine into lateral flexion. One advantage of this position is that it allows the surgeon to sit. Extravasated blood drains down, away from the operative field (see Fig. 6-1B).

For both positions, use a cold-light headlamp to illuminate the deepest layers around the spinal cord.

## Landmarks and Incision

### Landmarks

The *spinous processes* are easily palpable. Note that a line drawn between the highest points on the *iliac crest* is in the L4-5 interspace. The line is only a rough guide, however; the best means of determining the exact level is either to insert a small needle into the spinous process and obtain a radiograph or to carry the dissection distally and identify the sacrum.

### Incision

Make a midline longitudinal incision over the spinous processes, extending from the spinous process above to the spinous process below the pathologic level. The length of the incision depends on the number of levels to be explored (Fig. 6-2).

## Internervous Plane

The internervous plane lies between the two paraspinal muscles (erector spinae), each of which receives a segmental nerve supply from the posterior primary rami of the lumbar nerves.

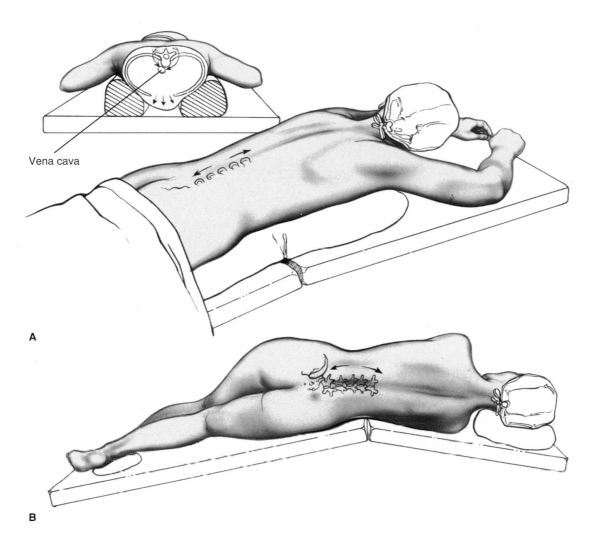

Vena cava

**A**

**B**

**Figure 6-1**   **(A)** The position of the patient for the posterior approach to the lumbar spine. **(B)** Alternatively, place the patient in the lateral position with the affected side up.

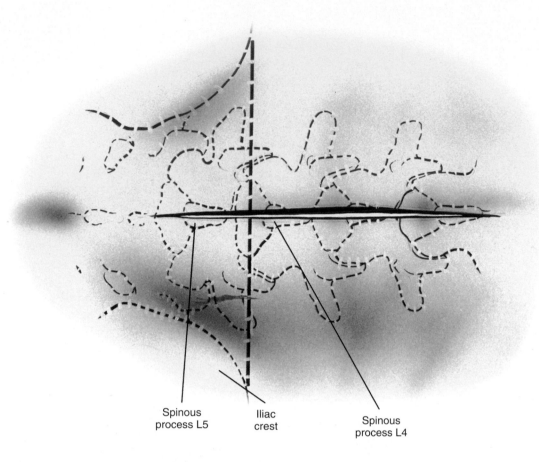

Spinous
process L5

Iliac
crest

Spinous
process L4

**Figure 6-2**   Make a longitudinal incision over the spinous processes extending from
the spinous process above to the spinous process below the level of pathology. A line
drawn across the highest point of the iliac crest is in the L4-5 interspace.

## Superficial Surgical Dissection

Deepen the incision through fat and fascia in line
with the skin incision until the spinous process itself
is reached. Detach the paraspinal muscles subperiosteally as one unit from the bone, using a dissector,
such as a Cobb elevator (Fig. 6-3). Dissect down the
spinous process and along the lamina to the facet
joint. In a young patient, the tip of the spinous
process is a cartilaginous apophysis; it can be split in
the midline, making subperiosteal muscle removal
easier (Fig. 6-4).

If necessary, dissection can be continued laterally,
stripping the facet joint capsule from the descending
and ascending facets. To do this, strip the joint capsule in a medial to lateral direction across the posterior aspect of the descending facet; then, continue
over the tip of the mamillary process of the more lateral ascending facet. If the transverse processes must

be reached, continue dissecting down the lateral side
of the ascending facet and onto the transverse
process itself (Fig. 6-5).

## Dangers

Close to the facet joints, in the area between the
transverse processes, are the vessels supplying the
paraspinal muscles on a segmental basis. These
branches of the lumbar vessels frequently bleed as
the dissection is carried out laterally. Vigorous cauterization of these vessels may be necessary to stop
the bleeding. Note that the posterior primary rami of
the lumbar nerves, which also supply the paraspinal
muscles segmentally, run with these vessels. Loss of
some of these nerves does not denervate the
paraspinal muscles totally, because they are innervated segmentally (see Fig. 6-5).

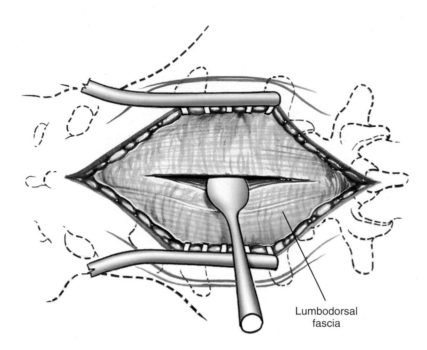

**Figure 6-3** Deepen the incision through the fat and fascia in line with the skin incision until the spinous process itself is reached. Detach the paraspinal muscles subperiosteally.

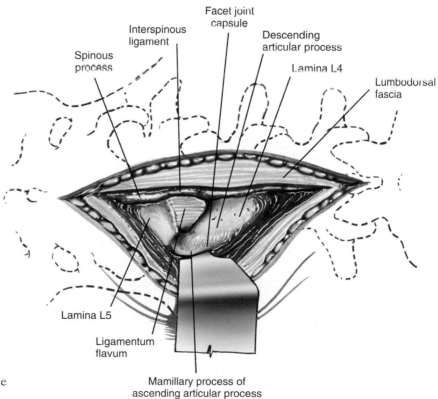

**Figure 6-4** Dissect the paraspinal muscles from the spinous process and lamina to the facet joint. Remove the paraspinal muscles subperiosteally as one unit from the bone.

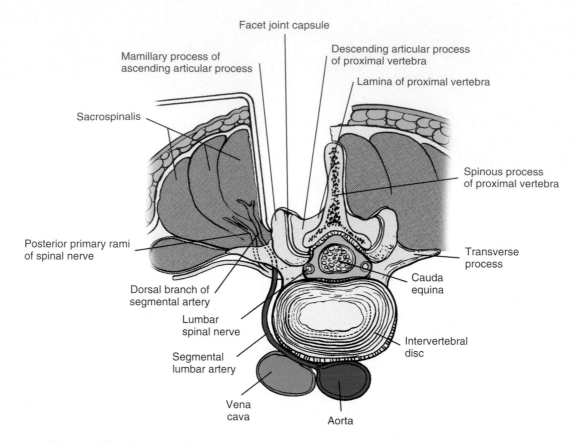

**Figure 6-5**    Continue dissecting laterally, stripping the joint capsule from the descending and ascending facets. Place the point of a Taylor retractor on the lateral side of the ascending facet, using it as a fulcrum to allow for greater retraction of the paraspinal muscles. Note the branches of the lumbar vessels that bleed during stripping of the muscles.

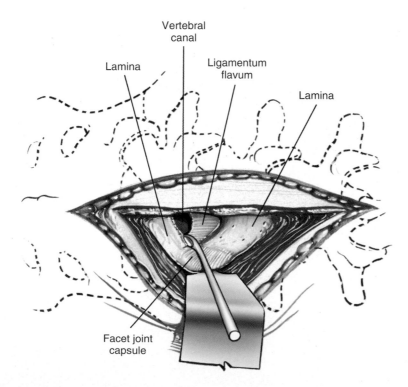

**Figure 6-6**    Remove the ligamentum flavum by cutting its attachment to the superior or leading edge of the inferior lamina.

## Deep Surgical Dissection

Remove the ligamentum flavum by cutting its attachments to the superior, or leading, edge of the inferior lamina using either a curet or sharp dissection. Immediately beneath are epidural fat and the blue-white dura. Using blunt dissection and staying lateral to the dura, carefully continue down to the floor of the spinal canal, retracting the dura and its nerve root medially (Figs. 6-6 through 6-10).

## Dangers

### Nerves

Each nerve root must be identified individually and protected. The more lateral the surgical field, the easier it is to identify the nerve root and retract it so the disc space can be seen. If a larger exposure is needed, incise part of the lamina on the distal portion of the involved vertebra.

**Figure 6-7** **(A)** Insert a blunt dissector under the cut edge of the ligamentum flavum. **(B)** Use a Kerrison Leskel to remove the distal end of the lamina. Note that the ligamentum flavum attaches halfway up the undersurface of the lamina. **(C)** Remove additional lamina and the remaining portion of the ligamentum flavum at its attachment to the undersurface of the lamina.

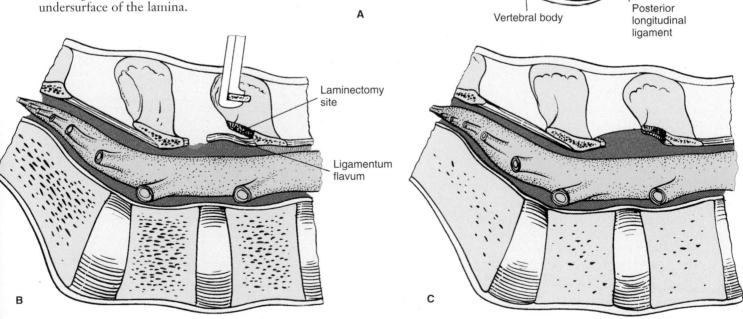
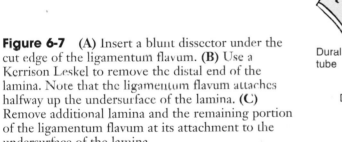

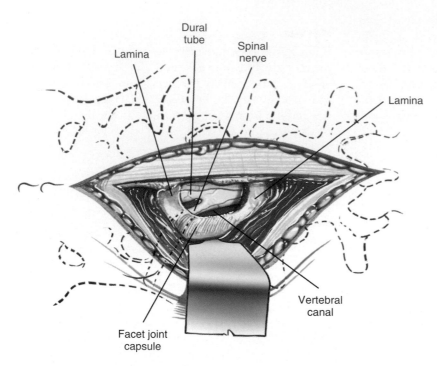

**Figure 6-8**   Immediately beneath the ligamentum flavum and epidural fat is the blue-white dura. Identify the nerve root. Note the overlying epidural veins.

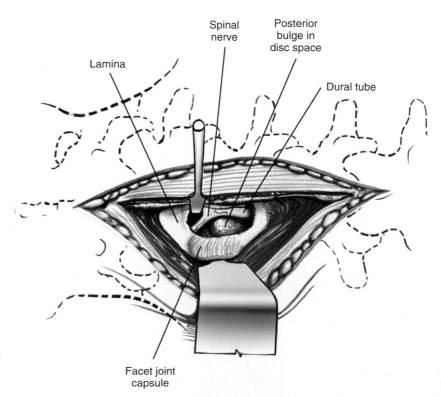

**Figure 6-9**   Using blunt dissection, carefully continue down the lateral side of the dura to the floor of the spinal canal; retract the dura and its nerve root medially. Reveal the posterior aspect of the disc space.

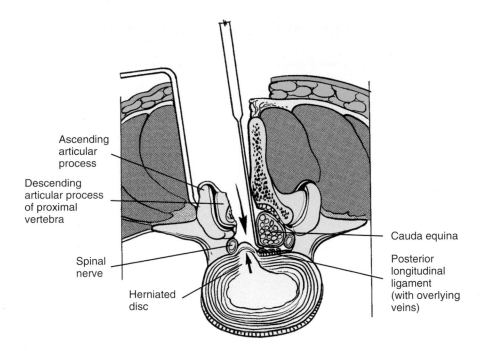

Ascending
articular
process

Descending
articular process
of proximal
vertebra

Spinal
nerve

Herniated
disc

Cauda equina

Posterior
longitudinal
ligament
(with overlying
veins)

**Figure 6-10** Cross section revealing the retraction of the dural tube and a herniated nucleus pulposus impinging on a nerve root.

## Vessels

The **venous plexus** surrounding the nerves and the floor of the vertebra may bleed during the blunt dissection needed to reach the disc (see Fig. 6-10). The bleeding can be stopped with Gelfoam or cotton patties soaked in thrombin. Bipolar Malis cautery also may be used, although it must be done with great care because of the proximity of the cord and nerve roots.

The **iliac vessels** lying on the anterior aspect of the vertebral bodies may be injured if instruments pass through the anterior portion of the annulus fibrosus (see Fig. 6-22).[6]

## How to Enlarge the Approach

### Local Measures

1. To gain better exposure of the dura, nerve root, and disc, remove additional portions of the lamina, both from the leading edge of the lamina below and from the caudal edge of the lamina above. A portion of the facet joint itself even can be removed. Remember that it is safer to remove bone than to retract nerve roots or dura excessively. If the wound is tight, dissect the paraspinal muscles off the posterior spinal elements above and below the exposed level to make the muscles easier to retract.

2. To gain access to other parts of the posterior aspect of the spine, carry the dissection as far laterally as possible, onto the transverse processes. Complete lateral dissection exposes the facet joints and transverse processes, permitting facet joint fusion and transverse process fusion, if necessary (see Fig. 6-5).

### Extensile Measures

To extend the approach, merely extend the skin incision proximally or distally and detach the posterior spinal musculature from the posterior spinal elements. The approach can be extended from C1 down to the sacrum.

# Applied Surgical Anatomy of the Posterior Approach to the Lumbar Spine

## Overview

The muscles of the lumbar spine are made up of superficial and deep layers. The superficial layer consists of the latissimus dorsi, a powerful muscle of the posterior axillary wall that originates from the spinous processes and inserts into the intertubercular groove of the humerus. The surgically important deep layer consists of the paraspinal muscles and itself is divided into two layers: the superficial portion, which contains the sacrospinalis muscles (erector spinae), and the deep portion, which consists of the multifidus and rotator muscles (Fig. 6-11).

This arrangement is not apparent during surgery, because the approach involves detaching all these muscles in a single mass.

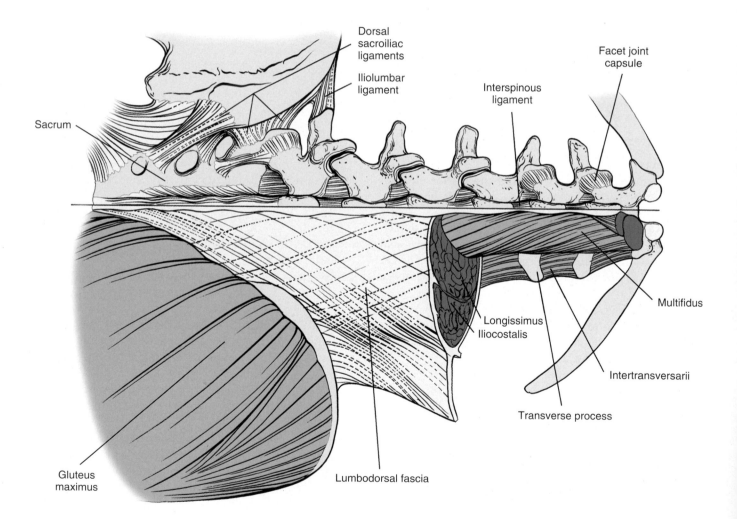

**Figure 6-11**    An overview of the musculature of the lumbosacral spine. In the lumbar spine, the sacrospinalis system is composed of the multifidi, longissimus, and iliocostalis muscles. Note the intertransversarii muscles located deeper. Note the dorsal sacroiliac ligaments.

## Landmarks and Incision

### Landmarks

*Spinous Processes.* The spinous processes in the lumbar area are thick. The distal end of the tip of the spinous process is bulbous and extends slightly caudally. Each process separates the paraspinal muscles on each side. In a growing patient, the processes are capped by cartilaginous apophyses, which, when split, make it easier to remove the paraspinal muscles subperiosteally.

*Posterior Superior Iliac Spine and Crest of the Ilium.* The broad iliac crests run posteriorly at a 45° angle toward the midline. Because muscles either take origin from or insert into the crest (none cross it), it has a palpable subcutaneous border. The palpable, visible dimples over the buttocks lie

directly over the posterior superior iliac spines. A line drawn between the two posterior superior iliac spines crosses the second part of the sacrum; a line drawn between the highest points of the iliac crest crosses between the spinous processes of L4 and L5 (Fig. 6-12).

### Incision
The midline incision follows the course of the spinous processes. It tends to heal with a fine, thin scar, because it is not under tension after suturing and is attached firmly to underlying fascia. No major cutaneous nerves cross the midline.

## Superficial Surgical Dissection and its Dangers

The dorsal lumbar fascia and the supraspinous (supraspinal) ligaments lie between the skin and the

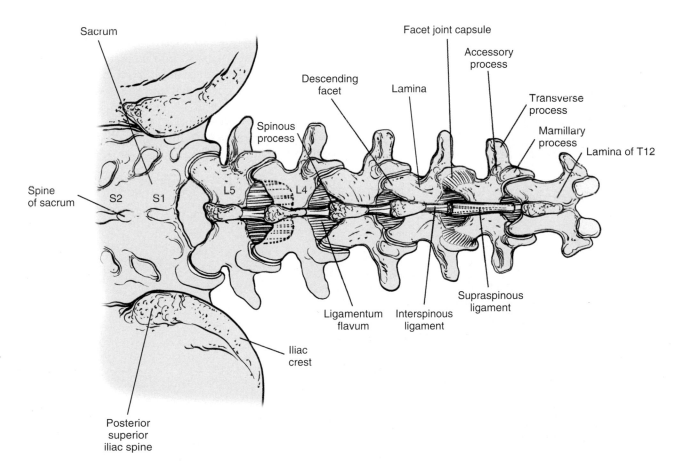

**Figure 6-12**   The bony anatomy of the lumbosacral spine and the posterosuperior aspect of the pelvis. The facet joint capsules, ligamentum flavum, and interspinous ligaments are shown. A line drawn across the crest of the ilium intersects the L4-5 interspinous space. A line crossing the posterior superior iliac spine intersects the second part of the sacrum.

spinous processes. The fascia is a broad, relatively thick, white sheet of tissue that forms a sheath for the sacrospinalis muscles and attaches to the spinous processes (see Fig. 6-11). It extends to the cervical spine, where it becomes continuous with the nuchal fascia of the neck. Medially, it is attached to the spinous processes of the vertebrae, the supraspinous ligaments, and the medial crest of the sacrum. Inferiorly, it is attached to the iliac crests. Laterally, it is continuous with the origin of the aponeurosis of the transversus abdominis and latissimus dorsi muscles.

The supraspinous ligaments extend from vertebra to vertebra, connecting the spinous processes. They blend intimately with the attachment of the dorsal lumbar fascia to the spinous processes (Fig. 6-13).

Further dissection consists of detaching the two layers of muscle from bone. Because these muscles are detached in a single mass, their critical feature, in regard to their surgical anatomy, lies in their blood supply and not in their structure. The segmental lumbar vessels branch directly from the aorta. They wrap around the waist of each vertebral body and then ascend close to the pedicle, where they divide into two branches. One supplies the spinal cord; the other, larger branch then comes directly posteriorly to supply the paraspinal musculature. During the approach, these vessels appear between the transverse processes, close to the facet joints (see Fig. 6-12). They often bleed as dissection is carried out. In addition, the arteries branch within the muscle bodies, frequently creating a very vascular field. For this reason, the dissection should be kept as close to the midline as possible; no major vessels cross the midline, and the plane is safe for use (Fig. 6-14; see Fig. 6-12).

## Deep Surgical Dissection and its Dangers

The ligamentum flavum is the most important structure in the deep layer. Consisting of yellow elastic tissue, the ligament takes origin from the leading edge of the lower lamina and inserts into the anterior surface of the lamina above, about halfway up onto a small ridge (see Fig. 6-13). The two ligamenta flava, one from each side, meet in the midline, but generally do not fuse; the plane between the ligamentum flavum and the underlying dura fat can be entered most easily at that point. Because of its attachments, the ligamentum flavum is removed best from the leading edge of the lower lamina through sharp dissection or curettage (see Fig. 6-6).

The major danger in the deep dissection involves damage to the dura. Once the ligamentum flavum is entered, a thin spatula should be placed beneath it to protect the underlying dura from being torn (see Fig. 6-7A). The cord itself and the nerve roots often are difficult to see as a result of bleeding from epidural veins. The veins, which are thin-walled and easy to rupture, even with blunt dissection, can be controlled by direct pressure using a pattie or by bipolar cautery.

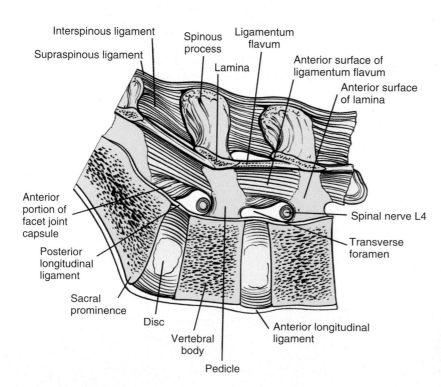

Interspinous ligament
Supraspinous ligament
Spinous process
Ligamentum flavum
Lamina
Anterior surface of ligamentum flavum
Anterior surface of lamina
Anterior portion of facet joint capsule
Posterior longitudinal ligament
Sacral prominence
Disc
Vertebral body
Pedicle
Anterior longitudinal ligament
Spinal nerve L4
Transverse foramen

**Figure 6-13**   A sagittal section through the lamina of a lumbar vertebra. Note the origin and insertion of the ligamentum flavum as well as the supraspinous and interspinous ligaments. The nerve roots exit at the inferior aspect of the pedicle.

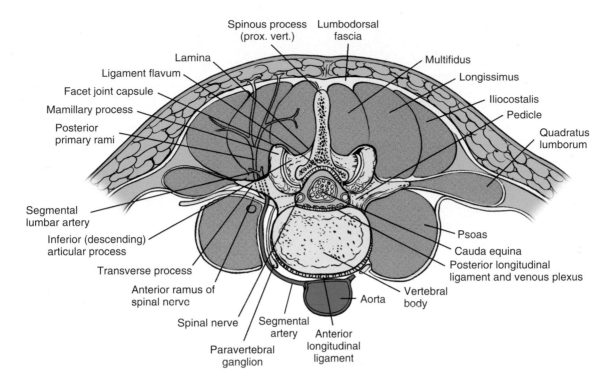

**LUMBAR REGION**

**Figure 6-14**   Cross section at the L3-4 disc space, looking distally. The segmental lumbar vessels branch directly from the aorta. They wrap around the waist of each individual vertebral body and then ascend close to the pedicle, where they divide into two branches. One branch supplies the cord; the other, larger branch proceeds directly posterior to supply the paraspinal musculature. During the surgical approach, these vessels appear between the transverse processes, close to the facet joints. Note that the posterior primary rami and the posterior branches of the lumbar vessels appear between the transverse processes close to the pedicle and descending facet.

# Anterior (Transperitoneal) Approach to the Lumbar Spine

The transperitoneal anterior approach to the lumbar spine usually is reserved for fusing L5 to S1. It also may be used for fusing L4 to L5, although it then involves mobilization of the great vessels. Although the approach is simple in concept, the occasional user may appreciate the assistance of a general surgeon who is more familiar with the area exposed.[7,8]

## Position of the Patient

Place the patient supine on the operating table (Fig. 6-15). Make sure that two areas remain bare for incision: one for the abdominal incision, and one for har-

vesting an anterior iliac crest bone graft. Insert a urinary catheter to keep the bladder empty. Pass a nasogastric tube, because ileus is common after the surgery. Use elastic stockings or mechanical calf stimulators to decrease the risk of thromboembolism.

## Landmarks and Incision

### Landmarks

The *umbilicus* normally is opposite the L3-4 disc space, but varies in level depending on how fat the patient is.

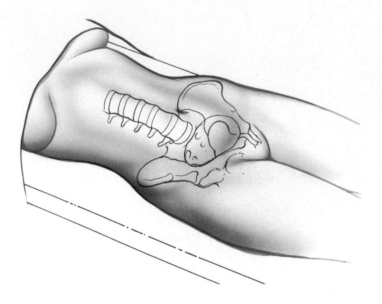

**Figure 6-15**    The position of the patient for the anterior (transperitoneal) approach to the lumbar spine.

Palpate the *pubic symphysis* at the lower end of the abdomen through the fatty mons pubis. The pubic tubercle, on the upper border of the pubis just lateral to the midline, may be easier to palpate than the superior surface of the symphysis itself.

**Incision**

Make a longitudinal midline incision from just below the umbilicus to just above the pubic symphysis. Extend it superiorly, curving it just to the left of the umbilicus and ending about 2 to 3 cm above it. Heavier patients will require longer incisions (Fig. 6-16).

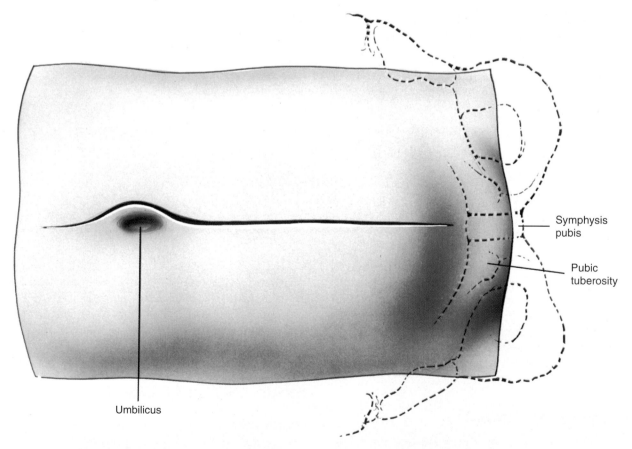

Symphysis pubis

Pubic tuberosity

Umbilicus

**Figure 6-16**    Make a longitudinal midline incision from just below the umbilicus to just above the pubic symphysis. Extend it superiorly, to the left of the umbilicus.

## Internervous Plane

The midline plane lies between the abdominal muscles on each side, segmentally supplied by branches from the seventh to the 12th intercostal nerves. Therefore, this incision can be extended from the xiphisternum to the pubic symphysis.

## Superficial Surgical Dissection

Deepen the wound in line with the skin incision by cutting through the fat to reach the fibrous rectus sheath. Incise the sheath longitudinally, beginning in the lower half of the incision, to reveal the two rectus abdominis muscles (Fig. 6-17). Separate the muscles with the fingers to expose the peritoneum (Fig. 6-18). Then, pick up the peritoneum carefully between two pairs of forceps and, after making sure that no viscera are trapped beneath it, incise it with a knife (Fig. 6-19). Extend the incision distally, but take care not to incise the dome of the bladder at the inferior end of the wound. With one hand inside the abdominal cavity to protect the viscera, carefully deepen the upper half of the incision, staying in the midline and cutting through the linea alba, the band of fibrous tissue that separates the two rectus abdominis muscles in the upper half of the abdomen. Complete the exposure by cutting through the peritoneum in the upper half of the wound (Fig. 6-20).

## Deep Surgical Dissection

Use a self-retaining Balfour retractor to retract the rectus abdominis muscles laterally and the bladder distally (Fig. 6-21). Perform a routine abdominal exploration. Next, put the operating table in Trendelenburg's position at 30° and carefully pack the bowel in a cephalad position, keeping it inside the abdominal cavity. Spread a moist lap pad (swab) over it to prevent loops of bowel from slipping free. It is much safer to keep the bowel within the abdominal cavity, but do not pack it so tightly that vascular compromise is induced. In women, the uterus may be retracted forward with a 0 silk suture placed in its fundus and tied to the Balfour retractor.

Infiltrate the tissue over the anterior surface of the sacral promontory with a few milliliters of saline

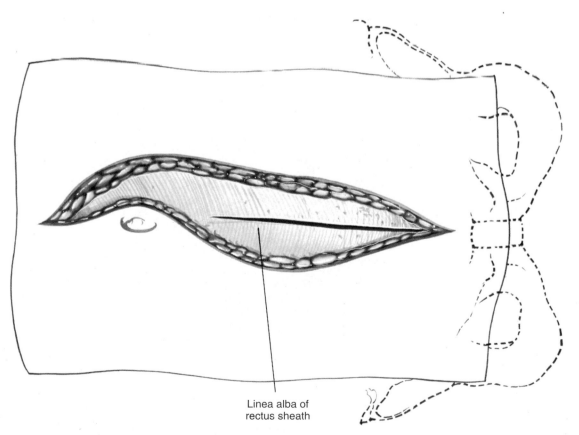

Linea alba of
rectus sheath

**Figure 6-17**  Deepen the wound in line with the skin incision by cutting through the fat to reach the fibrous rectus sheath. Incise the sheath longitudinally.

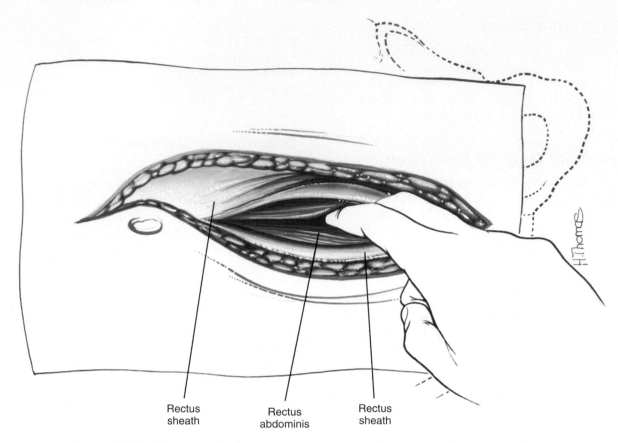

Rectus
sheath

Rectus
abdominis

Rectus
sheath

**Figure 6-18**   With your fingers, separate the rectus abdominis muscles in the midline
to expose the peritoneum.

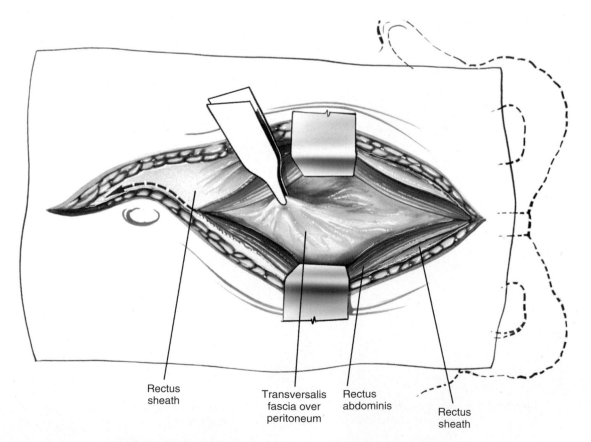

Rectus
sheath

Transversalis
fascia over
peritoneum

Rectus
abdominis

Rectus
sheath

**Figure 6-19**   Pick up the peritoneum with forceps and incise it.

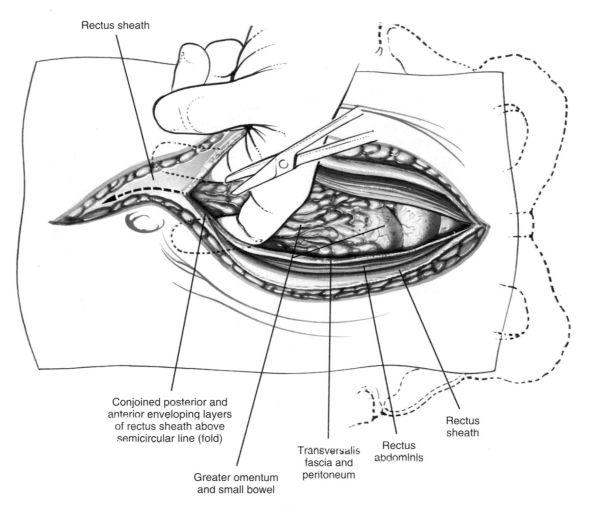

Rectus sheath

Conjoined posterior and
anterior enveloping layers
of rectus sheath above
semicircular line (fold)

Greater omentum
and small bowel

Transversalis
fascia and
peritoneum

Rectus
abdominis

Rectus
sheath

**Figure 6-20** With one hand inside the abdominal cavity to protect the viscera, carefully deepen the upper half of the incision, staying in the midline and cutting through the linea alba.

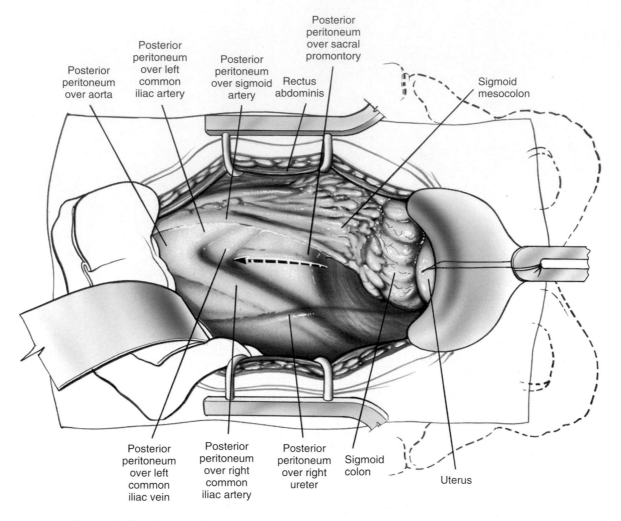

**Figure 6-21** Use a self-retaining retractor to retract the rectus abdominis muscles laterally and the bladder distally. Carefully mobilize and retract the bowel in a cephalad position, keeping it inside the abdominal cavity. Observe the posterior peritoneum overlying the bifurcation of the great vessels and the promontory of the sacrum. Incise the peritoneum longitudinally.

solution to make dissection easier and to allow identification of the presacral parasympathetic nerves that run down through this area. For the L5-S1 disc space, incise the posterior peritoneum in the midline over the sacral promontory. The sacral artery runs down along the anterior surface of the sacrum and must be ligated. The ureters should be well lateral to the surgical approach.

Preserve any small nerve fibers that are found. Identify the L5-S1 disc space either by palpating its sharp angle or by inserting a metallic marker and taking a radiograph. The L5-S1 disc space lies below the bifurcation of the aorta; it should be possible to expose it fully without mobilizing any of the great vessels (Figs. 6-22 and 6-23).

Operating on the L4-5 disc space requires a larger exposure; mobilizing the great vessels is necessary, unless the vascular bifurcation occurs much higher. Carefully incise the peritoneum at the base of the sigmoid colon and mobilize the colon upward and to the right to expose the bifurcation of the aorta, the left common iliac artery and vein, and the left ureter. Identify the aorta just above its bifurcation and gently begin blunt dissection on its left side. Identify and ligate the fourth and fifth left lumbar vessels, then divide them. Now, the aorta, vena cava, and left common iliac vessels can be moved to the right, exposing the L4-5 disc space. This exposure is difficult to achieve; a high incidence of venous thrombosis has been reported with anterior surgery at this level. Take care

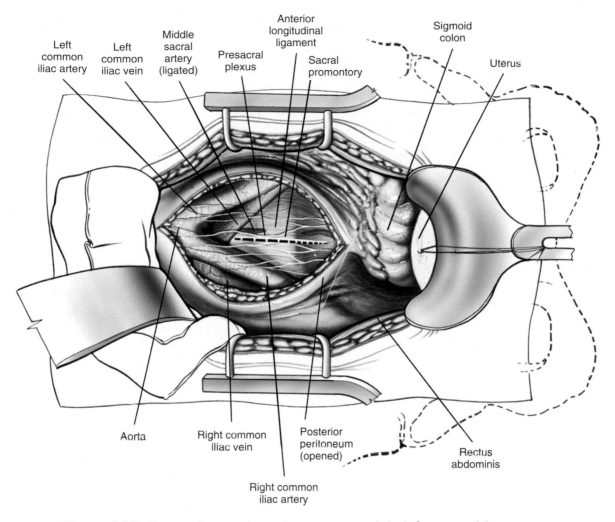

Left
common
iliac artery

Left
common
iliac vein

Middle
sacral
artery
(ligated)

Presacral
plexus

Anterior
longitudinal
ligament

Sacral
promontory

Sigmoid
colon

Uterus

Aorta

Right common
iliac vein

Posterior
peritoneum
(opened)

Rectus
abdominis

Right common
iliac artery

**Figure 6-22** Retract the posterior peritoneum to reveal the bifurcation of the aorta and vena cava. Ligate the middle sacral artery. Identify the presacral parasympathetic plexus overlying the aorta and the sacral promontory.

not to injure the left ureter, which crosses the left common iliac vessels roughly over the sacroiliac joint. The ureter may have to be moved laterally, but mobilize it only as much as necessary to reduce the risk of postoperative ischemic stricture formation.

An alternative method is to approach the L4-5 disc space from below, working upward into the apex of the vascular bifurcation. Isolate the left and right common iliac artery, placing umbilicus loops around them. Retract the two arteries cephalad and laterally to expose the common iliac veins. Dissect into the confluence of the veins and isolate the left common iliac vein with a loop. Gently retract the venous structures to expose the disc space. Use only minimal retraction to avoid injuring the intima, which may lead to venous thrombosis (see Fig. 6-23).

## Dangers

### Nerves

The **presacral plexus of parasympathetic nerves** is critically important to sexual function. Removing the entire plexus will cause retroejaculation and impotence in men. Therefore, dissection should be carried out carefully, and only with a blunt peanut dissector. The incision over the anterior part of the sacrum should be made in the midline, and it should be long enough to allow for lateral mobilization of these nerves with minimal trauma. Injecting saline solution into the presacral tissue aids in identifying and preserving these nerves (see Figs. 6-22 and 6-28).

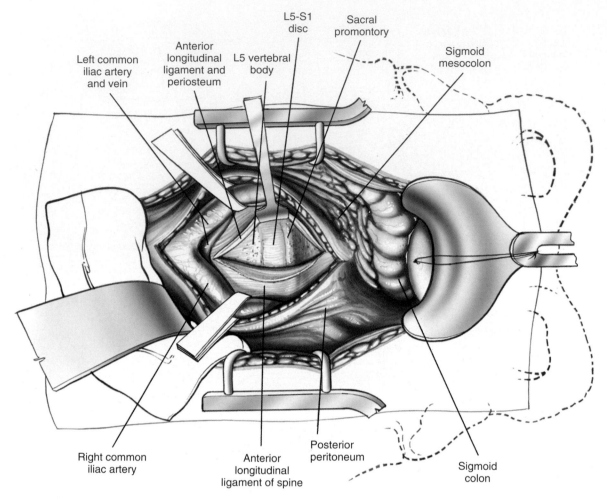

**Figure 6-23**    Mobilize the great vessels as needed for additional exposure. Expose the L5-S1 disc space subperiosteally.

## Arteries and Veins

The **middle sacral artery** can be a troublesome bleeder in the region of the L5-S1 disc space and must be tied off (see Fig. 6-22).

The **aorta** and **inferior vena cava** are tethered to the anterior surface of the lumbar vertebrae by the lumbar vessels. These smaller vessels must be ligated and cut to allow the great vessels to be lifted forward off the lumbar vertebrae, exposing the L4-5 disc space (see Fig. 6-14). It is important to dissect these vessels out carefully without cutting them flush with the aorta. If the vessels are cut flush, there will be, in effect, a hole in the aorta, and the bleeding may be extremely difficult to control. Mobilization of the venous structures should be undertaken very carefully, because they are fairly fragile and easily traumatized. Damage to these vessels may result in thrombosis; mobilization and retraction should be kept to a minimum.

## Special Structures

The **ureter** must be mobilized laterally, particularly for exposure of the L4-5 disc space. It can be identified easily by gently pinching it with a pair of nontoothed forceps to induce peristalsis (see Fig. 6-28).

## How to Enlarge the Approach

### Local Measures

Packing the bowel away carefully is the key to adequate exposure in the pelvis. Careful mobilization of the great vessels is crucial to exposure higher up (see Figs. 6-21 and 6-23).

### Extensile Measures

In theory, this exposure can be extended to the xiphisternum, but the exposure of higher discs almost always is performed better through a retroperitoneal approach.

# Applied Surgical Anatomy of the Anterior Approach to the Lumbar Spine

## Overview

The anterior approach to the lumbar spine involves three stages of dissection. The superficial stage consists of cutting the skin and subcutaneous tissues down to the bowel. Below the skin lies the linea alba, a fibrous structure in the midline that is identified most easily in the upper abdomen. Cutting the linea alba in the lower half of the abdomen exposes the rectus muscle, which can be separated by finger pressure. Beneath it is the posterior rectus sheath and peritoneum.

The anatomy of the intermediate stage, which involves packing away the bowel, is the anatomy of the bowel and is not included in this book.

The deep stage of dissection consists of mobilizing the retroperitoneal structures that lie anterior to the L4-5 and L5-S1 disc spaces. These structures include the aorta, vena cava, common iliac vessels, lumbar vessels, ureter, and presacral plexus.

## Landmarks and Incision

### Landmarks

The *umbilicus* lies superficial to the linea alba. It usually is about halfway between the pubic symphysis and the infrasternal notch, although it may be pulled lower in obese patients.

The *linea alba* is marked externally by a groove in the midline of the abdomen. It divides one side of the rectus abdominis muscle from the other. In the upper abdomen, it actually separates the two muscles; cutting through it leads directly down to the peritoneum, with neither muscle being exposed. Below the umbilicus, the linea alba is less distinct; it does not separate the two rectus muscles.

The *pubic symphysis* is the articulation between the two pubic bones in the midline of the body. It is a relatively immobile joint (diarthrodial; Fig. 6-24).

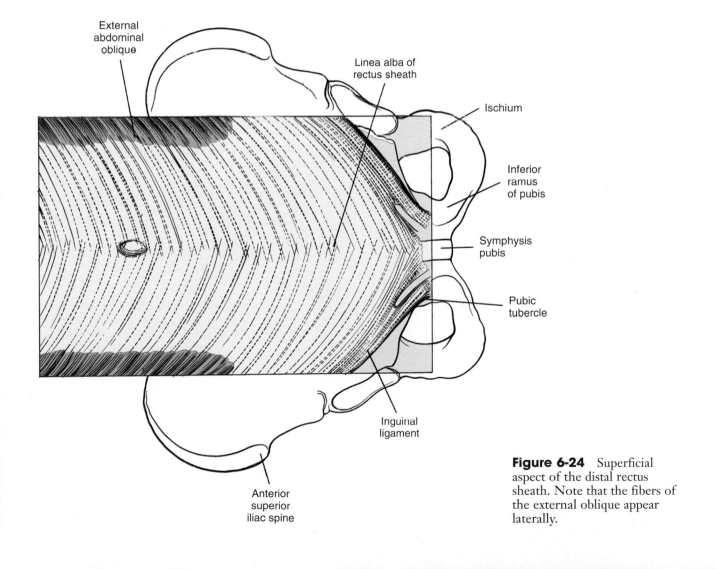

**Figure 6-24** Superficial aspect of the distal rectus sheath. Note that the fibers of the external oblique appear laterally.

## Incision

The midline longitudinal incision arches around the umbilicus. Because the skin is mobile and loosely attached to the tissues immediately beneath it, it heals with a thin scar. The cleavage or tension lines below the umbilicus appear in a chevron pattern, with the apex of the V in the midline.

The skin of the anterior abdominal wall is supplied segmentally from T7 in the region of the xiphoid to T12 just above the inguinal ligament. These segmental nerves do not cross the midline. Therefore, midline incisions do not cut any major cutaneous nerves.

## Superficial Surgical Dissection and Its Dangers

The long, flat rectus abdominis muscle extends along the length of the entire abdomen, split into two muscles in the upper half by the linea alba. The muscle is enclosed in a fascial sheath. Above the umbilicus, the sheath has three elements: the aponeurosis of the internal oblique splits to enclose the rectus muscle; the aponeurosis of the external oblique passes in front of the rectus to form part of the anterior sheath; and the aponeurosis of the transversus abdominis fascia passes behind to form part of the posterior sheath. The inferior margin of the posterior sheath is known as the semicircular line (semicircular fold of Douglas). Below the umbilicus, all three aponeuroses pass anteriorly, leaving a thin film of tissue posteriorly (Figs. 6-25 and 6-26).

The arrangement of the rectus sheath and the linea alba means that, in the upper half of the incision, the approach through fibrous tissue leads directly down to the peritoneum, whereas in the lower half, it leads to the rectus abdominis muscle. Because of this, it is easier to open the abdomen in the lower half of the incision (Fig. 6-27; see Fig. 6-26).

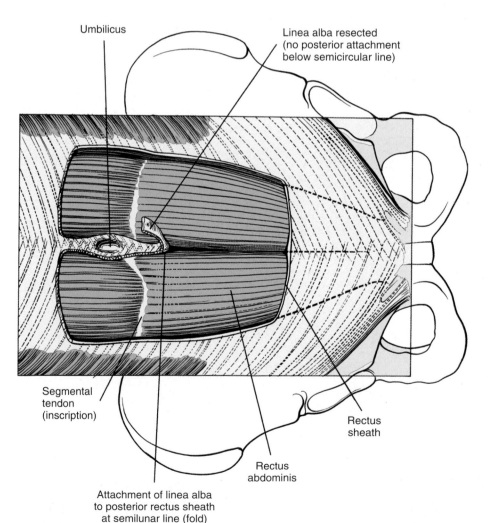

Umbilicus

Linea alba resected
(no posterior attachment
below semicircular line)

Segmental
tendon
(inscription)

Attachment of linea alba
to posterior rectus sheath
at semilunar line (fold)

Rectus
abdominis

Rectus
sheath

**Figure 6-25**   The anterior portion of the rectus sheath is resected, revealing the fibers of the rectus abdominis muscle. Distal to the semicircular line, the linea alba (which is shown elevated by sutures) overlies the muscle fibers of the rectus abdominis but does not separate them. Proximal to the semicircular line, the linea alba separates the rectus abdominis muscles by attaching to the posterior rectus sheath, which begins at the semicircular line.

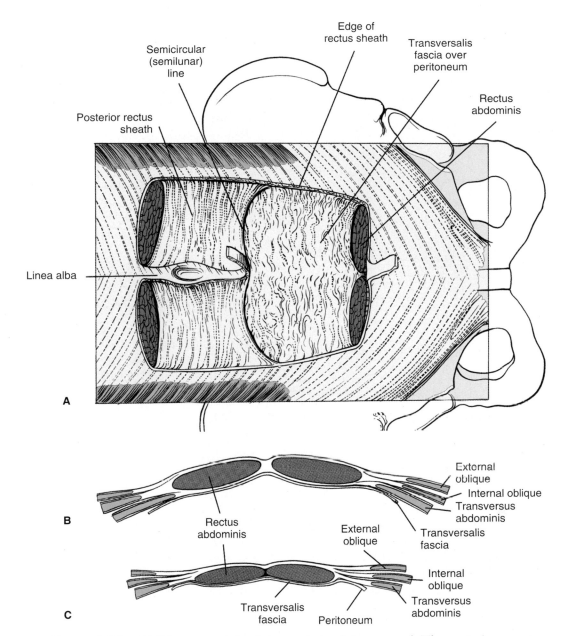

**Figure 6-26** **(A)** The rectus abdominis muscle has been resected. The posterior aspect of the rectus sheath ends just distal to the umbilicus. Its distal edge is called the semicircular line. The linea alba attaches to the posterior rectus sheath, thus separating the rectus abdominis muscles proximal to the semicircular line. **(B)** Cross section above the semicircular line. Note that the rectus abdominis muscles are enveloped by the posterior and anterior rectus sheaths and separated from each other by the linea alba. **(C)** Cross section below the semicircular line. The rectus sheath exists only anteriorly. Posteriorly is the transversalis fascia and peritoneum.

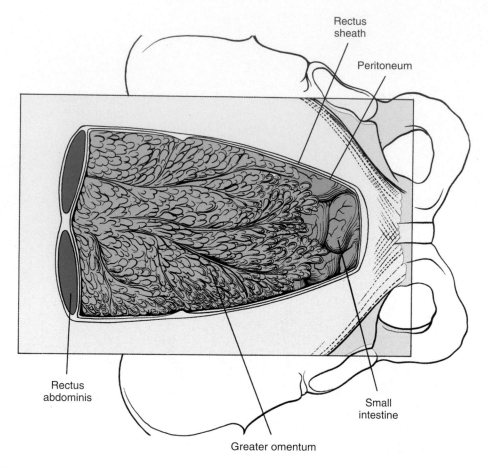

**Figure 6-27**   The posterior rectus sheath has been removed to reveal the peritoneum and the abdominal viscera.

The inferior epigastric artery supplies blood to the lower half of the rectus abdominis muscle. The artery lies between the muscle and the posterior part of the rectus sheath. If the surgical plane remains in the midline, this vessel should escape injury. If the artery is damaged when the rectus muscle is mobilized, it can be tied with impunity.

## Deep Surgical Dissection and Its Dangers

Deep surgical dissection consists of freeing the distal ends of the aorta and the vena cava from the vertebrae in the L4-5 vertebral area. The aorta divides on the anterior surface of the L4 vertebra into the two common iliac arteries. Just below this bifurcation, the common iliac vessels divide in turn at about the S1 level into the internal and external iliac vessels. The internal iliac is the more medial of the two (Fig. 6-28).

The aorta and vena cava are held firmly onto the anterior parts of the lower lumbar vertebrae by the lumbar vessels. These segmental vessels must be mobilized to permit the aorta and vena cava to be moved (see Fig. 6-14). Because the arterial structures are easier to dissect and more muscular than are the thin-walled venous structures, the preferred approach to the L4-5 disc space is from the left, the more arterial side. The median sacral artery originates from the aorta at its bifurcation at L4 and runs in the midline, over the sacral promontory and down into the hollow of the sacrum (see Fig. 6-28). The lumbosacral disc usually lies in the V that is formed by the two common iliac vessels. Nevertheless, the level at which the vessels bifurcate may vary; on rare occasions, they may have to be mobilized to expose the L5-S1 disc space.

Note that the left common iliac vein lies below the left common iliac artery, whereas the right com-

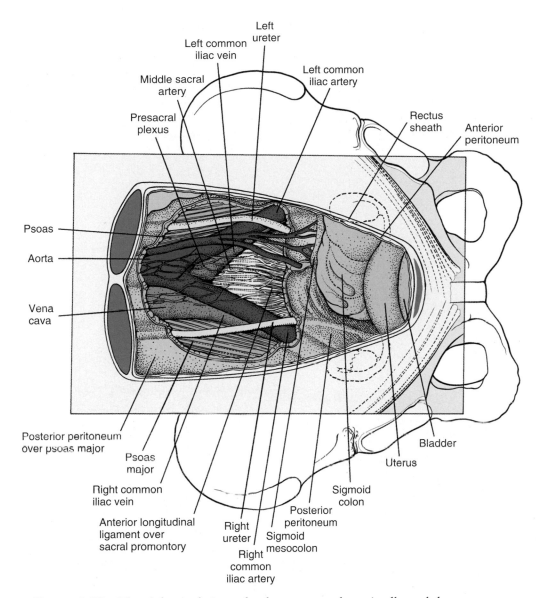

**Figure 6-28**   The abdominal viscera has been retracted proximally, and the retroperitoneum has been resected to reveal the great vessels at their bifurcation, the ureters, and the presacral parasympathetic plexus.

mon iliac artery lies below and medial to the right common iliac vein. Therefore, special care must be taken when mobilizing the left side of the vascular V, because the vessel closest to the surgery is the thin-walled vein, not the artery (Fig. 6-29; see Fig. 6-28).

The parasympathetic nerves in the presacral area exist as a diffuse plexus of nerves running around the aorta, heading inferiorly from the bifurcation and running along the anterior surface of the sacrum beneath the posterior peritoneum. They should be protected, if at all possible, to preserve adequate sex-

ual function and prevent retroejaculation in men. Because of the function of these nerves, this approach may be safer in women than in men (see Figs. 6-28 and 6-29).

The ureter runs down the posterior abdominal wall on the psoas muscle. At the bifurcation of the common iliac artery over the sacroiliac joint, it clings to the posterior abdominal wall, held there by the peritoneum, and should be well lateral to the approach to the L5-S1 disc space. It may have to be mobilized for exposure of the L4-5 disc space (Fig. 6-30; see Fig. 6-29).

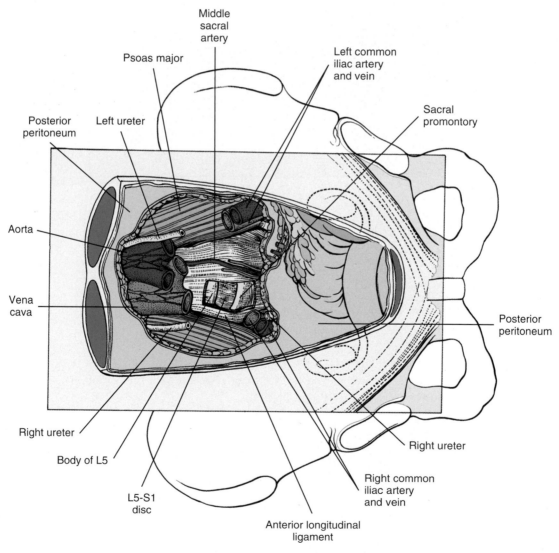

**Figure 6-29**  Portions of the major vessels have been resected to reveal the underlying L5-S1 disc space, the sacral promontory, and its overlying presacral plexus.

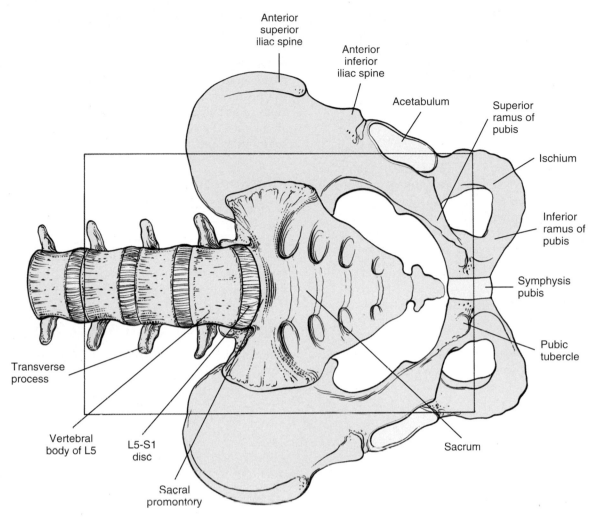

**Figure 6-30** Osteology of the anterior aspect of the pelvis and lumbosacral spine.

# Anterolateral (Retroperitoneal) Approach to the Lumbar Spine

The retroperitoneal approach to the anterior part of the lumbar spine has several advantages over the transperitoneal approach. First, it provides access to all vertebrae from L1 to the sacrum, whereas the transperitoneal approach is difficult to use above the level of L4. Second, it allows drainage of an infection, such as a psoas abscess, without the risk of a postoperative ileitis. Because of the arrangement of the vascular anatomy of the retroperitoneal space, however, it is slightly more difficult to reach the L5-S1 disc space using the retroperitoneal approach.

The uses of this approach include the following:

1. Spinal fusion
2. Drainage of psoas abscess and curettage of infected vertebral body
3. Resection of all or part of a vertebral body and associated bone grafting
4. Biopsy of a vertebral body when a needle biopsy is either not possible or hazardous

The most common use of the retroperitoneal approach is in general surgery, for exposure of the sympathetic chain.[9]

## Position of the Patient

Place the patient on the operating table in the semi-lateral position. The patient's body should be at about a 45° angle to the horizontal, facing away from the surgeon. Keep the patient in this position throughout the surgery by placing sandbags under the hips and shoulders or by using a kidney rest brace to hold the patient. The angle allows the peritoneal contents to fall away from the incision. Alternatively, place the patient supine on the operating table and tilt the table at 45° to the horizontal away from the surgeon. This position has the advantage of not putting the psoas muscle on stretch (Fig. 6-31).

For most procedures, have the left side up so that the "aortic" rather than the "caval" side is approached.

## Landmarks and Incision

### Landmarks

Palpate the *12th rib* in the affected flank and the *pubic symphysis* in the lower part of the abdomen. Palpate the lateral border of the *rectus abdominis muscle* about 5 cm lateral to the midline.

### Incision

Make an oblique flank incision extending down from the posterior half of the 12th rib toward the rectus abdominis muscle and stopping at its lateral border, about midway between the umbilicus and the pubic symphysis (Fig. 6-33).

## Internervous Plane

No internervous plane is available for use. The three muscles of the abdominal wall (the external oblique, internal oblique, and transversus abdominis) are divided in line with the skin incision. Because all three muscles are innervated segmentally, significant denervation does not occur (Fig. 6-32).

## Superficial Surgical Dissection

Deepen the incision through subcutaneous fat to expose the aponeurosis of the external oblique mus-

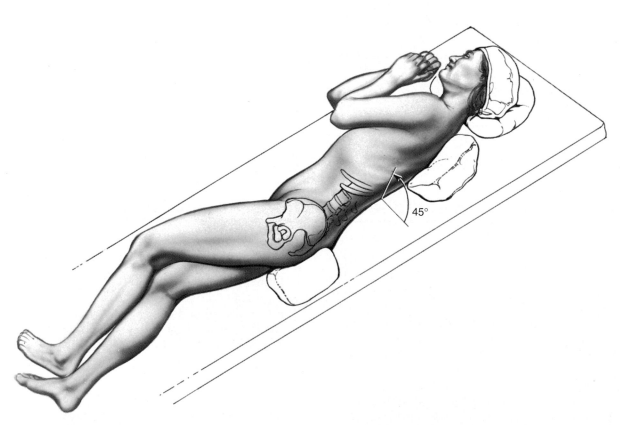

**Figure 6-31**  Place the patient in the semilateral position for the anterolateral (retroperitoneal) approach to the lumbar spine.

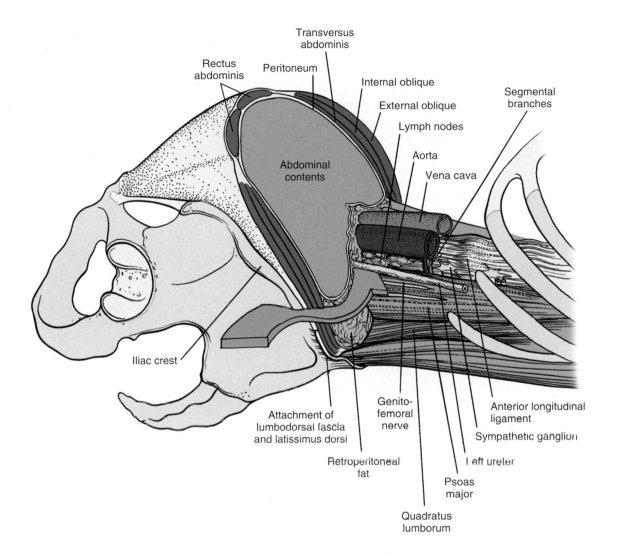

**Figure 6-32**   The anterior abdominal musculature and viscera have been transected and removed at the level of the iliac crest. The *arrow* indicates the route of surgery between the peritoneum anteriorly and the retroperitoneal structures posteriorly.

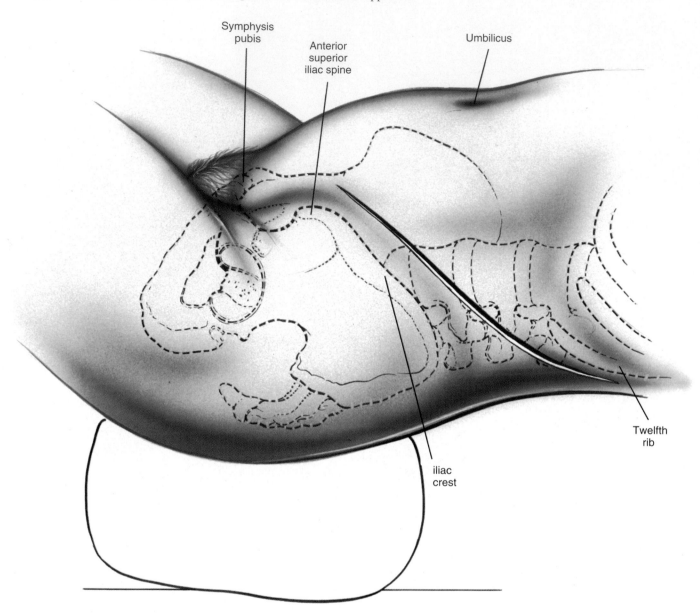

**Figure 6-33**   Make an oblique flank incision extending down from the posterior half of the 12th rib toward the rectus abdominis muscle.

cle. Divide the aponeurosis of this muscle in the line of its fibers, which is in line with the skin incision. The muscle fibers of the external oblique rarely appear below the level of the umbilicus except in very muscular patients. If they are found there, the muscle should be split in the line of its fibers (Fig. 6-34).

Next, divide the internal oblique muscle in line with the skin incision and perpendicular to the line of its muscular fibers. This division causes partial denervation, but if the muscle is closed properly, postoperative hernias can be avoided (Fig. 6-35). Under the internal oblique muscle lies the transversus abdo-

minis muscle. It, too, should be divided in line with the skin incision to expose the retroperitoneal space (Figs. 6-36, 6-37, 6-41, and 6-42).

Using blunt finger dissection, develop a plane between the retroperitoneal fat and the fascia that overlies the psoas muscle (Fig. 6-38). Gently mobilize the peritoneal cavity and its contents and retract them medially (Fig. 6-39). Carry out this dissection from either the left lower quadrant or the right upper quadrant, depending on the side that needs to be exposed.

Because the aorta is on the left, the exposure used for routine spinal fusion comes from the left side.

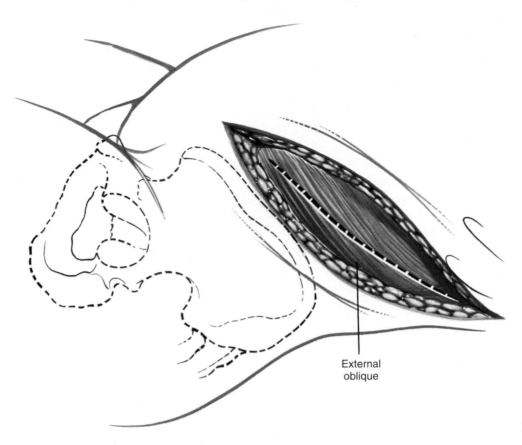

**Figure 6-34** Incise the external oblique muscle and aponeurosis in line with its fibers and in line with the skin incision.

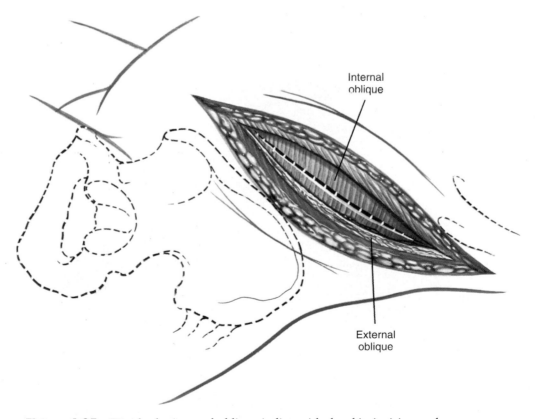

**Figure 6-35** Divide the internal oblique in line with the skin incision and perpendicular to the line of its muscular fibers.

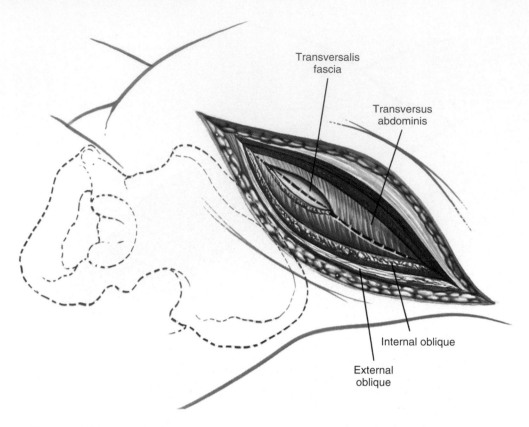

Transversalis fascia

Transversus abdominis

Internal oblique

External oblique

**Figure 6-36** Divide the underlying transversus abdominis muscle in line with the skin incision.

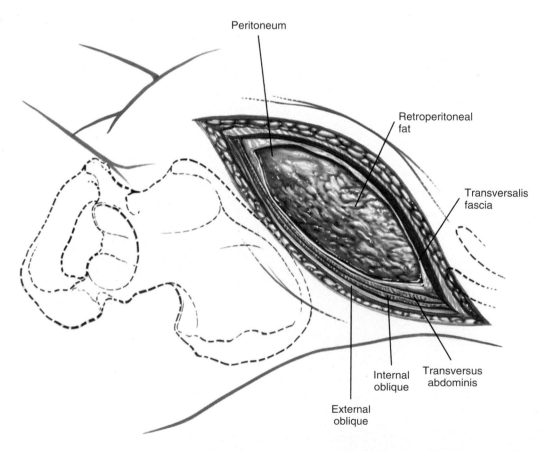

Peritoneum

Retroperitoneal fat

Transversalis fascia

Transversus abdominis

Internal oblique

External oblique

**Figure 6-37** In the anterior part of the wound, identify the peritoneum and its contents. Posteriorly, identify the retroperitoneal fat.

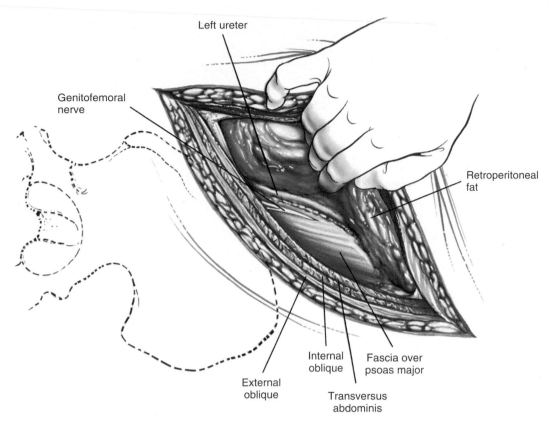

Left ureter

Genitofemoral
nerve

Retroperitoneal
fat

Internal
oblique

Fascia over
psoas major

External
oblique

Transversus
abdominis

**Figure 6-38**   Using blunt finger dissection, develop the plane between the retroperitoneal fat and fascia that overlie the psoas muscle.

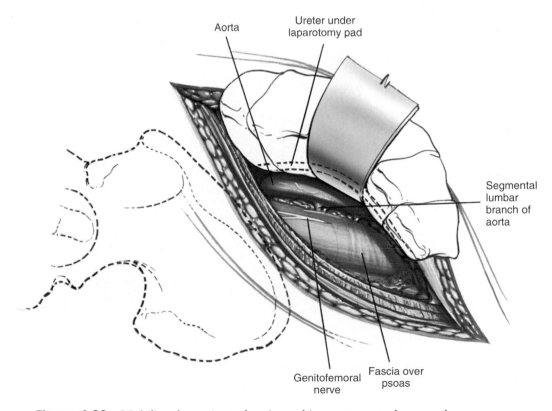

Aorta

Ureter under
laparotomy pad

Segmental
lumbar
branch of
aorta

Genitofemoral
nerve

Fascia over
psoas

**Figure 6-39**   Mobilize the peritoneal cavity and its contents, and retract them medially.

Place a Dever retractor over the peritoneal contents and retract them to the right upper quadrant. The ureter, which is attached loosely to the peritoneum, is carried forward with it.

## Deep Surgical Dissection

Identify the psoas fascia, but do not enter the muscle. Any existing psoas abscess is easily palpable at this point. If one is found, it should be entered from its lateral side with finger dissection. Follow the abscess cavity with a finger directly to the infected disc space or spaces. If there is no psoas abscess, follow the surface of the psoas muscle medially to reach the anterior lateral surface of the vertebral bodies.

The aorta and vena cava effectively are tied to the waist of the vertebral bodies by the lumbar arteries and veins. These smaller vessels must be located individually on the involved vertebrae and tied so that the aorta and vena cava can be mobilized and the anterior part of the vertebral body reached. Make sure that the lumbar vessels are not cut flush with the aorta; a slipped tie then would prove hard to deal with (Figs. 6-40 and 6-43).

Place a needle into the involved lumbar vertebra and take a radiograph to identify the exact location.

## Dangers

### Nerves

The **sympathetic chain** lies on the lateral aspect of the vertebral body and on the most medial aspect of the psoas muscle. It is easy to identify as the tissue is cleared from the front of the vertebrae.

The **genitofemoral nerve** lies on the anterior medial surface of the psoas muscle, attached to its fascia. Easily identifiable, it should be preserved (see Figs. 6-39 and 6-43).

### Vessels

The **segmental lumbar arteries and veins** must be tied or excessive bleeding will occur (see Fig. 6-43).

The **vena cava** may be injured if the peritoneal contents are retracted vigorously when the approach is made from the right side. That is why the left lateral approach is recommended; the aorta will be come down on, and it is a much tougher structure that is more resistant to injury.

The **aorta** is easy to identify. Its pulsating length can be palpated (see Fig. 6-43).

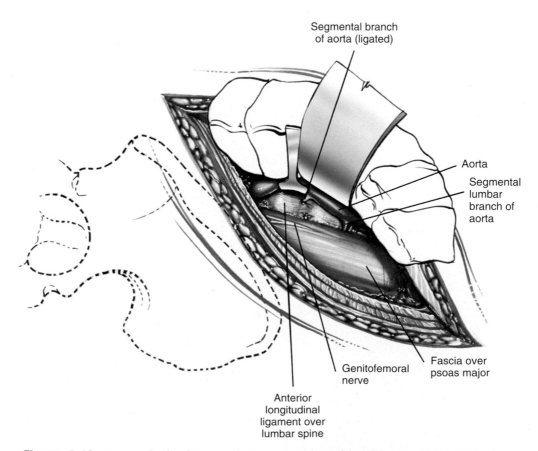

Segmental branch of aorta (ligated)

Aorta

Segmental lumbar branch of aorta

Genitofemoral nerve

Fascia over psoas major

Anterior longitudinal ligament over lumbar spine

**Figure 6-40** Ligate the lumbar vessels (segmental branches of the aorta). Mobilize the aorta and vena cava to reach the anterior part of the vertebral body.

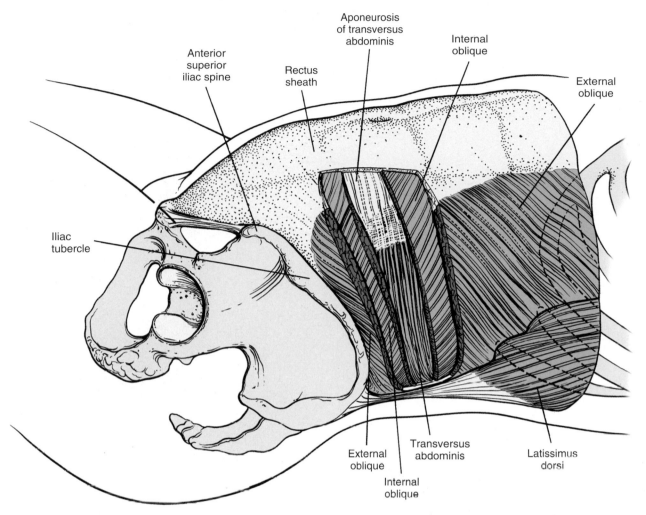

**Figure 6-41** The external and internal oblique have been resected to reveal their relationship to each other and to the transversus abdominis muscle.

## Ureter

The **ureters** run in the medial aspect of the field between the peritoneum and the psoas fascia. Because the ureter is attached not to the psoas fascia, but loosely to the peritoneum, it normally falls forward with the peritoneum and its contents, away from the operative field. If doubt exists regarding the identity of the ureter, it should be stroked gently to produce peristalsis (see Fig. 6-43).

## How to Enlarge the Approach

### Local Measures

Chest wound retractors are the key to providing good visibility. They are self-retaining and offer excellent cephalad and caudad exposure. If the incision does not comfortably expose the involved vertebra, continue dissecting more posteriorly, taking additional fibers of the latissimus dorsi, and even possibly the quadratus lumborum, to allow more posterior exposure.

### Extensile Measures

This incision generally is limited to the lower lumbar vertebrae. Parallel incisions may be made at higher levels for access to the upper lumbar vertebrae, but they involve rib resection and potentially are hazardous because of the proximity of the pleura and the kidney. They should be performed in conjunction with a general surgeon unless the orthopaedic surgeon has considerable experience in this area.

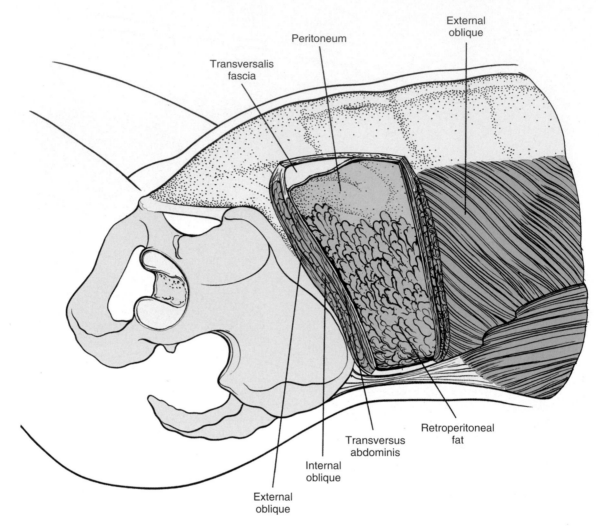

**Figure 6-42**   The transversus abdominis muscle is resected to reveal the peritoneum and the retroperitoneal fat.

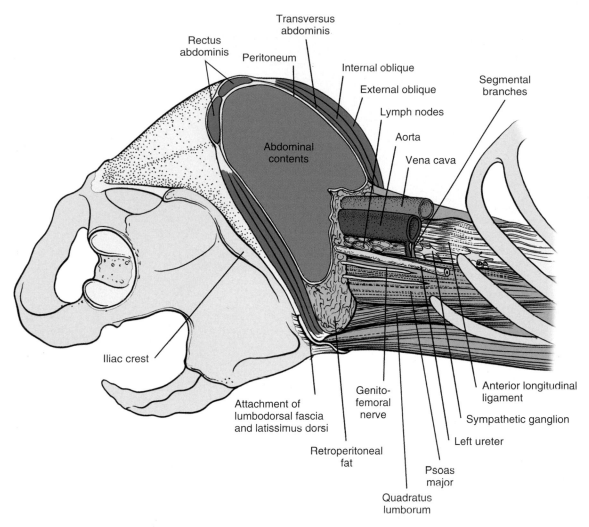

**Figure 6-43**   The abdominal muscles and viscera have been removed proximal to the level of the iliac crest to reveal retroperitoneal structures. Note the interval between the psoas muscle and the aorta. This interval provides access to the sympathetic chain and the anterior portion of the vertebral bodies.

# Posterior Approach to the Cervical Spine

The midline posterior approach is the most commonly used approach to the cervical spine, allowing quick and safe access to the posterior elements of the entire cervical spine. It is used for the following:

1. Posterior cervical spine fusion[10]
2. Excision of herniated discs
3. Treatment of tumors
4. Treatment of facet joint dislocations[11,12]
5. Nerve root exploration

## Position of the Patient

Place the patient in the prone position. Move the head into a few degrees of flexion to open the interspinous spaces. A special head brace or a padded ring may be used to control the position of the head during surgery, holding it in the midline (Fig. 6-44).

Alternatively, the patient may be seated upright, with the head held in a special brace. This position

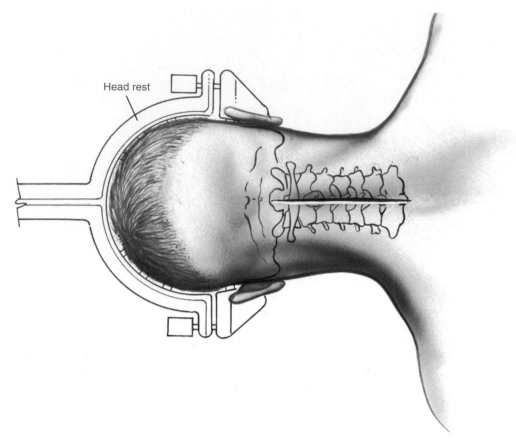

**Figure 6-44**     The position of the patient for the posterior approach to the cervical spine.

has the advantage of decreasing venous bleeding, but it has been implicated as a cause of air emboli.

Illumination is important; a cold-light headlamp adds significant clarity to the operative field.

## Landmarks and Incision

### Landmarks

The *spinous processes* are the most prominent landmarks in the vertebral arch. The C2 spinous process is one of the largest cervical spinous processes, as are C7 and T1. All three are quite palpable along the midline. Because it sometimes is difficult to distinguish between C7 and T1 during surgery, place a radiopaque marker (such as a needle) into the spinous process at the level of the pathology before making the incision, so that the exact location of the process can be identified. Sometimes placing a second marker into C7 may be helpful. Because the distance between the various cervical facet joints and interspaces is tiny, a significant portion of the neck may be dissected unnecessarily unless the vertebra being treated is identified, with the help of an x-ray film.

### Incision

Make a generous straight incision in the midline of the neck (Fig. 6-45). Use the needle that has been inserted into the spinous process as a guide to and center point of the incision. Note that the skin of the posterior cervical spine is thicker and less mobile than the skin of the anterior neck, and that the resultant scar usually is broader; however, hair usually covers most of the scar.

### Internervous Plane

The internervous plane is in the midline, between the left and right paracervical muscles (which are supplied segmentally by the left and right posterior rami of the cervical nerves).

### Superficial Surgical Dissection

Continue the incision down to the spinous processes. Minimal bleeding may come from venous plexuses that cross the midline; these should be cauterized (Figs. 6-46 and 6-47).

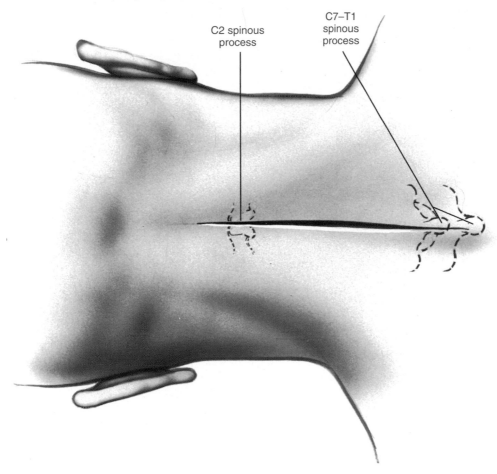

**Figure 6-45**  Make a straight incision in the midline of the neck, centering the incision over the area of pathology.

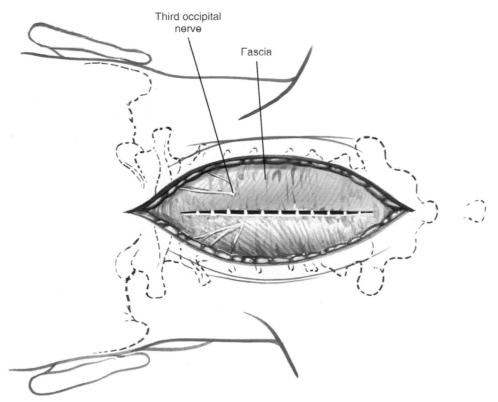

**Figure 6-46**  Retract the skin flaps and incise the fascia in the midline. Note the position of the third occipital nerve.

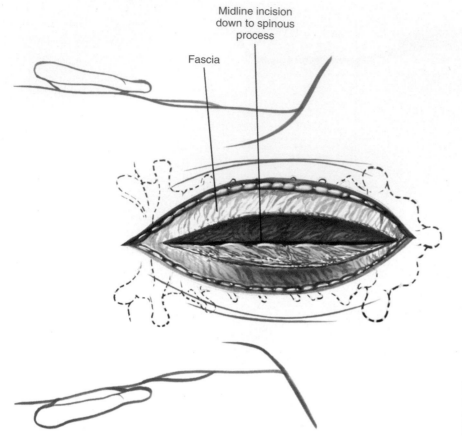

**Figure 6-47**  Continue the dissection down to the spinous processes through the nuchal ligament.

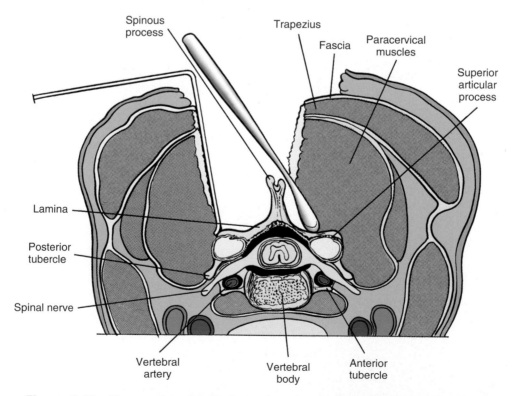

**Figure 6-48**    Remove the paraspinal muscles subperiosteally from the posterior aspect of the cervical spine either unilaterally or bilaterally, depending on the exposure needed. Note that the vertebral artery is considerably anterior to the posterior facet joints.

Remove the paraspinal muscles subperiosteally from the posterior aspect of the cervical spine either unilaterally or bilaterally, depending on the exposure needed; bilateral removal is done for a spine fusion and unilateral removal for a herniated disc. Use a Cobb elevator, which can remove the muscles from the bone without damaging them unduly (Fig. 6-48). Carry the dissection as far laterally as necessary to reveal the lamina, the facet joints, and the beginnings of the transverse processes (Figs. 6-49 and 6-50). If necessary, cauterize the segmental arterial vessel that runs between the transverse processes and close to the facets.

This dissection is quite safe. If it strays from the midline and cuts into muscles, however, notable bleeding can occur that will require immediate cauterization. If the patient has significant spina bifida, it is possible to enter the spinal canal, injuring neural tissue.

## Deep Surgical Dissection

Identify the ligamentum flavum that runs between the laminae. With a sharp blade, remove it from the leading edge of the lamina of the inferior vertebra. Place a flat, spatula-shaped instrument in the midline in the space between the two ligaments and cut down on the ligamentum flavum, with the metallic unit separating the ligamentum from the underlying dura. Perform a laminectomy, either partial or complete, removing as much of the lamina as necessary to see the blue-white dura, which lies immediately below it, probably covered by epidural fat. Next, gently retract the spinal cord medially and identify the posterior portion of the vertebral body, the disc space, and the possibly herniated disc (Figs. 6-51 and 6-52). Occasionally, the thin epidural veins surrounding the cord may bleed significantly. The veins can bleed anywhere; they are hardest to control between the anterior aspect of the cord and the posterior part of the vertebral body.

## Dangers

### Nerves

Take care never to retract the exposed **spinal cord and its nerve root** overzealously. If enough bone is removed during the laminectomy, both medially and laterally, the exposure should be large enough to minimize the need for cord retraction. The nerve roots themselves should be retracted gently to prevent unnecessary tethering from postoperative adhesions. Occasionally, the facet joint must be removed partially to expose the nerve root.

The **posterior primary rami** of the cervical nerve roots supply the paraspinal muscles and sensation to the overlying skin; they rarely are in danger. Even if a posterior ramus must be cauterized, the nerve supply to the paracervical muscles and skin is so rich that the denervation has no clinical effect.

### Vessels

The **venous plexus in the cervical canal** is plentiful and thin walled; when it is retracted, it may bleed profusely. Frequently, bipolar (or Malis) cau-

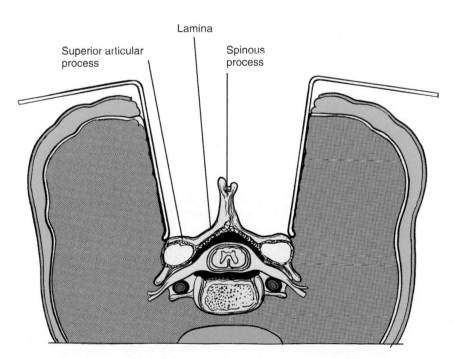

**Figure 6-49** Bilateral exposure of the posterior cervical spine.

Superior articular process

Lamina

Spinous process

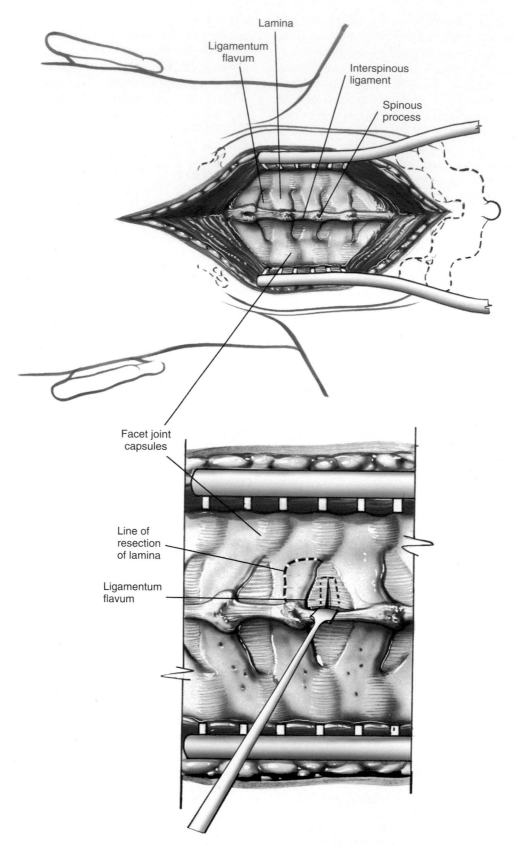

**Figure 6-50**   Carry the dissection as far laterally as necessary to reveal the lamina and facet joints, and the beginning of the transverse processes. Identify the ligamentum flavum and remove it *(inset)*. (Enlarged surgical field.)

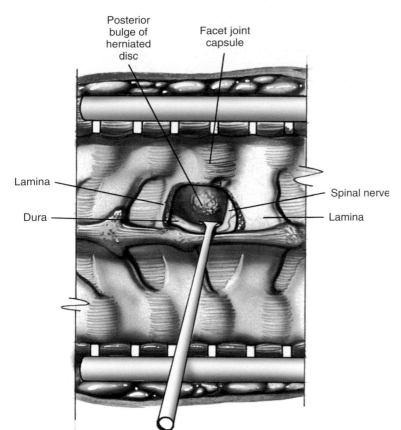

Posterior bulge of herniated disc

Facet joint capsule

Lamina

Dura

Spinal nerve

Lamina

**Figure 6-51** Perform a laminectomy, partial or complete, removing as much lamina as needed. Gently retract the nerve root and spinal cord medially to identify the posterior portion of the vertebral body.

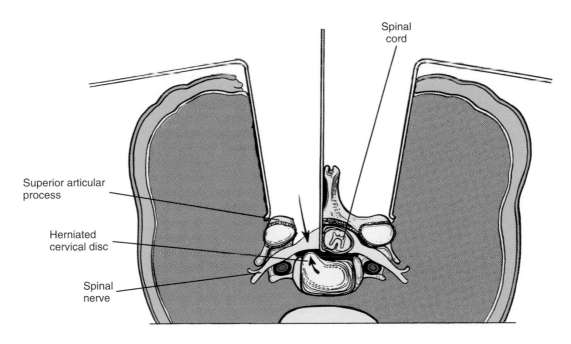

Spinal cord

Superior articular process

Herniated cervical disc

Spinal nerve

**Figure 6-52** Gently retract the cord medially. Identify the disc space and a possible herniated disc.

terization is the best way to control the venous bleeding.

The **segmental blood supply** to the paracervical muscles may be cut or stretched as the muscles are stripped past the facet joints. The muscles often contract, stopping the small amount of hemorrhage; however, if the torn vessels can be seen, they should be cauterized. The blood supply to the posterior cervical muscles is generous. Cauterization causes no problem and allows for a dry surgical field. Occasionally, a nutrient foramen of the spinous processes or lamina may bleed. This can be controlled easily with a dab of bone wax or cautery placed directly against the foramen.

The **vertebral artery** is enclosed in a bony canal running through the transverse process (transverse foramen). It is protected even if the transverse process is dissected onto. If the process is destroyed as a result of infection, tumor, or trauma, however, take great care not to enter the transverse foramen (see Figs. 6-48 and 6-56).

## How to Enlarge the Approach

### Local Measures
To enlarge the exposure, lengthen the skin incision. In addition, an extra vertebra may have to be dissected out proximally or distally. The exposure may be expanded laterally by drawing the muscles well out and past the facet joints and onto the transverse processes without causing damage. On occasion, the laminae even may be exposed bilaterally and the laminectomy extended both proximally and distally to improve exposure to the spinal cord and nerve roots.

### Extensile Measures
The cervical midline incision is very extensile. It may be extended proximally (staying in the midline plane) as high as the occiput of the skull and as far distally as the coccyx via subperiosteal removal of the paraspinal muscles.

# Applied Surgical Anatomy of the Posterior Approach to the Cervical Spine

## Overview

The muscles covering the posterior aspect of the cervical spine run longitudinally and are supplied segmentally. Although it is not critical to know the various individual posterior muscles of the cervical spine, being aware of these muscles and their layers is helpful. Because the approach itself is in the midline, it disturbs no vital structures and is relatively safe.

## Landmarks and Incision

### Landmarks
The spinous processes of the cervical spine, from C2 to C6, are bifid. C2 is the largest proximal cervical spinous process; the spinous processes of C3, C4, and C5 are relatively small. C7 is thicker, is not bifid, and has a tubercle at its end. Because it is the largest distal cervical spinous process, it is easy to palpate (see Fig. 6-57A).

All the spinous processes (except C7) are directed caudad and posteriorly, serving as points of attachment for the cervical muscles.

### Incision
The skin on the back of the neck is thicker and less mobile than is the skin on the throat; it is attached directly to the underlying fascia. The incision runs perpendicular to the tension line of the skin, causing thicker scarring. Nevertheless, the wound usually heals well, and, because the nape of the neck is covered with hair, cosmetic concerns seldom are a problem.

## Superficial Surgical Dissection

The ligamentum nuchae is a fibroelastic septum that takes origin from the occiput and inserts into the C7 spinous processes, sending septa down to each of the cervical spinous processes and dividing the more lateral paracervical muscles. The septum, which is almost vestigial in humans, is well developed in quadrupeds, because it helps the muscles support the head. It is the homologue of the supraspinous ligament in the rest of the spine. Dissection through it is safe, as long as it remains in the midline (see Fig. 6-57B).

The paracervical muscles in the cervical spine run in three layers. The most *superficial layer* consists of the trapezius muscle, which takes origin from the superior nuchal line and from all the spinous processes of the cervical spine. The trapezius covers the entire cervical area; in common with its counterpart in the lumbar spine, the latissimus dorsi, it is essentially an upper limb muscle (Fig. 6-53).

The *intermediate layer* is filled by the splenius capitis, a relatively large, flat muscle that takes origin from the midline (spine of C7, the lower half of the ligamentum nuchae, and the upper three thoracic

spinous processes) and inserts into the occipital bone (Fig. 6-54).

The *deep layer* is subdivided into three portions: superficial, middle, and deep. The superficial portion consists of the semispinalis capitis, a relatively large muscle that lies immediately beneath the splenius. The semispinalis capitis takes its origin from the transverse processes of the cervical vertebrae and inserts into the occipital bone. The middle portion of the deep layer is filled by the semispinalis cervicis, which originates from the transverse processes of the upper five or six thoracic vertebrae and inserts into the midline interspinous processes. The deepest portion of

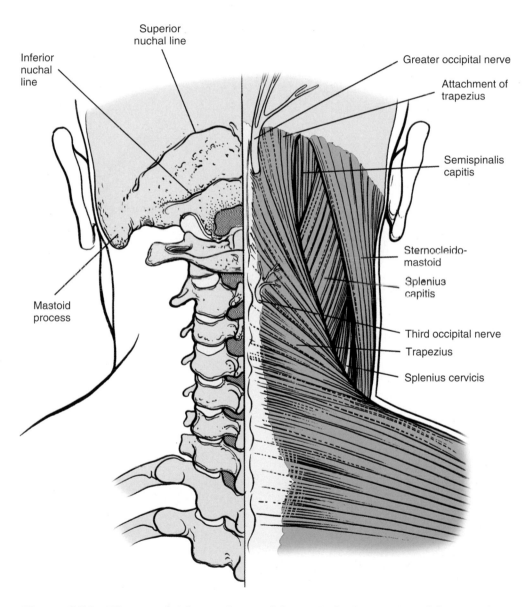

**Figure 6-53** The superficial musculature of the cervical spine consists of the trapezius and the sternocleidomastoid muscles. Between these and deeper levels lies the intermediate layer, the splenius capitis.

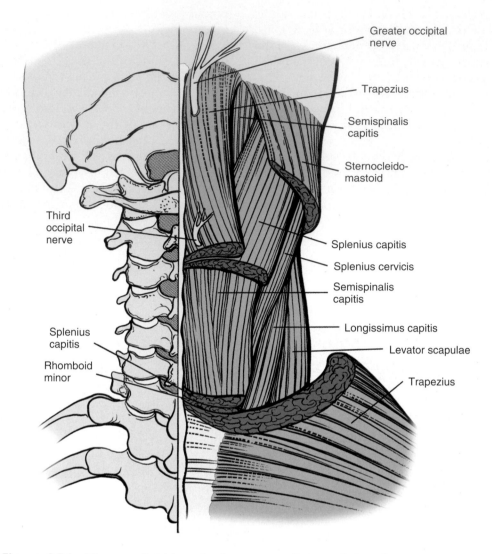

**Figure 6-54**   The superficial layer has been resected to reveal the splenius capitis, which also is resected partially. Deep to this are the semispinalis capitis, the longissimus capitis, the splenius cervicis, and, most laterally, the levator scapulae.

the deep layer consists of the multifidus muscles and the short and long rotator muscles (Fig. 6-55).

The laminae of the cervical vertebrae are angled from medial to lateral at 45°. Lateral to the laminae are the joint capsules, which completely surround the cervical facet joints. The facet joints are in a frontal plane (Figs. 6-57*B* and 6-58).

Unless the patient has a large spina bifida, the spinal canal is safe during this phase of the dissection. A wide, flat instrument (such as a Cobb dissector) held transverse to the lamina helps to protect the canal (see Fig. 6-48).

## Deep Surgical Dissection and its Dangers

As it does elsewhere in the spine, the ligamentum flavum connects the lamina on one vertebra to the adjacent vertebra, filling the space between the two. The ligaments are paired, one on each side, and may be separated in the midline by a tiny space. They take origin from the leading edge of the lower lamina and insert proximally into small ridges on the anterior surface of the higher vertebra, about one third up the anterior surface.

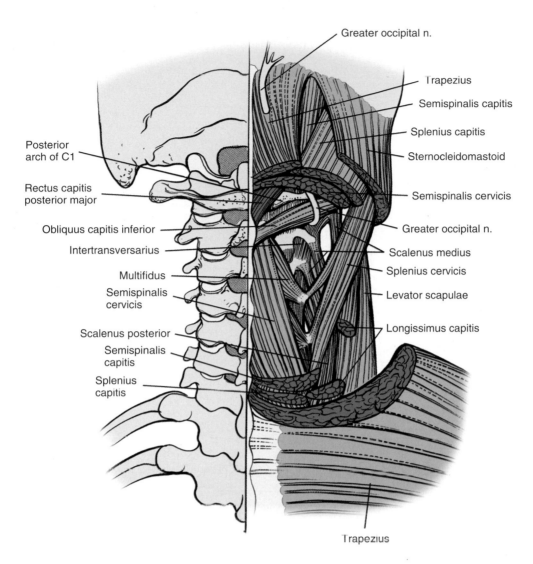

Greater occipital n.

Trapezius

Semispinalis capitis

Splenius capitis

Sternocleidomastoid

Semispinalis cervicis

Greater occipital n.

Scalenus medius

Splenius cervicis

Levator scapulae

Longissimus capitis

Posterior arch of C1

Rectus capitis posterior major

Obliquus capitis inferior

Intertransversarius

Multifidus

Semispinalis cervicis

Scalenus posterior

Semispinalis capitis

Splenius capitis

Trapezius

**Figure 6-55** The semispinalis capitis has been resected to reveal the deepest layer, the semispinalis cervicis, and the multifidi muscles.

Each ligamentum flavum extends from the midline laterally to the joint capsule. The spinal cord is directly beneath the ligamentum flavum. Therefore, the ligament must be removed carefully, so that the coverings of the cord (the outer dura, the middle arachnoid, the inner pia) do not tear. If the cord must be retracted medially to expose the disc space, it should be moved carefully so that its wrappings are not injured (see Fig. 6-51).

The posterior longitudinal ligament lies on the posterior surface of the cervical vertebral bodies, within the vertebral canal, and extends down through the entire spinal canal. The ligament attaches to each vertebra and disc; it is broadest in the cervical region.

Over the ligament, on the floor of the canal, lie large vertebral veins, comprising a nonvalvular venous plexus. These may bleed and require cauterization.

The key vascular structure in the deep dissection is the vertebral artery. The artery runs upward in the neck through a series of foramina in the transverse processes of the cervical vertebrae. Vigorous decortication may breach the posterior walls of these foramina and damage the artery, which carries a blood supply that is vital to the hindbrain. The risks are far greater when the transverse processes are involved in pathology. If the artery is damaged during dissection, no attempt should be made to repair it. It should be packed (see Figs. 6-56 and 6-58).

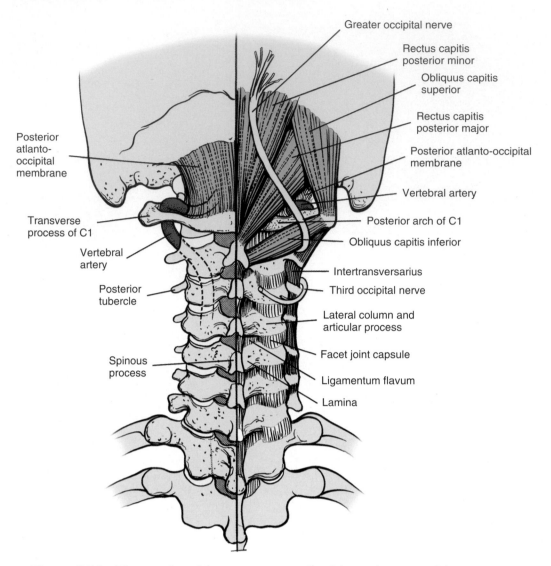

**Figure 6-56**   The muscles of the posterior triangle of the neck consist of the rectus capitis posterior minor and major, and the obliquus capitis superior and inferior. Note the course of the vertebral artery on the superior border of the arch of C1. It is lateral to the midline. The course of the vertebral artery in the transverse foramen distal to C1 is anterior to the facet joints.

**Rectus Capitis Posterior Major.** *Origin.* Tendinous, from spinous process of axis. *Insertion.* Into lateral part of inferior nuchal line of occipital bone and immediately below this line. *Action.* Extends head and rotates it to same side. *Nerve supply.* Nerve branch of posterior primary rami main line of suboccipital nerve.

**Rectus Capitis Posterior Minor.** *Origin.* Tendinous, from tubercle of posterior arch of atlas. *Insertion.* Into medial part of nuchal line of occipital bone and surface beneath it, and foramen magnum (only muscle to take origin from posterior arch of C1). *Action.* Extends head. *Nerve supply.* A branch of posterior primary main line of suboccipital nerve.

**Obliquus Capitis Inferior.** *Origin.* From apex of spinous process of axis. *Insertion.* Into inferoposterior part of transverse process of atlas. *Action.* Rotates atlas; turns head toward same side. *Nerve supply.* Branches of posterior primary rami main line of greater occipital nerve.

**Obliquus Capitis Superior.** *Origin.* From tendinous fibers from upper surface of transverse process of atlas. *Insertion.* Into occipital bone between superior inferior nuchal lines; lateral to the semispinalis capitis. *Action.* Extends head and bends it laterally. *Nerve supply.* A branch of posterior primary division of greater occipital nerve (first cervical nerve).

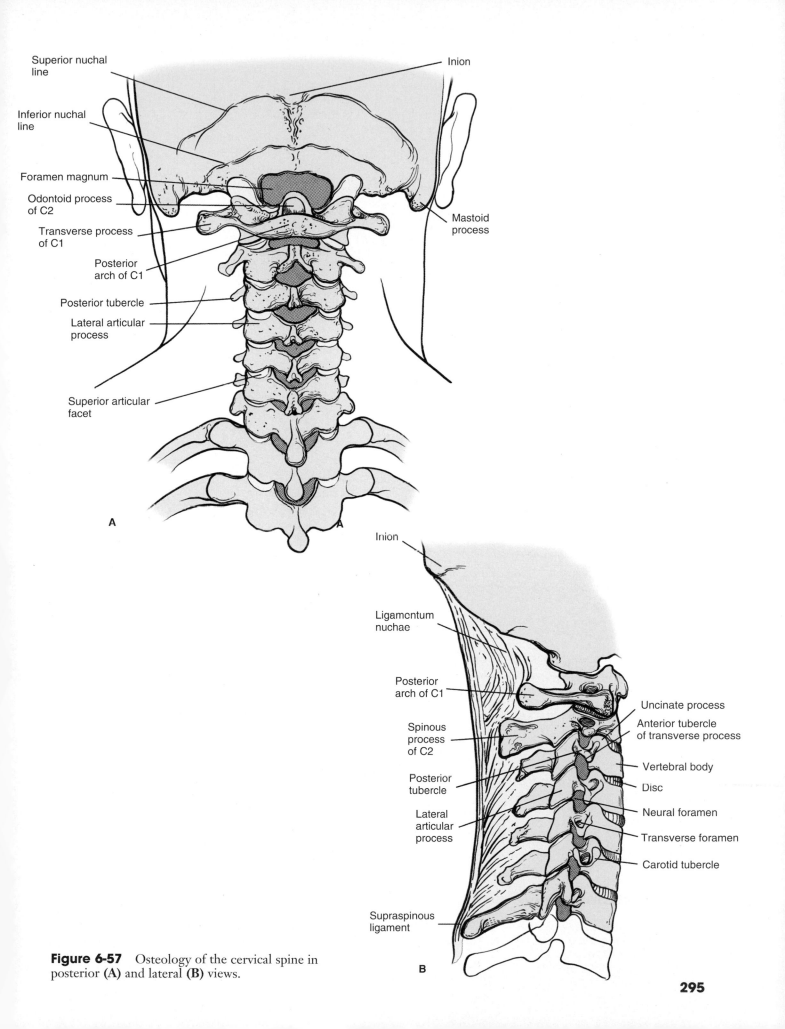

**Figure 6-57** Osteology of the cervical spine in posterior (**A**) and lateral (**B**) views.

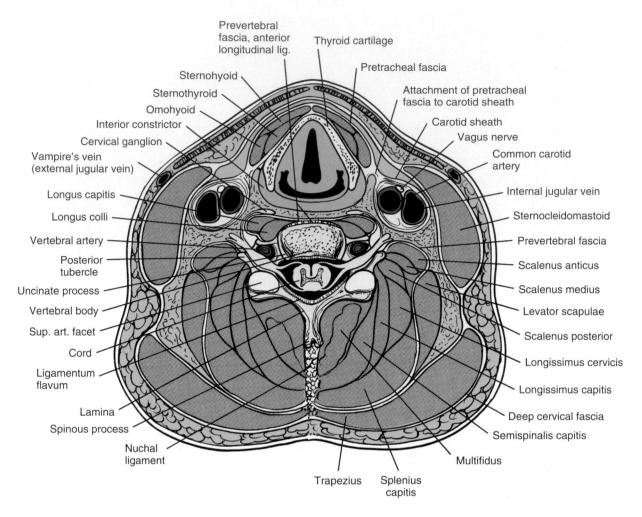

**Prevertebral fascia, anterior longitudinal lig.**

**Thyroid cartilage**

**Sternohyoid**

**Sternothyroid**

**Omohyoid**

**Interior constrictor**

**Cervical ganglion**

**Vampire's vein (external jugular vein)**

**Longus capitis**

**Longus colli**

**Vertebral artery**

**Posterior tubercle**

**Uncinate process**

**Vertebral body**

**Sup. art. facet**

**Cord**

**Ligamentum flavum**

**Lamina**

**Spinous process**

**Nuchal ligament**

**Pretracheal fascia**

**Attachment of pretracheal fascia to carotid sheath**

**Carotid sheath**

**Vagus nerve**

**Common carotid artery**

**Internal jugular vein**

**Sternocleidomastoid**

**Prevertebral fascia**

**Scalenus anticus**

**Scalenus medius**

**Levator scapulae**

**Scalenus posterior**

**Longissimus cervicis**

**Longissimus capitis**

**Deep cervical fascia**

**Semispinalis capitis**

**Multifidus**

**Trapezius**    **Splenius capitis**

**Figure 6-58**    Cross section of the cervical spine. Note that the vertebral artery is anterior to the nerve root.

# Posterior Approach to the C1-2 Vertebral Space

The posterior approach to the specialized cervical vertebrae C1 and C2, the atlas and the axis, is similar to that for the rest of the cervical spine. Because the two vertebrae differ slightly in their anatomy and function, however, they are discussed separately. The uses for this approach are the following:

1. Spinal fusion[13]
2. Decompression laminectomy
3. Treatment of tumors

## Position of the Patient

Place the patient prone, with the head and neck flexed to separate the occiput and the ring of the atlas (C1; see Fig. 6-44).

## Landmarks and Incision

### Landmarks

Palpate the *external occipital protuberance* high in the midline of the skull at the midpoint of the superior nuchal line. Although the *spinous process of C2* is the largest spinous process in the proximal part of the cervical spine, it is hard to palpate except as a resistance. C1 has no spinous process at all and is not palpable.

### Incision

Make an incision in the midline from the external occipital protuberance inferiorly for 6 to 8 cm (Fig. 6-59).

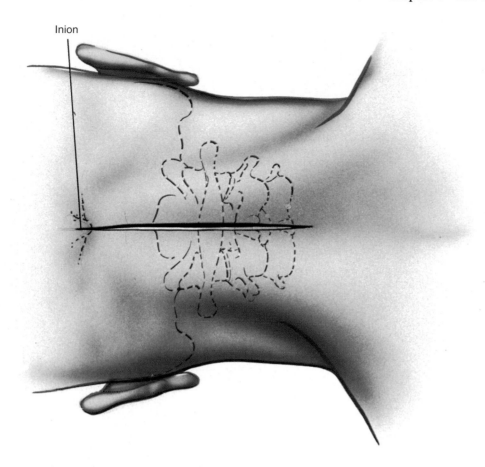

Inion

**Figure 6-59**   Make an incision in the midline from the external occipital protuberance inferiorly for 6 to 10 cm.

## Internervous Plane

The midline plane lies between paracervical muscles supplied by branches of the left and right posterior primary rami of the proximal cervical nerve roots. The plane is internervous and extensile.

## Superficial Surgical Dissection

Deepen the wound in line with the skin incision by incising the fascia and nuchal ligament in the midline of the neck, cutting down onto the large spinous process of C2 (Figs. 6-60 and 6-61). Extend this fascial incision distally onto the spinous process of C3 and then proximally onto the tubercle of C1. Continue proximally, cutting down onto the external occipital protuberance.

Carefully remove the paracervical muscles from the posterior elements of C1 and C2 (Fig. 6-62). Use a wide dissecting instrument (such as a Cobb elevator) to avoid inadvertently breaching the spinal canal. Note that the facet joints between C1 and C2 are about an inch further anterior than are those between C2 and C3. Carry the dissection up to the base of the occiput, if necessary, to expose the superior margin of the ring of C1 (see Fig. 6-62).

## Deep Surgical Dissection

If necessary, the ligamentum flavum (posterior atlantoaxial ligament) can be removed from between C2 and C1, and the posterior atlanto-occipital membrane can be removed from between C1 and the occiput (Fig. 6-63). This rarely is necessary. Usually, separating these membranes from bone is all that is needed to pass a wire underneath the arch of C1 so that the area can retain bone graft. Once these posterior ligaments have been removed, the dura of the cervical portion of the spinal cord is uncovered.

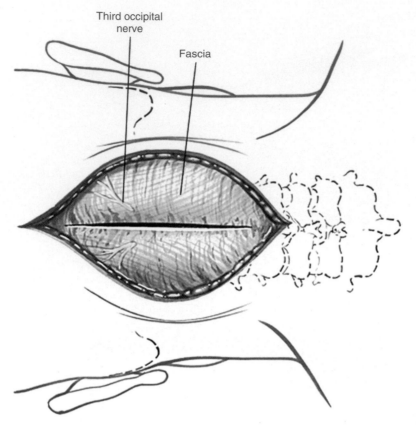

**Figure 6-60** Deepen the wound in line with the skin incision by incising the fascia and nuchal ligament in the midline of the neck.

## Dangers

### Nerves

In nontumorous conditions, a considerable gap exists between the dura and the bony ring at the level of C1-2, and the cord rarely has to be retracted. Retracting the cord is extremely hazardous, because overzealous retraction can cause death from respiratory paralysis; in principle, it simply should not be retracted.

Two large cutaneous nerves, **the greater occipital nerve** (C2) and the **third occipital nerve** (C3), cross the operative field (see Figs. 6-53 and 6-56). These nerves, which are branches from the posterior rami, supply a large area of skin at the back of the scalp. They run upward from a lateral position, and midline dissection does not damage them. Take care when dissecting laterally to stay on bone and avoid damaging these nerves.

### Vessels

The **vertebral artery** crosses the operative field. It passes from the transverse foramen of the atlas, immediately behind the atlanto-occipital joint, and pierces the lateral angle of the posterior atlanto-occipital membrane. It is vulnerable at that point during the approach (see Fig. 6-56).

## How to Enlarge the Approach

### Local Measures

Extend the skin incision proximally and dissect the paracervical muscles from their attachments to the skull. Extend the incision distally and strip the muscles off the posterior bony elements of C3.

### Extensile Measures

Extend the incision distally. Then continue the midline approach to the spinous processes of the remaining cervical vertebrae. Theoretically, the approach can be extended down to the coccyx.

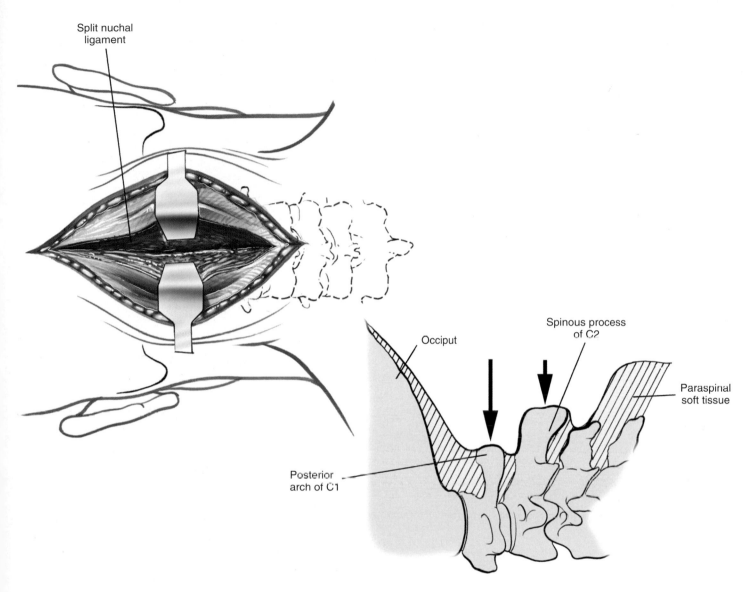

**Figure 6-61**   Incise the nuchal ligament down onto the large spinous processes of C2. Lateral view *(inset)*. Note that the ring of C1 is further anterior than the spinous process of C2.

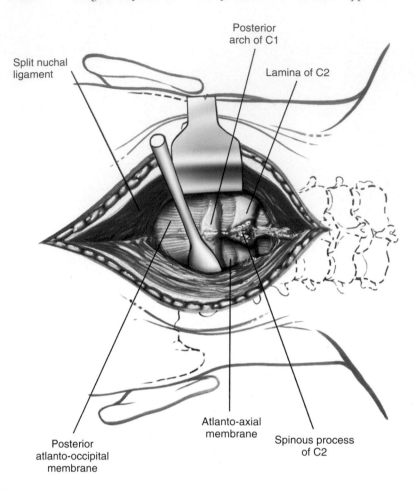

**Figure 6-62**    Remove the paracervical muscles from the posterior elements of C1 and C2. Carry the dissection up to the base of the occiput.

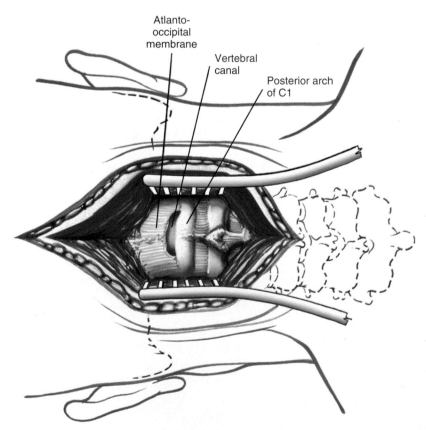

**Figure 6-63**    Remove the posterior atlanto-occipital membrane from between C1 and the occiput, if necessary.

# Applied Surgical Anatomy of the Posterior Approach to the C1-2 Vertebral Space

## Overview

C1 and C2 are specialized to permit the extreme motion of the upper cervical spine. As in other parts of the spine, the muscles covering C1 and C2 lie in three layers. The outer layer consists of the trapezius, a muscle of the upper limb. The intermediate layer is made up of the paraspinal muscles, in this case, the splenius capitis and the semispinalis capitis.

The anatomy of the area is unique in its deepest layer; there are four pairs of small muscles that drive the unusual movements that these joints are capable of. The riskiest part of surgery in the area occurs in the deepest plane. The vertebral artery, which runs through the foramen transversarium (still deeper) never should be seen during dissection, but its position always must be kept in mind.

## Landmarks and Incision

### Landmarks

The spinous process of C2 is large, bulbous, and bifid, accommodating the insertions of the semispinalis cervicis and multifidus, deep muscles that attach to it and stop, leaving the atlas with almost no muscle attachment so that it is free to rotate around the occiput. The posterior vertebral arch of C2 and its lamina, which ascends to the spinous processes, are massive enough to support the larger spinous process.

The *external occipital protuberance*, or inion, a large boss of bone in the center of the occiput, divides the superior nuchal line, which extends from it to each side. The superior nuchal line separates the scalp above from the area of insertion of the nuchal muscles (see Fig. 6-57).

### Incisions

Skin incisions heal well because of the area's rich blood supply. Because the incisions run along the midline, they suffer minimal tension. Cosmetically, they are difficult to see because of the hairline.

## Superficial Surgical Dissection

The ligamentum nuchae, the midline fibrous membrane, extends from the external occipital protuber-ance to the spinous process of the seventh cervical vertebra. A septum extends from its anterior border; it attaches to the posterior tubercle of the atlas and all the remaining spinous processes of the cervical spine (see Fig. 6-57B).

The muscles of the superficial and intermediate layers consist of the trapezius (in the superficial layer) and the splenius capitis, which covers the semispinalis capitis and the longissimus capitis (all in the intermediate layer; see Figs. 6-53 and 6-54).

The splenius capitis arises from the thoracic spinous processes before inserting into the base of the skull. Deep to it lies the semispinalis cervicis, which inserts onto the axis.

Detaching these muscles uncovers the four unique muscles of the suboccipital triangle, the rectus capitis posterior major and minor, and the oblique capitis inferior and superior (see Fig. 6-56).

## Deep Surgical Dissection

Because C1 has no spinous process, finding its bony ring posteriorly requires an especially deep dissection (see Fig. 6-57B).

The atlantoaxial and atlanto-occipital membranes, which form the remaining posterior coverings of the cord, are homologues of the original ligamentum flavum. The spinal canal at C1-2 is particularly spacious, allowing extensive motion (see Fig. 6-56).

Two important cutaneous nerves intrude into the lateral aspect of the suboccipital triangle: the greater occipital nerve (the posterior primary ramus of C2) and the third occipital nerve (the posterior primary ramus of C3; see Figs. 6-53 and 6-56). The most important structure in the suboccipital triangle is the *vertebral artery*. This key blood supply to the hindbrain ascends in the neck through a series of foramina in the transverse processes. At the level of the atlas, it pierces the foramen transversarium of the atlas and then turns medially behind the atlanto-occipital joint. To enter the spinal canal, it pierces the posterior atlanto-occipital membrane at its lateral angle; therefore, it is extremely vulnerable during dissection of the atlanto-occipital membrane (see Fig. 6-56).

# Anterior Approach to the Cervical Spine

The anterior approach to the cervical spine exposes the anterior vertebral bodies from C3 to T1. It also allows direct access to the disc spaces and uncinate processes in the region. It is used for the following:

1. Excision of herniated discs (R.B. Cloward, personal communication, 1969)[14]
2. Interbody fusion (see the section regarding the anterior approach to the iliac crest for bone graft)
3. Removal of osteophytes from the uncinate processes and from either the anterior or the posterior lip of the vertebral bodies
4. Excision of tumors and associated bone grafting
5. Treatment of osteomyelitis
6. Biopsy of vertebral bodies and disc spaces
7. Drainage of abscesses

The recurrent laryngeal nerve is the most important structure at risk during the anterior approach to the cervical spine. The left recurrent laryngeal nerve ascends in the neck between the trachea and the esophagus, having branched off from its parent nerve, the vagus, at the level of the arch of the aorta. The right recurrent laryngeal nerve runs alongside the trachea in the neck after hooking around the right subclavian artery. In the lower part of the neck, it crosses from lateral to medial to reach the midline trachea; therefore, it is slightly more vulnerable during the exposure than is the left recurrent laryngeal nerve. This is why some surgeons prefer left-sided approaches, whereas others simply approach from the side of pathology.

## Position of the Patient

Place the patient supine on the operating table with a small sandbag between the shoulder blades to ensure extension of the neck. Turn the patient's head away from the planned incision to provide good access to the side of the neck (Fig. 6-64). Install halter traction so that it can be used later if distraction is required. Elevate the table 30° to reduce venous bleeding and make the neck more accessible. Place the patient's arm at his or her side.

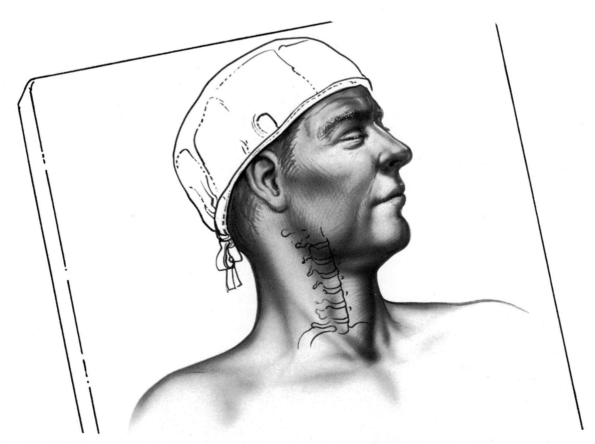

**Figure 6-64**    Place the patient supine on the operating table with a small sandbag between the shoulder blades to ensure an extended position of the neck. Turn the patient's head away from the planned incision.

## Landmarks and Incision

### Landmarks

Several palpable anterior structures in the midline help identify the vertebral level in the neck.

1. Hard palate–arch of the atlas
2. Lower border of the mandible–C2-3
3. Hyoid bone–C3
4. Thyroid cartilage–C4-5
5. Cricoid cartilage–C6
6. Carotid tubercle–C6

These landmarks make it possible to determine the approximate level of the incision (Fig. 6-65; see Fig. 6-76).

***Sternocleidomastoid Muscle.*** The sternocleidomastoid, an oblique muscle, runs from the mastoid process to the sternum, just lateral to the midline of the neck. To make it more prominent, turn the head away from the muscle in question, into the operating position.

***Carotid Artery.*** Place a finger over the leading edge of the sternocleidomastoid and press posteriorly and laterally to feel the carotid pulse. Palpate only one pulse at a time to avoid creating temporary brain ischemia.

***Carotid Tubercle (Chassaignac's Tubercle).*** Palpate deeper; note the large tubercle adjacent to the carotid pulse on the anterior part of the transverse process of C6.[15]

### Incision

If the level of pathology is localized, make a transverse skin crease incision at the appropriate level of the vertebral pathology (see above). The incision should extend obliquely from the midline to the posterior border of the sternocleidomastoid muscle. Such an incision has extreme cosmetic advantage (see Fig. 6-65).

## Internervous Plane

No internervous plane is available superficially, but incising or dividing the platysma muscle causes no significant problems; the muscle is supplied high up in the neck by branches of the facial (seventh cranial) nerve.

More deeply, the plane lies between the sternocleidomastoid muscle (which is supplied by the spinal accessory nerve) and the strap muscles of the neck (which receive segmental innervation from C1, C2, and C3; see Fig. 6-68, *cross section*).

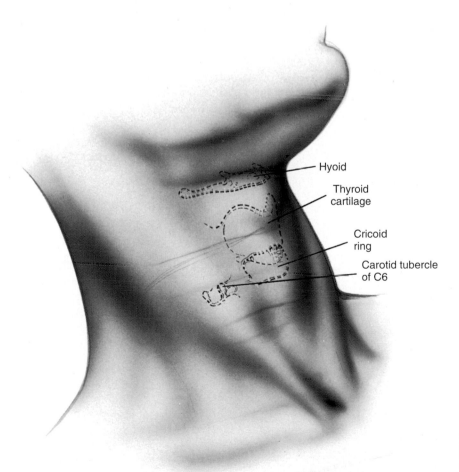

Hyoid

Thyroid cartilage

Cricoid ring

Carotid tubercle of C6

**Figure 6-65**  Make an oblique incision in the skin crease of the neck at the appropriate level of the vertebral pathology.

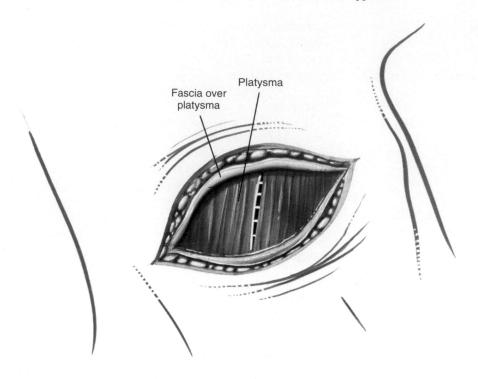

Fascia over platysma

Platysma

**Figure 6-66**   Incise the fascial sheath over the platysma in line with the skin incision. Split the platysma longitudinally, parallel to its long fibers.

Deeper still, the plane lies between the left and right longus colli muscles, which are supplied separately by segmental branches from the second to the seventh cervical nerves (see Fig. 6-70, *cross section*).

## Superficial Surgical Dissection

The skin and the platysma muscle are very vascular. For this reason, some surgeons inject the area with a dilute solution of epinephrine (Adrenalin) before incising the skin.

Incise the fascial sheath over the platysma in line with the skin wound (Fig. 6-66). Then, split the platysma longitudinally using the tips of the index fingers, dissecting parallel to the long fibers. Identify the anterior border of the sternocleidomastoid muscle and incise the fascia immediately anterior to it (Fig. 6-67). Using the fingers, gently retract the sternocleidomastoid muscle laterally. Retract the sternohyoid and ster-

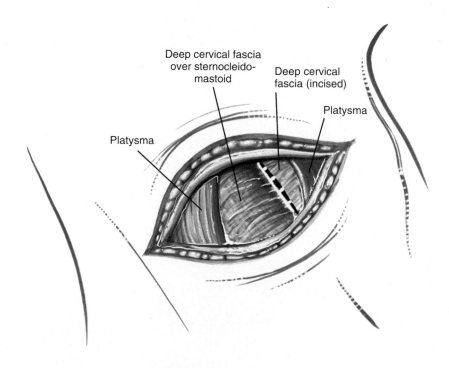

Deep cervical fascia over sternocleido-mastoid

Deep cervical fascia (incised)

Platysma

Platysma

**Figure 6-67**   Identify the anterior border of the sternocleidomastoid and incise the fascia medially anterior to it.

nothyroid strap muscles (with the associated trachea and underlying esophagus) medially.

The carotid sheath enclosing the common carotid artery, vein, and vagus nerve now can be exposed, if necessary (Fig. 6-68).

Palpate the artery. Develop a plane between the medial edge of the carotid sheath and the midline

structures (thyroid gland, trachea, and esophagus), cutting through the pretracheal fascia on the medial side of the carotid sheath. Retract the sheath and its enclosed structures laterally with the sternocleido-mastoid muscle (Fig. 6-69).

Two arteries connect the carotid sheath with the midline structures. These two vessels, the superior

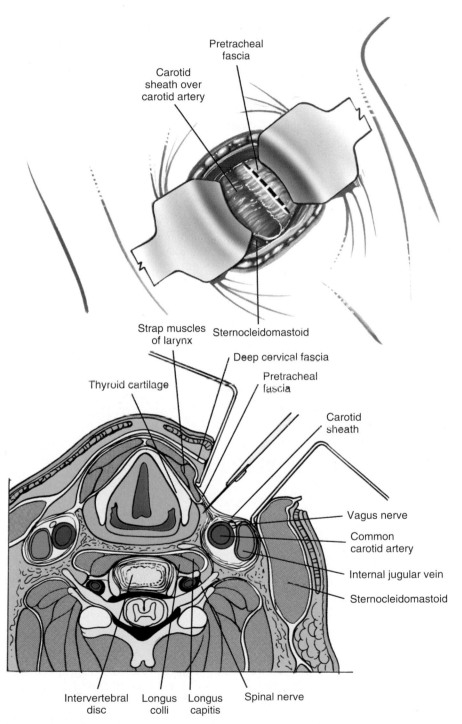

**Figure 6-68**   Retract the sternocleidomastoid laterally, and the strap muscles and thyroid structures medially. Cut through the exposed pretracheal fascia on the medial side of the carotid sheath. The cervical spine C3 through C5 *(cross section)*. Retract the sternocleidomastoid laterally and the strap muscles medially, and incise the pretracheal fascia immediately medial to the carotid sheath.

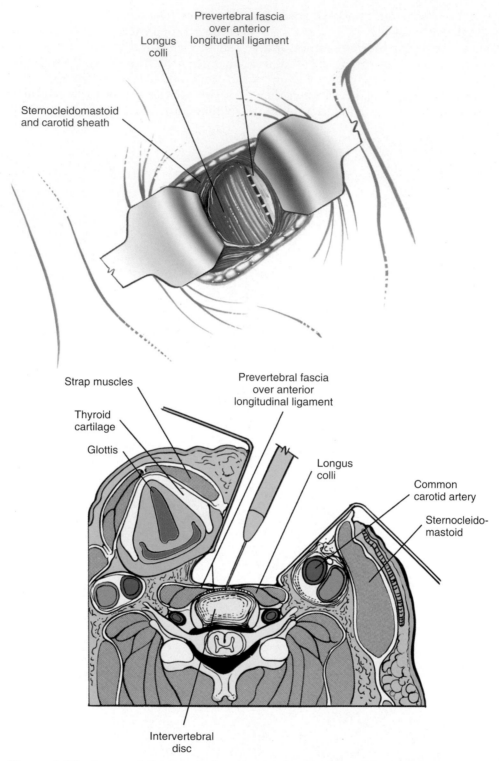

Longus
colli

Prevertebral fascia
over anterior
longitudinal ligament

Sternocleidomastoid
and carotid sheath

Strap muscles

Prevertebral fascia
over anterior
longitudinal ligament

Thyroid
cartilage

Glottis

Longus
colli

Common
carotid artery

Sternocleido-
mastoid

Intervertebral
disc

**Figure 6-69**   Retract the sternocleidomastoid and the carotid sheath laterally, and the strap muscles, trachea, and esophagus medially to expose the longus colli muscle and pretracheal fascia. Retract the sternocleidomastoid muscle and carotid sheath laterally, and the strap muscles and thyroid structures medially, then split the longus colli muscle longitudinally in the midline *(cross section)*.

**Figure 6-70**   Dissect the longus colli muscle subperiosteally from the anterior portion of the vertebral body and retract each portion laterally to expose the anterior surface of the vertebral body. The longus colli muscles are retracted to the left and right of the midline to expose the anterior surface of the vertebral body *(cross section)*.

and inferior thyroid arteries, may limit the extent to which this plane can be opened up above C3-4. Occasionally, either or both of them may have to be divided to open the plane.

Now, develop a plane deep to the cut pretracheal fascia by blunt dissection, proceeding carefully in a medial direction behind the esophagus, which is retracted from the midline.

The cervical vertebrae should be visible now, covered by the longus colli muscle and the prevertebral fascia. The anterior longitudinal ligament in the midline can be seen as a gleaming white structure.

The sympathetic chain lies on the longus colli, just lateral to the vertebral bodies (see Fig. 6-69).

## Deep Surgical Dissection

Using cautery, split the longus colli muscle longitudinally over the midline of the vertebral bodies that need to be exposed (see Fig. 6-69, *cross section*). Then, dissect the muscle subperiosteally with the anterior longitudinal ligament and retract each portion laterally (i.e., to the left and right of the midline) to expose the anterior surface of the vertebral body (Fig. 6-70). Obtain a lat-

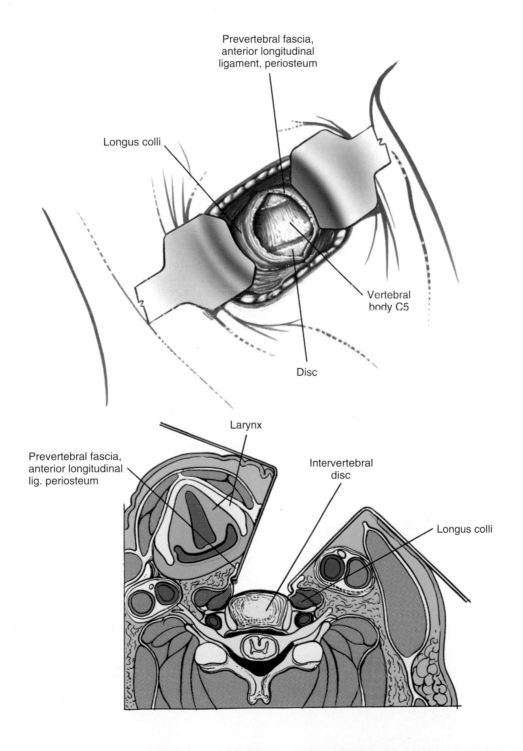

Prevertebral fascia, anterior longitudinal ligament, periosteum

Longus colli

Vertebral body C5

Disc

Larynx

Prevertebral fascia, anterior longitudinal lig. periosteum

Intervertebral disc

Longus colli

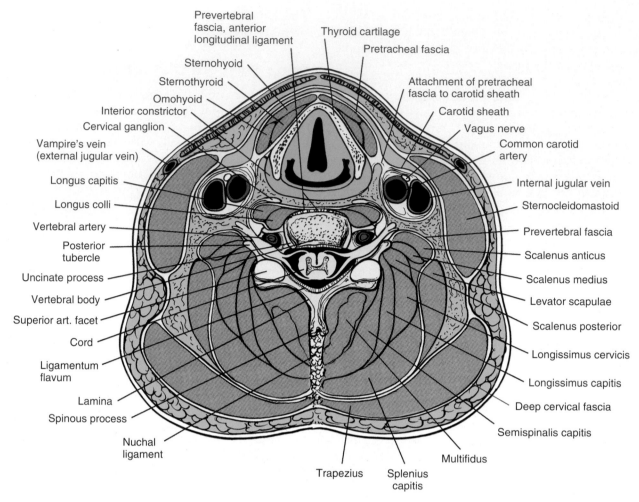

**Figure 6-71**   Cross section at the level of C5. Note the deep cervical fascia, the pretracheal fascia, and the prevertebral fascia. Note the relationship of the pretracheal fascia to the carotid sheath.

eral radiograph after placing a needle marker in the appropriate vertebral body to identify the level correctly. Make sure that the retractors are placed underneath each of the longus colli muscles, widening the exposure while protecting the recurrent laryngeal nerve, trachea, and esophagus.

## Dangers

### Nerves

The **recurrent laryngeal nerve** may be traumatized during the deepest layer of the approach. Protect it by placing the retractors well under the medial edge of the longus colli muscle (Fig. 6-73).

The **sympathetic nerves and stellate ganglion** may be damaged or irritated, causing Horner's syndrome. Protect them by making sure that dissection onto the bone is subperiosteal from the midline.

Avoid dissecting out onto the transverse processes (Fig. 6-74; see Fig. 6-69).

### Vessels

The **carotid sheath and its contents** are protected by the anterior border of the sternocleidomastoid muscle. Do not place self-retaining retractors in this area, or the sheath will be endangered. If additional retraction is necessary, use hand-held retractors with rounded ends (see Figs. 6-68, *cross section*, and 6-73).

The **vertebral artery,** which lies in the costo-transverse foramen on the lateral portion of the transverse processes, should not be visible during the approach unless the plane of operation strays well away from the midline (Fig. 6-75; see Fig. 6-70, *cross section*).

The inferior thyroid artery may cross the operative field in lower cervical approaches. If it is divided accidentally, it may retract behind the carotid sheath,

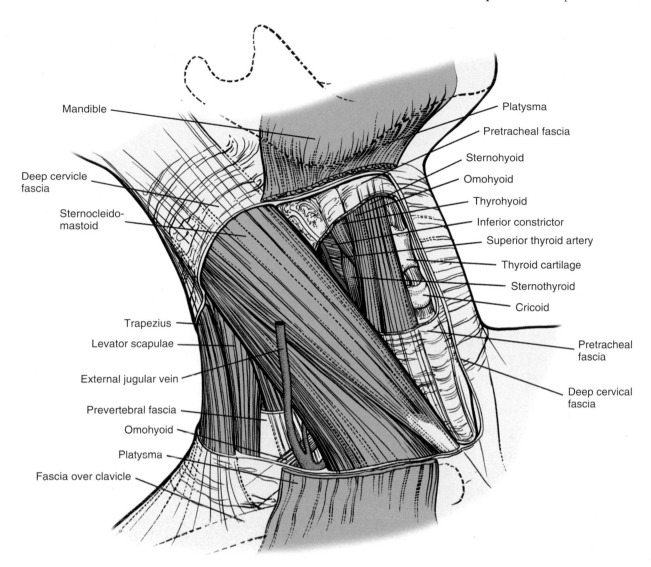

**Figure 6-72**   The platysma and deep cervical fascia have been removed. Note that the deep cervical fascia (investing fascia) encloses the sternocleidomastoid. The deeper pretracheal fascia encloses the strap muscles and thyroid structures.

where it is difficult to retrieve and tie off (see Fig. 6-74).

## Special Points

Poorly placed retractors endanger the trachea and esophagus. Unless they are placed underneath the longus colli muscle, the retractors used should be rounded and hand-held (see Fig. 6-70, *cross section*).

## How to Enlarge the Approach

### Local Measures

To enlarge the approach laterally, remove the origins of the longus colli muscle subperiosteally from the vertebral body. Take care not to proceed too far laterally to avoid damaging the sympathetic chain.

### Extensile Measures

This approach cannot be extended.

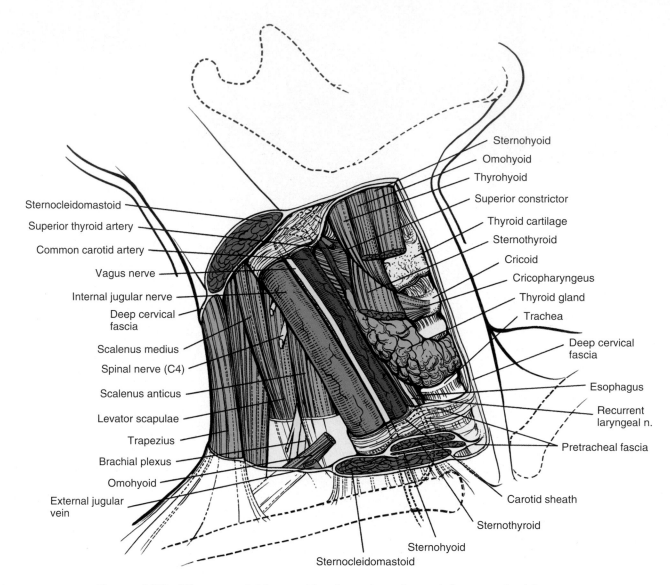

Sternocleidomastoid
Superior thyroid artery
Common carotid artery
Vagus nerve
Internal jugular nerve
Deep cervical fascia
Scalenus medius
Spinal nerve (C4)
Scalenus anticus
Levator scapulae
Trapezius
Brachial plexus
Omohyoid
External jugular vein

Sternohyoid
Omohyoid
Thyrohyoid
Superior constrictor
Thyroid cartilage
Sternothyroid
Cricoid
Cricopharyngeus
Thyroid gland
Trachea
Deep cervical fascia
Esophagus
Recurrent laryngeal n.
Pretracheal fascia
Carotid sheath
Sternothyroid
Sternohyoid
Sternocleidomastoid

**Figure 6-73** The sternocleidomastoid and strap muscles, and the pretracheal fascia have been resected. The carotid sheath and its contents have been exposed. The thyroid gland, cartilage, and trachea are seen. Note the course of the recurrent laryngeal nerve.

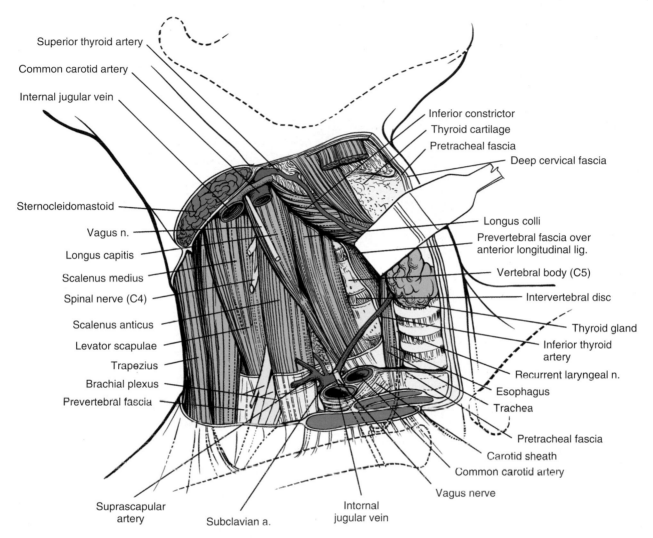

**Figure 6-74**   The carotid sheath and its contents have been resected. The larynx and its related structures are retracted medially. The longus colli and scalenus muscles with their overriding prevertebral fascia are seen. The sympathetic chain lies on the lateral border of the longus colli muscle. Note the position of the recurrent laryngeal nerve between the trachea and esophagus.

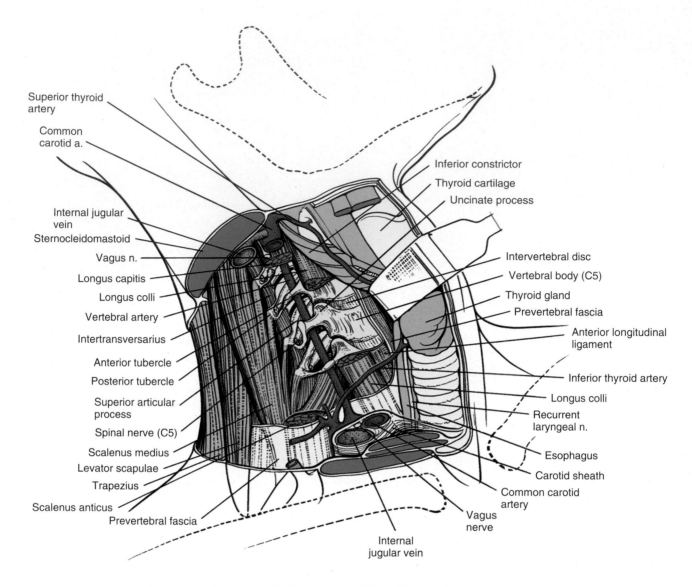

**Figure 6-75**   The longus colli, the longus capitis, and the scalenus anticus muscles have been resected to reveal the anterior portion of the vertebral bodies and transverse processes. Note the course of the vertebral artery through the transverse processes anterior to the nerve root. Note the course of the superior and inferior thyroid vessels.

# Applied Surgical Anatomy of the Anterior Approach to the Cervical Spine

## Overview

The key to understanding the anatomy of the anterior approach to the cervical spine lies in appreciating the three fascial layers of the neck. The most superficial fascial layer is the investing layer of *deep cervical fascia*. The fascia surrounds the neck like a collar, but splits around the sternocleidomastoid and trapezius muscles to enclose them. Posteriorly, it joins with the ligamentum nuchae (nuchal ligament). The superficial layer is incised along the anterior border of the sternocleidomastoid muscle. Dividing the layer of fascia allows the sternocleidomastoid to be retracted laterally and separated from the underlying strap muscles. The only structures that lie superficial to it are the platysma muscle (a remnant of the old panniculus carnosus, or muscle of the skin) and the external jugular vein, which can be divided safely if it intrudes into the operative field (Figs. 6-71 and 6-72).

The next fascial layer is the *pretracheal fascia*, which forms a layer between sliding surfaces. It invests the strap muscles and runs from the hyoid bone down into the chest (see Fig. 6-72). Its key relationship is with the carotid sheath, which encloses the common carotid artery, the internal jugular vein, and the vagus nerve. The pretracheal fascia is continuous with the carotid sheath at the sheath's lateral margin (see Figs. 6-71 and 6-73). Hence, the pretracheal fascia must be divided on the medial border of the carotid sheath so that the carotid sheath can be retracted laterally and the midline structures can be retracted medially. Two sets of vessels, the superior and inferior thyroid vessels, run from the carotid sheath through the pretracheal fascia into the midline. On rare occasions, the thyroid vessels have to be

divided to enlarge the exposure (see Fig. 6-74). The superior laryngeal nerve, however, which runs with the superior thyroid vessels, must be preserved.

The deepest layer of fascia is the *prevertebral fascia*, a firm, tough membrane that lies in front of the prevertebral muscles. On its surface runs the cervical sympathetic trunk, which lies roughly over the transverse processes of the cervical vertebrae. Beneath the prevertebral fascia are the left and right longus colli muscles (see Figs. 6-71 and 6-74).

## Landmarks and Incision

### Landmarks

The *carotid tubercle* is the enlargement of the anterior tubercle of the transverse process of C6. It is larger than all other vertebral tubercles (there is no anterior tubercle of C7) and may be palpable. The tubercle of C6 is the key surgical landmark in the anterior incision (Fig. 6-76).

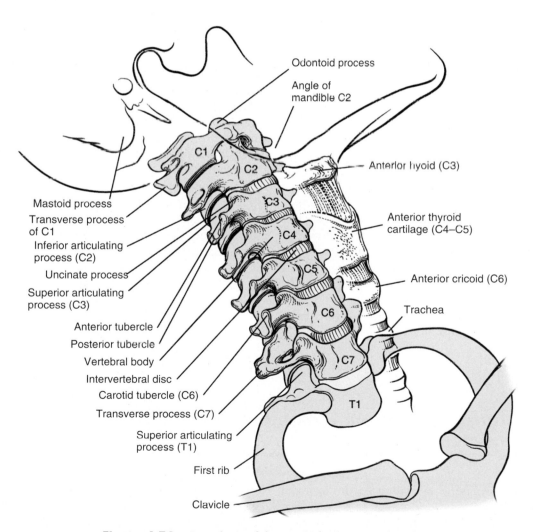

**Figure 6-76** Osteology of the cervical spine, anterior view.

The *cricoid ring* is easily palpable just beneath the thyroid cartilage. The only complete ring of the trachea, it is opposite the C6 vertebral body (see Figs. 6-65 and 6-72).

The *sternocleidomastoid muscle* runs obliquely down the side of the neck from the mastoid process to the sternum and clavicle. It is enclosed in fascia, which must be divided on the medial side before the muscle can be retracted laterally. The nerve supply of the sternocleidomastoid comes from the accessory nerve, which innervates the muscle from its posterior and lateral surfaces. There is no danger of neurologic damage as long as the dissection remains on the medial or anteromedial side of the muscle. If it strays to the posterior side, however, the spinal accessory nerve, which supplies not only the sternocleidomastoid, but also the trapezius, can be damaged (see Fig. 6-72).

### Incision

Ideally, the skin incision should run parallel to the cleavage lines of the skin of the neck. Inferiorly and anteriorly, these lines run transversely, making the skin crease incision advantageous. The skin on the anterior part of the neck is thinner and more mobile than is the skin on the back of the neck, because of both the loose subcutaneous tissue and the superficial fascia that remains unconnected to the investing fascia of the neck. As a result, skin retraction is easy; the skin incision can be moved to accommodate the needs of the surgery.

## Superficial Surgical Dissection and its Dangers

The platysma muscle is split in line with its fibers. The muscle is difficult to denervate, because most of its nerve supply comes from the cervical branch of the facial nerve and begins in the region of the mandible. In any case, the muscle is not of great functional importance; sewing it carefully during closure can improve the cosmetic appearance of the scar.

Dividing the fascia on the anterior border of the sternocleidomastoid muscle reveals the carotid sheath (see Fig. 6-68, *cross section*). The sheath contains the common carotid artery, which divides at the upper border of the thyroid cartilage into internal and external carotid arteries. It also contains the internal jugular vein and the vagus nerve (see Fig. 6-73). After the plane between the carotid sheath and the trachea and esophagus has been entered, it is easy to develop by blunt dissection. The esophagus, however, is a fragile structure that is damaged easily by injudicious retraction.

## Deep Surgical Dissection and its Dangers

The longus colli muscles lie on the anterior surface of the vertebral column, between C1 and T3. The muscles are pointed at their ends and broad in the middle. They must be removed from the vertebral bodies to expose the vertebrae. Removal does not denervate them, because they are innervated segmentally and laterally from their posterior surfaces. Running on the anterolateral surfaces of the longus colli muscles is the cervical sympathetic trunk, with its numerous ganglia. These must be avoided (see Figs. 6-71 and 6-74).

### Recurrent Laryngeal Nerves

The two recurrent laryngeal nerves are branches of the vagus nerve. The left recurrent laryngeal nerve descends into the thorax within the carotid sheath. It curves around the aortic arch and ascends back in the neck, running between the trachea and esophagus to supply the larynx. The right recurrent laryngeal nerve descends within the carotid sheath and curves around the subclavian artery before ascending into the neck at a higher level than the left recurrent laryngeal nerve. In addition, the right recurrent laryngeal nerve is, on rare occasions, aberrant, leaving the carotid sheath at a higher level and crossing the operative field at the level of the thyroid gland (see Figs. 6-73 and 6-74). Thus, left-sided approaches often are preferred. The nerves usually are safe as long as retractors are placed correctly underneath the longus colli muscles.

# Posterolateral (Costotransversectomy) Approach to the Thoracic Spine

The classic posterolateral approach to the thoracic spine was developed for the drainage of tuberculous abscesses in this part of the spine. Its major advantage is that it does not involve entering the thoracic cavity, which was a potentially fatal event in the era before antibiotics. The approach is less extensive than a formal thoracotomy and offers a poorer exposure. It probably is best for limited exposures in patients who are at high risk.

Its uses include the following:

1. Abscess drainage[16,17]
2. Vertebral body biopsy
3. Partial vertebral body resection
4. Limited anterior spinal fusion
5. Anterolateral decompression of the spinal cord

## Position of the Patient

Place the patient prone on the operating table, with bolsters positioned longitudinally on each side of the rib cage to allow for chest expansion. Drape widely over the rib cage area so that the rib cage can be exposed laterally (see Fig. 6-95).

## Landmarks and Incision

### Landmarks

Palpate the *spinous processes* in the area. If the patient has a gibbous deformity, use it as a landmark for surgery. In any case, a needle should be placed into the spinous process of the vertebra to be exposed so that a lateral x-ray film can pinpoint the position. Remember that the spinous processes of the thoracic area are long and slender, and tend to overlap the vertebrae below. Note that the rib in the area to be exposed often is more prominent.

### Incision

Make a curved linear incision about 8 cm lateral to the appropriate spinous process and 10 to 13 cm long. Center the incision over the rib that is involved in the pathologic process (Fig. 6-77).

## Internervous Plane

There is no true internervous plane in this approach; it involves splitting the trapezius muscle and cutting through the paraspinal muscles. Because the paraspinal muscles are innervated segmentally, no sig-

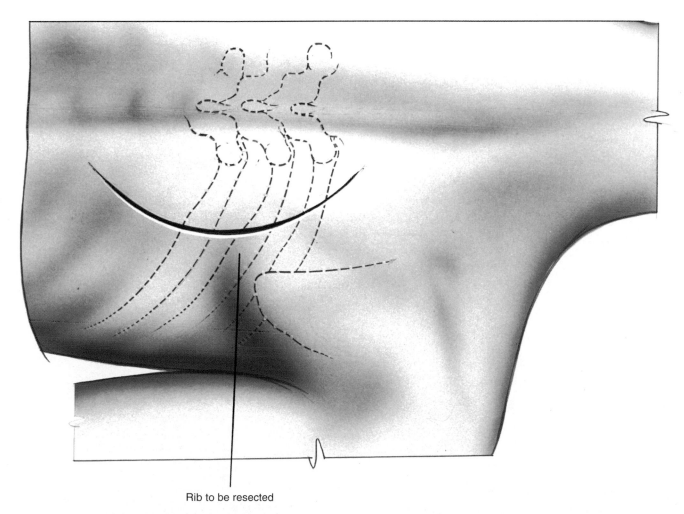

Rib to be resected

**Figure 6-77**    Make a curved linear incision lateral to the appropriate spinous process. Center the incision over the rib involved in the pathologic process.

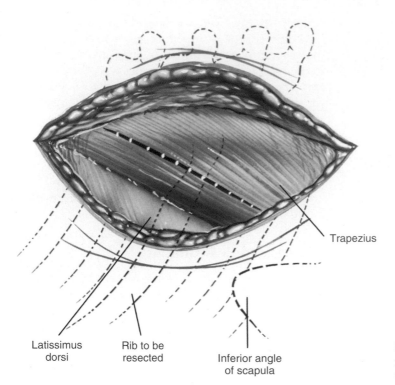

Latissimus
dorsi

Rib to be
resected

Inferior angle
of scapula

Trapezius

**Figure 6-78**   Incise the subcutaneous fat and fascia in line with the skin incision. Incise the trapezius muscle parallel with its fibers.

nificant denervation occurs. The trapezius receives its supply from the spinal accessory nerve higher up.

## Superficial Surgical Dissection

Incise the subcutaneous fat and fascia in line with the skin incision, cutting through the trapezius muscle parallel with its fibers close to the transverse processes. Deep to it are the paraspinal muscles (Fig. 6-78).

Cut down onto the posterior aspect of the rib to be resected all the way to bone. The plane often is bloody; a cutting cautery (diathermy) is useful (Fig. 6-79).

## Deep Surgical Dissection

Carefully separate all the muscle attachments from the rib that has been approached, using subperiosteal dissection with a periosteal elevator (Fig. 6-80). Dis-

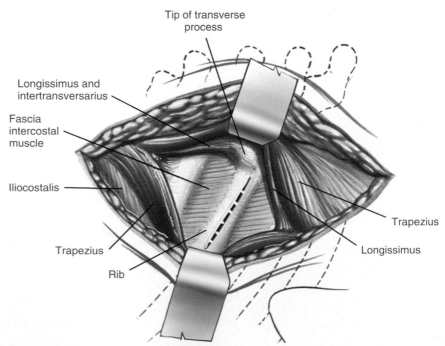

Tip of transverse
process

Longissimus and
intertransversarius

Fascia
intercostal
muscle

Iliocostalis

Trapezius

Rib

Trapezius

Longissimus

**Figure 6-79**   Cut down onto the posterior aspect of the rib to be resected. Strip the muscles laterally and medially onto the transverse process. Incise the periosteum over the rib.

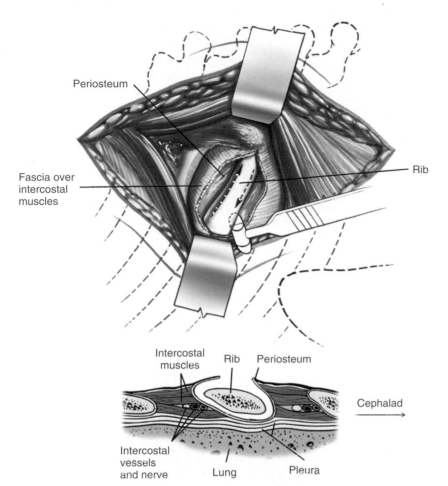

Figure 6-80   Separate all the muscle attachments from the rib, using subperiosteal dissection.

sect laterally along the superior border of the rib and medially along the inferior border. Continue dissection subperiosteally on to the anterior surface of the rib. Divide the rib about 6 to 8 cm from the midline. Then, lift it up and carefully cut any remaining mus-

cle attachments and the costotransverse ligament. Twist the rib's medial end to complete the resection (Figs. 6-81 and 6-82). At this point, the field may flood with a gush of pus from the opened abscess cavity.

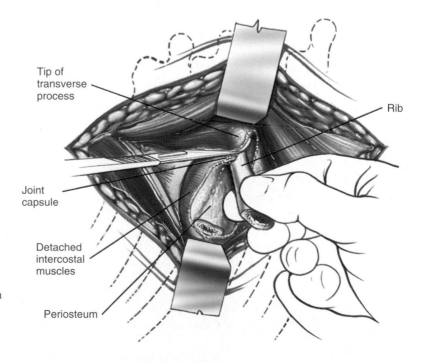

**Figure 6-81**   Divide the rib about 6 to 8 cm from the midline. Lift it up and carefully cut any remaining muscle attachments and the costotransverse ligament.

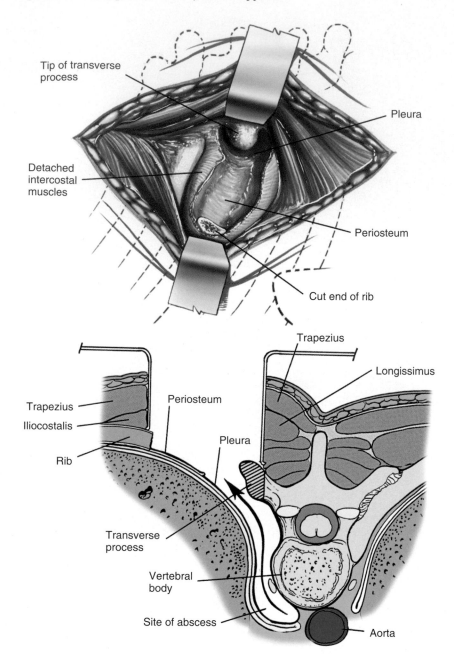

**Figure 6-82** Twist the rib's medial end to complete the resection and remove the rib. The abscess cavity now is exposed. The abscess cavity may extend along the lateral and anterior borders of the vertebra *(cross section)*. Resect the transverse process if greater exposure is necessary.

Remove all muscle attachments from the transverse process; divide the process at its junction with the lamina and pedicle, using a rongeur biting instrument. Remove the transverse process to gain wider exposure (see Fig. 6-82, *cross section*).

Carefully enter the retropleural space by digital palpation and dissection, removing the parietal pleura from the vertebral body. Note that this plane is safe only if the pleura is thickened by disease. Careful blunt dissection is essential to avoid entering the pleural cavity. At this point, the ver-

tebral body and disc space should have been exposed.

## Dangers

### Nerves
If dissection is extensive around the vertebral body, the central canal can be entered accidentally. If the **dura** is damaged, it must be closed to prevent spinal fluid leaks.

### Vessels

The segmental **intercostal arteries** often are damaged when the ribs are stripped. They lie on the inferior border of the rib and should be ligated if they are cut (see Fig. 6-88).

### Lungs

The **pleura** often is thickened by infections of the underlying lung. As dissection proceeds, damage to the pleura can be minimized by using blunt dissection to strip the pleura from the anterolateral surface of the affected vertebral body. The approach can cause a **pneumothorax,** however. If there is a sucking sound or a tear in the pleura, it should be treated by inserting a chest tube after closure.

## How to Enlarge the Approach

### Local Measures

If the musculature is too tight, divide the paraspinal muscles transversely in line with the transverse process to facilitate retraction.

### Extensile Measures

The incision cannot be extended, but it can be enlarged to include adjacent ribs and vertebrae either cephalad or caudad.

---

# Anterior (Transthoracic) Approach to the Thoracic Spine

The transthoracic approach to the thoracic spine offers unrivaled exposure of the anterior portions of the vertebral bodies, from T2 to T12. Nevertheless, this approach seldom is used, mainly because of its dangers. A surgeon who uses the transthoracic approach only occasionally should operate with a thoracic surgeon who is accustomed to dealing with the hazards of the area.[18,19]

The approach is effective in the following situations:

1. Treatment of infections, such as tuberculosis of the thoracic vertebral bodies[20]
2. Fusion of the vertebral bodies
3. Resection of the vertebral bodies for tumor and reconstruction with bone grafting
4. Correction of scoliosis (Dwyer instrumentation technique and rods)
5. Correction of kyphosis
6. Osteotomy of the spine
7. Anterior spinal cord decompression
8. Biopsy

## Position of the Patient

Place the patient on his or her side on the operating table, stabilizing the patient with a kidney rest or sandbags. Move the hand and arm on the side to be approached above the patient's head or onto an airplane splint. Place a small pad in the axilla of the dependent side to avoid compression of the axillary artery and vein. Feel for a radial pulse after positioning; make sure that there is no venous obstruction in the arm. The surgeon should be positioned behind the patient (Fig. 6-83).

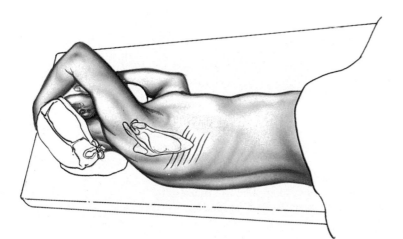

**Figure 6-83** Place the patient on his or her side for the anterior transthoracic approach to the spine. On the side to be approached, move the patient's hand and arm above his or her head.

Although the thoracic vertebrae can be approached from either side, approaching from the right side is easier because the aortic arch and aorta can be avoided.

## Landmarks and Incision

### Landmarks

Palpate the *tip of the scapula* with the patient in the lateral position. Remember that the scapula is mobile and the position of the tip will vary from patient to patient. Palpate the *spines of the thoracic vertebrae.* They are long and slender. Observe the *inframammary crease* on the anterior chest wall.

### Incision

Begin the incision two fingerbreadths below the tip of the scapula and curve it forward toward the inframammary crease. Complete the incision by extending it backward and upward toward the thoracic spine, ending at a point halfway up the medial border of the scapula and halfway between the spine and the scapula. The incision usually overlies the seventh or eighth rib (Fig. 6-84).

## Superficial Surgical Dissection

Divide the latissimus dorsi muscle posteriorly in line with the skin incision (Fig. 6-85). Then, divide the

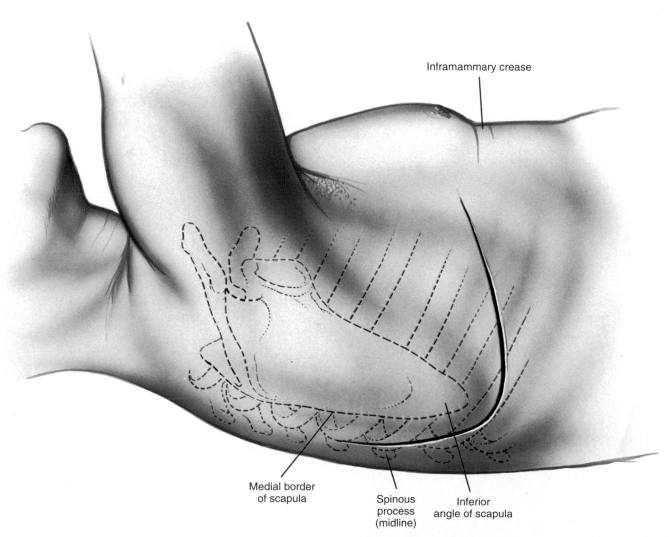

**Figure 6-84** Begin the incision two fingerbreadths below the tip of the scapula. Curve the incision forward toward the inframammary crease. Complete the incision by extending it backward and upward toward the thoracic spine. The incision usually overlies the seventh rib.

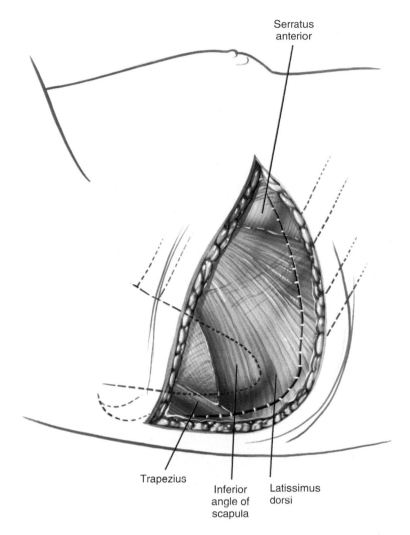

Serratus
anterior

Trapezius

Inferior
angle of
scapula

Latissimus
dorsi

**Figure 6-85** Divide the latissimus dorsi posteriorly in line with the skin incision.

serratus anterior muscle along the same line, down to the ribs (Fig. 6-86). This allows the scapula to be elevated and muscles to be cut proximally to expose the underlying ribs (Fig. 6-87). It seldom is necessary to cut the more posterior rhomboid muscles. Because the operation is not performed in an intermuscular plane, bleeding is a problem; cutting cautery (diathermy) can be used to control it (see Figs. 6-92 and 6-93).

The thoracic cavity can be reached either through an intercostal space or by resection of one or more ribs. Rib resection creates a better exposure, and the cut ribs can be used for bone grafting.

The level at which the chest is entered depends on the location of the pathology to be treated. Unless the vertebrae involved are low (between T10 and T12), use the fifth intercostal space (between the fifth and sixth ribs) for entering the chest, because

the scapula easily *overrides the healing site* and will not cause clicking. For pathology at T10 to T12, use the sixth intercostal space, which provides better exposure of the lower vertebral bodies. During its range of motion, however, the scapula may have to jump over the callus formed at the healing site, causing a click.

To use an intercostal approach, cut down onto the rib with cutting diathermy. Cut the periosteum on the upper border of the rib and into the pleura in this line. Entering the pleura from above the ribs avoids damage to the intercostal nerve and vessels, which lie along its lower border (Fig. 6-88; see Fig. 6-87). For greater exposure, strip all muscular attachments from either the cephalad or the caudad rib (usually the fifth), using a periosteal elevator or cautery, and resect the posterior three fourths of the rib as far posterior as necessary (Fig. 6-89).

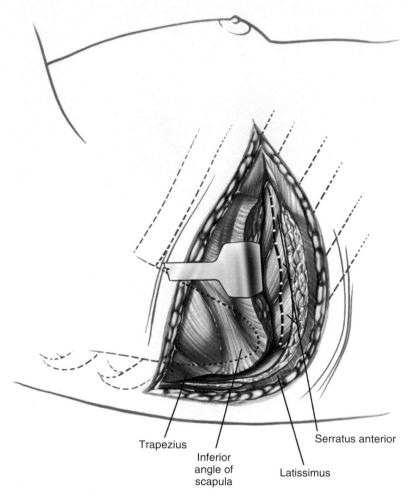

Trapezius

Inferior
angle of
scapula

Serratus anterior

Latissimus

**Figure 6-86**     Divide the serratus anterior along the line of the skin incision down to
the ribs.

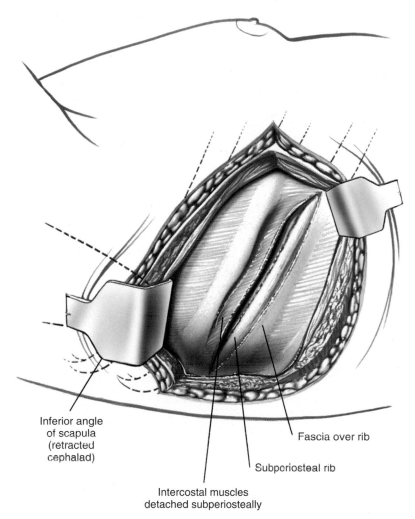

Inferior angle
of scapula
(retracted
cephalad)

Fascia over rib

Subperiosteal rib

Intercostal muscles
detached subperiosteally

**Figure 6-87** Elevate the scapula with the cut attached muscles proximally to expose the underlying ribs. Cut the periosteum on the upper border of the rib.

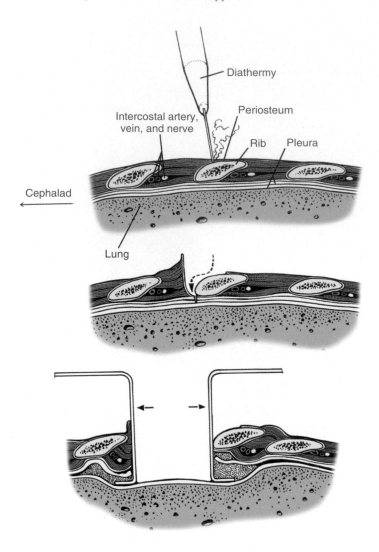

**Figure 6-88**   Enter the pleura from above the rib to avoid damage to the intercostal nerve and vessels that lie along this lower border. Insert a rib spreader to hold the ribs apart.

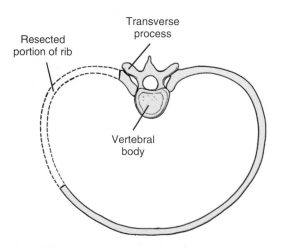

**Figure 6-89**   Resect the posterior three fourths of the ribs as far posterior as necessary for greater exposure.

Insert a rib spreader during either approach to hold the ribs apart; spread the ribs slowly to allow the muscles to adapt. Incising the paraspinal muscles seldom is necessary. Ensure complete hemostasis, especially in the posterior angle, before proceeding.

## Deep Surgical Dissection

Ask the anesthesiologist to deflate the lung. Then, gently retract it anteriorly, using moist lap pads to protect it. Under it lies the posterior mediastinum. Identify the esophagus over the vertebral bodies by palpating a previously placed large Levin's tube or esophageal stethoscope. These make identification easier. Incise the pleura over the lateral side of the esophagus so that the esophagus can be retracted and the anterior part of the spine reached (Fig. 6-90). The esophagus is easy to mobilize with finger dissection; retract it from the anterior surface of the spine with two Penrose drains. The intercostal vessels cross the operative field; one or more may have to be tied off (Fig. 6-91). Tying off more intercostal vessels than is necessary should be avoided, however, because the blood supply to the spinal cord from these vessels varies. Damage from ischemia may occur on rare occasions if more than two sequential intercostal vessels are ligated close to the vertebral bodies. Approaching the vertebral body from the right side obviates the need to ligate both the left and right segmental intercostal arteries. Approaching the vertebrae from the right side is safer and simpler than is trying to move the aorta itself (Fig. 6-94*B*).

## Dangers

### Vessels

The **intercostal vessels** are vulnerable at two stages. They are damaged most often during rib resection, when they run along the undersurface of the rib; they also may be damaged during exposure to the vertebrae within the chest and must be tied off carefully before they are transected and allowed to retract (see Figs. 6-88 and 6-94*A*).

### Lungs

About every 30 minutes, ask the anesthesiologist to expand the **lungs** to help prevent microatelectasis postoperatively. Before closing, make sure that the lung is expanded fully. Inform the anesthesiologist when sharp instruments are in the chest so that he or

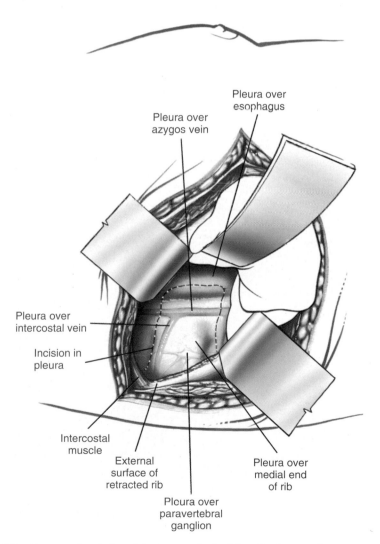

Pleura over azygos vein

Pleura over esophagus

Pleura over intercostal vein

Incision in pleura

Intercostal muscle

External surface of retracted rib

Pleura over paravertebral ganglion

Pleura over medial end of rib

**Figure 6-90**   Retract the deflated lung anteriorly. Identify the esophagus over the vertebral bodies. Incise the pleura over the lateral side of the esophagus to enable it to be retracted.

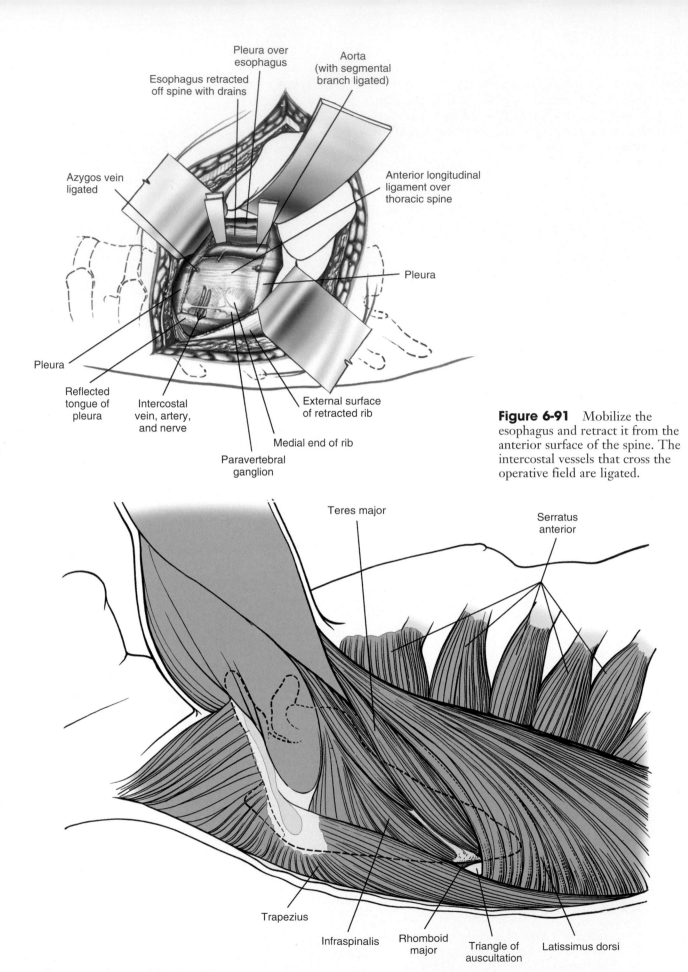

Pleura over
esophagus

Esophagus retracted
off spine with drains

Aorta
(with segmental
branch ligated)

Azygos vein
ligated

Anterior longitudinal
ligament over
thoracic spine

Pleura

Pleura

Reflected
tongue of
pleura

Intercostal
vein, artery,
and nerve

External surface
of retracted rib

Medial end of rib

Paravertebral
ganglion

**Figure 6-91** Mobilize the esophagus and retract it from the anterior surface of the spine. The intercostal vessels that cross the operative field are ligated.

Teres major

Serratus
anterior

Trapezius

Infraspinalis

Rhomboid
major

Triangle of
auscultation

Latissimus dorsi

**Figure 6-92** The superficial muscles of the posterolateral aspect of the thorax.

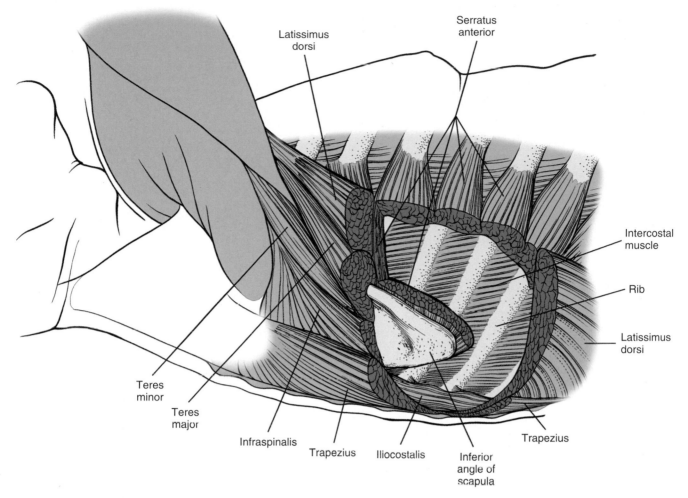

**Figure 6-93** The superficial muscles of the posterior wall of the thorax (the trapezius, serratus anterior, latissimus dorsi, and teres major) have been resected to reveal the rib cage and the intercostal muscles.

she does not ventilate the patient excessively or do so jerkily.

## How to Enlarge the Approach

### Local Measures
If the intercostal incision is inadequate, dissect the rib below it, resect it, and spread the rib cage further apart.

### Extensile Measures
This incision cannot be extended, although it can provide good access to vertebrae from T2 to T12. In the lower part of the incision, part of the diaphragm may need to be resected to enhance the exposure. To accomplish this, remove the arcuate ligament from its origin on the transverse process of L1. Note that the risks of surgery increase in this area, because two major body cavities may be entered. Reattach the diaphragm before closing.

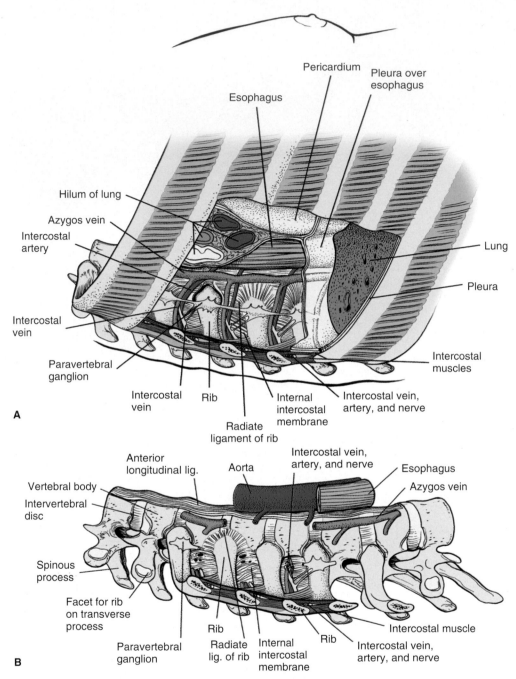

**Figure 6-94**   **(A)** The ribs and lung have been resected, as well as the posterior pleura, to reveal the esophagus, azygos vein, and intercostal arteries and nerves. Note the position of the sympathetic chain. **(B)** A detailed view of the anterolateral aspect of the thoracic spine. It is surgically significant that the azygos vein and esophagus overlie the vertebral bodies and must be mobilized to expose them.

# Posterior Approach to the Thoracic and Lumbar Spines for Scoliosis

The posterior approach to the thoracic and lumbar spines is the approach used most frequently for the surgical treatment of scoliosis.[21–25] The approach is safe, avoiding vital structures, and allows direct approach to the posterior aspect of the vertebral bodies in an internervous plane.

This approach is used for the following:

1. Scoliosis surgery (see the section regarding rib resection and the posterior approach to the iliac crest for bone graft)
2. Posterior spine fusions (extensive and limited; see the section regarding the posterior approach to the iliac crest for bone graft)
3. Removal of tumors of the posterior aspect of the vertebrae
4. Open biopsy
5. Stabilization of fractured vertebrae (see the section regarding the posterior approach to the iliac crest for bone graft)

## Position of the Patient

Place the patient prone on the operating table, with bolsters along each side so that the anterior chest wall clears the table and the chest can expand. The bolsters should be long enough to reach and support the anterior superior iliac spine so that the anterior abdominal wall clears the table as well; this allows emptying of the nonvalvular vertebral venous plexus into the vena cava, reducing operative bleeding (Fig. 6-95).

## Landmarks and Incision

### Landmarks
The *gluteal cleft* and the *C7-T1 spinous processes* mark the midline. The beginning of the gluteal cleft should be draped with a clear plastic drape so that it still can be seen. The spinous processes of C7 and T1 are the largest spinous processes in the lower cervical

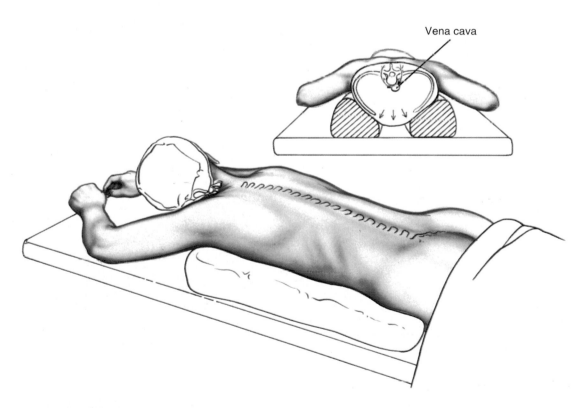

**Figure 6-95** The position of the patient on the operating table for the posterior approach to the thoracic and lumbar spines. Place the bolsters so that the anterior abdominal wall clears the table; this allows emptying of the vertebral venous plexus to the vena cava.

and upper thoracic spines. They offer a guide to the location and level of the incision if the spinous processes are counted down from C7.

### Incision

Make a straight midline incision above the thoracic and lumbar spines that require surgery. Use the spinous processes of C7 and T1 and the gluteal cleft as guides. A scalpel drawn along a straightedge between these two points leaves an exact midline incision (Fig. 6-96). (Frequently, the spinous processes are rotated away from the midline in association with scoliosis; nevertheless, for cosmetic reasons, the incision should be placed along the midline.)

### Internervous Plane

The paraspinal muscles are innervated segmentally by the posterior primary rami of the individual nerve roots in the thoracic and lumbar spines. Because the incision is in the midline, it is truly internervous; the nerves do not cross the midline.

### Superficial Surgical Dissection

Palpate the individual spinous processes. Determine whether they have deviated from the midline as they rotate in scoliosis. Continue dissecting down to the middle of the spinous processes and move the muscle origins to either side of the surface. In children, split the spinous process apophyses longitudinally and dis-

sect them to each side of the processes with a Cobb elevator (Fig. 6-97).

### Deep Surgical Dissection

Remove the paraspinal muscles from the spinous processes and partially from the laminae by subperiosteal dissection (Fig. 6-98). In the thoracic area, work in a distal to proximal direction, in the direction of the muscle fibers along the spinous process. After the paraspinal muscles have been stripped from the spinous processes and laminae, keep the dissection open with self-retaining retractors (Fig. 6-99).

Now, still using the Cobb instruments, remove the short rotators from the base of the spinous processes to the leading edges of the laminae. Then, strip the muscles from the rest of the laminae laterally, onto the transverse processes (Figs. 6-100 and 6-101).

### Dangers

The **posterior primary rami** emerge posteriorly from between the transverse processes, close to the facet joints. Because of the significant overlap of innervation in the paraspinal muscles, loss of an individual posterior primary ramus is not harmful (see Figs. 6-100*B* and 6-105).

**Segmental vessels** coming directly off the aorta appear between the transverse processes and supply the paraspinal muscles. They bleed when muscles are stripped from the transverse processes and must be

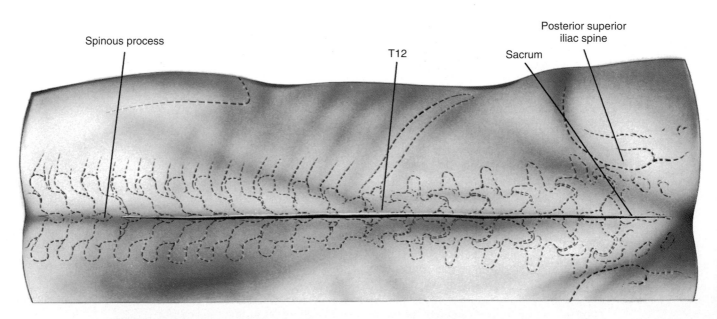

**Figure 6-96**   Make a straight midline incision over the thoracic and lumbar spines that require surgery.

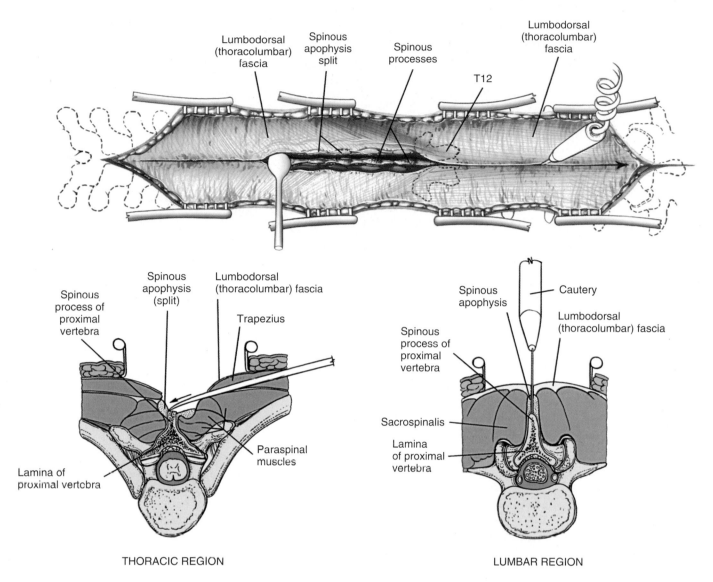

THORACIC REGION         LUMBAR REGION

**Figure 6-97** Dissect down onto the middle of the spinous processes. In children, split the spinous apophyses longitudinally and dissect them to either side with a Cobb elevator *(inset)*.

cauterized. The posterior primary rami are close to these vessels (see Figs. 6-100*B* and 6-105).

## How to Enlarge the Approach

### Local Measures
To widen the exposure, use self-retaining retractors and carry the dissection out onto the tips of the transverse processes. If the area being worked in is tight, extend the incision one vertebra higher or lower, whichever is appropriate.

### Extensile Measures
This incision can be extended. It may be used to dissect the entire spine, from the cervical area to the

coccyx. Because no nerves cross the midline of the body, the nerves that segmentally supply the paraspinal muscles remain safe.

## Special Points

To determine a precise anatomic location, identify the 12th (last) rib and dissect one level distal to it to locate the transverse process of L1. Note that the last rib is mobile, a floating rib without sternal attachment, whereas the transverse process of L1 is quite rigid and firm, and does not yield to pressure. The rib also is longer and more tubular than the transverse process (see Fig. 6-100). After the last rib has been found, identify the nearby facet joints. The descending facet joint of T12 is a lumbar facet joint, set in the sagittal

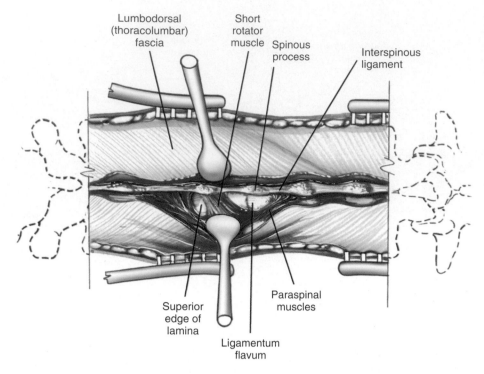

**Figure 6-98**   Remove the paraspinal muscles from the spinous processes and partially from the laminae by subperiosteal dissection.

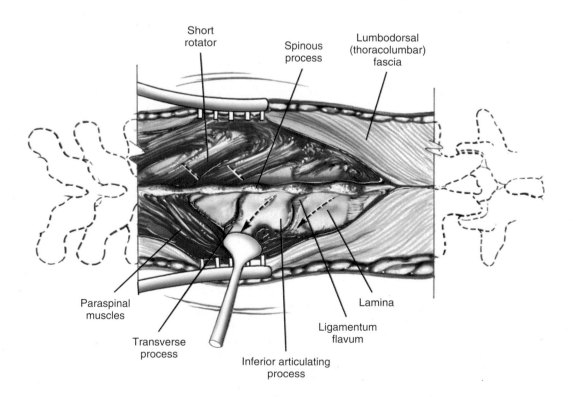

THORACIC REGION

**Figure 6-99**   In the thoracic area, work from distal to proximal, in the direction of the muscle fibers along the spinous processes. With the use of Cobb elevators, remove the short rotators from the base of the spinous processes to the leading edges of the laminae. Then, strip the muscles from the rest of the laminae laterally onto the transverse processes.

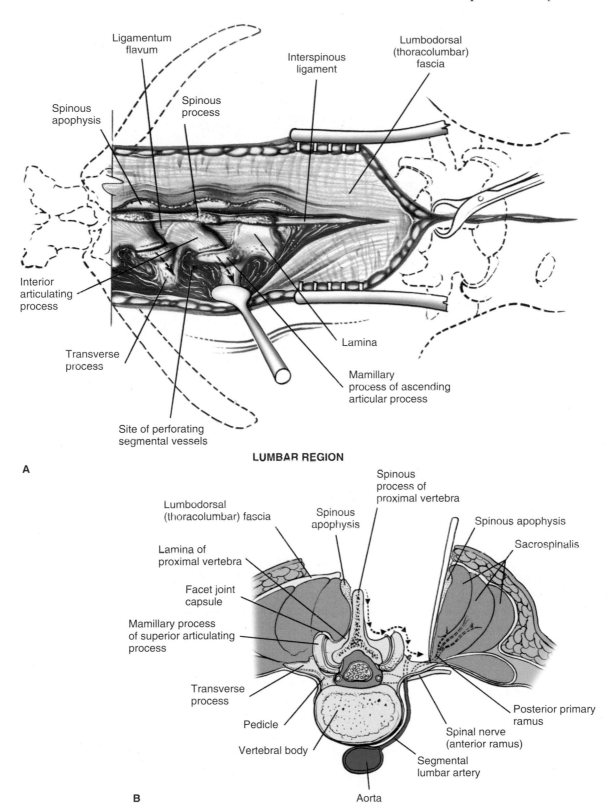

**LUMBAR REGION**

A

B

**Figure 6-100** **(A)** In the lumbar area, strip the paraspinal muscles from proximal to distal. Remove the joint capsule from medial to lateral. After crossing the mamillary process on the tip of the ascending facet, dissect laterally and caudally onto the transverse process. Be prepared to cauterize the segmental vessels that appear between the transverse processes. **(B)** Note that the transverse process is further anterior and distal than the mamillary process.

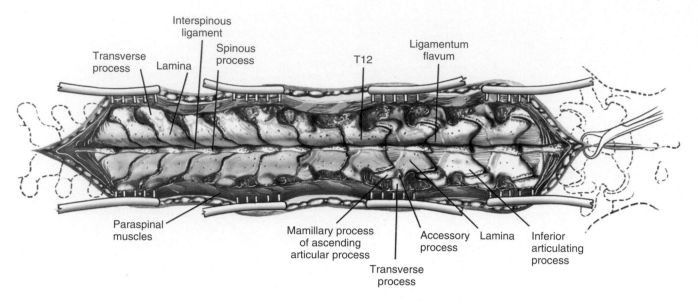

**Figure 6-101** After you have stripped the paraspinal muscles from the spinous processes, laminae, and transverse processes, keep the dissection open with self-retaining retractors.

plane, whereas the ascending facet joint at the upper end of T12 is a thoracic facet joint, set in a frontal plane (see Fig. 6-104). Identifying the direction of facets, the last rib, and the first lumbar transverse process provides a precise anatomic location. The only alternative is to place markers in the spinous processes in the lumbar area and to obtain a radiograph, or to carry the dissection distally and identify the sacrum.

The musculature in the lumbar area may be stripped at each vertebral level, either in a proximal to distal direction or in a distal to proximal direction. A half-inch osteotome may be used in conjunction with the Cobb elevator to strip the facet joint capsules from the ascending and descending facets, and to continue the dissection laterally onto the transverse processes (see Fig. 6-100B).

# Applied Surgical Anatomy of the Posterior Approach to the Thoracic and Lumbar Spines

## Overview

The posterior muscles of the thoracic and lumbar spines are arranged in three layers:

1. Superficial layer: the mooring muscles that attach the upper extremity to the spine
2. Intermediate layer: the muscles of accessory respiration
3. Deep layer: the paraspinal muscle system, the intrinsic muscles of the back

These distinct layers are not actually seen during surgical exposure of the spine, but the layering concept clarifies how the anatomy relates to the dissection.

The *superficial layer* of muscles can be subdivided into two layers: the most superficial layer consists of the trapezius and latissimus dorsi; the deeper layer is composed of the rhomboid major and minor.

The *intermediate layer* consists of the serratus posterior superior and the serratus posterior inferior, which are small, laterally placed muscles that attach to the spine.

The *deep layer* includes the sacrospinalis muscles (erector spinalis) and a deep, obliquely running layer consisting of the semispinalis, multifidus, and rotator muscles.

The muscles of the superficial layer are supplied by the peripheral nerves: the trapezius by the spinal accessory nerve, the rhomboids by the nerve to them from C5, and the latissimus dorsi by the thoracodorsal nerve. They are not affected by a midline dissection.

The muscles of the intermediate layer are supplied by the anterior primary rami; they, too, are unaffected by the dissection.

The muscles of the deep layer are supplied segmentally at each level of the spine by the posterior rami of the thoracic and lumbar nerves. Their nerve supplies usually are safe, but they may be denervated partially by excessive lateral dissection.

## Landmarks and Incision

The C7 and T1 spinous processes are the largest processes in the region, with T1 being slightly larger. They point directly posteriorly, with minimal caudal angulation, and are easily palpable. The large L5 spinous process, which also has minimal caudal angulation, can be palpated, but it cannot be differentiated from the other equally large lumbar spinous processes. The gluteal cleft, which runs between the protuberances of the gluteal (cluneal) muscles, is easy to see.

The skin on the posterior aspect of the spine is thicker than that on the anterior chest wall and abdomen. It usually heals with a fine line scar because there is so little tension across the sutured incision. The skin in the lumbar region (which is dissected subcutaneously to leave the iliac crest accessible for a bone graft) and the skin in the thoracic region (which is dissected subcutaneously to reach the ribs) heal well, despite the subcutaneous dissection. Dimpling of the skin over the iliac crest or ribs does not occur as long as the thick, subcutaneous, fatty tissue layer is taken with the skin to prevent it from adhering to the cut bony surfaces.

## Superficial Surgical Dissection and its Dangers

The tips of the spinous processes in the thoracic region are much narrower than are those in the lumbar area, and more muscles attach directly to their tips. As a result, dissection must approach the tips of the spinous processes exactly in the midline, without straying to either side. More bleeding occurs in the thoracic region, mainly because of the direct attachment of muscle fibers from the trapezius and rhomboid muscles; in the lumbar area, only the relatively avascular lumbodorsal fascia attaches to the tips of the lumbar and lower thoracic processes (Fig. 6-102). If the patient has scoliosis with extensive vertebral body rotation, the paraspinal muscles on the convex side of the curve may bunch up and roll over the tips of the spinous processes, causing further bleeding if the muscles are cut inadvertently during dissection.

## Intermediate Surgical Dissection

The deep layer of the back consists of a superficial portion and a deep portion. The superficial portion is made up of the sacrospinalis muscle (the erector spinae), which runs longitudinally. In the lumbar area, the muscle is a single mass; in the thoracic region, it divides into three units, namely, from medial to lateral, the spinalis, the longissimus, and the iliocostalis (see Figs. 6-102 and 6-105).

The deep portion of the deep layer itself has three layers: superficial, intermediate, and deep groups. The superficial group consists of the semispinalis muscles, which span about five segments from origin to insertion. The intermediate group, the multifidus muscles, spans about three segments. The deep group, the rotator muscles, spans adjacent segments (Figs. 6-103 and 6-104; see Fig. 6-102). The rotator muscles pass in a lateral to medial direction, with the distal end of the muscle being more lateral. The resulting angle between the muscle and its insertion makes stripping the muscles in a caudad to cephalad direction in the thoracic region easier (see Figs. 6-99 and 6-102 through 6-104). In addition, because the spinous processes are angled more caudally in the thoracic area than in the lumbar area (where they stand erect, almost directly over the vertebral bodies), it is easier to dissect the paraspinal muscles free from the thoracic spinous processes in a distal to proximal direction. Finally, the short rotators take origin from the caudal end of the spinous processes and are detached easily and dissected out laterally onto the transverse processes (see Figs. 6-99 and 6-104).

The transverse processes themselves should be stripped of musculature in a distal to proximal direction. The transverse processes become larger from T12 to T1.

Intermediate surgical dissection avoids the middle layer of back muscles, the muscles of respiration; these are placed more laterally.

The posterior primary rami of the paired thoracic and lumbar nerves may be injured during dissection of the muscles, particularly laterally between the transverse processes where the rami are located. Although the loss of one or two posterior primary rami may denervate the paraspinal muscles partially, the significant overlap of the segmental nerve supply to these muscles prevents total denervation. Excessive lateral retraction and cauterization at each level, however, can cause muscle denervation.

Segmental vessels come directly off the aorta in the lumbar and thoracic areas; they are located between the transverse processes, close to the posterior primary rami. The vessels constitute the main blood supply to the paraspinal muscles. Cauterizing

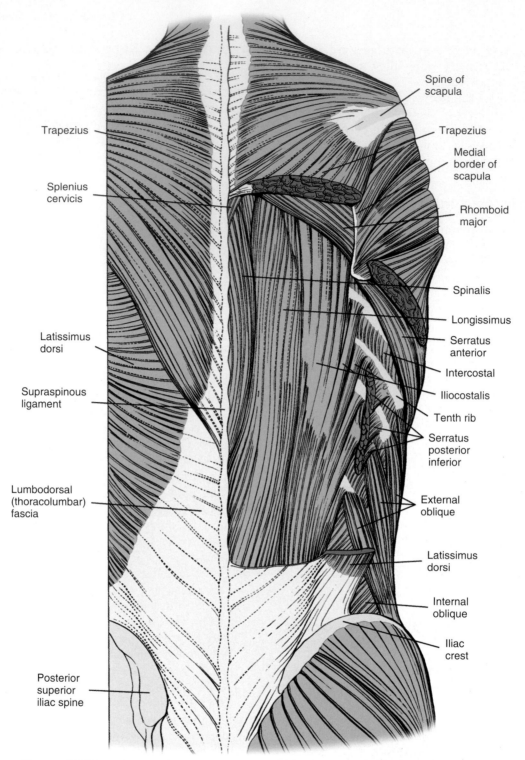

**Figure 6-102** The musculature of the back. The most superficial layer is seen, including the trapezius, the latissimus dorsi, and the lumbodorsal fascia *(left)*. The trapezius and latissimus dorsi have been resected to reveal the deep layer, the sacrospinalis muscles, including the spinalis, longissimus, and iliocostalis muscles *(right)*. A portion of the rhomboid major muscle of the superficial layer is seen inserting into the medial border of the scapula.

**Trapezius.** *Origin.* From all spinous processes of cervical spine except C1; from all spinous processes of thoracic vertebrae (T1-T12); and from superior nuchal line. Attachment to cervical spine is indirect, via ligamentum nucha. *Insertion.* Upper fibers from upper third of muscle, passing laterally and inferiorly to flattened posterior border of lateral third of clavicle and its upper surface. Intermediate muscle fibers pass laterally in a horizontal direction to adjacent part of upper surface of acromion and to associated upper lip of crest of spine of scapula. Lower fibers ascend, passing superiorly and laterally, inserting into tubercle on lower lip of spine of scapula. *Action.* Stabilizing muscle of shoulder girdle. *Nerve supply.* Spinal accessory nerve; cranial nerve XI.

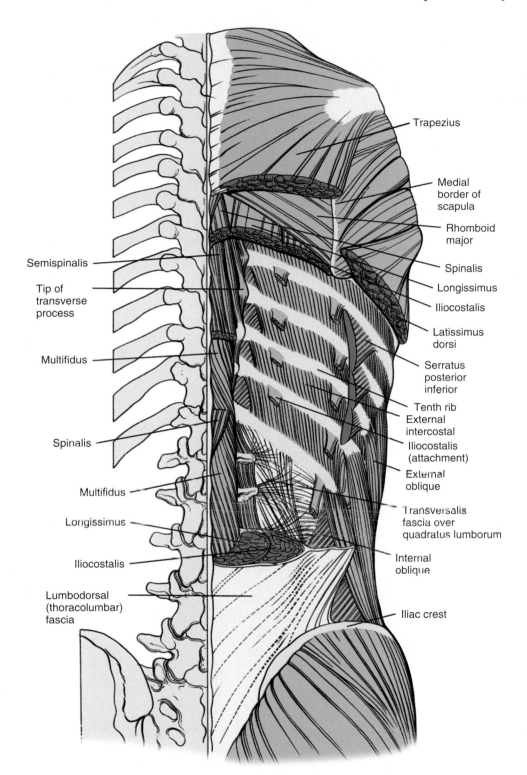

Trapezius

Medial border of scapula

Rhomboid major

Spinalis

Longissimus

Iliocostalis

Latissimus dorsi

Serratus posterior inferior

Tenth rib
External intercostal
Iliocostalis (attachment)
External oblique

Transversalis fascia over quadratus lumborum

Internal oblique

Iliac crest

Semispinalis

Tip of transverse process

Multifidus

Spinalis

Multifidus

Longissimus

Iliocostalis

Lumbodorsal (thoracolumbar) fascia

**Figure 6-103**   The sacrospinalis system has been resected to reveal the deep portion of the deep layer, which consists of the semispinalis and multifidi. Note the intertransversarii muscles and the insertion of the iliocostalis muscles into the borders of the ribs.

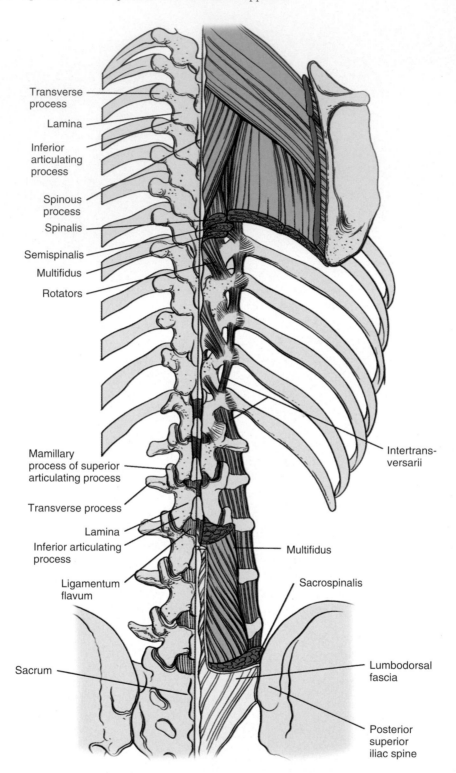

Transverse process

Lamina

Inferior articulating process

Spinous process

Spinalis

Semispinalis

Multifidus

Rotators

Mamillary process of superior articulating process

Transverse process

Lamina

Inferior articulating process

Ligamentum flavum

Sacrum

Intertransversarii

Multifidus

Sacrospinalis

Lumbodorsal fascia

Posterior superior iliac spine

**Figure 6-104**    The muscles are resected further to reveal the deep muscles of the deep layer (i.e., the short rotators as well as the intertransversarii muscles and the interspinous muscles) and the facet joint capsules.

**Figure 6-105**    **(A)** Cross section through the level of a thoracic vertebra. Superficial and deep layers of the thoracic spine are visualized, as well as their nerve and blood supply. **(B)** Cross section through the level of a lumbar vertebra. Note that the individual muscles of the sacrospinalis musculature are one paravertebral mass at this level. Note that the medial end of the cup-shaped ascending articulating process is closest to the lumbar nerve root.

them does not appear to cause significant loss of blood supply to the muscles. If they are cut, they must be cauterized or tied off; they branch directly from the aorta and may cause postoperative bleeding under pressure (Fig. 6-105; see Figs. 6-99 and 6-100*B*).

## Deep Surgical Dissection

The lumbar facet joints and their capsules are much larger than their thoracic counterparts and protrude further posteriorly. Their size is mainly the result of their large articulating processes and large mamil-

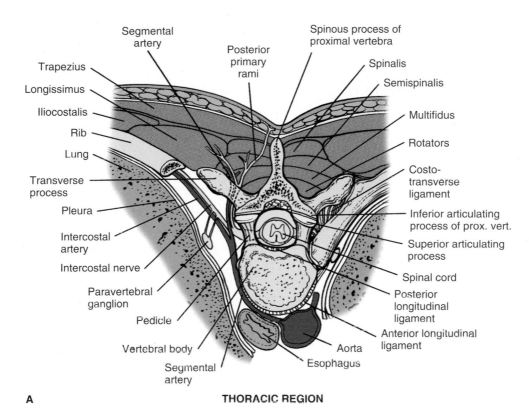

Segmental artery

Trapezius

Longissimus

Iliocostalis

Rib

Lung

Transverse process

Pleura

Intercostal artery

Intercostal nerve

Paravertebral ganglion

Pedicle

Vertebral body

Segmental artery

Posterior primary rami

Spinous process of proximal vertebra

Spinalis

Semispinalis

Multifidus

Rotators

Costo-transverse ligament

Inferior articulating process of prox. vert.

Superior articulating process

Spinal cord

Posterior longitudinal ligament

Anterior longitudinal ligament

Aorta

Esophagus

**A** **THORACIC REGION**

Spinous process (prox. vert.)

Lamina

Ligament flavum

Facet joint capsule

Mamillary process

Posterior primary rami

Segmental lumbar artery

Inferior (descending) articular process

Transverse process

Anterior ramus of spinal nerve

Spinal nerve

Paravertebral ganglion

Segmental artery

Lumbodorsal fascia

Multifidus

Longissimus

Iliocostalis

Pedicle

Quadratus lumborum

Psoas

Cauda equina

Posterior longitudinal ligament and venous plexus

Aorta

Vertebral body

Anterior longitudinal ligament

**B** **LUMBAR REGION**

lary processes that sit on the posterior aspect of the ascending processes, extending the bone even further posteriorly. The lumbar facet joints lie in the sagittal plane (see Fig. 6-105*B*). The joint capsules themselves are shiny, usually quite white, and are continuous with the ligamentum flavum, which is yellow-white. In the thoracic region, the joints are smaller, do not protrude as far posteriorly, are flatter, and are placed in the frontal plane (see Fig. 6-105*A*). The facet joints are vulnerable during removal of the joint capsules. Surgical injury may lead to traumatic arthritis, unless the joints are fused (see Fig. 6-100*B*).

The ligamentum flavum, which originates from the leading edge of the inferior vertebra and extends upward to a ridge under the lamina of the next vertebra, covers the blue-white dura and its layer of epidural fat. The dura must be protected; any epidural tear must be closed off (see Figs. 6-12 and 6-13).

The cup-shaped ascending articulating process is closest to the lumbar nerve root. Arthritis of the medial end of the ascending facet can cause compression of the nerve in the foramen. The nerve root is safe during the foraminotomy if the anatomic arrangement of the facet joints to the nerve root is appreciated. The nerve root should be protected while the medial portion of the ascending process, the portion that is close to the nerve root, is being removed (see Fig. 6-105*B*).

# Approach to the Posterior Lateral Thorax for Excision of Ribs

After scoliosis surgery has been completed, portions of the ribs on the posterolateral aspect of the rib cage may have to be resected to flatten out a hump caused by ribs that still protrude.

## Position of the Patient

Place the patient prone on the operating table. Position bolsters longitudinally on either side of the patient from the anterior superior iliac spine to the shoulders to allow room for chest expansion (see Fig. 6-95).

## Landmarks and Incision

### Landmarks
The best landmarks are the *prominent ribs*, usually on the right posterior thoracic region. They may be so distorted that they produce a "razorback" deformity.

### Incision
The standard incision for scoliosis surgery, the longitudinal midline incision, also is used for the removal of ribs (see Fig. 6-96).

## Internervous Plane

The internervous plane lies between the trapezius and latissimus dorsi muscles. The trapezius is innervated by the spinal accessory nerve and the latissimus dorsi is innervated by the long thoracic (thoracodorsal) nerve. The deeper muscle, the iliocostalis portion of the sacrospinalis, is innervated segmentally and, therefore, is not denervated when it is split longitudinally.

## Superficial Surgical Dissection

With retractors, lift the skin and its thick subcutaneous tissue. Free them from the underlying fascia and retract them laterally. Center the dissection over the most prominent, or apical, rib. Extend it laterally to at least 12 cm from the midline, and then proximally and distally to expose all the deformed ribs (Fig. 6-106).

## Intermediate Surgical Dissection

The fibers of the trapezius muscle run obliquely downward toward the midline as far as the spinous process of T12. Identify this muscle by its rolled, lateral free border. Dissect along the lateral border and retract the muscle medially. The medial portion of the fibers of the latissimus dorsi muscle and its aponeurosis run almost perpendicular to and under the trapezius muscle; it takes origin from the lower six thoracic spinous processes, as well as from the lumbodorsal fascia. Dissect the muscle free with cautery and retract it laterally (see Fig. 6-106).

## Deep Surgical Dissection

Below the retracted trapezius and latissimus dorsi muscles lies the iliocostalis, a longitudinal muscle with flattened tendons in its musculature that insert into the lower borders of the ribs. Split the iliocostalis muscle longitudinally over each of the deformed portions of the ribs that are being removed, then dissect and retract it medially and laterally in line with the ribs (Fig. 6-107).

Incise the periosteum along the posterior aspect of the rib in the rib's own plane. Use an Alexander dis-

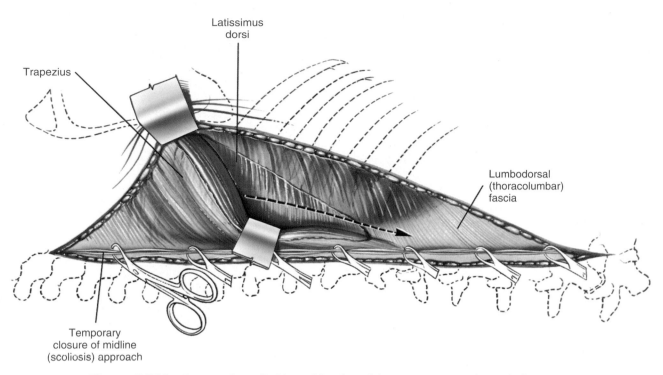

**Figure 6-106**   Retract the rolled lateral border of the trapezius muscle medially to expose the thin, aponeurotic medial portion of the latissimus dorsi. Incise the aponeurotic medial portion of the latissimus dorsi perpendicular to its fibers.

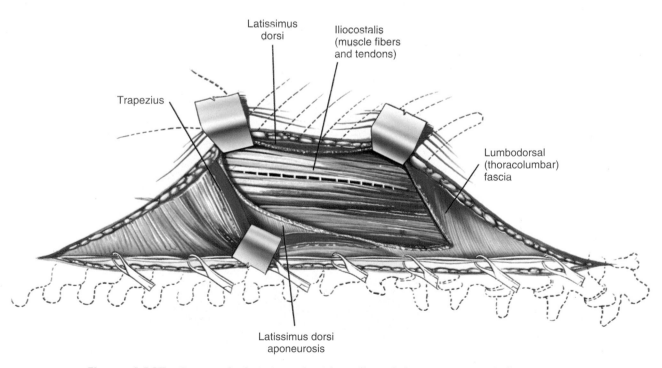

**Figure 6-107**   Retract the latissimus dorsi laterally and the trapezius medially to expose the underlying iliocostalis muscle. Incise the muscle longitudinally, parallel to its fibers.

sector to push the split periosteum to the upper and lower borders of the rib. With the special end of the dissector, strip the intercostal muscles off the upper end of the rib in a medial to lateral direction in the angle formed by the intersection of the external intercostal muscles and the rib. Then, strip the intercostal muscles from the lower end of the rib in a lateral to medial direction, remaining in the angle formed by the origin of the external intercostal muscle and the rib to discourage bleeding. By keeping the dissection in a subperiosteal location, the neurovascular bundle, which will have been freed from the lower border of the rib with the intercostal muscles, will be avoided (Fig. 6-108).

Before continuing, have the anesthesiologist stop the patient's breathing so that the visceral pleura can fall away from the rib, minimizing the danger to the pleura during anterior dissection. When the ribs have been uncovered completely, begin to resect them.

## Dangers

The **neurovascular bundle** lies along the lower edge of the rib in the neurovascular groove. Unless the dissection is kept in a subperiosteal location, it may be cut inadvertently during the resection and the intercostal vessels will have to be cauterized, causing possible segmental chest wall numbness (see Fig. 6-108, *inset*).

Violating the pleura may result in a **pneumothorax.** If that happens, plan to insert a chest tube immediately after the wound is closed, while the patient is still in the operating room.

Connecting the midline wound with that of the rib resection may cause a **hemothorax,** with blood flowing from the area of the spinal fusion into the lung. If the two areas of dissection are connected, be prepared to insert a chest tube to drain the blood.

The **skin** may adhere to the cut ends of the ribs, causing unsightly dimpling. To prevent this, take a

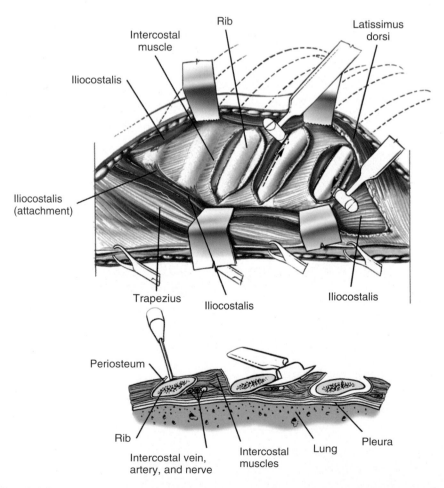

**Figure 6-108**   Dissect and retract the iliocostalis muscles laterally and medially from their insertion to expose the posterior aspect of the ribs. Incise the periosteum over the rib. Push the split periosteum to the upper and lower borders of the rib. With a special dissector, strip the intercostal muscles off the borders of the rib as well as anteriorly.

thick subcutaneous layer with the skin and, during closure, suture the fascia of the trapezius muscle to that of the latissimus dorsi muscle.

## How to Enlarge the Approach

### Local Measures

Continue subcutaneous dissection further laterally, proximally, and distally to ensure a complete view of the distorted ribs.

Occasionally, in more proximal rib resections, the lower portion of the rhomboid major muscle may have to be dissected to expose the rib area more fully. Distally, the muscular belly of the iliocostalis muscle may have to be split as it splits from the sacrospinalis muscle.

### Extensile Measures

This incision cannot be extended; deciding which ribs to remove depends on the size and extent of the rib hump.

## Special Points

When removing ribs, resect each one from the point just lateral to its maximum deformity to the most medial end, without removing its head and neck. The lateral portion of the resected rib will drop forward, reducing the rib hump, but the medial portion, held rigidly in place by the costotransverse and costovertebral ligaments, will not move. That is why the rib should be resected as medially as possible. Otherwise, the medial end of the rib will continue to stick out posteriorly, causing continued deformity.

The removal of more than four ribs may cause a sympathetic effusion of a lung field. If this occurs, insert a chest tube to drain the fluid.

Treat the cut ends of the ribs with bone wax to prevent continued oozing of blood. The wax does not prevent the ribs from regenerating.

The resected portions of the ribs can be cut into small, matchstick-sized pieces and used as graft material in a midline spine fusion.

If the vertebral body has rotated up under the rib, resecting the ribs will not produce a significant reduction in the rib hump deformity.

## REFERENCES

1. MIXTER WJ, BARR JS: Rupture of the intervertebral disc and involvement of the spinal cord. N Engl J Med 211:210, 1934
2. SEIMON L: Low back pain: clinical diagnosis and management. New York, Appleton-Century-Crofts, 1983
3. HIBBS RA: An operation for progressive spinal deformities. N Y Med J 93:1013, 1911
4. HIBBS RA: A report of 59 cases of scoliosis treated by fusion operation. J Bone Joint Surg 6:3, 1924
5. ROTHMAN HR, SIMEONE FA: The spine. Philadelphia, WB Saunders, 1975
6. HOLSCHER EC: Vascular complication of disc surgery. J Bone Joint Surg [Am] 30:968, 1948
7. SACKS S: Anterior interbody fusion of the lumbar spine: indications and results in 200 cases. Clin Orthop 44:163, 1966
8. MICHELE AA, KRUEGER FJ: Surgical approach to the vertebral body. J Bone Joint Surg [Am] 31:873, 1949
9. PEARL FL: Muscle-splitting extra peritoneal lumbar ganglionectomy. Surg Gynecol Obstet 65:197, 1937
10. JOHNSON RM, SOUTWICK WO: Surgical approaches to the cervical spine, p 133
11. ROGERS WA: Treatment of fracture dislocation of the cervical spine. J Bone Joint Surg 24:245, 1942
12. HOLDSWORTH FW: Fractures, dislocations and fracture dislocations of the spine. J Bone Joint Surg [Br] 45:6, 1963
13. WILLARD DP, NICHOLSON JT: Dislocations of the first cervical vertebra. Ann Surg 113:464, 1941
14. ROBINSON RA, SMITH GW: Anterolateral cervical disc removal and interbody fusion for cervical disc syndrome. Bull Johns Hopkins Hosp 96:223, 1955
15. HOPPENFELD S: Physical examination of the spine and extremities. New York, Appleton-Century-Crofts, 1976:107
16. CAPENER N: The evolution of lateral rhachotomy. J Bone Joint Surg [Br] 36:173, 1954
17. WILKINSON MC: Curettage of tuberculous vertebral disease in treatment of spinal caries. Proc R Soc Med 43:114, 1950
18. BURCH BH, MILLER AC: Atlas of pulmonary resections. Springfield, Ill, Charles C Thomas, 1965:8
19. COOK WA: Trans-thoracic vertebral surgery. Ann Thorac Surg 12:54, 1971
20. HODGSON AR, STOCK FE, FANG HSY ET AL: Anterior spinal fusion: the operative approach and pathological findings in 412 patients with Pott's disease of the spine. Br J Surg 48:172, 1980
21. HOPPENFELD S: A manual of concept and treatment. Philadelphia, JB Lippincott, 1967:96
22. WINTER RB: Congenital deformities of the spine. New York, Grune & Stratton, 1983
23. MOE J, WINTER RB, BRADFORD LONSTEIN J: Scoliosis and spinal deformities. Philadelphia, WB Saunders, 1978
24. KEIM H: The adolescent spine. New York, Grune & Stratton, 1976:159
25. HARRINGTON PR: Treatment of scoliosis: correction and internal fixation by spine instrumentation. J Bone Joint Surg [Am] 44:591, 1962

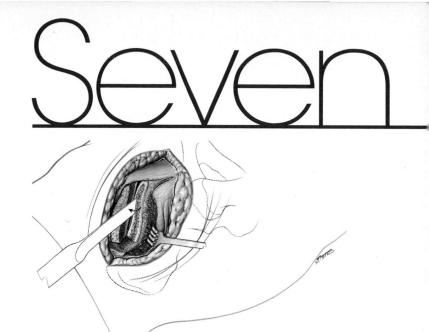

# The Pelvis

The pelvis is a complex bony structure with interconnecting ligaments. It consists of the two innominate bones, which articulate anteriorly with each other at the pubic symphysis and posteriorly with the body of the sacrum at the sacroiliac joint. The bones are covered on each side by muscles, and the intraabdominal contents make surgical exposure potentially complex. The presence of a large subcutaneous surface (the iliac crest), however, allows safe access.

Five approaches to the pelvis are described in this chapter, all of which provide access to the bone via its subcutaneous portion. The anterior and posterior approaches to the iliac crest are used almost exclusively for bone grafting. The anterior approach to the pubic symphysis, and the anterior and posterior approaches to the sacroiliac joints are performed rarely; their use is associated almost exclusively with the open reduction and internal fixation of pelvic ring fractures. A description of acetabular approaches may be found in the chapter on hip approaches.

## Anterior Approach to the Iliac Crest for Bone Graft

Anterior iliac crest bone grafts are the most commonly used grafts in orthopaedic surgery. The iliac crest is subcutaneous, and cortical or cortical cancellous grafts can be taken from it with ease and safety for grafting in all parts of the body, including the spine. It also is possible to remove pieces of the iliac crest, including both cortices, for major bone reconstructions, especially in the head and neck. For posterior spinal fusion work on conditions such as scoliosis, the bone graft usually is taken from the posterior aspect of the iliac crest.

### Position of the Patient

Place the patient supine on the operating table. Because the graft usually is taken in conjunction with other procedures, the iliac crest should be draped as a separate unit. There is much to be said for preparing this area routinely in all cases of open reduction and internal fixation of long-bone fractures. Place a small sandbag under the gluteal (cluneal) area of the side from which the graft will be taken to elevate the crest and rotate it internally, making it more accessible.

### Landmarks and Incision

#### Landmarks
The subcutaneous *anterior superior iliac spine*, the most important landmark, is easily palpable. Continue palpating along the crest of the ilium until its widest portion is reached, at the iliac tubercle. The *iliac tubercle* marks the anterior portion of the ilium, the area containing the largest amount of cortical cancellous bone for graft material.

#### Incision
The length of incision depends on the amount of bone graft that is required. For an extensive bone graft make an 8-cm incision parallel to the iliac crest and centered over the iliac tubercle (Fig. 7-1).

### Internervous Plane

Muscles either take origin from or insert onto the iliac crest, but do not cross it. Therefore, the crest offers a truly internervous plane.

The tensor fasciae latae, gluteus minimus, and gluteus medius are the muscles affected most directly by grafts taken from the anterior portion of the crest, because they originate from the outer portion of the ilium and are supplied by the superior gluteal nerve. The abdominal muscles take their origin directly from the iliac crest and are supplied segmentally.

### Superficial Surgical Dissection

Retract the skin and identify the iliac crest. Incise the crest before releasing the muscle attachments. Cut down onto the iliac crest with a scalpel (Fig. 7-2). In children, the crest still may be an avascular apophysis. If so, incise it and remove the muscle through the crest in either direction with a Cobb elevator. No apophysis will be present in adults.

Take care not to carry the incision from the apophysis or iliac crest onto the anterior superior iliac spine itself; if this occurs, the origin of the inguinal ligament may be detached and an inguinal hernia may result.

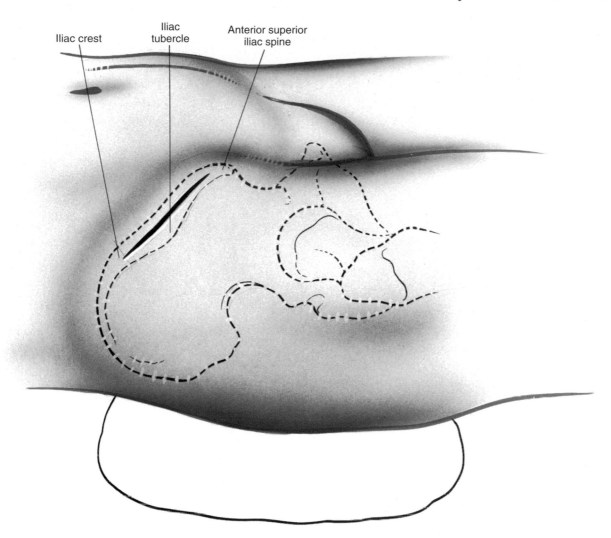

Iliac crest

Iliac
tubercle

Anterior superior
iliac spine

**Figure 7-1**   Make an 8-cm incision parallel to the iliac crest and centered over the iliac tubercle.

## Deep Surgical Dissection

The muscles may be stripped off either the inner or the outer wall of the ilium. Initially, cut down onto the bone using a scalpel. Follow the contour of the bone, sticking to it rigidly (Fig. 7-3). Below the crest itself, the ilium narrows considerably, so the sharp dissection will need to follow the contour of the bone carefully to avoid straying out of plane and into trouble. After coming around the corner of the crest onto the ilium, continue the dissection using blunt instruments such as a Cobb elevator. The muscles will come away from the bone easily. Alternatively, push a swab into the plane between the iliac wing and the overlying muscles. Using a blunt instrument, introduce more and more of the swab into the plane. The swab will act as a tissue expander, pushing the muscle away from the bone, while at the same time protecting the soft tissues. Corticocancellous strips may be taken from either side of the bone, or a complete block of the ilium can be removed. Pure cancellous bone can be taken by elevating a small piece of the cortex of the crest. Be aware that the largest supply of cancellous bone is directly underneath the subcutaneous surface of the crest.

## Dangers

Both the crest of the ilium and the anterior superior iliac spine should be left intact to preserve the normal appearance of the pelvis. If the anterior superior iliac spine is taken as graft material, the inguinal ligament might retract, causing an inguinal hernia.

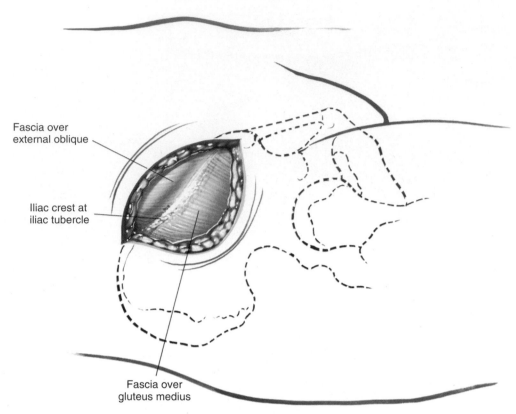

Fascia over
external oblique

Iliac crest at
iliac tubercle

Fascia over
gluteus medius

**Figure 7-2**   Retract the skin, identify the iliac crest, and incise the soft tissues overlying the iliac crest down to bone.

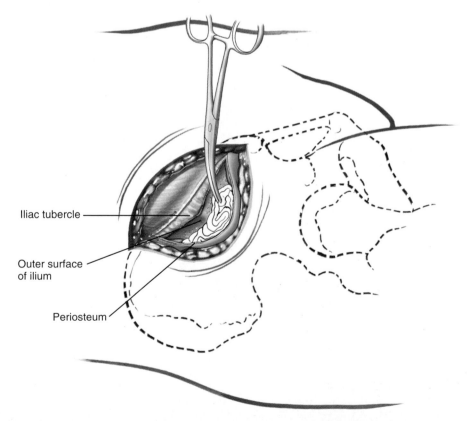

Iliac tubercle

Outer surface
of ilium

Periosteum

**Figure 7-3**   Remove the origins of the gluteus minimus and medius muscles subperiosteally from the outer cortex of the ilium.

## How to Enlarge the Approach

### Local Measures

Place a sharp-tipped retractor onto the bone to retract either the gluteal muscles from the outer cortex or the iliacus muscle from the inner cortex. Placing a swab between the retractor and the muscles creates a bloodless field and prevents little pieces of bone graft from being lost in the depth of the wound. Great care must be taken, however, to remove this swab before undertaking closure. The incision may have to be lengthened on the iliac crest and additional amounts of gluteus medius or iliacus stripped off to provide a better view of the outer or inner cortex of the anterior portion of the ilium.

### Extensile Measures

This approach is extensile as part of the extended iliofemoral approach to the acetabulum. This is not really relevant, however, because the approach has been described in this section merely as a means of obtaining bone graft.

# Posterior Approach to the Iliac Crest for Bone Graft

Posterior iliac crest bone grafts usually are taken during any posterior spine surgery that requires additional autogenous bone to supplement the area to be fused. The grafts also may be used as corticocancellous grafts for any part of the skeleton that needs fusion or refusion.

## Position of the Patient

Place the patient prone on the operating table, with bolsters running longitudinally to support the chest wall and pelvis, allowing the chest wall and abdomen to expand without touching the table. Place drapes distally enough so that the beginning of the gluteal cleft and the posterior superior iliac spine can be seen (see Fig. 6-77).

## Landmarks and Incision

### Landmarks

Palpate the *posterior superior iliac spine* under the dimpling of the skin above the buttock. The subcutaneous iliac crest also is palpable.

### Incision

Make an 8-cm oblique incision, centered over the posterior superior iliac spine and in line with the iliac crest (Fig. 7-4, *inset*).

If scoliosis surgery or lumbar surgery is being performed, the midline incision can be extended distally to the sacrum. Then, the skin and a thick, fatty, subcutaneous layer can be retracted laterally. Using a Hibbs retractor, the flap should be dissected free from the underlying lumbodorsal fascia until the posterior superior iliac spine and crest can be palpated and seen (see Fig. 7-4).

## Internervous Plane

Muscles insert into or take origin from the iliac crest, but do not cross it. Therefore, the outer border of the iliac crest is truly an internervous plane. The gluteus medius, minimus, and maximus muscles take their origins from the outer surface of the ilium (the gluteus medius and minimus are supplied by the superior gluteal nerve and the gluteus maximus is supplied by the inferior gluteal nerve). The segmentally supplied paraspinal muscles take their origin from the iliac crest itself, as does the latissimus dorsi, which is supplied proximally by the long thoracic nerve. Thus, an incision into the iliac crest does not denervate muscles, even if it is not placed exactly on the outer lip of the crest.

## Superficial Surgical Dissection

The subcutaneous tissues should be dissected until the iliac crest is reached. In children, the iliac apophysis is white and quite visible; it may be incised or split in line with the iliac crest, using it as an avascular plane. In adults, the apophysis is ossified and fused to the crest; the incision lands directly on the crest itself.

The Cobb elevator should be used to remove the apophysis or muscles from the iliac crest both medially and laterally, to bare the surface of the posterior portion of the crest.

## Dangers

### Nerves

The **cluneal nerves** cross the iliac crest. They can be avoided by placing the incision no more than 8 cm anterolateral to the posterior superior iliac spine. The nerves supply sensation to the skin over the

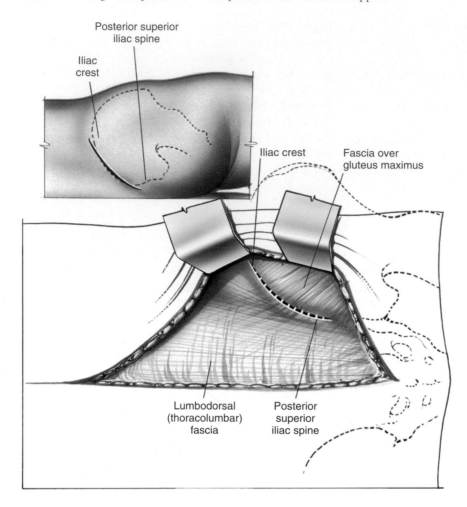

Iliac crest

Posterior superior iliac spine

Iliac crest

Fascia over gluteus maximus

Lumbodorsal (thoracolumbar) fascia

Posterior superior iliac spine

**Figure 7-4** If lumbar spine surgery is being performed, extend the midline incision distally, retracting the skin laterally until the posterior superior iliac spine and crest can be palpated and seen. Incise the soft tissues overlying the crest down to bone. Make an 8-cm oblique incision, centered over the posterior superior iliac spine and in line with the iliac crest *(inset).*

cluneal (gluteal) area. They are composed of the posterior primary rami of L1, L2, and L3. Their loss does not cause problems for the patient.

## Deep Surgical Dissection

Strip the musculature completely off the posterior portion of the lateral surface of the ilium so that a large enough graft can be obtained. Take care to stay in a subperiosteal plane while passing from the iliac crest to the outer cortex of the ilium. Proceeding 1.5 cm down the ilium in the area of the posterior superior spine, the elevated posterior gluteal line can be seen and felt; pass subperiosteally up over the line and then down its other side. Do not err by letting the line direct the incision outward from bone into muscle. A Taylor retractor will help the exposure by holding the muscles laterally. Note that the posterior gluteal line separates the origins of the gluteus maximus (posterior) from the gluteus medius (anterior; Fig. 7-5).

## Dangers

### Nerves

It is remotely possible that an osteotome will hit the **sciatic nerve,** which runs close to the distal end of

the wound deep to the sciatic notch; however, if an imaginary line is drawn from the posterior superior iliac spine perpendicular to the operating table, and all work is performed cephalad to it, both the notch and the nerve will be avoided completely. If a larger graft is necessary, palpate the sciatic notch itself before taking the graft (see Fig. 7-5*B*).

### Vessels

The **superior gluteal vessel,** a branch of the internal iliac (hypogastric) artery, leaves the pelvis via the sciatic notch, staying against the bone and proximal to the piriformis muscle. If a graft is taken too close to the sciatic notch, the vessel may be cut and may retract into the pelvis. Nutrient vessels from the artery supply the iliac crest bone along the midportion of the anterior gluteal line, and the vessel may become an osseous bleeder as it enters bone via the nutrient foramen. To control bone bleeding, use bone wax on the raw cancellous surface of the pelvis after the graft has been removed.

### Bone

Avoid the **sciatic notch.** Breaking through the thick portion of the bone that forms the notch disrupts the

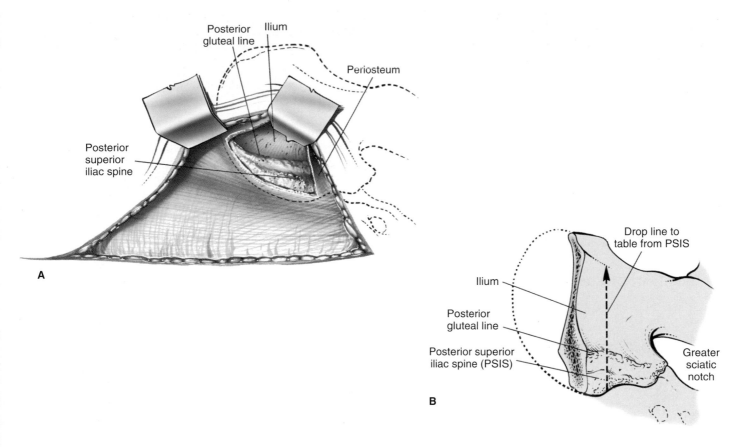

**Figure 7-5** **(A)** Subperiosteally, strip the musculature off the posterior portion of the lateral surface of the ilium. **(B)** Proceeding down the outer surface of the ilium in the area of the posterior superior spine, the elevated posterior gluteal line can be seen and felt; pass subperiosteally up and over the line and then down its other side. Do not err by letting the line direct you outward from bone to muscle. If you draw an imaginary line from the posterior superior iliac spine perpendicular to the operating table and stay cephalad to it, you will avoid the sciatic notch and its contents.

stability of the pelvis. Removal of bone from the false pelvis proximal to the notch does not cause loss of stability (see Fig. 7-5B).

## How to Enlarge the Approach

### Local Measures
Place a sharp-tipped, right-angled Taylor retractor into the bone to retract the gluteal muscles away from the bone and increase the exposure. To increase the exposure further, lengthen the iliac crest incision and strip more of the gluteal muscles from the outer cortex to avoid working through a "keyhole."

### Extensile Measures
This incision cannot be extended. It is designed specifically for removing bone for graft material from the posterior outer cortex of the ilium. Inner cortex also may be taken, but soft tissues should not be stripped off the anterior (deep) aspect of the ilium.

# Anterior Approach to the Pubic Symphysis

The anterior approach to the pubic symphysis is a direct approach that is used almost exclusively for the open reduction and internal fixation of a ruptured symphysis. Other uses include biopsy of tumors and treatment of chronic osteomyelitis.

Because widely displaced symphysis injuries often are associated with urologic damage, obtaining a urologic assessment is advisable before undertaking open surgery. A urethral catheter must be inserted before surgery. A full bladder will seriously interfere with the surgical approach.

## Position of the Patient

Place the patient supine on the operating table.

## Landmarks and Incision

### Landmarks
The *superior pubic ramus* and *pubic tubercles* are easily palpable in all but the most obese patients. The pubic symphysis will be palpable (as a gap) only in cases of rupture.

### Incision
Make a 15-cm curved incision in the line of the skin crease, centering it about 1 cm above the pubic symphysis (Fig. 7-6). The patient should have an indwelling catheter in place.

## Internervous Plane

An internervous plane is not available for use in this approach. Because the rectus abdominis muscles receive a segmental nerve supply, they are not denervated, even though they are divided by this approach.

## Superficial Surgical Dissection

Incise the subcutaneous fat in the line of the skin incision, deepening the incision down to the anterior portion of the rectus sheath (Fig. 7-7). Identify, lig-

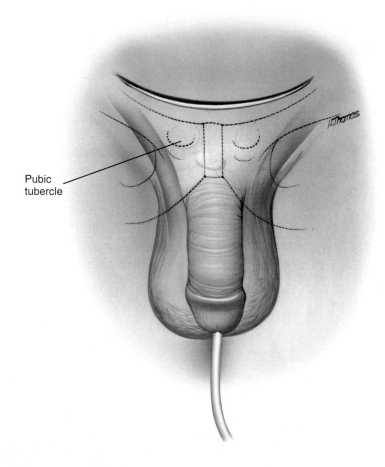

Pubic tubercle

**Figure 7-6**    Palpate the pubic tubercles. Make a curved incision in the line of the skin crease, centering it 1 cm above the pubic symphysis.

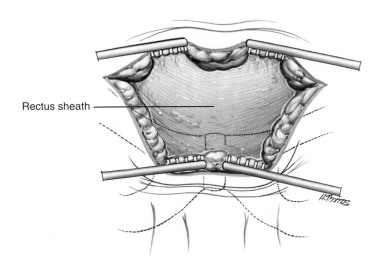

Rectus sheath

**Figure 7-7** Incise the fat in the line of the skin incision and retract the skin edges to reveal the anterior portion of the rectus sheath.

ate, and divide the superficial epigastric artery and vein that run up from below across the operative field. Then, divide the rectus sheath transversely, about 1 cm above the symphysis pubis. The two rectus abdominal muscles now are visible (Fig. 7-8). In most cases of rupture of the symphysis pubis, one of these muscles will have been detached from its insertion into the pubic symphysis. Divide the remaining muscle a few millimeters above its insertion into the bone.

## Deep Surgical Dissection

Retract the cut edges of the rectus abdominal muscles superiorly to reveal the symphysis and pubic crest (Fig. 7-9). If access to the back of the symphysis

is required, use the fingers to push the bladder gently off the back of the bone. This dissection is very easy to perform unless adhesions have formed due to damage to the bladder. Such adhesions make it difficult to open up this potential space (the preperitoneal space of Retzius) (Fig. 7-10). The pubic symphysis and superior pubic rami now are exposed adequately for internal fixation.

## Dangers

### Bladder
The **bladder** may have been damaged during the trauma. If so, adhesions will have developed between the damaged bladder and the back of the pubis. Mobilization of the space of Retzius, therefore, may

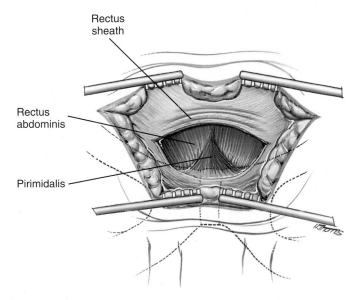

Rectus sheath

Rectus abdominis

Pirimidalis

**Figure 7-8** Divide the rectus sheath transversely 1 cm above the symphysis pubis to reveal the rectus abdominis muscles and pyramidalis.

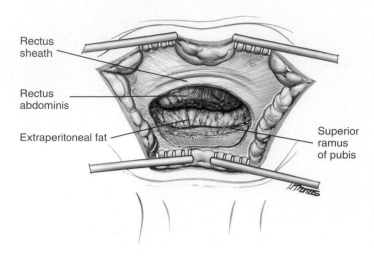

**Figure 7-9**  Divide the rectus muscles 1 cm above their insertion and retract their cut edges superiorly to reveal the superior ramus of the pubis.

lead to inadvertent bladder rupture. If fixation is considered in the presence of urologic damage, it is best to operate in conjunction with an experienced urologic surgeon.

## How to Enlarge the Approach

### Local Measures
Because of the considerable amount of subcutaneous fat in this area, it may be necessary to extend the skin incision and superficial dissection in both directions to allow better visualization of the deep structures in obese patients.

### Extensile Measures
The approach can be extended laterally to expose the entire anterior column of the acetabulum and the inner wall of the ilium. This extended ilioinguinal approach is discussed in Chapter 8.

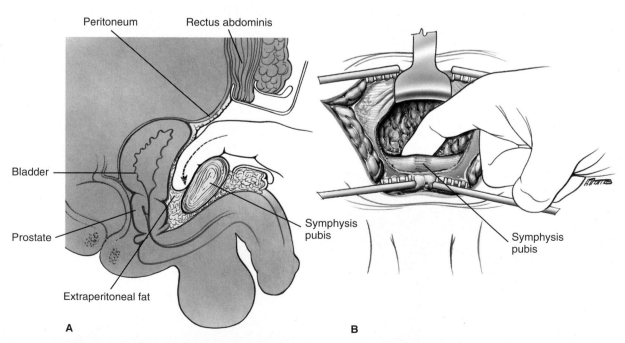

**Figure 7-10**  **(A)** Open the plane behind the symphysis pubis, using your finger as a blunt dissector. **(B)** The pubic symphysis and superior pubic rami now are exposed.

# Anterior Approach to the Sacroiliac Joint

The anterior approach to the sacroiliac joint offers safe, reliable access to that structure and allows anterior plates to be positioned accurately across the joint. It also permits the exposure of the inner wall of the ala of the ilium, allowing fixation of associated iliac fractures. Paradoxically, although the sacroiliac joint is one of the most posterior structures in the entire pelvic ring, the anterior approach allows greater exposure and control than does the seemingly more logical posterior approach, because of the shape of the joint. Anteriorly, the joint is flat and directly available, whereas posteriorly it is overhung by the posterior iliac crest.

## Position of the Patient

Place the patient in a supine position on the operating table and put a large sandbag under the buttock. The iliac crest should be pushed up toward the surgeon. Support the opposite iliac wing with a support attached to the operating table and then tilt the table 20° away, allowing the mobile contents of the pelvis to fall away.

## Landmarks and Incision

### Landmarks

The *anterior superior iliac spine* and the *anterior third of the iliac crest* are subcutaneous and easy to palpate.

### Incision

Make a long, curved incision over the iliac crest, beginning 7 cm posterior to the anterior superior iliac spine (at about the level of the iliac tubercle). Curve the incision forward until the anterior superior iliac spine is reached. Continue the incision anteriorly and medially along the line of the inguinal ligament for an additional 4 to 5 cm (Fig. 7-11).

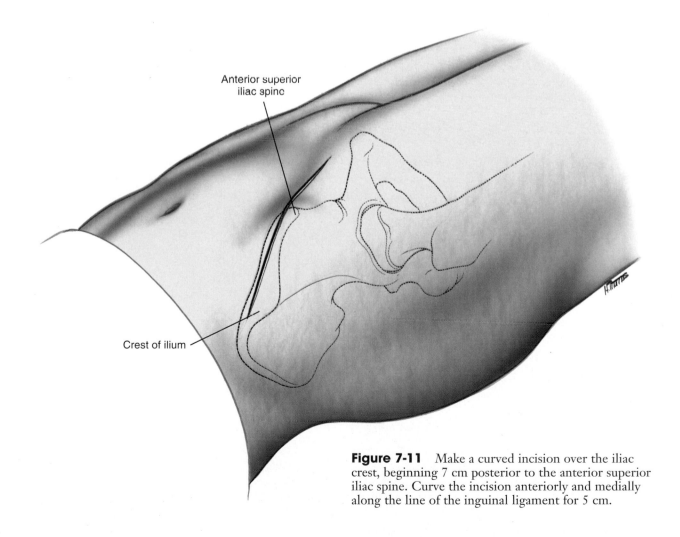

Anterior superior iliac spine

Crest of ilium

**Figure 7-11**   Make a curved incision over the iliac crest, beginning 7 cm posterior to the anterior superior iliac spine. Curve the incision anteriorly and medially along the line of the inguinal ligament for 5 cm.

## Internervous Plane

No true internervous plane is available for use. The approach consists simply of stripping muscles off the pelvis; because the bone is being approached via its subcutaneous surface, no muscle is denervated.

## Superficial Surgical Dissection

Deepen the skin incision through the subcutaneous fat. Expose the deep fascia overlying the glutei and tensor fasciae latae muscles at the point where it attaches to the outer lip of the iliac crest. Next, incise the periosteum of the entire anterior third of the iliac crest and gently strip the muscles off the outer wall of the pelvis to expose about 1 cm of the outer surface below the crest of the ilium. Predrill the iliac crest for easy reattachment. Using an oscillating saw, transect the wing of the ilium at this level, cutting only the outer cortex and the cancellous bone underneath (Fig. 7-12). Next, crack the inner cortex with

an osteotome. This allows the anterior superior iliac spine to be detached along with the transected portion of the iliac wing (Fig. 7-13).

## Deep Surgical Dissection

The iliacus muscle arises from the inner wall of the ilium; detach it by blunt dissection. As the dissection is deepened, the detached anterior superior iliac spine, which still is attached to the lateral end of the inguinal ligament, must be mobilized. This block of bone and muscle must be moved medially; to accomplish this, divide some fibers of both the tensor fasciae latae and sartorius muscles (Fig. 7-14). Note that the lateral cutaneous nerve of the thigh is very close to the anterior superior iliac spine and may have to be divided to permit this mobilization.

Remaining strictly in a subperiosteal plane, strip the iliacus muscle off the inner wall of the pelvis to expose the underlying sacroiliac joint (see Fig. 7-14). The distance is surprisingly short. As the muscle is

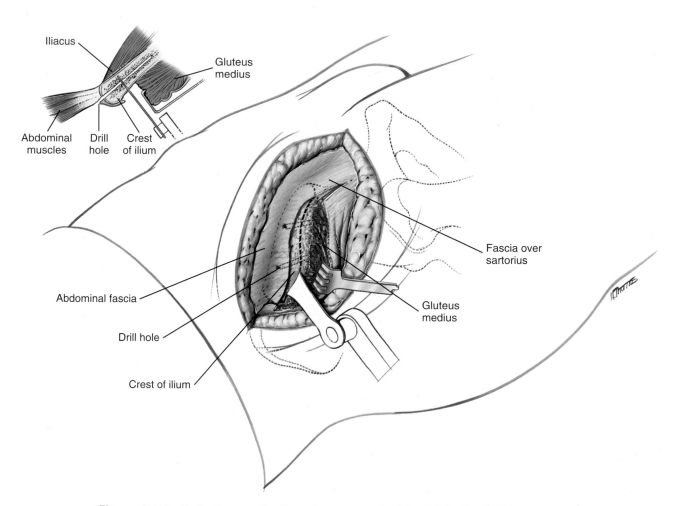

**Figure 7-12** Strip the muscles from the outer wall of the pelvis. Predrill the iliac crest. Divide the outer cortex 1 cm below the crest using an oscillating saw.

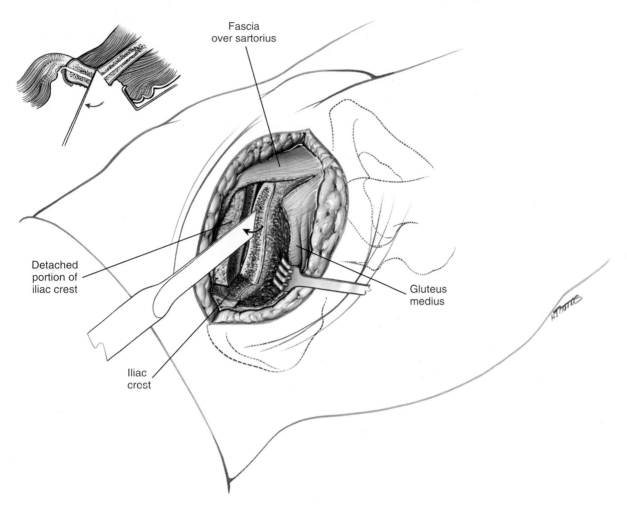

Fascia
over sartorius

Detached
portion of
iliac crest

Gluteus
medius

Iliac
crest

**Figure 7-13**   Crack the inner cortex using an osteotome to complete the iliac osteotomy.

stripped off, some nutrient vessels will have to be detached from the inner wall of the pelvis. Bleeding usually can be controlled by bone wax. Mobilizing the iliacus muscle off the inside of the pelvis with a large bone block allows the muscles to be reattached securely with screws during closure. The muscle then resumes its anatomic position, and the dead space beneath it is obliterated.

## Dangers

### Nerves
The **lateral cutaneous nerve** of the thigh may have to be divided during the mobilization of the anterior superior iliac spine. This will cause some numbness of the lateral aspect of the thigh.

### Sacral Nerve Roots
The sacral nerve roots can be damaged at the point where they arise from the sacral foramina. For this

reason, the dissection cannot be carried further medially than the sacral foramina. The sacral nerve roots are not usually exposed during this approach. They can be at risk at two stages of the operation. If sharp pointed retractors such as Homans are used medially, great care should be taken that the point of these retractors is not inadvertently inserted into a sacral foramen. Sacral nerve roots can also be entrapped under the medial end of plates applied to the anterior surface of the sacroiliac joint. Meticulous preoperative planning will allow you to know exactly how many screw holes can be inserted safely into the sacrum without endangering the sacral nerve root.

### Vessels
Relatively large nutrient vessels often are avulsed from the inner wall of the ilium. Bleeding from these vessels can be controlled by pressure or bone wax.

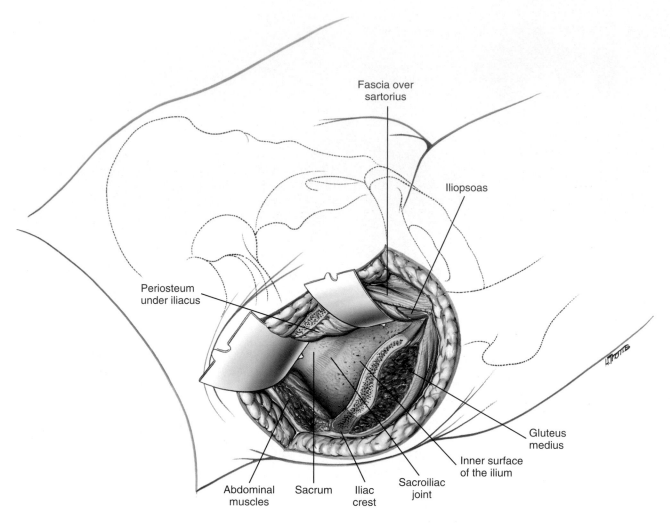

**Figure 7-14**   Strip the iliacus from the inner wall of the pelvis to expose the underlying sacroiliac joint.

## How to Enlarge the Approach

### Local Measures
Paradoxically, the key to adequate exposure of the posteriorly placed sacroiliac joint is adequate anterior dissection. The lateral end of the inguinal ligament and its attached anterior superior iliac spine must be mobilized to visualize the sacroiliac joint adequately.

### Extensile Measures
The approach may be enlarged into an extended ilioinguinal approach that provides access to the entire anterior column of the acetabulum. This approach is discussed in Chapter 8.

## Posterior Approach to the Sacroiliac Joint

The posterior approach to the sacroiliac joint is a simple, safe approach that does not endanger any vital structures. Its uses include open reduction and internal fixation of disruptions of the sacroiliac joint, open reduction and internal fixation of fractures of the ilium near the joint, and treatment of infections of the sacroiliac joint or surrounding bones.

Achieving fixation of these fractures is technically demanding because of the shape of the joint and the presence of the sacral nerve roots arising from the sacral foramina. Practice the direction of screw placement on a bone model before surgery is attempted. During surgery, strict radiological control of screw fixation using two plane C-arm imaging is mandatory. Safe screw fixation can also be facilitated by the use of computer-assisted surgery, if such technology is available to the operating surgeon.

## Position of the Patient

Place the patient prone on the operating table. Position bolsters longitudinally to support the chest wall and pelvis; the bolsters should allow the chest wall and abdomen to expand without touching the table. Take great care during preparation and draping to exclude the contaminated anal region from the operative field.

## Landmarks and Incision

Palpate the *subcutaneous posterior iliac crest*, which terminates in the posterior superior iliac spine.

### Incision

Make a curved incision overlying the posterior iliac crest, beginning 3 cm distal and lateral to the posterior superior iliac spine. Extend the incision from this spot to the posterior superior iliac spine and then continue along the crest to its highest point (Fig. 7-15).

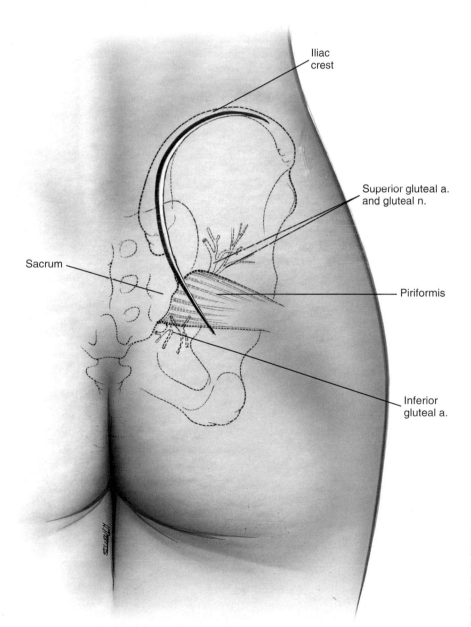

Iliac crest

Superior gluteal a. and gluteal n.

Sacrum

Piriformis

Inferior gluteal a.

**Figure 7-15** Make a curved incision, beginning 3 cm distal and lateral to the posterior superior iliac spine. Cross the posterior superior iliac spine and continue along the crest to its highest point.

## Internervous Plane

No internervous plane is available for use. Both the gluteus maximus and gluteus medius muscles must be detached partially from their origins, but their individual neurovascular pedicles are preserved easily.

## Superficial Surgical Dissection

Divide the subcutaneous tissues in line with the skin incision. Anteriorly, small cutaneous nerves (the superior cluneal nerves) may have to be cut, but they are of little clinical significance. Cut down into the outer border of the subcutaneous surface of the iliac crest to reveal the layer of fascia that covers the gluteus maximus muscle. Detach the origin of the gluteus maximus from the crest and carefully reflect the muscle downward and laterally (Fig. 7-16). Two vital structures penetrate this muscle from its deep surface. First, branches from the inferior gluteal artery, which emerge from the pelvis and with the piriformis muscle and through the greater sciatic notch, penetrate the muscle. In addition, the inferior gluteal nerve emerges from the notch beneath the piriformis to supply the muscle. Because it is imperative that these two structures be preserved, they limit the inferior mobilization of the muscle. As the gluteus maximus muscle is reflected, the gluteus medius and piriformis muscles will be uncovered as they emerge through the greater sciatic notch.

## Deep Surgical Dissection

Gently elevate the gluteus medius muscle from the outer wing of the ilium. The muscle cannot be elevated much anteriorly because its deep surface is tethered by its neurovascular bundle—the superior gluteal nerves and vessels (Fig. 7-17). In cases of trauma, the ruptured sacroiliac joint or fracture is easily visible, but reduction is extremely difficult. To

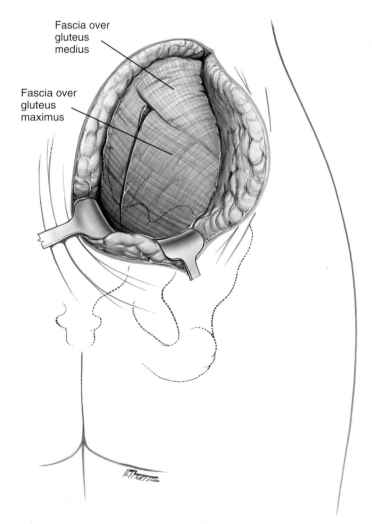

Fascia over gluteus medius

Fascia over gluteus maximus

**Figure 7-16**   Divide the subcutaneous fat and reflect the skin flap to reveal the fascia overlying the gluteus maximus and gluteus medius.

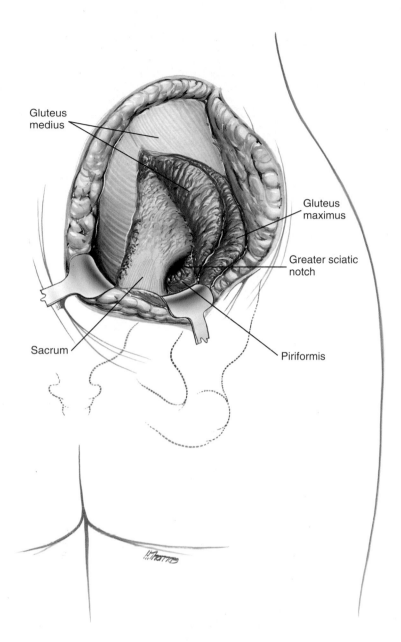

Gluteus medius

Gluteus maximus

Greater sciatic notch

Piriformis

Sacrum

**Figure 7-17** Reflect the gluteus maximus muscle and the gluteus medius from the outer surface of the pelvis.

evaluate any reduction, detach part of the origin of the piriformis muscle from around the greater sciatic notch and insert a finger through the notch to palpate the joint from its anterior surface. The surface of the joint will feel smooth if it has been reduced (Fig. 7-18).

## Dangers

### Nerves

The **inferior gluteal nerve** enters the deep surface of the gluteus maximus muscle. Overzealous downward retraction of the muscle can cause a traction injury to this nerve.

The **superior gluteal nerve** also enters the deep surface of the gluteus medius muscle. This limits the forward retraction of this muscle, restricting the exposure of the outer wing of the ilium. Excessive retraction of the muscle will injure the superior gluteal nerve.

The **sacral nerve roots** are not endangered by the surgical approach but can be injured by inaccurate screw fixation across the sacroiliac joint. Accurate x-ray control of screw placement is mandatory.

### Vessels

Branches of the superior and inferior gluteal arteries run with their respective nerves and also are in danger.

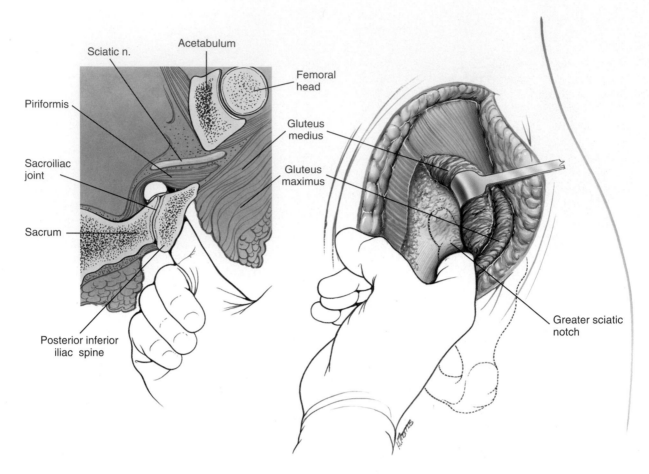

**Figure 7-18**  Detach part of the origin of the piriformis and insert a finger through the greater sciatic notch to palpate the sacroiliac joint from its anterior surface.

## How to Enlarge the Approach

### Local Measures
There are no local measures for enlarging this approach.

### Extensile Measures
The skin incision can be extended anteriorly and the gluteus medius and gluteus minimus muscles elevated from the outer side of the iliac wing. This will enable more extensive fractures of the wing and the ilium to be dealt with.

# Applied Surgical Anatomy of the Bony Pelvis

## Overview

The approaches described in this chapter all obtain access via a subcutaneous portion of the bony pelvis. Thereafter, access is afforded by stripping the muscular coverings off the bone while remaining in a strictly subperiosteal plane. Using this technique, the approaches avoid vital structures and, therefore, are extremely safe. More muscles must be stripped and the view becomes poorer, however, the further one proceeds from a subcutaneous part of the bone. For

this reason, these approaches are limited in the exposure they provide. They cannot be extended and afford only limited access to certain portions of the bony skeleton. Access to the deepest parts of the innominate bone, the acetabulum, is afforded by the modification of hip joint approaches, which are considered in the next chapter.

Two superficial parts of the innominate bones are used for access. The iliac crest has the external oblique and transversus abdominis muscle arising from its surface. The wing of the ilium itself is sandwiched between two masses of muscles, the glutei and tensor fasciae latae muscles on the outer side, and the iliacus muscle on the inner side. The pubic tubercles and upper parts of the superior pubic rami have the rectus abdominis muscle attached to them, and these must be detached for access to the superior surface of the structures.

## Landmarks and Incisions

### Landmarks

The *anterior superior iliac spine* is the site of insertion of the inguinal ligament and the sartorius muscle. The anterior third of the iliac crest is the site of origin for the external oblique, transversus abdominis, and tensor fasciae latae muscles.

The posterior iliac crest is easily palpable and is the site of origin of the external oblique muscle. The pos-

terior superior iliac spine is marked by an overlying dimple. A line connecting these dimples crosses the sacroiliac joint at the level of S2. The pubic tubercle is the medial attachment of the inguinal ligament and the most lateral part of the body of the pubis.

### Incisions

All the incisions described roughly parallel the lines of cleavage. Scars can be broad and ugly, however, but this rarely is of clinical significance because they usually are covered with clothing.

## Superficial Surgical Dissection

In all approaches, superficial surgical dissection consists of incising down onto the superficial portion of the bone. In the iliac crest, this merely involves divid-

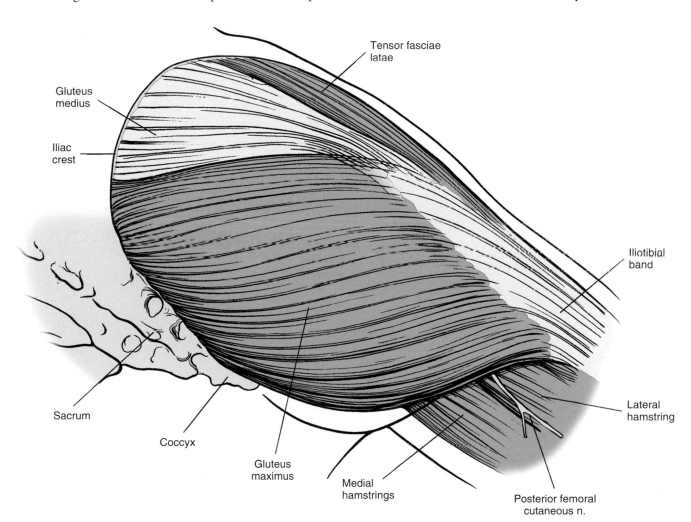

**Figure 7-19**  The superficial musculature of the posterior approach to the hip joint. The gluteus maximus predominates.

**Gluteus Maximus.** *Origin.* From posterior gluteal line of ilium and that portion of the bone immediately above and behind it; from posterior surface of lower part of sacrum and from side of coccyx; and from fascia covering gluteus medius. *Insertion.* Into iliotibial band of fascia lata and into gluteal tuberosity. *Action.* Extends and laterally rotates thigh. *Nerve supply.* Interior gluteal nerve.

ing the overlying fat. In the symphysis pubis, the rectus sheath must be opened. The rectus sheath is a tough fibrous structure derived from all three muscles of the anterior abdominal wall. It forms a tough anterior covering to the underlying rectus muscle, which is easy to repair (see Fig. 7-8).

## Deep Surgical Dissection

Muscles can be stripped safely off both aspects of the anterior third of the iliac crest, but only from the outer aspect of the posterior third of the crest.

Dissection of the outer side of the ilium involves detaching the origin of the tensor fasciae latae. Covering this muscle is a thick layer of fascia that is continuous with the fascia covering the gluteus maximus muscle. The tensor fascia latae, or gluteus maximus and fascia, therefore, can be thought of as an outer layer of the buttock anatomy (Fig. 7-19). This is analogous to the position of the deltoid muscle in the shoulder. Deep to the structures are the origins of the gluteus medius and gluteus minimus muscles from the outer wing of the ilium. These can be lifted off the bone entirely to provide a view of the wing of the ilium. It is important to realize, however, that the rectus femoris muscle still remains between the surgeon and the hip joint, thus limiting the approach.

The inner surface of the ilium serves as origin for the iliacus muscle. This can be lifted off the bone safely, providing access down to the brim of the true pelvis.

The sacroiliac joint is a paradox. It is a true synovial joint in which any movement is very difficult to demonstrate. The joint is reinforced heavily by anterior and posterior supporting ligaments. Approached from the front, the sacroiliac joint is perpendicular to the plane of dissection. Approached from the rear, the joint is overhung by the posterior iliac crest, making it oblique to the plane of dissection. It is critically important to appreciate this obliquity when planning the insertion of any screws that may be used to cross the joint.

In contrast, the pubic symphysis is not a synovial joint, but a secondary cartilaginous joint. Its superior surface is readily accessible once the insertion of the rectus abdominis muscle has been detached. Behind the symphysis pubis is a potential space filled with loose areola tissue; this is known as the cave of Retzius. This potential space lies between the symphysis pubis and the bladder, and allows access to the inner surface of the pubis down to the muscles of the pelvic floor. This access rarely is required, however.

# Eight

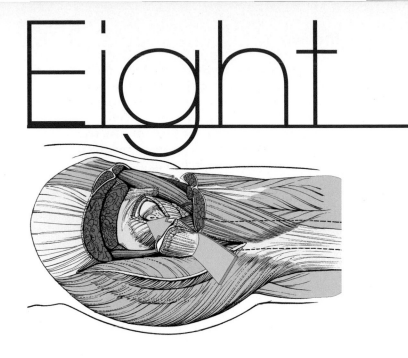

# The Hip and Acetabulum

## The Hip

Operations on the hip joint are among the most common surgical procedures performed in orthopaedics. Total joint replacement for degenerative joint disease has revolutionized the lives of millions of patients. Open approaches to the hip joint are also required for hemiarthroplasties, tumor surgery, and for the treatment of infection around the hip joint.

Four basic approaches expose the entire hip. The *anterior approach*, less common for total joint replacements, allows good access to the pelvis as well as to the hip joint. The *anterolateral approach*, the most common approach for total hip replacement, has many variations because of the different requirements of the several prosthetic designs that can be inserted. The standard anterolateral approach is described; readers are advised to consult the original papers of the

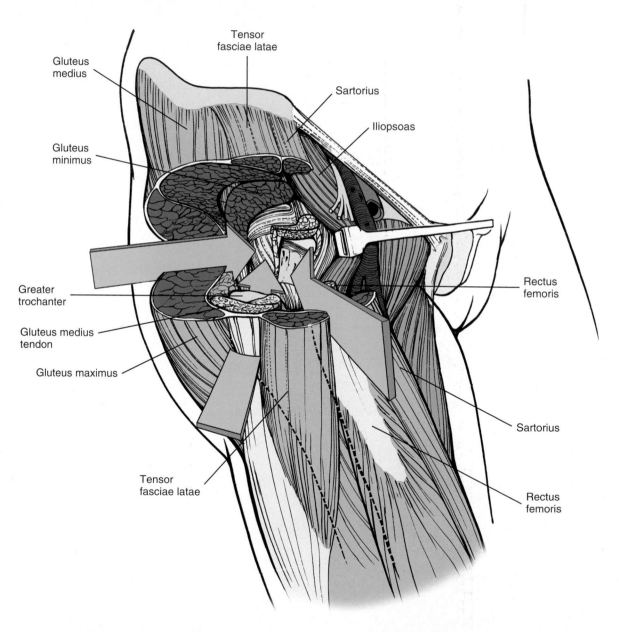

**Figure 8-1**  The intermuscular intervals used in the anterior, anterolateral, and posterior approaches to the hip.

designers of the arthroplasty before performing a particular joint replacement. The *posterior approach*, which is used extensively for hemiarthroplasty as well as for total hip joint replacement, is probably the most common approach performed around the hip joint. It is both safe and easy to perform with only one assistant. The *medial approach* is rarely used, and then mainly for local procedures on the lesser trochanter and surrounding bone.

These four basic approaches to the hip take advantage of the muscular intervals that surround the joint. The anterior approach uses the interval between the sartorius and the tensor fasciae latae; the anterolateral approach uses the interval between the tensor fasciae latae and the gluteus medius; the posterior approach gains access either through the interval between the gluteus medius and the gluteus maximus or by splitting the gluteus maximus; and the medial approach exploits the interval between the adductor longus and the gracilis (Fig. 8-1).

Three anatomical sections augment the description of the approaches. Because the anterior and anterolateral approaches share so much anatomy, they are grouped together. The anatomy for the posterior and medial approaches follows the appropriate approach.

## Acetabulum

Approaches to the acetabulum are the most complex and demanding approaches a surgeon can be asked to perform. They are most often used for the reconstruction of the acetabulum following fractures. Because each approach only gives access to a limited part of the acetabulum, it is critically important that the correct approach is used for each fracture pattern (Fig. 8-2). This requires accurate assessment of the anatomy of the fracture using radiographic techniques, including computerized tomography.[1-3]

The anterior approach to the acetabulum allows access to the anterior column and anterior lip of the acetabulum. When extended, it gives limited access to the posterior column. It does not allow access to the medial aspect of the acetabulum (see Fig. 8-19).[4]

The ilioinguinal approach to the acetabulum allows access to the anterior column and medial aspect of the acetabulum. It also allows visualization of the inner

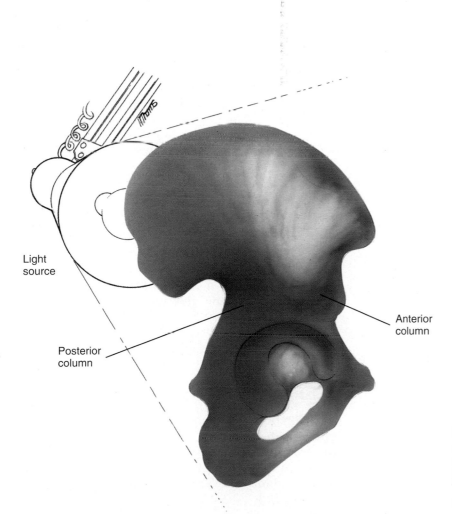

Light source

Posterior column

Anterior column

**Figure 8-2**   To appreciate the anatomy of the anterior and posterior columns of the acetabulum, hold a hemipelvis up against a light source. These two massive columns can then be appreciated in contrast to the thin central area of the wing of the ilium.

aspect of the pelvis from the sacroiliac joint to the symphysis pubis. It does not allow access to the posterior column or posterior lip (see Fig. 8-49).

The posterior approach to the acetabulum allows access to the posterior column, posterior lip and dome segment of the acetabulum. It allows very limited access to the anterior column of the acetabulum and no access to the medial aspect of the acetabulum (see Fig. 8-73).

Because each approach only provides limited access to the acetabulum, complex fractures may require the use of more than one approach.

Most acetabular fractures occur as a result of extremely violent trauma. The tissues are, therefore, contused, and muscle planes are often difficult to develop. The fractures themselves are difficult to reduce, and control and specialized instruments are necessary to ensure anatomical reduction and stable fixation. There is rarely, if ever, indication to perform these approaches in an emergency situation. Acetabular fractures are rare. Understanding of the anatomy of the fracture is difficult. Surgical approaches are technically demanding. The results of acetabular reconstruction depend largely on the accuracy of the reduction of the fracture. For these reasons, acetabular surgery should, if at all possible, be performed by experienced surgeons working in centers large enough to attract a sufficient volume of patients.

# Anterior Approach to the Hip

The anterior approach, also known as the Smith-Petersen[5,6] approach, gives safe access to the hip joint and ilium. It exploits the internervous plane between the sartorius (femoral nerve) and the tensor fasciae latae (superior gluteal nerve) to penetrate the outer layer of the joint musculature. Its uses include the following:

1. Open reduction of congenital dislocations of the hip when the dislocated femoral head lies anterosuperior to the true acetabulum[7]
2. Synovial biopsies
3. Intraarticular fusions
4. Total hip replacement
5. Hemiarthroplasty
6. Excision of tumors, especially of the pelvis

The upper part of the approach may also be used for the following:

7. Pelvic osteotomies

The approach does not expose the acetabulum as completely as other incisions unless muscles are extensively stripped off the pelvis.

## Position of the Patient

Place the patient supine on the operating table. If the approach is to be used for pelvic osteotomy, place a small sandbag under the affected buttock to push the affected hemipelvis forward (Fig. 8-3).

## Landmarks and Incision

### Landmarks

The *anterior superior iliac spine* is subcutaneous and is easily palpable in thin patients. In obese patients, it is covered by adipose tissue and is more difficult to find. You can locate it most easily if you bring your thumbs up from beneath the bony protuberance.

The *iliac crest* is subcutaneous and serves as a point of origin and insertion for various muscles. However, none of these muscles cross the bony crest; it remains available for palpation (Fig. 8-4).

### Incision

Make a long incision following the anterior half of the iliac crest to the anterior superior iliac spine. From there, curve the incision down so that it runs vertically for some 8 to 10 cm, heading toward the lateral side of the patella (see Fig. 8-4).

## Internervous Plane

Two internervous planes are used: the superficial plane lies between the *sartorius* (femoral nerve) and the *tensor fasciae latae* (superior gluteal nerve); the deep plane lies between the *rectus femoris* (femoral nerve) and the *gluteus medius* (superior gluteal nerve) (Fig. 8-5*A,B*).

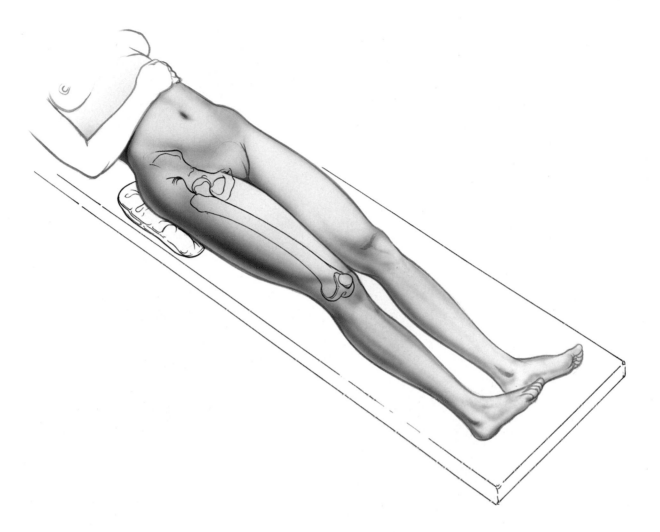

**Figure 8-3**    Position of the patient on the operating table for the anterior approach to the hip.

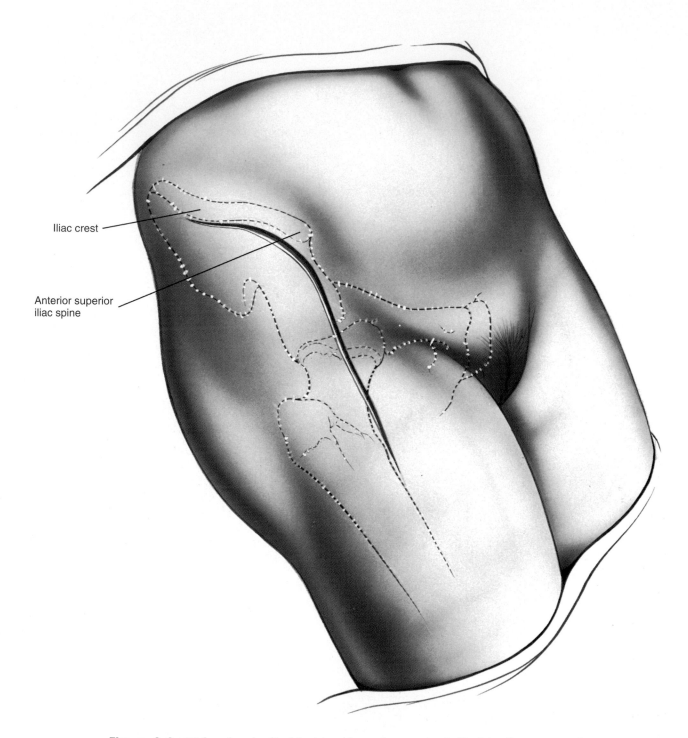

Iliac crest

Anterior superior
iliac spine

**Figure 8-4**    Make a longitudinal incision along the anterior half of the iliac crest to the anterior superior iliac spine. From there, curve the incision down so that it runs vertically for some 8 to 10 cm.

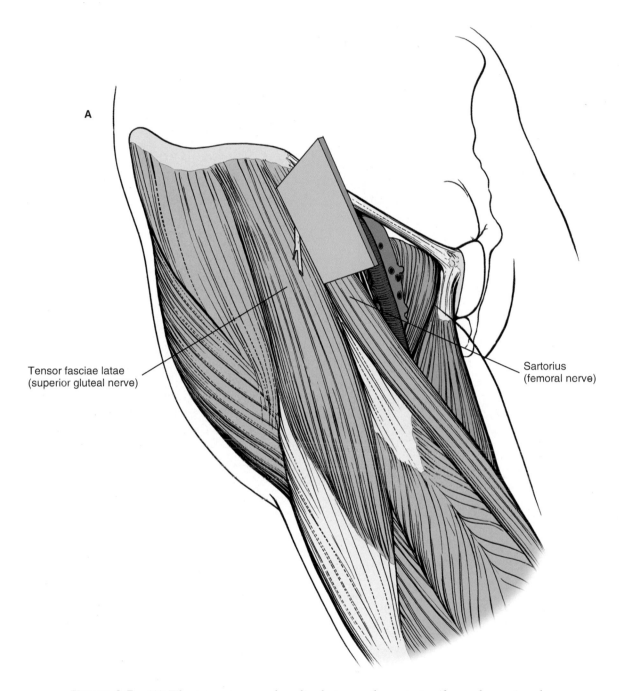

Tensor fasciae latae
(superior gluteal nerve)

Sartorius
(femoral nerve)

**Figure 8-5**   **(A)** The internervous plane lies between the *sartorius* (femoral nerve) and the *tensor fasciae latae* (superior gluteal nerve).

*(continued on next page)*

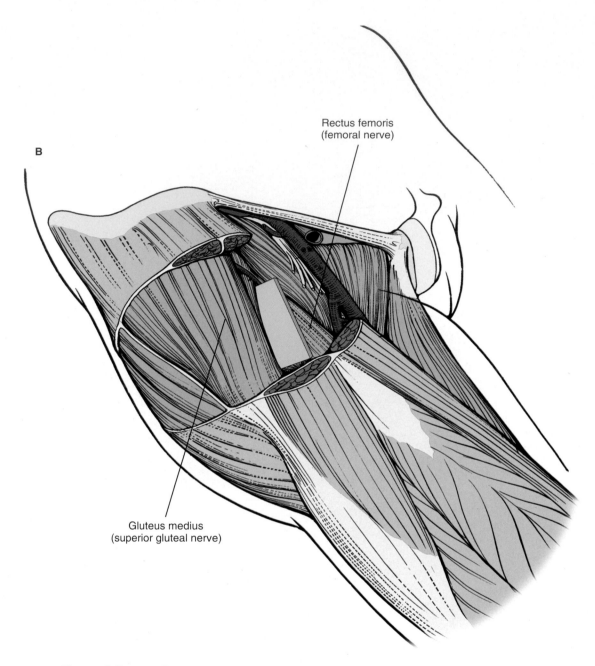

**Figure 8-5 (continued)** **(B)** The deeper internervous plane lies between the *rectus femoris* (femoral nerve) and the *gluteus medius* (superior gluteal nerve).

## Superficial Surgical Dissection

Externally rotate the leg to stretch the sartorius muscle, making it more prominent. Identify the gap between the tensor fasciae latae and the sartorius by palpation (Fig. 8-7). The best place to find it is some 2 to 3 inches below the anterior superior iliac spine, since the fascia that covers both muscles just below the spine makes the interval difficult to define at its highest point. With scissors, carefully dissect down through the subcutaneous fat along the intermuscular interval. Avoid cutting the lateral femoral cutaneous nerve (lateral cutaneous nerve of the thigh), which pierces the deep fascia of the thigh close to the intermuscular interval (Fig. 8-6).

Incise the deep fascia on the medial side of the tensor fascia latae. Staying within the fascial sheath of this muscle will protect you from damaging the lateral femoral cutaneous nerve because the nerve runs over the fascia of the sartorius. Retract the sar-

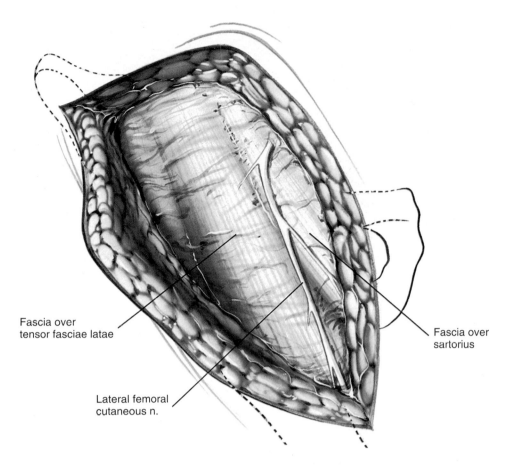

Fascia over
tensor fasciae latae

Fascia over
sartorius

Lateral femoral
cutaneous n.

**Figure 8-6** The lateral femoral cutaneous nerve (lateral cutaneous nerve of the thigh) pierces the deep fascia close to the intermuscular interval between the tensor fasciae latae and the sartorius.

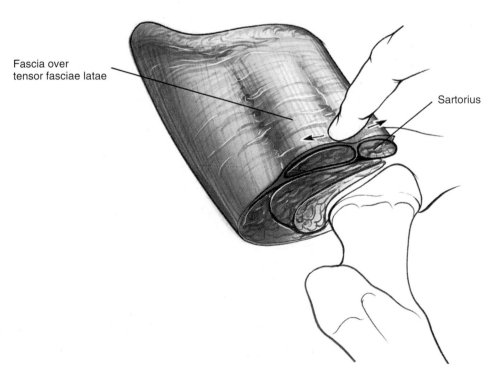

Fascia over
tensor fasciae latae

Sartorius

**Figure 8-7** Identify the gap between the tensor fasciae latae and the sartorius by palpation.

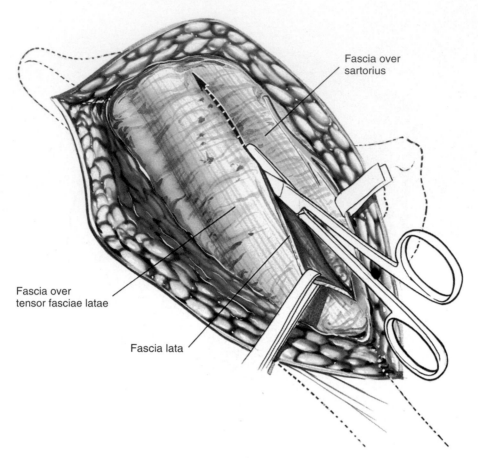

Fascia over
sartorius

Fascia over
tensor fasciae latae

Fascia lata

**Figure 8-8**   Incise the deep fascia on the medial side of the tensor fasciae latae. Retract the sartorius upward and medially and the tensor fascia downward and laterally.

torius upward and medially and the tensor fascia latae downward and laterally (Fig. 8-8).

Detach the iliac origin of the tensor fasciae latae to develop the internervous plane. The large ascending branch of the lateral femoral circumflex artery crosses the gap between the two muscles below the anterior superior iliac spine. It must be ligated or coagulated.

## Deep Surgical Dissection

Retracting the tensor fasciae latae and the sartorius brings you on to two muscles of the deep layer of the hip musculature, the rectus femoris (femoral nerve) and the gluteus medius (superior gluteal nerve) (Fig. 8-9).

The rectus femoris originates from two heads: the direct head, from the anterior inferior iliac spine, and the reflected head, from the superior lip of the acetabulum. The reflected head also takes origin from the anterior capsule of the hip joint. It is intimate with the capsule, making dissection between the two structures difficult.

If you have difficulty identifying the plane between the rectus femoris and the gluteus medius, palpate the femoral artery. The femoral pulse is well medial to the intermuscular interval; if you dissect near it, you are out of plane. Detach the rectus femoris from both its origins and retract it medially. Retract the gluteus medius laterally (Fig. 8-10).

The capsule of the hip joint is now exposed. Inferomedially, you can see the iliopsoas as it approaches the lesser trochanter: Retract it medially (Figs. 8-11 and 8-12). The iliopsoas is often partly attached to the inferior aspect of the hip joint capsule and must be released from it. Inferolaterally, the shaft of the femur lies under cover of the vastus lateralis.

Adduct and fully externally rotate the leg to put the capsule on stretch; define the capsule with blunt dissection. Incise the hip joint capsule as the surgery requires, with either a longitudinal or a T-shaped capsular incision (Fig. 8-13). Dislocate the hip by external rotation after the capsulotomy.

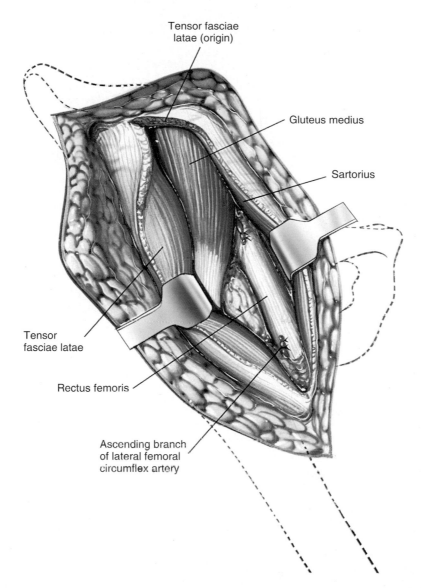

**Figure 8-9**   The deep layer of musculature, consisting of the rectus femoris and the gluteus medius, is now visible. The ascending branch of the lateral femoral circumflex artery must be ligated.

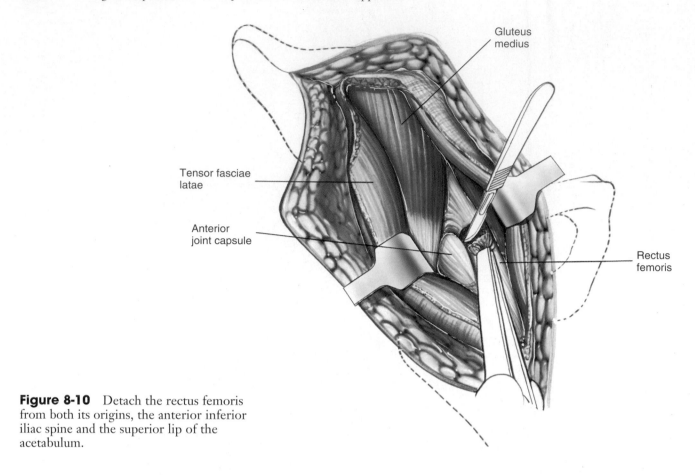

**Figure 8-10**   Detach the rectus femoris from both its origins, the anterior inferior iliac spine and the superior lip of the acetabulum.

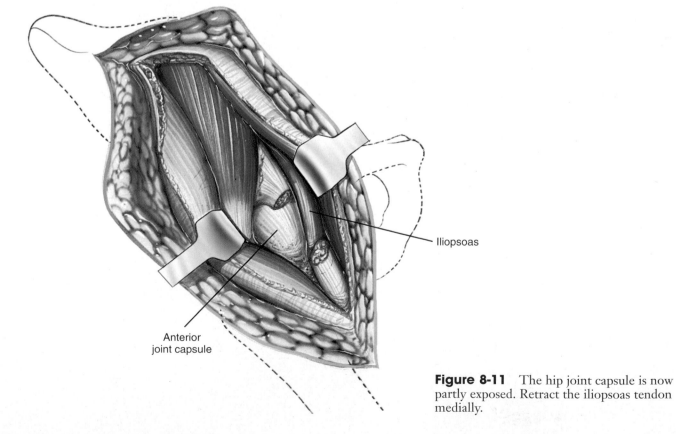

**Figure 8-11**   The hip joint capsule is now partly exposed. Retract the iliopsoas tendon medially.

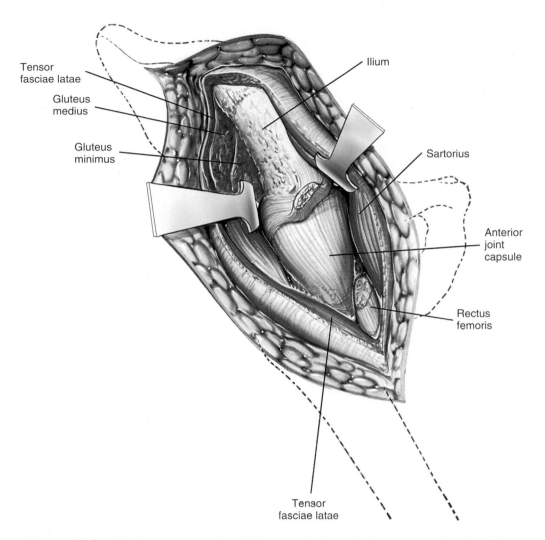

Tensor
fasciae latae

Gluteus
medius

Gluteus
minimus

Ilium

Sartorius

Anterior
joint
capsule

Rectus
femoris

Tensor
fasciae latae

**Figure 8-12**    The hip joint capsule is fully exposed. Detach the muscles of the ilium if
further exposure is needed.

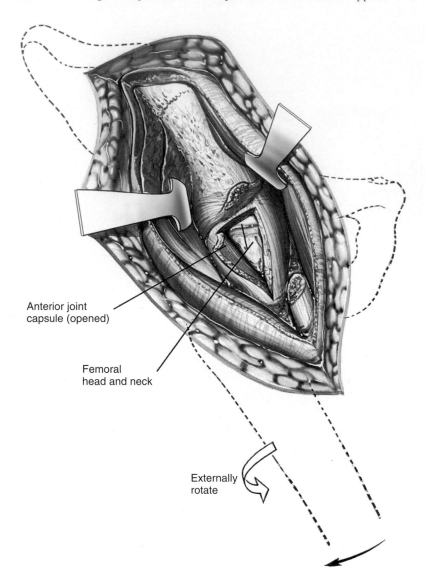

Anterior joint
capsule (opened)

Femoral
head and neck

Externally
rotate

**Figure 8-13**    Incise the hip joint capsule.

## Dangers

### Nerves

The **lateral femoral cutaneous nerve (lateral cutaneous nerve of the thigh)** reaches the thigh by passing over, behind, or through—usually over—the sartorius muscle, about 2½ cm below the anterior superior iliac spine. The nerve must be preserved when you incise the fascia between the sartorius and the tensor fasciae latae; cutting it may lead to the formation of a painful neuroma and may produce an area of diminished sensation on the lateral aspect of the thigh (Fig. 8-15; see Fig. 8-6).

The **femoral nerve** lies almost directly anterior to the hip joint itself, within the femoral triangle.

Because the nerve is well medial to the rectus femoris, it is not really in danger unless you stray far out of plane to the wrong side of the sartorius and the rectus femoris. If you lose the correct plane during deep dissection, locate the femoral pulse by palpation. Within the femoral triangle, the artery lies medial to the nerve (Figs. 8-16 and 8-17).

### Vessels

The **ascending branch of the lateral femoral circumflex artery** crosses the operative field, running proximally in the internervous plane between the tensor fasciae latae and the sartorius. Ligate or coagulate it when you separate the two muscles (see Figs. 8-9, 8-16, and 8-17).

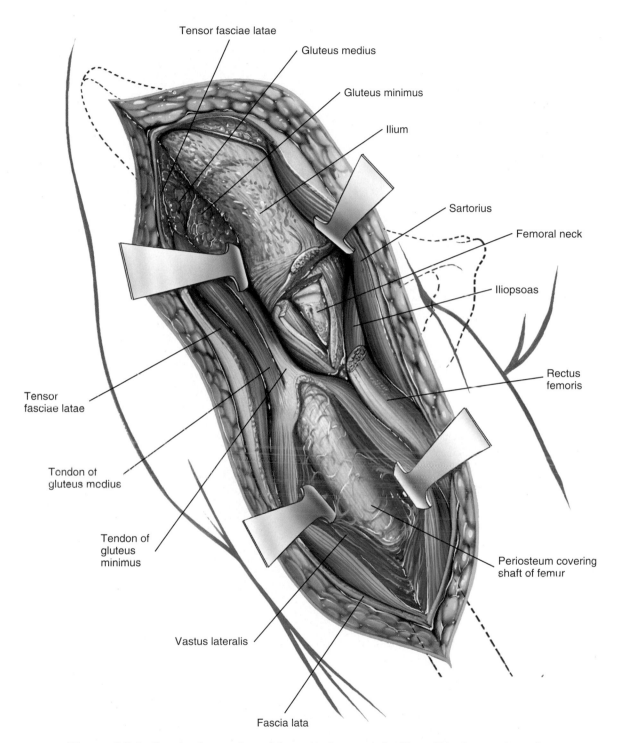

Tensor fasciae latae

Gluteus medius

Gluteus minimus

Ilium

Sartorius

Femoral neck

Iliopsoas

Rectus femoris

Tensor fasciae latae

Tendon of gluteus medius

Tendon of gluteus minimus

Periosteum covering shaft of femur

Vastus lateralis

Fascia lata

**Figure 8-14** Proximal extension of the wound exposes the ilium. Distal extension of the incision exposes the anterior aspect of the femur in the interval between the vastus lateralis and the rectus femoris. It may be necessary to split muscle fibers to actually expose the lateral aspect of the femur.

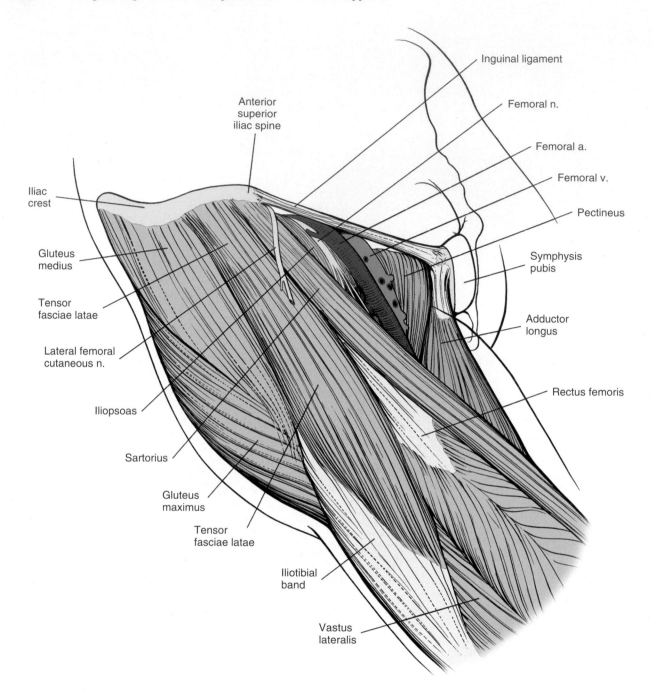

**Figure 8-15** Superficial view of the muscles of the anterior region of the hip, including the femoral triangle and its contents.

**Sartorius.** *Origin.* Anterior superior iliac spine and upper half of iliac notch. *Insertion.* Upper end of subcutaneous surface of tibia. *Action.* Flexor of thigh and knee and external rotator of hip. *Nerve supply.* Femoral nerve (L2-L4).

**Tensor Fasciae Latae.** *Origin.* From outer aspect of iliac crest between the anterior superior iliac spine and the tubercle of the iliac crest. *Insertion.* By iliotibial tract into *Gerdy's tubercle of the tibia. Action.* Maintains stability of extended knee and extended hip. *Nerve supply.* Superior gluteal nerve.

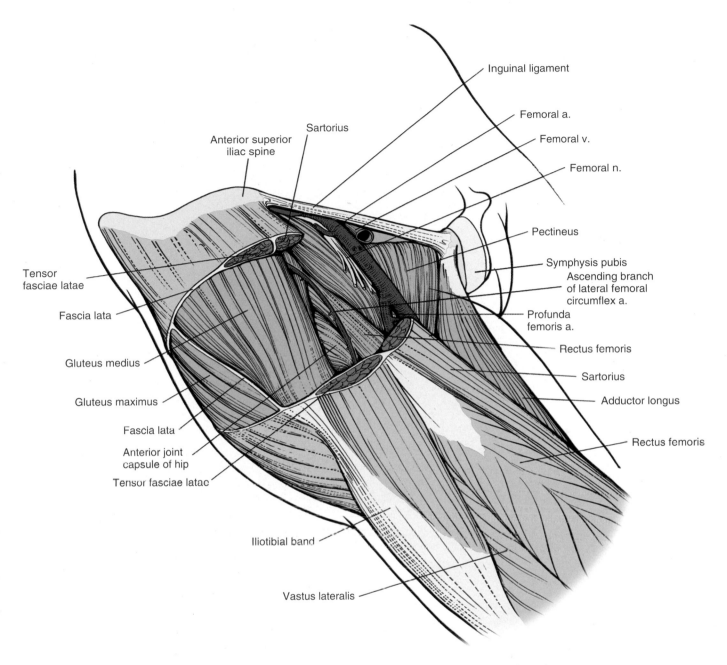

**Figure 8-16** The tensor fasciae latae, the sartorius, and the fascia lata have been resected on the anterior aspect of the hip to reveal the gluteus medius, the rectus femoris, and the ascending branch of the lateral femoral circumflex artery. The hip joint capsule is visible between these two muscles. Medially, note the relationship between the iliopsoas and the rectus femoris.

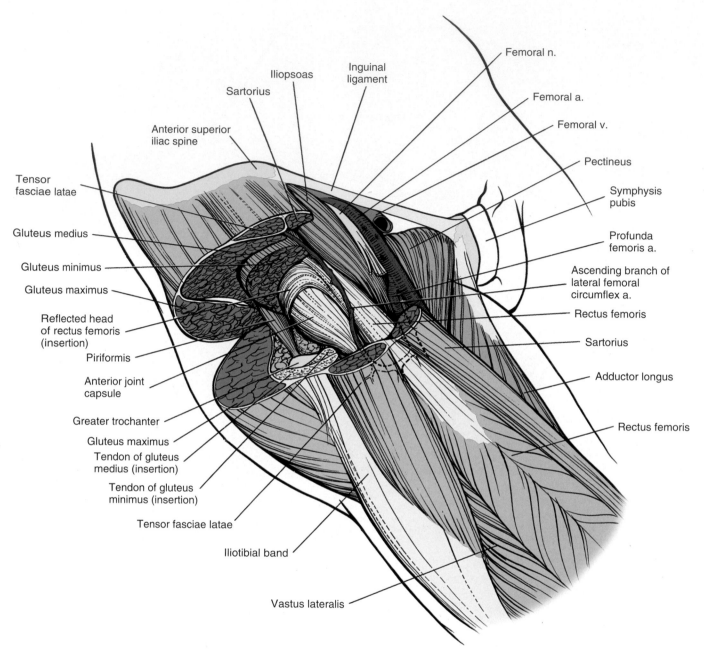

**Figure 8-17**   The gluteus minimus, medius, and maximus have been resected to reveal the hip joint capsule and the reflected head of the rectus femoris.

## How to Enlarge the Approach

### Local Measures

***Superficial Surgical Dissection.*** Detach the origins of the tensor fasciae latae and the sartorius.

***Deep Surgical Dissection.*** Detach the origins of the gluteus medius and minimus from the outer wing of the ilium by blunt dissection. (This procedure is always necessary during pelvic osteotomies.) Bleeding from the raw exposed surface of the ilium can be controlled if you pack the wound with gauze sponges. Individual bleeding points can be controlled by the application of bone wax. There is no other way to stop bleeding.

### Extensile Measures
The skin incision may be extended posteriorly along the iliac crest to expose that bone. In theory, the

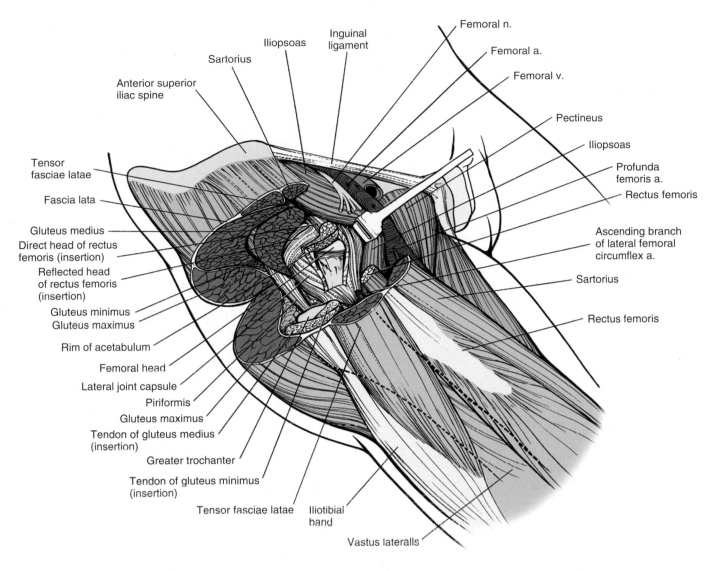

**Figure 8-18** The iliopsoas tendon has been retracted medially; the rectus femoris has been resected and the joint capsule opened to reveal the joint.

extension allows the taking of bone graft, but it is rarely used.

To extend the approach distally, lengthen the skin incision downward along the anterolateral aspect of the thigh. Incise the fascia lata in line with the skin incision; underneath it lies the interval between the vastus lateralis and the rectus femoris. Try to stay in the interval; you will have to split muscle fibers to expose the anterior aspect of the femur. This extension gives excellent exposure of the entire shaft of the femur (see Fig. 8-14).

The approach can be extended to allow visualization of both the inner and outer walls of the pelvis at the level of the hip joint to allow pelvis osteotomy. To obtain visualization of the outer part of the ilium, gently strip the muscular coverings from the bone at the level of the origin of the reflected head of rectus. Using blunt instruments stay in contact with bone. This dissection will lead you into the sciatic notch. Take great care that any instrument inserted into the notch remains firmly on the bone, since the sciatic nerve is also emerging through the notch. Detach the straight head of the rectus femoris from the anterior inferior iliac spine, and carefully lift off the iliacus muscle from the inside of the pelvis, again sticking very carefully to the bone. A blunt instrument will gradually lead you into the greater sciatic notch. At this stage, both instruments should be in contact with each other and with the bone of the sciatic notch. Retraction on both instruments will allow visualization of the entire thickness of the pelvis at the level of the top of the acetabulum, permitting an accurate osteotomy to be carried out.

# Anterior Approach to the Acetabulum

The anterior approach to the acetabulum, or the extended iliofemoral approach, provides exposure of almost all anterior column fractures (Fig. 8-19). It is also useful for the exposure of transverse fractures of the acetabulum. Additionally, the approach provides good exposure of some of the posterior column of the acetabulum and is therefore useful for double column fractures. As in other acetabular approaches, this is a technically demanding approach, and predissection of cadaveric material is advisable for the occasional user. A large amount of soft-tissue stripping is inherent in this approach. There is a risk of devitalizing the gluteal muscles. For these reasons, this approach is now rarely performed in acetabular reconstructive surgery. Two approach techniques utilizing the posterior approach to the acetabulum and the ilioinguinal approach to the acetabulum may be preferable in most fracture types.

## Position of the Patient

See Anterior Approach to the Hip.

## Landmarks and Incision

### Landmarks
See Anterior Approach to the Hip.

### Incision

*Skin Incision.* Extend the skin incision used for the anterior approach to the hip by curving the proximal end posteriorly 5 cm further over the iliac crest. Extend the distal end of the incision inferiorly 5 cm down the lateral part of the thigh that overlies the femur.

## Internervous Plane

See Anterior Approach to the Hip.

## Superficial Surgical Dissection

See Anterior Approach to the Hip.

## Deep Surgical Dissection

Strip the gluteus medius muscle from its origin by blunt dissection, peeling back the muscle from the bone (Fig. 8-20). By staying in this plane you will also elevate the gluteus minimus muscle from the outer wing of the ilium. Continue this dissection as far posteriorly as necessary to expose the fracture.

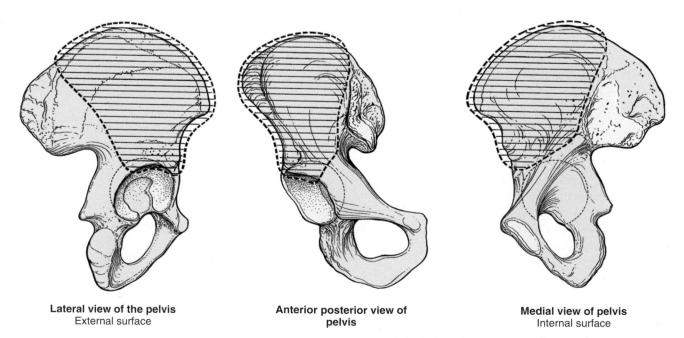

**Lateral view of the pelvis**
External surface

**Anterior posterior view of pelvis**

**Medial view of pelvis**
Internal surface

**Figure 8-19**    The anterior approach to the acetabulum allows access to the anterior column and anterior lip of the acetabulum. It also gives limited access to the posterior column.

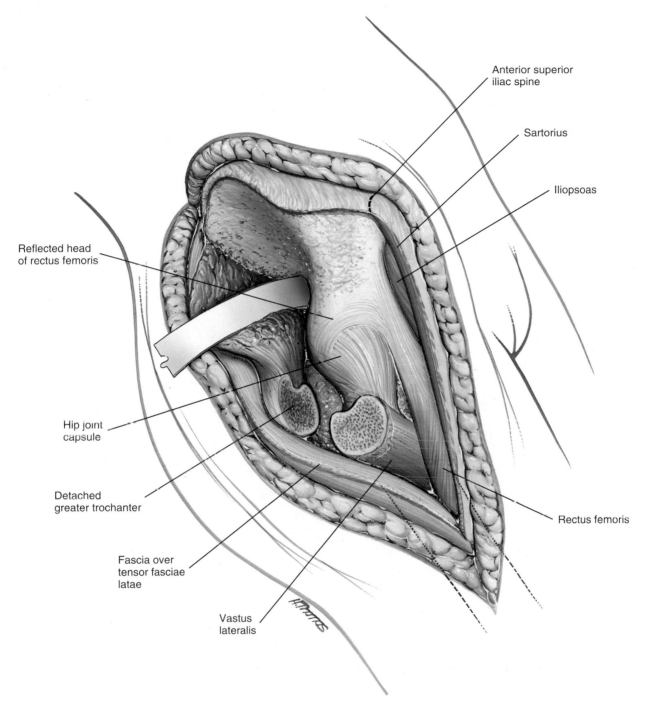

Anterior superior
iliac spine

Sartorius

Iliopsoas

Reflected head
of rectus femoris

Hip joint
capsule

Detached
greater trochanter

Rectus femoris

Fascia over
tensor fasciae
latae

Vastus
lateralis

**Figure 8-20**    Strip the gluteus medius muscle from its origin by blunt dissection.
Perform a trochanteric osteotomy and elevate the gluteal mass from the outer surface of
the pelvis to reveal the posterior column.

For exposure of the posterior column, detach the insertion of the glutei from the greater trochanter. This can be done either by dividing this insertion with a knife or by performing a trochanteric osteotomy. Trochanteric osteotomy may well ensure a better quality of reattachment of the muscle. At this point, it is critical to realize that the gluteus medius and minimus muscles are suspended by their neurovascular bundle (the superior gluteal nerve and artery), which is emerging through the greater sciatic notch. Great care must be taken of this artery to avoid massive muscle necrosis. You must ensure that the vessels are not put on a stretch for any period of time or thrombosis will occur. Part of the posterior column of the acetabulum and the lateral aspect of the iliac crest are now exposed (see Fig. 8-20).

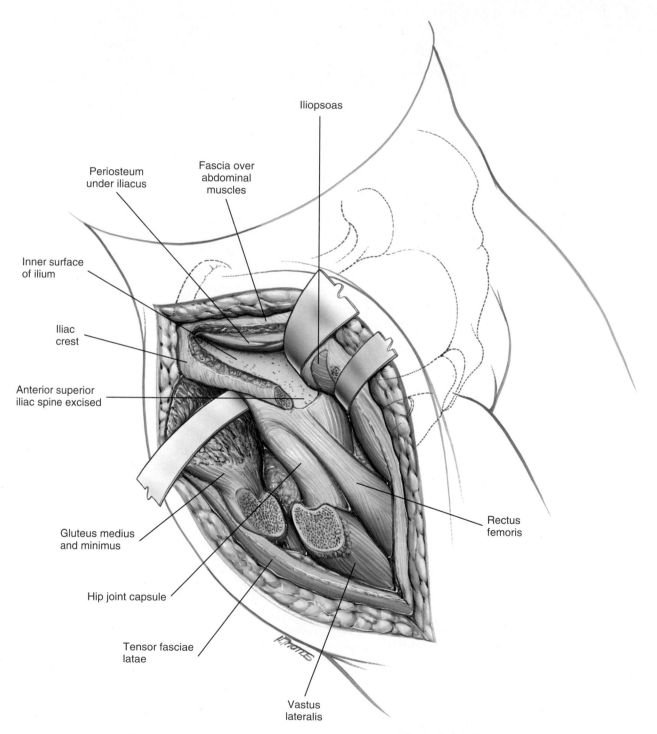

**Figure 8-21**   Detach the origin of the abdominal muscle from the iliac crest, and lift off the underlying iliacus muscle for access to the inner surface of the pelvis.

If you wish to gain access to the inner part of the iliac wing, detach the origins of the abdominal muscles from the iliac crest and lift off the underlying iliacus muscle by blunt subperiosteal dissection. This allows you to access the area from the inner side of the pelvis to the sacroiliac joint (Fig. 8-21).

## Dangers

See Anterior Approach to the Hip.

## Additional Dangers

### Vessels

The **superior gluteal artery** and vein form the neurovascular bundle that supplies the gluteus medius and minimus. These vessels are at most risk at the point where they emerge from the greater sciatic notch. Since this approach involves the detachment of both the origin and the insertion of these glutei, it is critical to preserve the neurovascular bundle to avoid muscle necrosis.

## How to Enlarge the Approach

### Extensile Measures

The skin incision may be extended distally along the lateral border of the thigh (see Fig. 8-14). By splitting the underlying vastus lateralis, you will then be allowed access to the anterolateral aspect of the entire shaft of the femur. The approach cannot be usefully extended proximally.

# Anterolateral Approach to the Hip

The anterolateral approach is the approach most commonly used for total joint replacements. It combines an excellent exposure of the acetabulum with safety during reaming of the femoral shaft. Popularized by Watson-Jones (D. Hirsh, personal communication, 1981) and modified by Charnley,[8] Harris,[9] and Müller,[10] it exploits the intermuscular plane between the tensor fasciae latae and the gluteus medius. It also involves partial or complete detachment of some or all of the abductor mechanism so that the hip can be adducted during reaming of the femoral shaft and so that the acetabulum can be more fully exposed (Fig. 8-23).

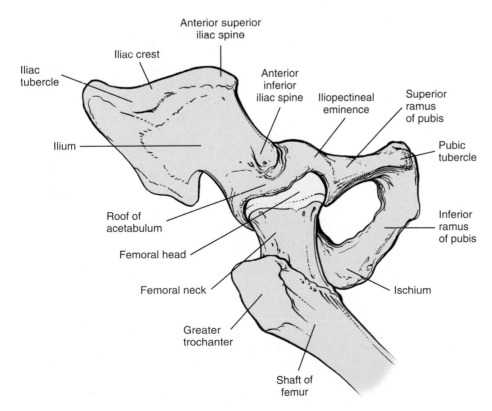

**Figure 8-22**   Osteology of the hip.

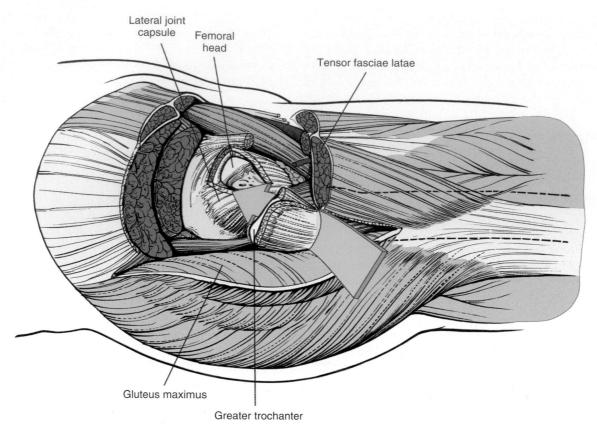

Lateral joint
capsule    Femoral
head

Tensor fasciae latae

Gluteus maximus

Greater trochanter

**Figure 8-23**    The route of the anterolateral approach to the hip joint.

The abductor mechanism can be released either by a trochanteric osteotomy[11] or by cutting the anterior part of the gluteus medius and the whole gluteus minimus off the trochanter.[10] The two methods seem to offer different approaches, but they are actually variations on a theme. The differences should not obscure the fundamental fact that all anterolateral approaches exploit the same intermuscular plane, between the tensor fasciae latae and the gluteus medius.

The uses of the anterolateral approach include the following:

1. Total hip replacement[10,11]
2. Hemiarthroplasty
3. Open reduction and internal fixation of femoral neck fractures
4. Synovial biopsy of the hip
5. Biopsy of the femoral neck

## Position of the Patient

Place the patient supine on the operating table, so close to the edge that the buttock of the affected side hangs over (Fig. 8-24). Tilt the table away from you as the patient lies flat. Both maneuvers allow the buttock skin and fat to fall posteriorly, away from the operative plane, and lift the skin incision clear of the table, making it easier to drape the patient. Either way, you must take into account the position of the pelvis when you insert the acetabular portion of a total joint replacement, since the guides used to position the acetabular prosthesis usually take the ground as their reference plane.

Drape the patient so that the limb can be moved during surgery.

## Landmarks and Incision

### Landmarks

The *anterior superior iliac spine* is subcutaneous. It is easy to palpate in all but the most obese patients, who have a thick layer of adipose tissue covering it. To palpate it, bring your thumbs up from beneath the bony protuberance.

The *greater trochanter* is a large mass of bone that projects up and back from the junction of the shaft of the femur and its neck (see Fig. 8-12).

The *shaft of the femur* can be felt as a resistance through the massive vastus lateralis on the lateral side of the thigh (see Fig. 8-12).

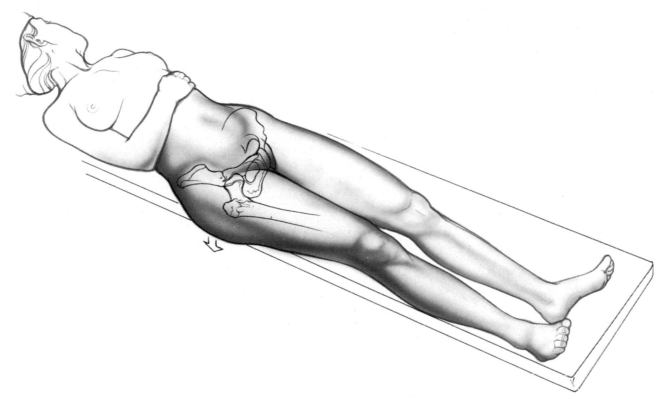

**Figure 8-24**   Position of the patient on the operating table for the anterolateral approach to the hip. Bring the greater trochanter to the edge of the table, and allow the buttocks, skin, and fat to fall posteriorly, away from the operative plane.

The *vastus lateralis* ridge, a rough line that marks the fusion site of the greater trochanter to the lateral surface of the shaft of the femur, is easiest to palpate from distal to proximal. It is not palpable in obese patients.

### Incision

Flex the leg about 30°, and adduct it so that it is lying across the opposite knee both to bring the trochanter into greater relief and to move the tensor fasciae latae anteriorly. Make a 15-cm straight longitudinal incision centered on the tip of the greater trochanter. The incision crosses the posterior third of the trochanter before running down the shaft of the femur (Fig. 8-25).

Note the importance of the position of the limb for this—and all—hip approaches. Flexion, adduction, and subsequent external rotation put the anterior capsule on stretch. The capsule itself is easier to dissect and the structures anterior to the joint relax so that you can develop a plane between them and the capsule. The position also moves the neurovascular bundles anteriorly, lessening the risk that they will be injured during surgery.

### Internervous Plane

There is no true internervous plane for this approach, since the gluteus medius and the tensor fasciae latae have a common nerve supply, the superior gluteal nerve. However, the superior gluteal nerve enters the tensor fasciae latae very close to its origin at the iliac crest; therefore, the nerve remains intact as long as the plane between the gluteus medius and the tensor fasciae latae is not developed up to the origins of both muscles from the ilium (see Fig. 8-23).

### Superficial Surgical Dissection

Incise the fat in the line of the skin incision to reach the deep fascia of the thigh. Using a sponge, gently push back subcutaneous fat off the fascia lata until you can reach the fascia at the posterior margin of the greater trochanter. Incise the fascia lata at this point, entering the bursa that underlies it (Fig. 8-26). Now, divide the fascia lata in the line of its fibers superiorly, heading proximally and anteriorly in the direction of the anterior superior iliac spine.

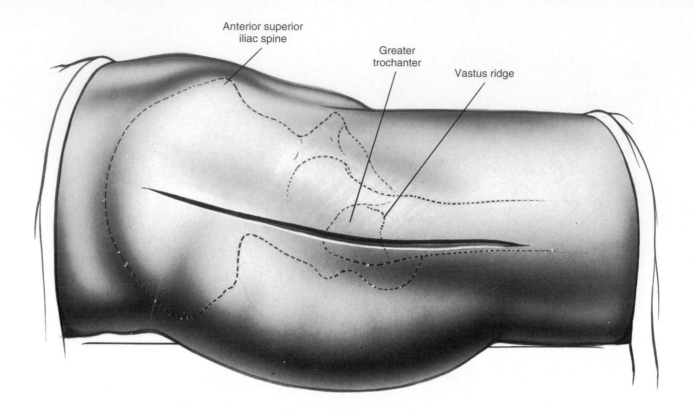

**Figure 8-25**  Incision for the anterolateral approach to the hip.

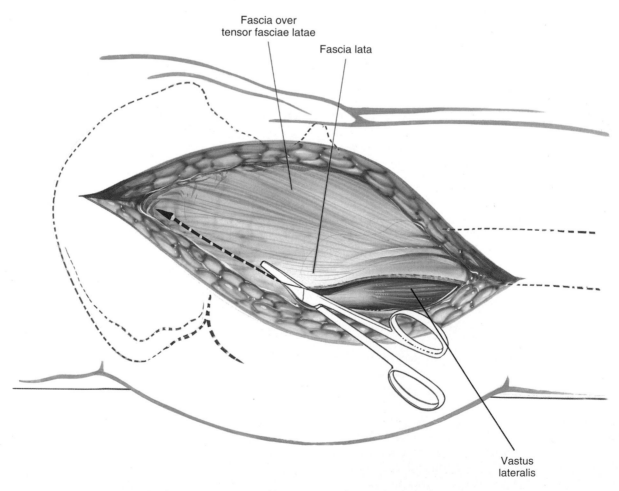

**Figure 8-26**  Incise the fascia lata posterior to the tensor fasciae latae.

Finally, complete the fascial incision by extending the cut distally and slightly anteriorly to expose the underlying vastus lateralis muscle. Elevate this flap anteriorly by getting your assistant to retract it forward, using a tissue-holding forcep. Now, detach the few fibers of gluteus medius that arise from the deep surface of this fascial flap and locate the interval between the tensor fasciae latae (which is being lifted anteriorly by the assistant) and the gluteus medius. This is best done by blunt dissection using your fingers. A series of vessels cross the interval between the tensor fasciae latae and the gluteus medius. These act as a guide to the interval, but require ligation (Fig. 8-27).

Now, place a right angled retractor deep to the gluteus medius and minimus, and retract these muscles proximally and laterally away from the superior margin of the joint capsule that covers the femoral neck (Fig. 8-28).

Fully externally rotate the hip to put the capsule on stretch. Identify the origin of the vastus lateralis at the vastus lateralis ridge. Incise the origin using a cautery knife, and reflect the muscle inferiorly for about 1 cm. Under it is the anterior aspect of the joint capsule, at the junction of the femoral neck and

shaft. Bluntly dissect up the anterior part of the joint capsule, lifting off the fat pad that covers it. The fat pad can reduce postoperative scarring and adhesions and should be preserved even though it intrudes into the operative field (Fig. 8-29).

## Deep Surgical Dissection

Deep surgical dissection consists in detaching part or all of the abductor mechanism and then dissecting up the femoral neck superficial to the capsule of the joint until a suitable retractor can be placed over the anterior lip of the acetabulum.

Two techniques improve exposure of the acetabulum by neutralizing the abductor mechanism, allowing the femur to fall posteriorly. They also permit adduction of the leg for safe femoral reaming and accurate positioning of prosthetic stems within the femoral shaft. The technique chosen depends on the prosthesis to be used.

1. *Trochanteric osteotomy.* Performing a trochanteric osteotomy allows complete mobilization of the gluteus medius and minimus muscles, which in turn allows excellent exposure of the shaft of the

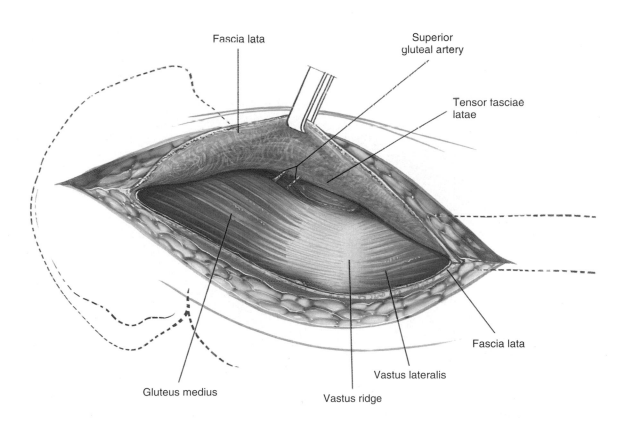

**Figure 8-27**   Retract the fascia lata and the tensor fasciae latae muscle, which it envelopes, anteriorly, revealing the gluteus medius and a series of vessels that cross the interval between the tensor fasciae latae and the gluteus medius.

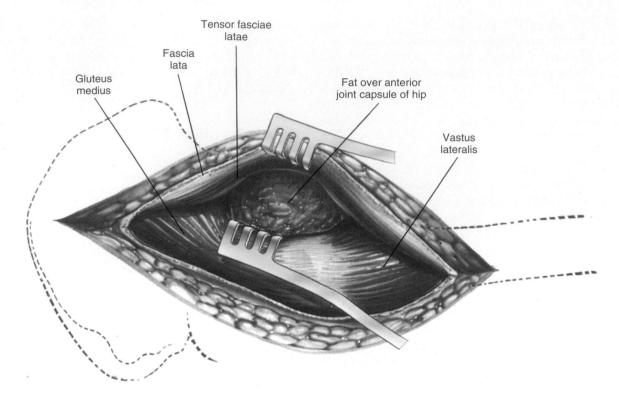

**Figure 8-28**   Retract the gluteus medius posteriorly and the tensor fasciae latae anteriorly, uncovering the fatty layer directly over the joint capsule.

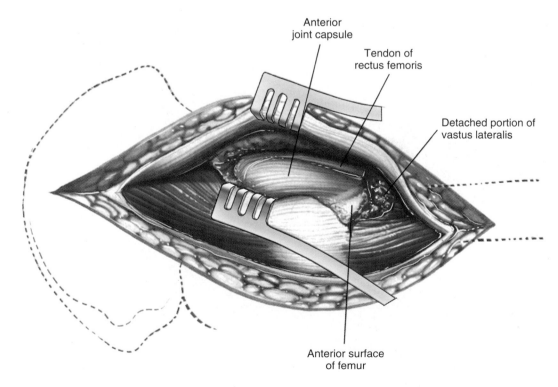

**Figure 8-29**   Bluntly dissect the fat pad off the anterior portion of the joint capsule to expose it and the rectus femoris tendon.

femur during femoral reaming. Palpate the vastus lateralis ridge on the lateral border of the femur, from distal to proximal. Osteotomize the trochanter, using either an oscillating saw or a Gigli saw, and reflect it upward with the attached gluteus medius and minimus muscles. The base of the osteotomy should be at the base of the vastus lateralis ridge. The upper end of the osteotomy may be either intracapsular or extracapsular; the thickness of the osteotomized portion of bone varies considerably, depending on the prosthesis you intend to use. Alternatively, detach the trochanter using two cuts at right angles to one another. This will leave the trochanter looking like the roof of a Swiss chalet. This technique maximizes the bone-to-bone contact surface area and, because of its shape, also is inherently more stable after fixation than a straight osteotomy.

Reflect the osteotomized trochanter upward. To free it completely, release some soft tissues (including the tendon of the piriformis muscle) from its posterior aspect (Figs. 8-30 and 8-31).

2. *Partial detachment of the abductor mechanism.* Place a stay suture in the anterior portion of the gluteus medius just above its insertion into the greater trochanter. Cut the insertion of this anterior portion off the trochanter. Identify the thick white tendon of the gluteus minimus as it inserts onto the anterior aspect of the trochanter and incise it. The exact amount of the gluteus medius that must be detached varies considerably from case to case (Fig. 8-32). In thin, non-muscular people, you may even be able to preserve the whole of the gluteus medius attachment.

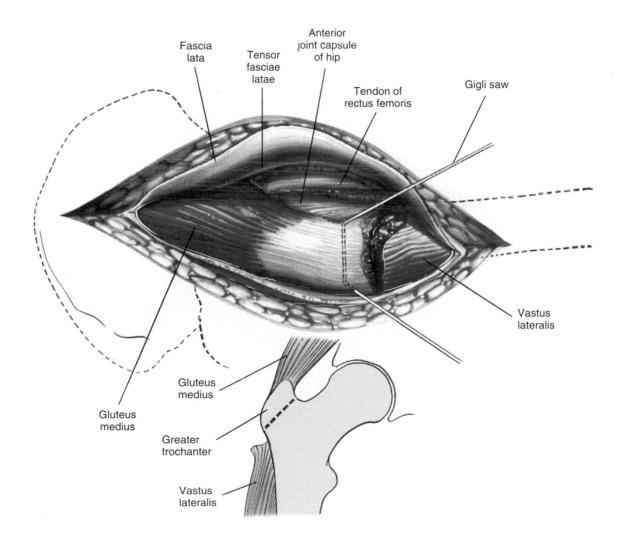

**Figure 8-30**   Osteotomize the greater trochanter.

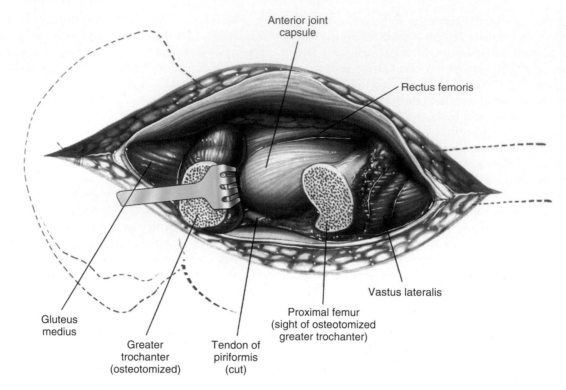

Anterior joint
capsule

Rectus femoris

Gluteus
medius

Greater
trochanter
(osteotomized)

Tendon of
piriformis
(cut)

Proximal femur
(sight of osteotomized
greater trochanter)

Vastus lateralis

**Figure 8-31**   Reflect the osteotomized portion of the trochanter superiorly (with the attached gluteus medius) to reveal the joint capsule.

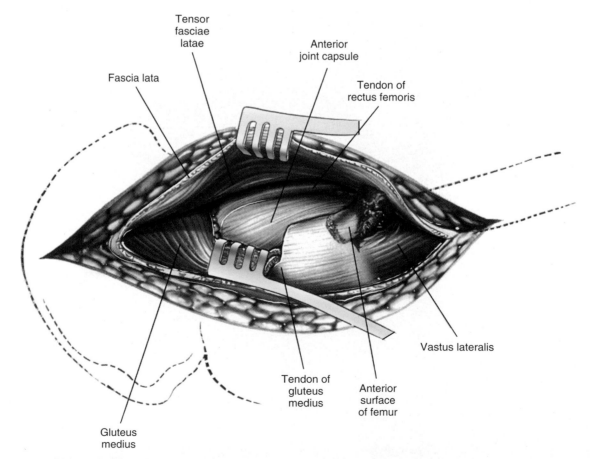

Tensor
fasciae
latae

Fascia lata

Anterior
joint capsule

Tendon of
rectus femoris

Gluteus
medius

Tendon of
gluteus
medius

Anterior
surface
of femur

Vastus lateralis

**Figure 8-32**   The joint capsule may also be exposed by partial resection of the gluteus medius tendon from the anterior portion of the trochanter.

Bluntly dissect up the anterior surface of the hip joint capsule in line with the femoral neck and head. Detach the reflected head of the rectus femoris from the joint capsule to expose the anterior rim of the acetabulum (Fig. 8-33, and *inset*). (This plane is easier to open up if the leg is partly flexed, since the rectus femoris remains relaxed. Flexing the leg also keeps the femoral nerves and vessels off the stretch and farther from the operative field.) Elevate part of the psoas tendon from the capsule. Because both the rectus femoris and the psoas may insert into the capsule, the plane between muscle and capsule is often difficult to establish.

Place a Homan retractor on the anterior rim of the acetabulum. Make certain that the dissection and

the insertion of retractors remain beneath the rectus femoris and iliopsoas, because the neurovascular bundle lies anterior to the psoas. If you cannot develop a plane between the psoas and the capsule, incise the capsule and insert a retractor around the femoral head so that you can see the joint better.

Incise the anterior capsule of the hip joint with a longitudinal incision. Develop this into a T-shaped incision by cutting the attachment of the capsule to the acetabulum as far around as you can reach. Now incise the capsule transversely at the base of the neck to convert the T-shaped incision into an H-shaped one (Fig. 8-34, and *inset*). Dislocate the hip by externally rotating it after you have performed an adequate capsulotomy (Fig. 8-35).

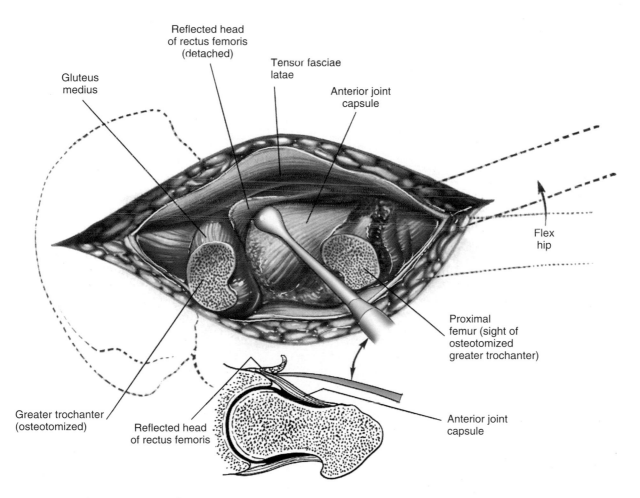

**Figure 8-33**   Reflect the head of the rectus femoris from the anterior portion of the joint capsule.

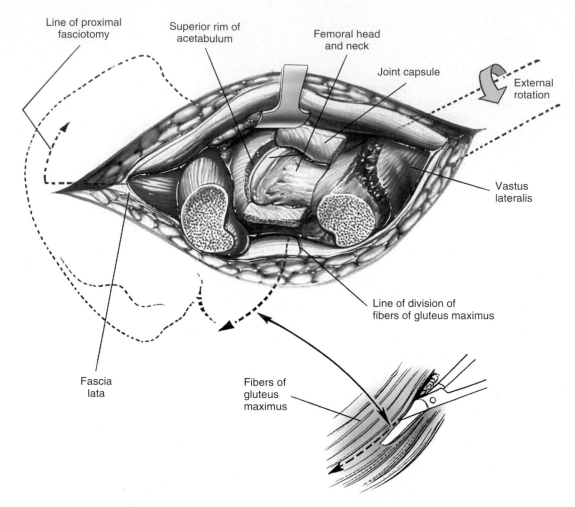

**Figure 8-34**    Incise the anterior joint capsule to reveal the femoral head and neck and the acetabular rim. If further proximal exposure is needed, incise the fascia lata proximally toward the iliac crest and along the iliac crest anteriorly. To facilitate dislocation of the hip, incise the tight fascia lata and the fibers of the gluteus maximus *(inset)*.

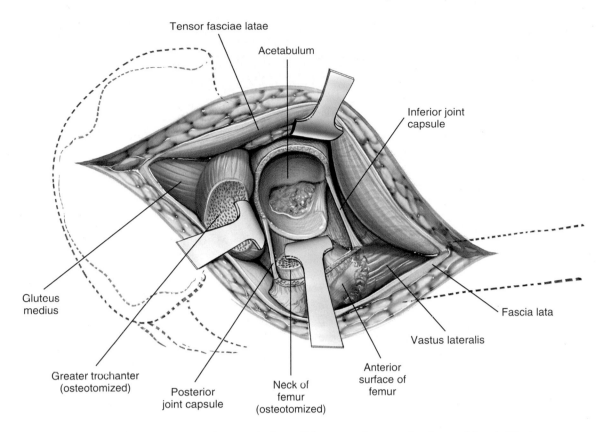

Figure 8-35   To expose the acetabulum, dislocate and resect the femoral head. Placing three or four Homan-type retractors around the lip of the acetabulum provides excellent exposure.

## Dangers

### Nerves

The **femoral nerve** is the most laterally placed structure in the neurovascular bundle in the femoral triangle, thus the structure closest to the operative field and most at risk. The most common problem is compression neurapraxia, caused by overexuberant medial retraction of the anterior covering structures of the hip joint. Less frequently, the nerve is directly injured by retractors placed in the substance of the iliopsoas (see Figs. 8-38 and 8-39).

### Vessels

The **femoral artery and vein** may be damaged by incorrectly placed acetabular retractors that penetrate the iliopsoas, piercing the vessels as they lie on the surface of the muscle. You can avoid this complication by making sure that the tip of the retractor is placed firmly on bone, with no intervening tissue. The anterior retractor should be placed in the 1-o'clock position for the right hip and in the 11-o'clock position for the left hip. Finding the correct plane between the rectus femoris and the anterior part of the hip joint capsule is easier if the limb is in about 30° of flexion.

The **profunda femoris artery** lies on the psoas muscle, deep to the femoral artery. It has also been damaged by poorly placed retractors.

### Fractures of the Femoral Shaft

Femoral shafts have been known to fracture while hips are being dislocated. For that reason, it is critical that you do an adequate capsular release before attempting dislocation. To dislocate the joint, lever the femoral head out of the acetabulum with a skid (such as a Watson-Jones) while your assistant gently externally rotates the limb. Your assistant has a considerable lever arm during this procedure; if he rotates the leg too forcibly, he can cause a spiral fracture of the femur.

In severe protrusion of the hip, you may have to osteotomize the rim of the acetabulum, which often has an osteophyte, to achieve dislocation.

If you cannot dislocate the hip without resorting to extreme force, it is safer to perform a double osteotomy of the femoral neck, excising a 1-cm portion of it: then remove the femoral head (which is lying free) with a corkscrew.

Fractures of the femoral shaft also can occur when the limb is placed in full adduction and external rotation for reaming of this femoral shaft. In order for the operator to gain a good enough view of the cut surface of the femur, the femoral shaft must be adducted. If the incision in the fascia lata has been placed too far anteriorly, then the fascia lata will resist adduction and enthusiastic assistants may cause femoral shaft fracture. This is the reason why the fascia lata should be incised initially at the posterior border of the greater trochanter. If the fascia lata gets in your way when attempting to adduct the leg, it is safest to incise it along the lines of fibers of gluteus maximus (see Fig. 8-34).

## How to Enlarge the Approach

### Local Measures

The posterior flap of the fascia lata, created during your superficial dissection, may prevent the adduction of the leg and complete dislocation of the hip needed for femoral reaming because it impinges on the trochanter. If it does, make an incision into the posterior flap of the tensor fasciae latae, heading obliquely upward and backward in line with the fibers of the gluteus maximus, which also inserts into the iliotibial tract (see Fig. 8-34).

If anterior retraction of the tensor fasciae latae proves difficult, use a pair of scissors to incise the fascia on the muscle's anterior aspect close to its origin from the ilium (see Fig. 8-34). Alternatively, continue the fascial incision farther down the lateral aspect of the femoral shaft. These maneuvers are seldom necessary.

The key to a full exposure of the acetabulum lies in correctly placing the retractors. Different approaches use different retractors, but three or four Homan-type retractors placed around the lip of the acetabulum, directly on bone, give as good an exposure as any (see Fig. 8-35).

### Extensile Measures

Extend the skin incision down the lateral aspect of the thigh, and incise the deep fascia in line with the skin incision. Split the vastus lateralis to gain access to the lateral aspect of the femur. In this way, you can usefully extend the approach to include the entire length of the femur. Distal extension is often needed when the approach is used for open reduction and internal fixation of fractures of the femoral neck (Fig. 8-36).

The approach cannot usefully be extended proximally.

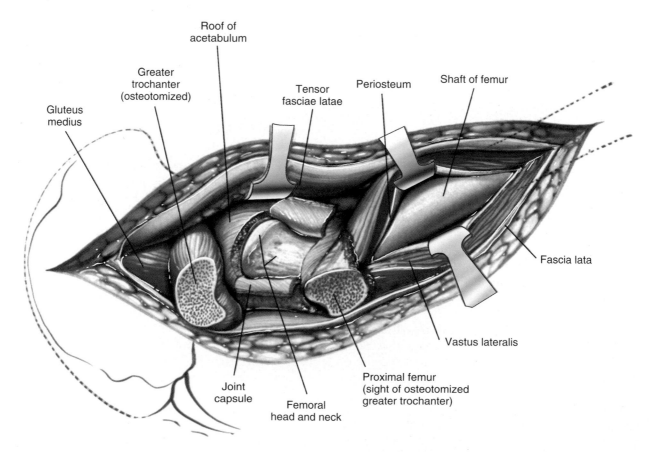

**Figure 8-36**    Extend the incision down the lateral aspect of the thigh, incising the deep fascia and splitting the vastus lateralis in line with its musculature to reach the lateral aspect of the femur.

# Applied Surgical Anatomy of the Anterior and Anterolateral Approaches to the Hip

## Overview

The fascia lata covers all the thigh and hamstring muscles around the hip joint. In hip surgery, its importance lies in its relationship to three muscles: the sartorius, the tensor fasciae latae, and the gluteus maximus. The fascia lata covers the sartorius; it also splits into a deep and superficial layer to enclose the tensor fasciae latae and gluteus maximus (Fig. 8-37). If the iliac crest is viewed from the lateral side, the outer layer of the covering seems to consist of the fascia lata of the thigh and the muscles that it encloses. The sartorius lies farther anteriorly. The gluteus medius, which arises from the outer wing of the ilium, is covered by the fascia lata, not enclosed by it (Fig. 8-38).

The key to the **anterolateral approach** to the hip lies in the relationship between the tensor fasciae latae and the gluteus medius. The tensor fasciae latae, a superficial structure, arises from the anterior portion of the outer lip of the iliac crest. The gluteus medius arises from the outer wall of the ilium, between the anterior and posterior gluteal lines. The origins of the two muscles are, therefore, almost continuous, but the tensor fasciae latae is slightly more superficial (lateral) and anterior than the gluteus medius (Fig. 8-39).

The tensor fasciae latae inserts into the iliotibial tract, the thickening of the deep fascia of the thigh, while the gluteus medius inserts into the anterior and lateral part of the greater trochanter. Thus, as the muscles run from origins to insertions, the tensor fasciae latae rises to an even more superficial position in relation to the gluteus medius (see Figs. 8-38 and 8-39).

To exploit the intermuscular plane between the gluteus medius and the tensor fasciae latae, incise the fascia lata posterior to the posterior margin of the

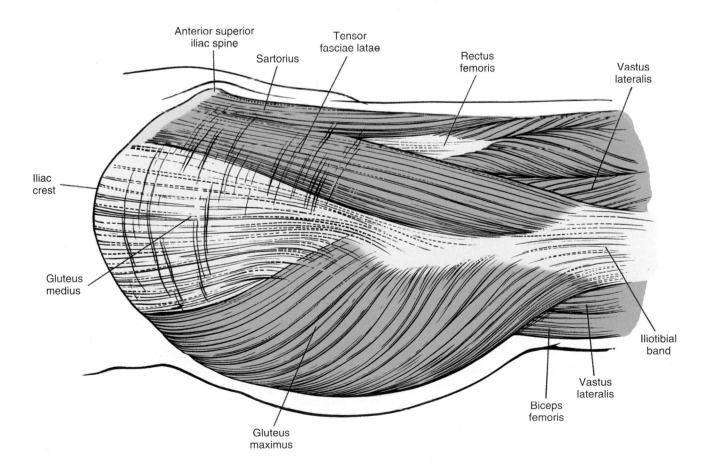

**Figure 8-37**   Superficial musculature of the lateral aspect of the hip.

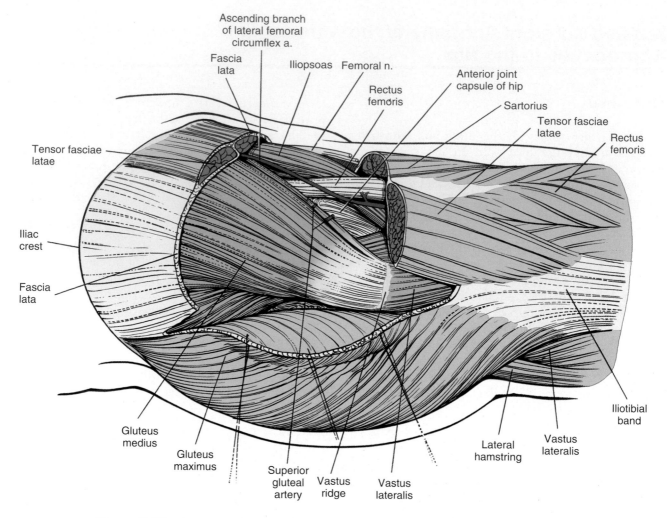

**Figure 8-38**   Resecting the sartorius, tensor fasciae latae, and fascia lata and reflecting the anterior portion of the gluteus maximus posteriorly reveal the gluteus medius and more anterior structures of the hip region. The fascia lata splits to envelop the tensor fasciae latae, but it only covers the gluteus medius muscle.

**Gluteus Medius.** *Origin.* Outer aspect of ilium between anterior and posterior gluteal lines and its overlying fascia. *Insertion.* Lateral surface of greater trochanter. *Action.* Abductor and medial rotator of hip. *Nerve supply.* Superior gluteal nerve.

tensor fasciae latae and retract the cut fascial edge anteriorly. Because the fascia lata actually encloses the tensor fasciae latae, the muscle is retracted with the fascia (see Fig. 8-38).

All anterolateral approaches use this one intermuscular plane to reach the femoral neck; then they follow the joint capsule medially to expose the anterior rim of the acetabulum. The techniques used in this approach differ mainly in how they detach the abductor mechanism to allow adduction of the femur for femoral reaming and retraction of the femoral neck posteriorly for adequate exposure of the acetabulum.

The **anterior approach** is more straightforward: Two distinct muscle layers must be incised. The *outer layer* consists of the tensor fasciae latae (superior gluteal nerve) and the sartorius (femoral nerve) (see Fig. 8-15). The interval between them forms a true internervous plane. Two structures, the lateral femoral cutaneous nerve and the ascending branch of the lateral femoral circumflex artery, lie between them; they must be identified and avoided during the dissection (see Figs. 8-15 and 8-16).

The *deep layer* of muscle consists of the rectus femoris (femoral nerve) and the gluteus medius (superior gluteal nerve). The interval between them

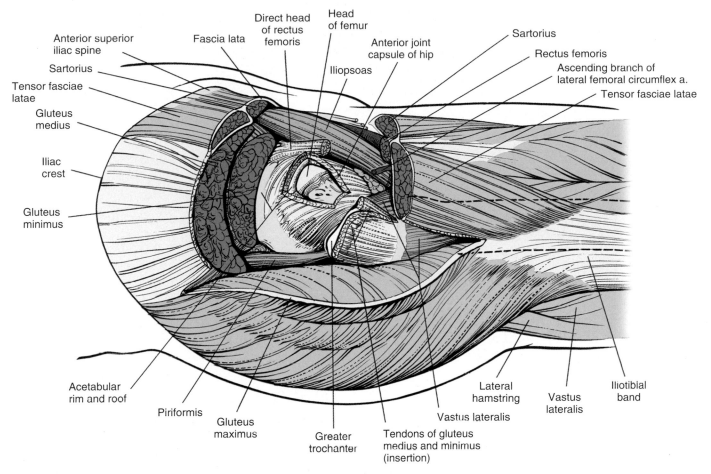

**Figure 8-39**   The gluteus medius, gluteus minimus, and rectus femoris have been resected to reveal the muscular layers down to the hip joint capsule. Resection of the joint capsule exposes the acetabulum and the femoral head and neck.

is also an internervous plane; exploiting it is difficult, mainly because the short head of the rectus femoris originates partly from the anterior capsule of the hip joint, where the iliopsoas partly inserts (see Figs. 8-16 and 8-17).

## Landmarks and Incision

### Landmarks

The *anterior superior iliac spine* is the site of attachment of two important structures. The sartorius takes its origin from it, and the inguinal ligament uses it as a lateral attachment. The anterior superior iliac spine is rarely used as a bone graft because the lateral cutaneous nerve of the thigh lies so close to it.

The *anterior third of the iliac crest* serves as the origin for the following three muscles:

1. The *external oblique* forms the outer layer of the muscles of the anterior abdominal wall. It originates from the outer strip of the anterior half of the iliac crest.

2. The *internal oblique* forms the middle layer of the muscles of the anterior abdominal wall. It originates from the center strip of the anterior half of the iliac crest.

3. The *tensor fasciae latae* arises from the outer lip of the anterior half of the iliac crest.

The origins of the external oblique and internal oblique are not detached during the anterior approach; the tensor fasciae latae is.

The *greater trochanter* is the traction apophysis of the proximal femur and the site of the insertion of the gluteus medius and minimus muscles.

The *vastus lateralis ridge* results partly from the pull of the aponeurosis of the vastus lateralis during growth and partly from the fusion of the trochanter apophyses of the shaft of the femur (Fig. 8-40; see Fig. 8-38).

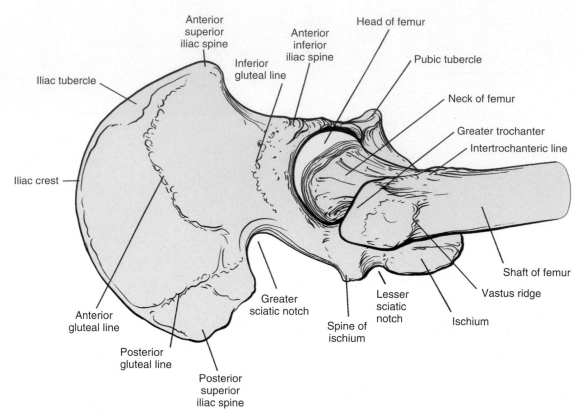

**Figure 8-40**    Osteology of the lateral aspect of the hip and pelvis.

### Incisions

Both anterior and anterolateral incisions largely ignore the lines of cleavage in the skin, but the scars are seldom broad and are nearly always hidden by clothing.

## Superficial Surgical Dissection and its Dangers

Both approaches use planes that involve the *tensor fasciae latae*. The anterior approach passes in front of it; the anterolateral approach passes behind it (Fig. 8-41).

### Anterior Approach

The tensor fasciae latae and the sartorius run side by side from an almost continuous line of origin along the anterior end of the iliac crest. The two muscles diverge a short distance below the anterior superior iliac spine so that the rectus femoris can emerge from between them (see Fig. 8-15).

The *tensor fasciae latae* itself is triangular. In cross section, it is unusually slim at its origin and thick just before it inserts into the iliotibial tract. Its action is difficult to interpret, because another large muscle, the gluteus maximus, also inserts into the iliotibial tract. In cases of poliomyelitis, dividing the iliotibial tract relieves flexion and abduction contractures of the hip joint.

Evidence suggests that the tensor fasciae latae may be important in standing in a one-legged stance, waiting in a bus line, for instance, where the muscle may maintain the stability of the extended knee and hip.[12]

The muscle fibers of the tensor fasciae latae are considerably finer than those of the gluteus medius, but the difference in the quality of fibers rarely makes it easier to identify the plane between the two muscles.

The *sartorius* is the longest muscle in the body, crossing both the hip and the knee. The individual fibers within the muscle are also the longest in the body; they leave the sartorius weak but capable of extraordinary contraction.

Two structures cross the plane between the tensor fasciae latae and the sartorius. Both complicate the superficial surgical dissection of the anterior approach.

1. The *ascending branch of the lateral femoral circumflex artery* is a comparatively large artery that often requires ligation. It is one of a series of ves-

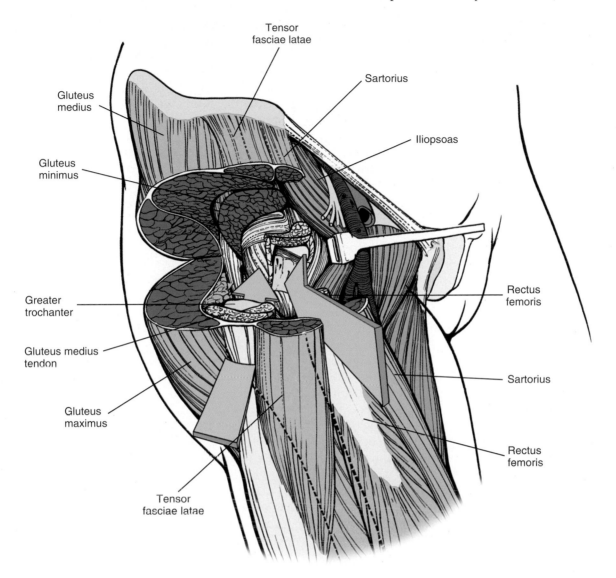

**Figure 8-41**   The anterior and anterolateral approaches to the hip joint, showing their muscular boundaries.

sels that run circumferentially around the thigh (see Anterior Approach to the Hip above). This is one of the rare instances in which a vessel crosses an internervous plane (see Figs. 8-16 and 8-17).

2. The *lateral femoral cutaneous nerve (lateral cutaneous nerve of the thigh)* arises from the lumbar plexus or, occasionally, from the femoral nerve itself. From there, it descends through the pelvis on the surface of the iliacus muscle. It enters the thigh under the inguinal ligament anywhere between the anterior superior iliac spine and the mid-inguinal point. The nerve pierces the fascia lata just below and medial to the anterior superior iliac spine. The path it takes may vary consider-

ably, as it can pass either around or through the sartorius muscle (see Fig. 8-15).

Compression syndromes (meralgia paresthetica) of the lateral femoral cutaneous nerve have been reported, particularly from the section that runs behind the inguinal ligament and from the point where the nerve pierces the fascia lata. These syndromes consist of painful paresthesias on the lateral side of the thigh, conditions that may be relieved by decompressing the nerve. Occasionally, decompression may have to extend into the pelvis, since the nerve may be compressed on the surface of the iliacus.

## Anterolateral Approach

One muscle, the *gluteus medius*, runs through both the superficial and the deep surgical dissection, mainly because its origin is relatively superficial while its insertion is deep (see Figs. 8-37 through 8-39). From an anterior approach, the gluteus medius appears to be one of the muscles of the inner layer over the hip joint. From an anterolateral approach, it occupies a more superficial position.

There are two important points about the structure of this muscle, knowledge of which prevents confusion during the anterolateral approach to the hip. First, fibers of the gluteus medius commonly arise from the deep surface of the fascia latae. This means that when you elevate the fascial flap to gain access to the anterior border of gluteus medius, you often have to detach muscular fibers from the inner surface of the fascia. Although the fascia lata encloses the tensor fasciae latae muscle and covers the gluteus medius, in many cases the fascia lata actually serves as part of the origin of the gluteus medius muscle. Second, there is often a thin fascial layer covering the gluteus medius muscle on its outer aspect just above the greater trochanter. In order to pick up the anterior border of the muscle for dissection, you frequently need to incise this fascial layer. If you do not do this, it is difficult to pick up the anterior border of the muscle since this fascial layer is continuous with the fascia covering the outer aspect of the greater trochanter.

The gluteus medius is the strongest abductor of the hip. Paralysis leads to a Trendelenburg gait, in which the patient cannot prevent his hip from adducting when he puts weight on the affected leg during walking.

Note that a bursa lies between the anterior part of the muscle and the anterior part of the greater trochanter. It may become inflamed, producing pain.

One nerve, the *superior gluteal nerve*, crosses the intermuscular plane between the gluteus medius and the tensor fasciae latae and must be cut if the dissection extends up to the pelvis. Whether denervation of the tensor fasciae latae muscle is clinically significant is a moot point.

## Deep Surgical Dissection and its Dangers

Perhaps the most difficult part of deep dissection is finding the plane between the joint capsule and the surrounding structures, because every muscle that crosses the hip joint directly sends some of its fibers to insert into the capsule.

## Anterior Approach

The deep layer of muscles consists of the rectus femoris and the gluteus medius. The rectus femoris has two heads of origin, both of which must be detached. The straight head arises from the anterior inferior iliac spine; the reflected head arises from just above the acetabulum and from the joint capsule itself. The gluteus medius arises from the outer aspect of the ilium, between the middle and posterior gluteal lines. While the intermuscular plane between the two muscles is easy to define and develop, the rectus is difficult to mobilize from the anterior joint capsule because part of it actually originates from the capsule itself (see Figs. 8-16 through 8-18).

The *iliopsoas muscle*, which intrudes into the inferomedial portion of the operative field, must be retracted medially to expose the anterior part of the joint. The iliopsoas crosses the hip joint directly; it sends some of its fibers to insert into the joint capsule (see Fig. 8-18).

The iliopsoas tendon is actually the tendon for two muscles, the psoas major and the iliacus. The iliopectineal bursa separates part of the tendon from the hip joint. The bursa, which may communicate with the joint itself, is usually obliterated in degenerative disease of the hip, leaving the tendon anchored to the anterior and medial portions of the joint capsule.

## Anterolateral Approach

The *femoral vessels* enter the thigh beneath the inguinal ligament. They lie on the psoas major muscle, halfway between the anterior superior iliac spine and the pubic tubercle, the midinguinal point. The femoral artery is thus directly anterior to the hip joint, with the psoas muscle interposed. The femoral nerve lies lateral, and the femoral vein medial, to the artery. (This arrangement can be remembered through the mnemonic "VAN"—*v*ein, *a*rtery, *n*erve.)

Retractors that are placed correctly on the anterior lip of the acetabulum do not damage any of these structures, although a neurapraxia of the femoral nerve (the most lateral of the triad) may occur if retraction is prolonged and forceful.

Retractors placed more anteriorly and not directly on bones are probably biting into the substance of the psoas; they can damage any of the neurovascular structures that lie in the femoral triangle. Avoiding these complications depends on keeping to the bone of the acetabular margin and staying beneath the reflected head of the rectus femoris and the iliopsoas.

## Lateral Approach to the Hip

The direct lateral approach (or transgluteal approach) allows excellent exposure of the hip joint for joint replacement. It avoids the need for trochanteric osteotomy. Because the bulk of the gluteus medius muscle is preserved intact, it permits early mobilization of the patient following surgery. However, the approach does not give as wide an exposure as the anterolateral approach with trochanteric osteotomy. It is therefore difficult to perform revision surgery using this approach.

### Position of the Patient

Place the patient supine on the operating table with the greater trochanter at the edge of the table. This allows the buttock muscles and gluteal fat to fall posteriorly away from the operative plane (see Fig. 8-24).

### Landmarks and Incision

#### Landmarks
Palpate the anterior superior iliac spine upwards from below. Palpate the lateral aspect of the greater trochanter and, below that, the line of the femur that feels like a resistance against the examining hand.

#### Incision
Begin the incision 5 cm above the tip of the greater trochanter. Make a longitudinal incision that passes over the center of the tip of the greater trochanter and extends down the line of the shaft of the femur for approximately 8 cm (Fig. 8-42).

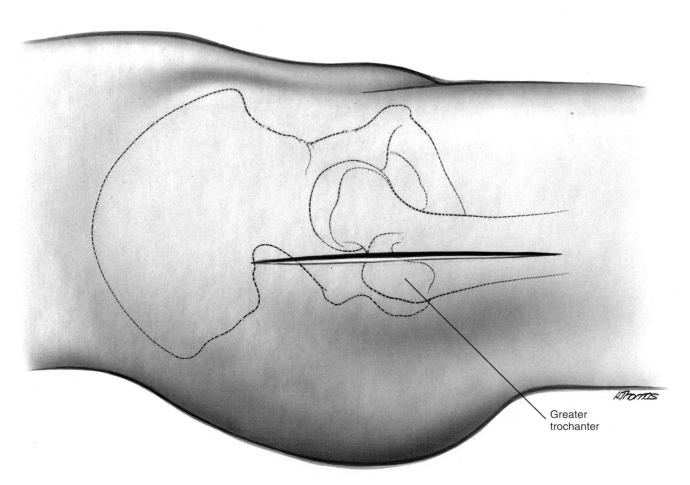

Greater
trochanter

**Figure 8-42**   Make a longitudinal incision centered over the tip of the greater trochanter in the line of the femoral shaft.

## Internervous Plane

There is no true internervous plane. The fibers of the gluteus medius muscle are split in their own line distal to the point where the superior gluteal nerve supplies the muscle. The vastus lateralis muscle is also split in its own line lateral to the point where it is supplied by the femoral nerve.

## Superficial Surgical Dissection

Incise the fat and underlying deep fascia in line with the skin incision. Retract the cut edges of the fascia to pull the tensor fasciae latae anteriorly and the gluteus maximus posteriorly. Detach any fibers of the gluteus medius that attach to the deep surface of this fascia by sharp dissection. The vastus lateralis and the gluteus medius are now exposed (Fig. 8-43).

## Deep Surgical Dissection

Split the fibers of the gluteus medius muscle in the direction of their fibers beginning in the middle of the trochanter. Do not go more than 3 cm above the upper border of the trochanter because more proximal dissection may damage branches of the superior gluteal nerve. Split the fibers of the vastus lateralis muscle overlying the lateral aspect of the base of the greater trochanter. Next, develop an anterior flap that consists of the anterior part of the gluteus medius muscle with its underlying gluteus minimus and the anterior part of the vastus lateralis muscle (Fig. 8-44). You will need to detach the muscles from the greater trochanter either by sharp dissection or by lifting off a small flake of bone. Continue developing this anterior flap—following the contour of the bone onto the

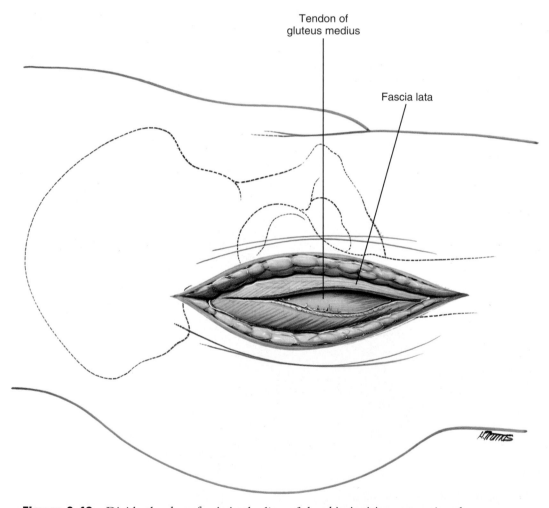

Tendon of
gluteus medius

Fascia lata

**Figure 8-43**    Divide the deep fascia in the line of the skin incision, retracting the fascial edges to pull the tenso-fasciolate anteriorly.

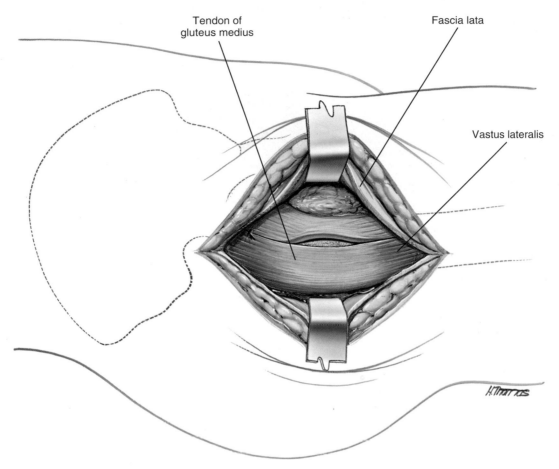

Tendon of
gluteus medius

Fascia lata

Vastus lateralis

**Figure 8-44**   Split the fibers of gluteus medius above the tip of the greater trochanter and extend this incision distally on the lateral aspect of the trochanter until 2 cm of the vastus lateralis is also split.

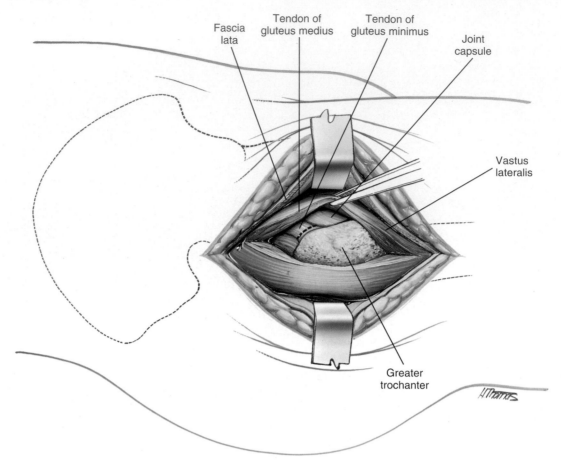

**Figure 8-45**  Develop this anterior flap and divide the tendon of the gluteus minimus muscle to reveal the anterior aspect of the hip joint capsule.

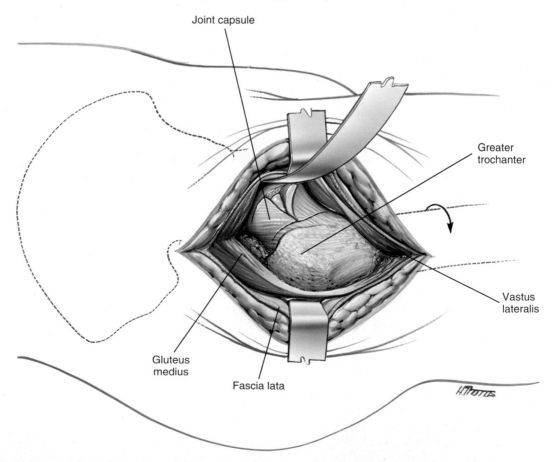

**Figure 8-46**  Enter the capsule using a longitudinal T-shaped incision.

femoral neck—until the anterior hip joint capsule is fully exposed. You will need to detach the insertion of the gluteus minimus tendon to the anterior part of the greater trochanter (Fig. 8-45). Enter the capsule using a longitudinal T-shaped incision (Fig. 8-46). Osteotomize the femoral neck (Fig. 8-47). Extract the femoral head using a cork screw. Complete the exposure of the acetabulum by inserting appropriate retractors around the acetabulum (Fig. 8-48).

## Dangers

### Nerves

The **superior gluteal nerve** runs between the gluteus medius and minimus muscles approximately 3 to 5 cm above the upper border of the greater trochanter. More proximal dissection may cut this nerve or may produce a traction injury. For this reason, insert a stay suture at the apex of the gluteus medius split. This will ensure that the split does not inadvertently extend itself during the operation (see Fig. 8-44).

The **femoral nerve,** the most lateral structure in the anterior neurovascular bundle of the thigh, is vulnerable to inappropriately placed retractors. Anterior retractors should be placed strictly on the bone of the anterior aspect of the acetabulum and should not infringe on the substance of the psoas muscle.

### Vessels

The **femoral artery and vein** are also vulnerable to inappropriately placed anterior retractors.

The transverse branch of the **lateral circumflex artery** of the thigh is cut as the vastus lateralis is mobilized. It must be cauterized during the approach.

## How to Enlarge the Approach

### Extensile Measures

The approach can easily be extended distally. To expose the shaft of the femur, split the vastus lateralis muscle in the direction of its fibers (see Lateral Approach in Chapter 9). The incision cannot be extended proximally.

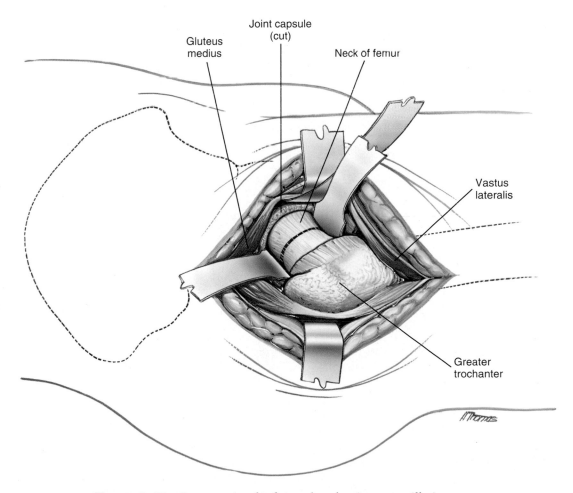

**Figure 8-47**   Osteotomize the femoral neck using an oscillating saw.

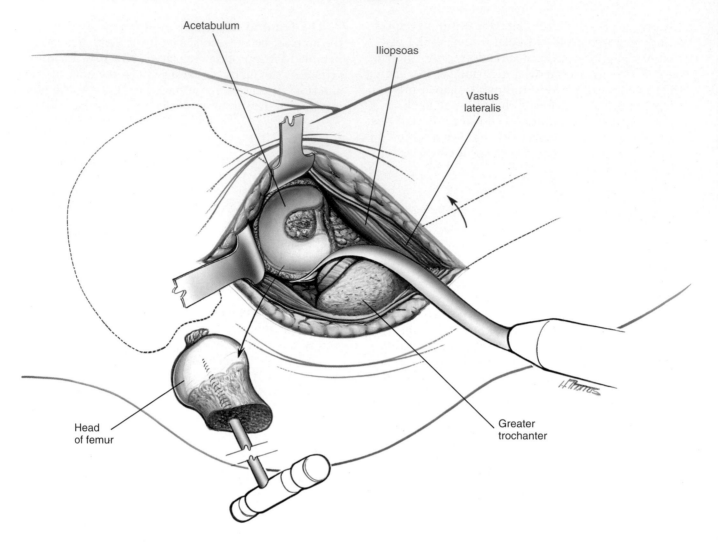

Acetabulum

Iliopsoas

Vastus
lateralis

Head
of femur

Greater
trochanter

**Figure 8-48**   Extract the femoral head. Insert appropriate retractors to reveal the
acetabulum.

# Ilioinguinal Approach to the Acetabulum

The ilioinguinal approach allows exposure of the inner surface of the pelvis from the sacroiliac joint to the pubic symphysis (Fig. 8-49). It allows visualization of the anterior and medial surfaces of the acetabulum and is, therefore, suitable for exposure of anterior column fractures of the acetabulum. The dissection involves isolating and mobilizing the femoral vessels and nerve, as well as the spermatic cord in the male and the round ligaments in the female. Because orthopaedic surgeons do not usually operate in this area, operating in conjunction with a general surgeon may be advisable. Alternatively, cadaveric dissection should be performed before embarking on this exposure.

## Position of the Patient

Place the patient supine on the operating table with the greater trochanter at the edge of the table. This allows the buttock muscles and gluteal fat to fall posteriorly away from the operative plane. Insert a urinary catheter. A full bladder will obscure vision.

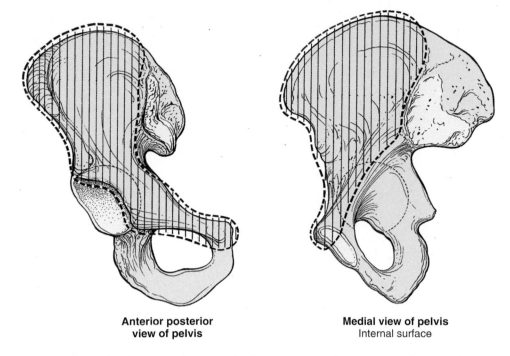

**Anterior posterior
view of pelvis**

**Medial view of pelvis**
Internal surface

**Figure 8-49** The ilioinguinal approach allows access to the anterior column and medial aspect of the acetabulum. It also allows visualization of the inner aspect of the pelvis from the sacroiliac joint to the symphysis pubis.

## Landmarks and Incision

### Landmarks
Palpate the anterior superior iliac spine by bringing your fingers up from below.

### Pubic Tubercles
With your fingers anchored on the trochanter, move your thumbs medially along the inguinal creases and obliquely downward until you can feel the pubic tubercle.

### Incision
Make a curved anterior incision beginning 5 cm above the anterior superior iliac spine. Extend the incision medially, passing 1 cm above the pubic tubercle to end in the midline (Fig. 8-50).

### Internervous Plane
There is no true internervous plane. The dissection consists essentially of lifting off muscular, nervous, and vascular structures from the inner wall of the pelvis.

## Superficial Surgical Dissection

Dissect down through the subcutaneous fat to expose the aponeuroses of the external oblique muscle (Fig. 8-51). The lateral cutaneous nerve of the thigh will appear in the lateral edge of the dissection. In most cases, the nerve will need to be divided. Divide the aponeurosis of the external oblique muscle in the line of its fibers from the superficial inguinal ring to the anterior superior iliac spine (Fig. 8-52). This will expose the spermatic cord in the male and the round ligament in the female. Carefully isolate these structures in a sling (Fig. 8-53). Continue the dissection medially, dividing the anterior part of the rectus sheath to expose the underlying rectus abdominis muscle. Strip the iliacus muscle from the inside of the wing of the ilium. Initially, you will need to use sharp dissection, but once inside the pelvis, use blunt dissection.

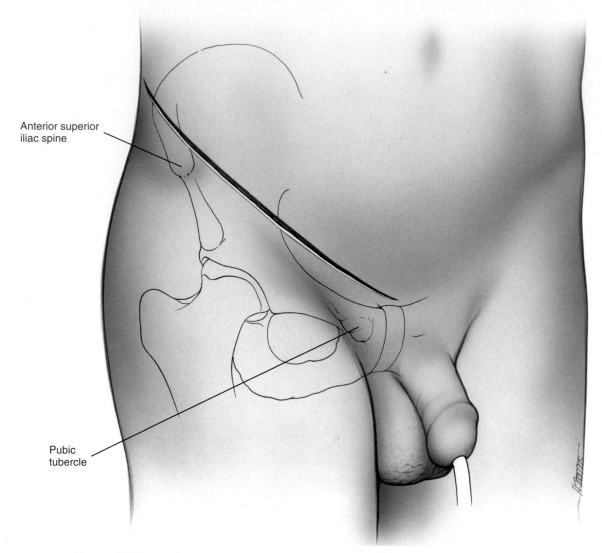

Anterior superior
iliac spine

Pubic
tubercle

**Figure 8-50**    Make a curved anterior incision beginning 5 cm above the anterior superior iliac spine. Extend the incision medially, passing just above the pubic tubercle to end in the midline.

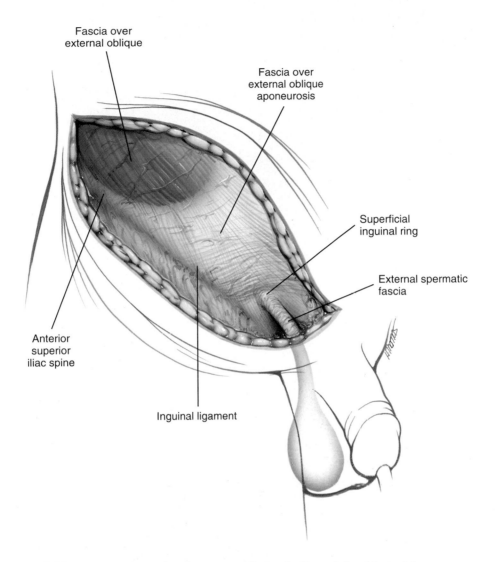

**Figure 8-51**  Dissect through subcutaneous fat in the line of the skin incision to expose the aponeurosis of the external oblique muscle.

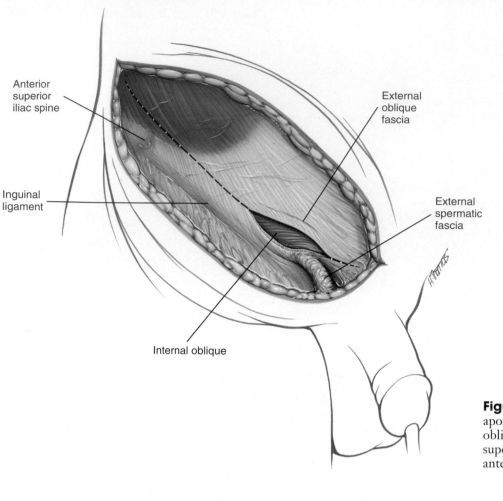

Anterior superior iliac spine

Inguinal ligament

External oblique fascia

External spermatic fascia

Internal oblique

**Figure 8-52** Divide the aponeurosis of the external oblique muscle from the superficial inguinal ring to the anterior superior iliac spine.

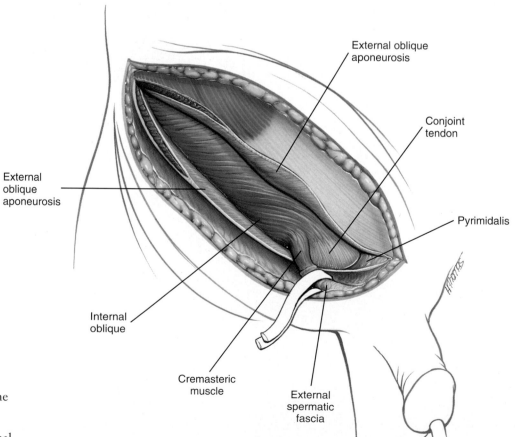

External oblique aponeurosis

Conjoint tendon

Pyrimidalis

External oblique aponeurosis

Internal oblique

Cremasteric muscle

External spermatic fascia

**Figure 8-53** Mobilize the spermatic cord or round ligament in a sling. The posterior wall of the inguinal canal is now exposed.

## Deep Surgical Dissection

Divide the rectus abdominal muscle transversely 1 cm proximal to its insertion into the symphysis pubis. Using blunt dissection, develop a plane between the back of the symphysis pubis and the bladder. This space (the Cave of Retzius) is easily developed with a finger.

Cut through those fibers of the internal oblique and transversus abdominus muscles that form the posterior wall of the inguinal canal (Fig. 8-54). Take care when approaching the deep inguinal ring; the inferior epigastric artery crosses the posterior wall of the canal at the medial edge of the deep inguinal ring and must be ligated at that point. Now divide those

fibers of the transversus abdominus and internal oblique muscles that arise from the lateral half of the inguinal ligament (Fig. 8-55).

The peritoneum covered with extraperitoneal fat is now exposed. Using a swab, push the peritoneum upward to reveal the femoral vessels, the femoral nerve and the tendon of iliopsoas (Fig. 8-56). Isolate the femoral vessels together in the femoral sheath and protect them with a rubber sling. Pass a second sling around the tendon of iliopsoas with the femoral nerve lying on top of it (Fig. 8-57). Retract these structures either medially or laterally to gain access to the underlying medial surface of the acetabulum and superior pubic ramus (Fig. 8-58).

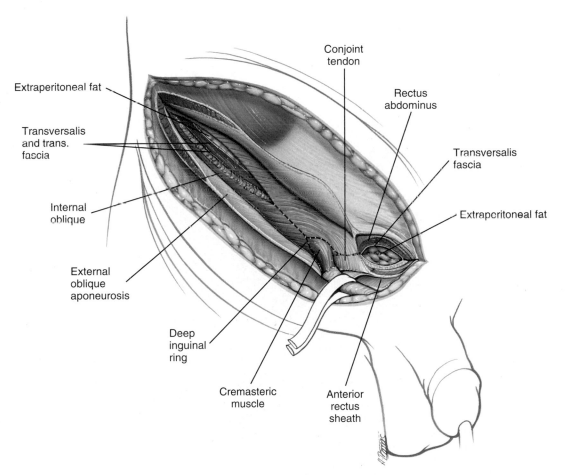

**Figure 8-54** Divide the rectus abdominal muscle 1 cm proximal to its insertion into the symphysis pubis. Divide the muscles forming the posterior wall of the inguinal canal.

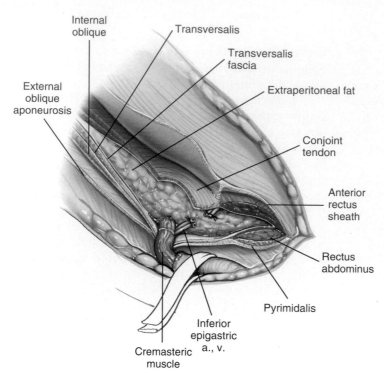

Internal oblique
External oblique aponeurosis
Transversalis
Transversalis fascia
Extraperitoneal fat
Conjoint tendon
Anterior rectus sheath
Rectus abdominus
Cremasteric muscle
Inferior epigastric a., v.
Pyrimidalis

**Figure 8-55** Ligate and divide the inferior epigastric vessels. Complete the division of the muscular structures of the posterior wall of the inguinal canal.

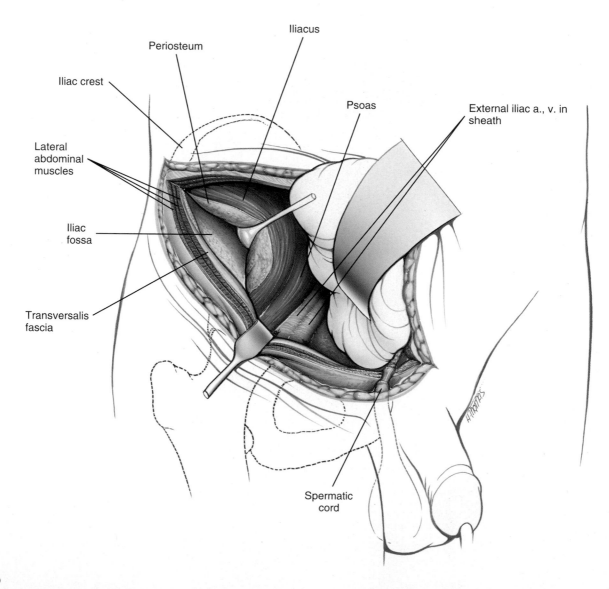

Periosteum
Iliacus
Psoas
External iliac a., v. in sheath
Iliac crest
Lateral abdominal muscles
Iliac fossa
Transversalis fascia
Spermatic cord

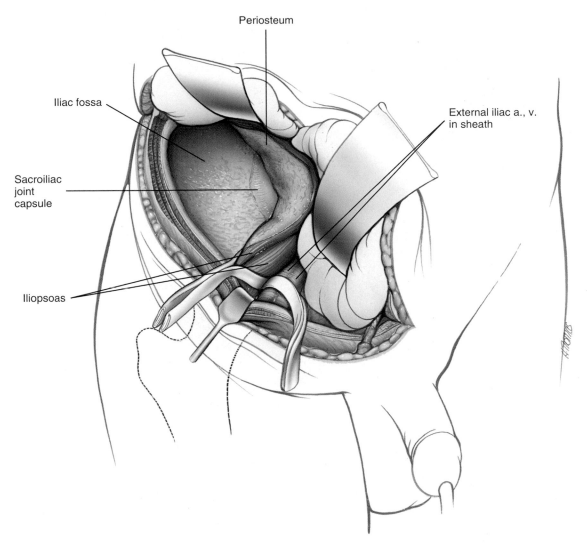

Periosteum

Iliac fossa

Sacroiliac
joint
capsule

Iliopsoas

External iliac a., v.
in sheath

**Figure 8-57**   Continue stripping off the iliacus from the inner wall of the ilium to
reveal the sacroiliac joint. Pass the sling around the femoral sheath.

## Dangers

### Nerves

The **femoral nerve** runs beneath the inguinal canal
lying on the iliopsoas muscle. Take care to avoid vigorous retraction, as stretching the nerve will result in
a paralysis of the quadriceps muscle.

The **lateral cutaneous nerve** of the thigh will
almost certainly have to be divided around the
anterior superior iliac spine at this stage of dissection. If it is possible to retract it without compromising the exposure, do so. Dividing the nerve will
leave a patch of numbness on the outer side of the
thigh.

### Vessels

The **femoral vessels** as they pass beneath the
inguinal ligament are surrounded by a funnel-shaped
fascial covering called the femoral sheath. It is this
sheath that should be mobilized and held between
slings rather than dissecting out the artery and vein
separately. Care should be taken on retraction of
these structures to minimize the risk of deep vein
thrombosis. The femoral sheath contains the femoral
artery and vein, and medial to the vein is a space
known as the femoral canal. The femoral canal contains efferent lymph vessels, but also provides a dead
space into which the femoral vein can expand. This
space can also, however, contain a femoral hernia,

**Figure 8-56**   Using a swab, push the peritoneum upwards to reveal the femoral vessels.
Mobilize the iliacus muscle from the inner aspect of the ilium.

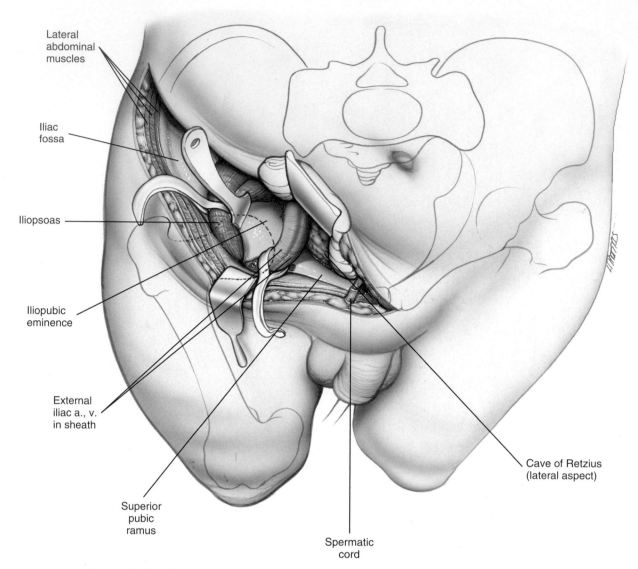

Lateral
abdominal
muscles

Iliac
fossa

Iliopsoas

Iliopubic
eminence

External
iliac a., v.
in sheath

Superior
pubic
ramus

Spermatic
cord

Cave of Retzius
(lateral aspect)

**Figure 8-58** Retract the iliopsoas and the femoral sheath either medially or laterally to reveal the medial surface of the acetabulum, the superior pubic ramus, and the inner surface of the ilium round to the sacroiliac joint.

and this should be remembered when mobilizing the structure.

The **inferior epigastric artery** crosses the operative field passing medial to the deep inguinal ring. It will need to be ligated to allow access to the deeper structures. The **inferior epigastric vein** may be damaged during dissection at the medial end of the approach. It is usually avulsed from the side of the femoral vein. This causes a profuse hemorrhage and requires the sewing of the resultant vascular defect in the side of the vein.

### Other Dangers
The **spermatic cord** contains the vas deferens and testicular artery. Although it is easily mobilized, it must be treated gently during the approach and the closure to avoid ischemic damage to the testicle.

The **bladder** is easily mobilized off the back of the symphysis pubis. Be aware that fractures of the lower half of the anterior column may have caused bladder damage and adhesions.

## How to Enlarge the Approach

### Extensile Measures
This approach can be extended proximally to expose the sacroiliac joint. Extend the skin incision posteriorly, following the iliac crest. Using sharp dissection, cut down onto the bone. Then strip off the origins of the iliacus from the inside of the ilium using blunt dissection. Retract this iliacus medially to expose the inner wall of the ilium and the sacroiliac joint (see Fig. 8-58).

This approach cannot be extended distally.

# Applied Surgical Anatomy of the Ilioinguinal Approach to the Acetabulum

## Overview

The applied anatomy of this approach is conveniently divided into two parts.

1. *Lateral and posterior to the anterior superior iliac spine.* The dissection consists of detaching those muscles that arise from or insert into the iliac crest and the inner wall of the ilium using subperiosteal dissection.
2. *Medial and anterior to the anterior superior iliac spine.* The applied anatomy of the approach is that of the inguinal canal and its related structures. Because pathology in this area nearly always relates to herniae, both inguinal and femoral, it is usually an unfamiliar ground for orthopaedic surgeons and, thus, is potentially hazardous.

## Landmarks and Incision

### Landmarks

The *anterior superior iliac spine* is the site of attachment to two important structures. The *sartorius* takes its origin from it, and the inguinal ligament uses it as a lateral attachment.

The *anterior third of the iliac crest* serves as the origin of the following three muscles.

1. The *external oblique* forms the outer layer of the muscles of the anterior abdominal wall. It originates from the outer strip of the anterior half of the iliac crest.
2. The *internal oblique* forms the middle layer of the muscles of the anterior abdominal wall. It originates from the center strip of the anterior half of the iliac crest.
3. The *tensor fasciae latae* arises from the outer lip of the anterior half of the iliac crest.

The pubic tubercle is not easily palpated because it is covered by the spermatic cord in the male and the round ligament in the female.

### Incision

This curved incision roughly follows the lines of cleavage in the skin. However, the extensive dissections involved may leave rather broad scars. They are nearly always hidden by clothing.

## Superficial Surgical Dissection and its Dangers

The dissection consists of the division of the fascia of the external oblique muscle and anterior rectus sheath. The *external oblique*, which is the outer layer of the abdominal muscles, arises from the lower eight ribs. It inserts as fleshy fibers into the anterior half of the iliac crest. However, from the anterior superior iliac spine, it becomes aponeurotic. The aponeurosis attaches to the pubic tubercle and medially becomes fused with the aponeurosis of the opposite external oblique muscle to form the anterior part of the rectus sheath. Therefore, the splitting of the fibers of the external oblique muscle and the incision of the anterior rectus sheath are both in the same plane. There is a free lower border of this muscle between the anterior superior iliac spine and the pubic tubercle. This free edge is called the inguinal ligament. The aponeurosis curls back on itself to form a gutter, and the free edge of this gutter is the origin of part of the internal oblique and transversus abdominis muscles.

Just above the pubic tubercle, there is a gap in this aponeurosis to allow the passage of the *spermatic cord* in the male and the *round ligament* in the female. This gap is known as the superficial inguinal ring (Fig. 8-59). Dividing the fascia of the external oblique opens up the inguinal canal, which is an oblique intramuscular slit running from the deep to the superficial inguinal rings. These contain the spermatic cord in the male and the round ligament in the female (Fig. 8-60).

The rectus abdominis muscle is enclosed in a sheath of fascia. In the region of this approach, however, the posterior layer of fascia is inferiorly deficient. The anterior rectus sheath also receives some tissue from both the internal oblique and transversus abdominis muscles.

The spermatic cord consists of the vas deferens accompanied by its artery and the testicular artery and vein. As these structures emerge through the abdominal wall, they get coverings from each layer they pass through (Fig. 8-61). The transversalis fascia covers the cord with a thin layer of tissue known as the internal spermatic fascia. Passing through the transversus abdominis and internal oblique, the cord gets covered with a layer of muscle known as the cremasteric muscle. As it passes through the external oblique at the superficial inguinal ring, it is covered by a thin layer

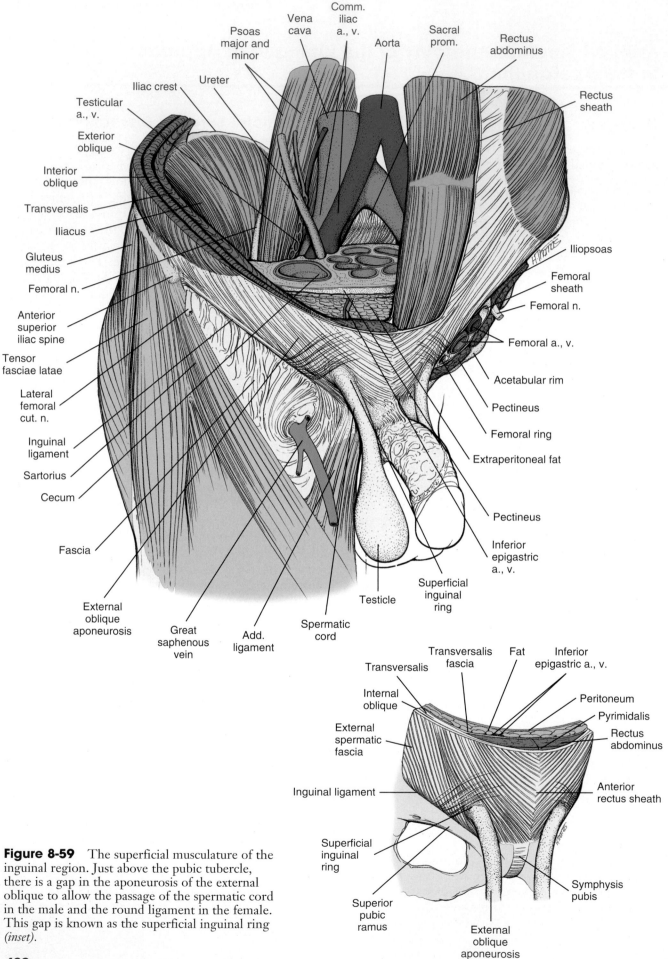

**Figure 8-59** The superficial musculature of the inguinal region. Just above the pubic tubercle, there is a gap in the aponeurosis of the external oblique to allow the passage of the spermatic cord in the male and the round ligament in the female. This gap is known as the superficial inguinal ring *(inset)*.

**420**

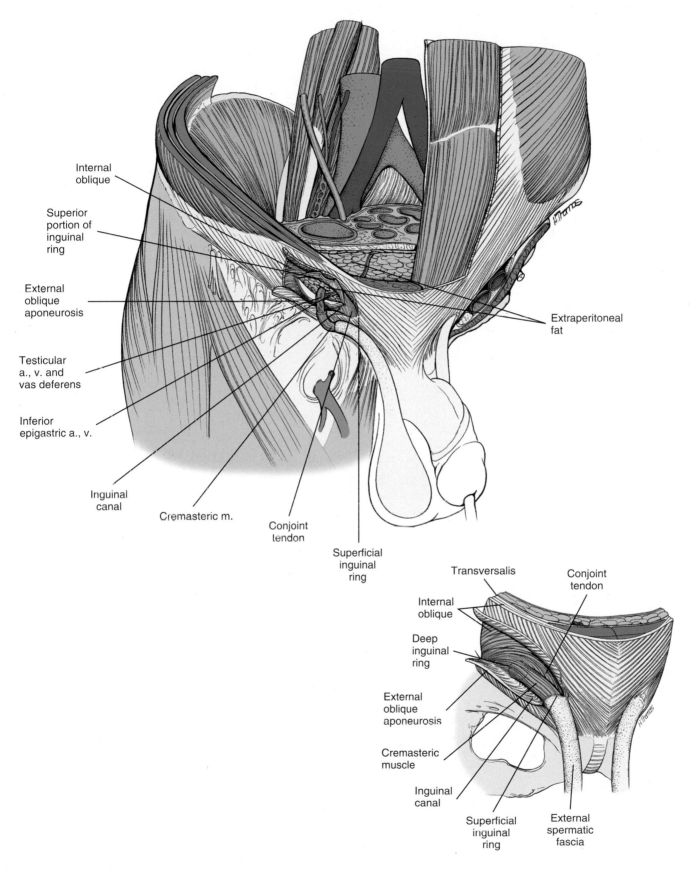

**Figure 8-60**   Dividing the external oblique muscle opens up in the inguinal canal. The spermatic cord is revealed covered by the cremasteric muscle, a muscle derived from the internal oblique muscle *(inset)*.

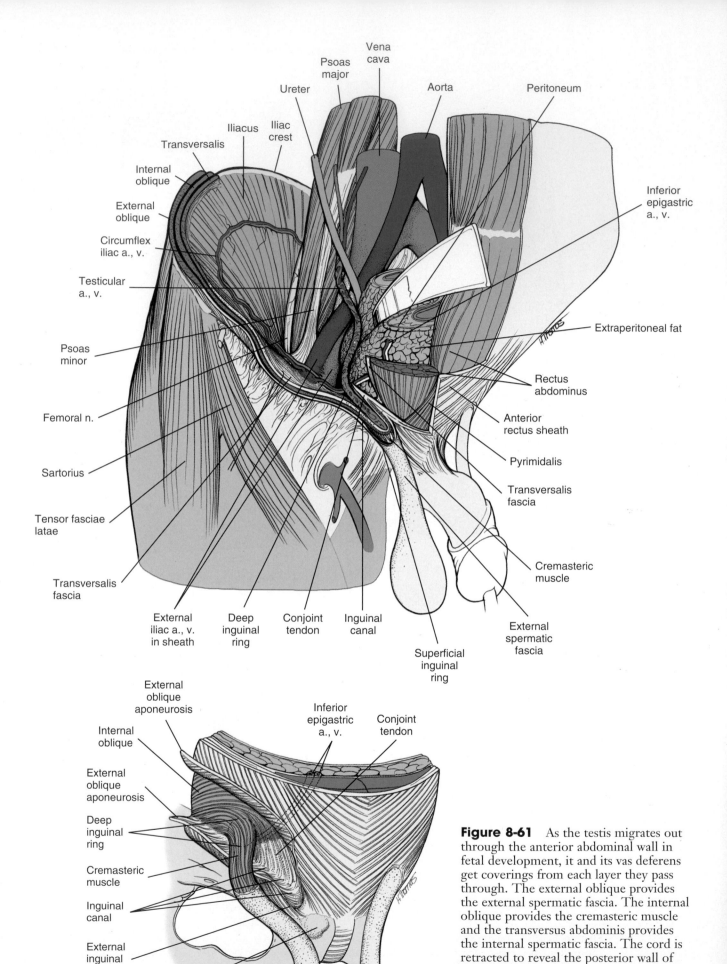

**Figure 8-61** As the testis migrates out through the anterior abdominal wall in fetal development, it and its vas deferens get coverings from each layer they pass through. The external oblique provides the external spermatic fascia. The internal oblique provides the cremasteric muscle and the transversus abdominis provides the internal spermatic fascia. The cord is retracted to reveal the posterior wall of the inguinal canal formed by the conjoint tendons (inset).

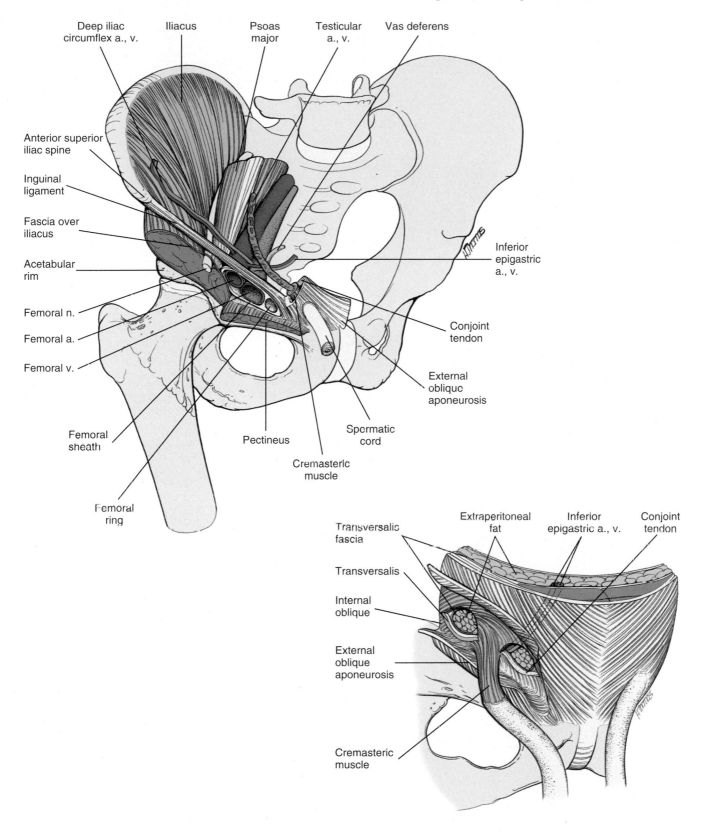

**Figure 8-62**   Deep to the inguinal ligament run the femoral nerve, the femoral vessel, as well as the psoas and iliacus muscles. Medial to the deep inguinal ring lies the inferior epigastric vessels *(inset)*.

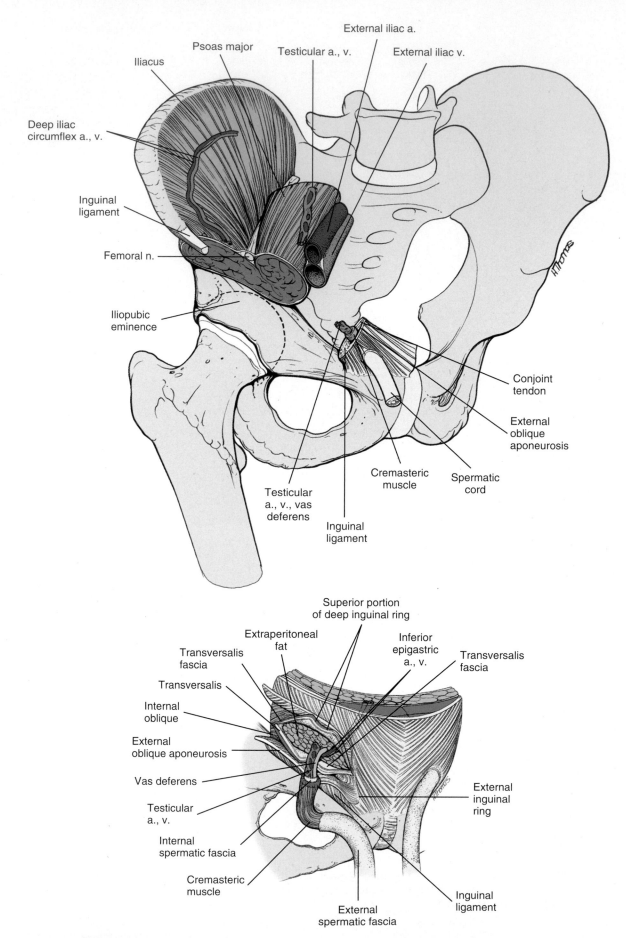

**Figure 8-63** Division of the posterior wall of the inguinal canal reveals the extraperitoneal fat.

known as the external spermatic fascia. The round ligament in the female is also covered by these three fascial layers. Both the spermatic cord and round ligament can be mobilized easily in the inguinal canal during the superficial surgical dissection.

## Deep Surgical Dissection and its Dangers

Once the spermatic cord has been mobilized, the posterior wall of the inguinal canal is seen. In the lateral half of the inguinal canal, the rolled free edge of the external oblique aponeurosis gives origin to muscle fibers from both the internal oblique and the transversus abdominis. These muscle fibers arch up over the spermatic cord and fuse to form a conjoint tendon that is attached posterior to the spermatic cord into the pubic crest. Therefore, in the medial half of the inguinal canal, its posterior wall consists of this conjoint tendon, which needs to be divided for access to the underlying structures. The spermatic cord exits from the abdominal cavity through the deep inguinal ring to enter the inguinal canal. Lateral to the deep inguinal ring, fibers of the internal oblique and transversus abdominis arise from the inguinal ligament and also have to be divided (see Fig. 8-61). Medial to the deep inguinal ring lies the *inferior epigastric artery*, which usually requires ligation. Deep to these muscles lies the thin transversalis fascia, extraperitoneal fat, and finally the peritoneum (Fig. 8-63).

The dissection completely disrupts the anatomy of the inguinal canal. Careful repair of all these structures on a layer-by-layer basis is important to prevent the development of an inguinal hernia.

Passing under the inguinal ligament from the abdomen into the thigh are the *femoral nerve*, the *femoral artery*, and the *femoral vein*, as well as the psoas and iliacus muscles (Fig. 8-62). The *iliacus* arises from the hollow of the iliac fossa, and runs into the thigh underneath the lateral part of the inguinal ligament. The *psoas muscle* arises from the anterior aspect of the lumbar spine and passes into the thigh below the middle of the inguinal ligament. Between these two muscles, the femoral nerve runs down into the thigh. It is intimately related to the iliopsoas and is mobilized with the muscle to avoid excessive retraction. Medial to the nerve, the femoral artery and vein enter the thigh. As these vessels leave the abdomen, they take with them a fascial layer derived from the extraperitoneal fascia. This is known as the femoral sheath. In addition to the artery and vein, the femoral sheath has a space in it, medial to the vein, known as the femoral canal. This is used for the passage of lymphatic vessels and also allows the vein to expand at times when the blood return from the leg becomes increased.

It is also, however, the site of a femoral hernia. Because the femoral artery and vein are enclosed in a common fascial sheath, they should be mobilized together. Separate mobilization of the femoral vein will traumatize it, leading to possible thrombosis.

The *bladder* is separated from the pubic bones by a space known as the Cave of Retzius. It is occupied by very thin tissue, the bladder, and, in the case of the male, the prostate. The prostate can be easily mobilized from the back of the pubis. However, in cases of fracture, there may be pathological adhesions in this area, and great care should be taken not to accidentally produce a bladder rupture. A full bladder will make safe access to this area impossible, and a urinary catheter inserted preoperatively is vital (Fig. 8-64).

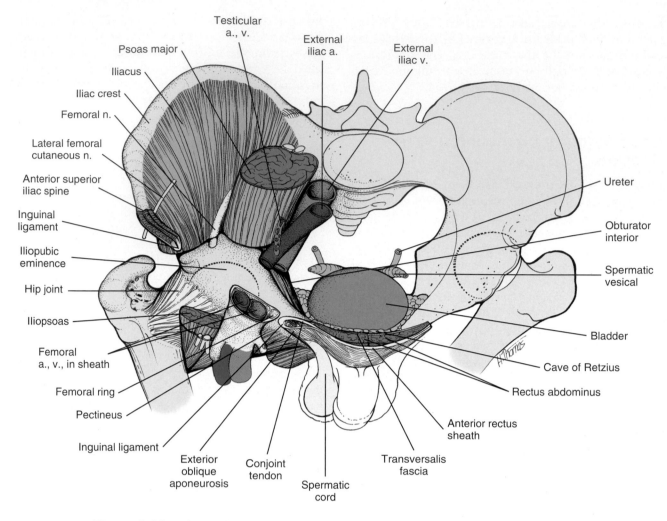

**Figure 8-64** The medial aspect of the acetabulum can be exposed by retraction of the iliopsoas and the femoral sheath. The inner aspect of the superior pubic ramus can only be visualized by careful mobilization of the bladder.

# Posterior Approach to the Hip

The posterior approach is the most common and practical of those used to expose the hip joint. Popularized by Moore,[13] it is often called the southern approach.

All posterior approaches allow easy, safe, and quick access to the joint and can be performed with only one assistant. Because they do not interfere with the abductor mechanism of the hip, they avoid the loss of abductor power in the immediate postoperative period. Posterior approaches allow excellent visualization of the femoral shaft, thus are popular for revision joint replacement surgery in cases in which the femoral component needs to be replaced.

Their uses include the following:

1. Hemiarthroplasty[14-16]
2. Total hip replacement, including revision surgery
3. Open reduction and internal fixation of posterior acetabular fractures
4. Dependent drainage of hip sepsis
5. Removal of loose bodies from the hip joint
6. Pedicle bone grafting[17]
7. Open reduction of posterior hip dislocations

## Position of the Patient

Place the patient in the true lateral position, with the affected limb uppermost. Because most patients requiring surgery are elderly and have delicate skin, it is important to protect the bony prominences of the legs and pelvis with pads placed under the lateral malleolus and knee of the bottom leg and a pillow between the knees. Drape the limb free to leave room for movement during the procedure (Fig. 8-65).

## Landmarks and Incision

### Landmarks
Palpate in detail the *greater trochanter* on the outer aspect of the thigh. The posterior edge of the trochanter is more superficial than the anterior and lateral portions, and, as such, it is easier to palpate (see Fig. 8-29).

### Incision
Make a 10-cm to 15-cm curved incision centered on the posterior aspect of the greater trochanter. Begin your incision some 6 cm to 8 cm above and posterior to the posterior aspect of the greater trochanter. The part of the incision that runs from this point to the posterior aspect of the trochanter is in line with the fibers of the gluteus maximus. Curve the incision across the buttock, cutting over the posterior aspect of the trochanter, and continue down along the shaft of the femur (Fig. 8-67*A*). If you flex the hip 90° and make a straight longitudinal incision over the poste-

rior aspect of the trochanter, it will curve into a "Moore-style" incision when the limb is straight. The final incision is curved and 10 to 15 cm long, centered on the posterior aspect of the greater trochanter.

## Internervous Plane
There is no true internervous plane in this approach. However, the gluteus maximus, which is split in the line of its fibers, is not significantly denervated because it receives its nerve supply well medial to the split (Fig. 8-66).

## Superficial Surgical Dissection
Incise the fascia lata on the lateral aspect of the femur to uncover the vastus lateralis. Lengthen the fascial incision superiorly in line with the skin incision, and split the fibers of the gluteus maximus by blunt dissection (Fig. 8-67*B*). (The fascial covering of the gluteus maximus varies considerably in its thickness. In the elderly, it is quite thin.)

The gluteus maximus receives its blood supply from the superior and inferior gluteal arteries, which enter the deep surface of the muscle and ramify outward like the spokes of a bicycle wheel;

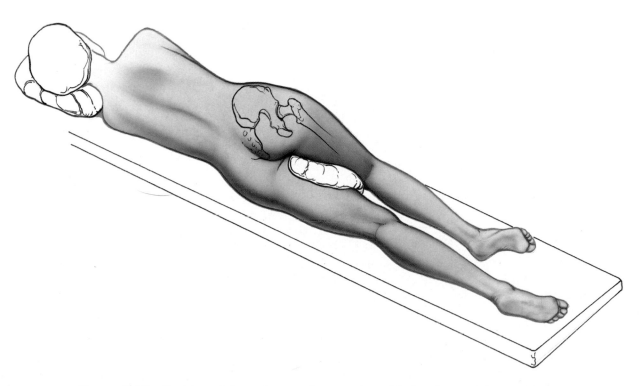

**Figure 8-65**  Position of the patient on the operating table for the posterior approach to the hip joint.

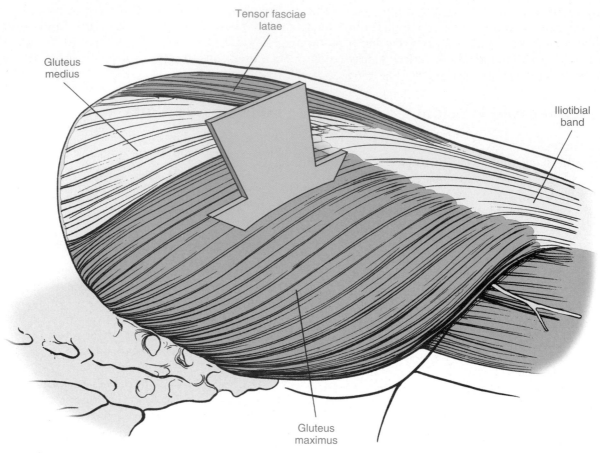

**Figure 8-66** There is no true internervous plane. Split the fibers of the gluteus maximus, a procedure that does not cause significant denervation of the muscle.

hence, splitting the muscle inevitably crosses a vascular plane. In addition to the arterial bleeding, venous bleeding must be anticipated. If you split the muscle gently, you may be able to pick up, coagulate, and cut the crossing vessels before they are stretched and avulsed by the blunt dissection of the split. Obviously, vessels that are torn when stretched retract into the muscle and are more difficult to control.

## Deep Surgical Dissection

Retract the fibers of the split gluteus maximus and the deep fascia of the thigh. Underneath is the posterolateral aspect of the hip joint, still covered by the short external rotator muscles, which attach to the upper part of the posterolateral aspect of the femur (Fig. 8-68).

Remember that the sciatic nerve leaves the pelvis through the greater sciatic notch and runs down the back of the thigh on the short external rotator muscle, encased in fatty tissue. The nerve crosses the obturator internus, the two gemelli, and the quadratus femoris before disappearing beneath the femoral attachment of the gluteus maximus. You can find the nerve lying on the short external rotators, and it can be easily palpated. Do not dissect to see the nerve; you may cause unnecessary bleeding from the vessels lying in the fat around it (Fig. 8-69).

Internally rotate the hip to put the short external rotator muscles on a stretch (making them more prominent) and to pull the operative field farther from the sciatic nerve (Fig. 8-70A,B).

Insert stay sutures into the piriformis and obturator internus tendons just before they insert into the greater trochanter. Detach the muscles close to their femoral insertion and reflect them backward, laying them over the sciatic nerve to protect it during the rest of the procedure (Fig. 8-70C). (The upper part of the quadratus femoris may also have to be divided to fully expose the posterior aspect of the joint capsule, but the muscle contains troublesome vessels that arise from the lateral circumflex artery. Normally, it should be left alone.)

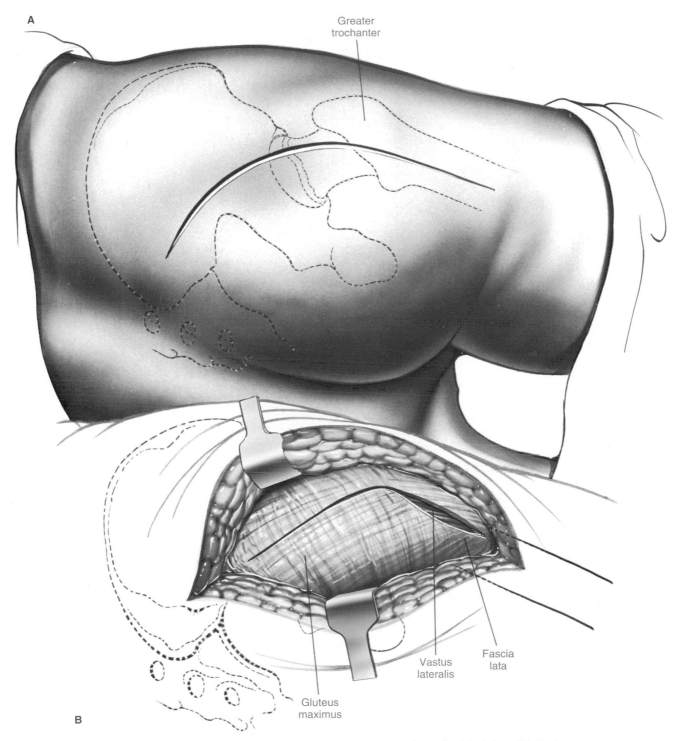

**Figure 8-67**   **(A)** Skin incision for the posterior approach to the hip joint. **(B)** Incise the fascia lata.

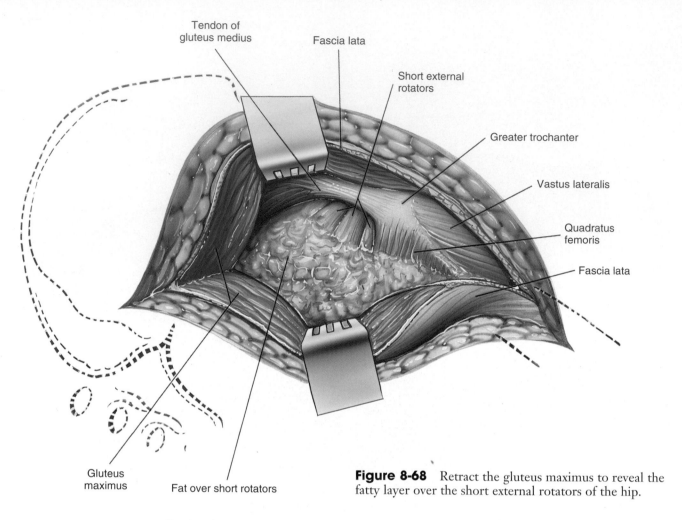

Tendon of
gluteus medius

Fascia lata

Short external
rotators

Greater trochanter

Vastus lateralis

Quadratus
femoris

Fascia lata

Gluteus
maximus

Fat over short rotators

**Figure 8-68** Retract the gluteus maximus to reveal the fatty layer over the short external rotators of the hip.

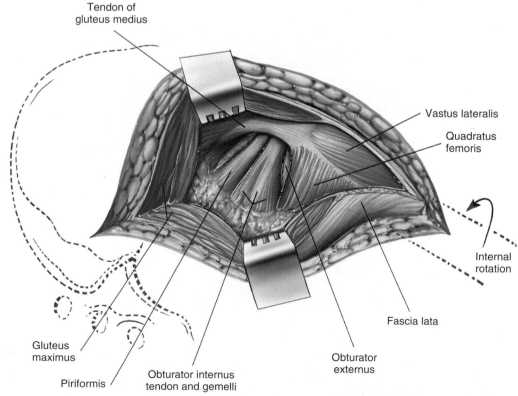

Tendon of
gluteus medius

Vastus lateralis

Quadratus
femoris

Fascia lata

Internal
rotation

Gluteus
maximus

Piriformis

Obturator internus
tendon and gemelli

Obturator
externus

**Figure 8-69** Push the fat posteromedially to expose the insertions of the short rotators. Note that the sciatic nerve is not visible; it lies within the substance of the fatty tissue. Place your retractors within the substance of the gluteus maximus superficial to the fatty tissue.

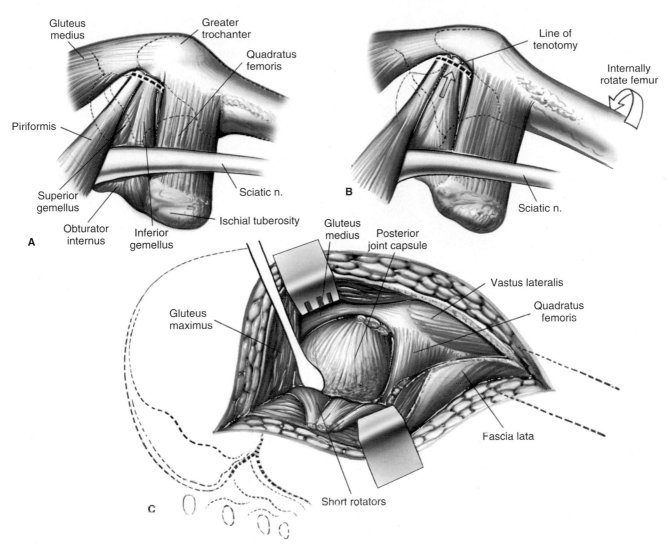

**Figure 8-70** (Λ, B) Internally rotate the femur to bring the insertion of the short rotators of the hip as far lateral to the sciatic nerve as possible. (C) Detach the short rotator muscles close to their femoral insertion and reflect them backward, laying them over the sciatic nerve to protect it.

The posterior aspect of the hip joint capsule is now fully exposed. The hip joint capsule can be incised with a longitudinal or T-shaped incision. Dislocation of the hip is achieved by internal rotation after capsulotomy (Fig. 8-71). Posterior joint capsulotomy will have exposed the femoral head and neck.

## Dangers

### Nerves
The **sciatic nerve** is rarely exposed or transected during this approach. However, it is sometimes involved in major complications. It can be damaged if it is compressed by the posterior blade of a self-retaining retractor used to split the gluteus maximus. Always keep the retractors on the cut surfaces of the rotators; the muscles will protect the nerve.

The sciatic nerve sometimes divides into its tibial and common peroneal branches within the pelvis; on occasion, you may expose these two "sciatic nerves" during this approach. If you have identified the sciatic nerve but think that it looks too small, search for the nerve's other branch; it is in danger if it is overlooked.

### Vessels
The **inferior gluteal artery** leaves the pelvis beneath the piriformis. It spreads cephalad to supply the deep surface of the gluteus maximus. Its branches are inevitably cut when the gluteus maximus is split; you can identify and coagulate them before they are avulsed if you are dissecting carefully.

The main trunk of the artery is vulnerable as it emerges from beneath the lower border of the piriformis when pelvic fractures involve the greater sci-

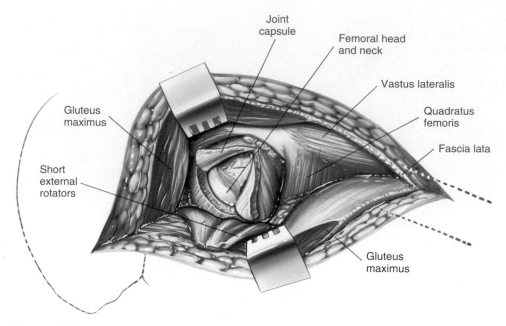

**Figure 8-71**   Incise the posterior joint capsule to expose the femoral head and neck.

atic notch. If it retracts into the pelvis and bleeding is brisk, turn the patient over into the supine position, open the abdomen, and tie off the artery's feeding vessel, the internal iliac artery.

## How to Enlarge the Approach

### Local Measures

1. Enlarge the skin incision. Obese patients may have a considerable layer of subcutaneous tissue over the buttock that restricts deep exposure; lengthening the skin incision and dissecting subcutaneously can compensate for this problem.
2. Extend the fascial incision superiorly and inferiorly.
3. Detach the upper half of the quadratus femoris. Because the muscle contains troublesome vessels, it should be divided about 1 cm from its insertion to make hemostasis easier. Its excellent blood sup-

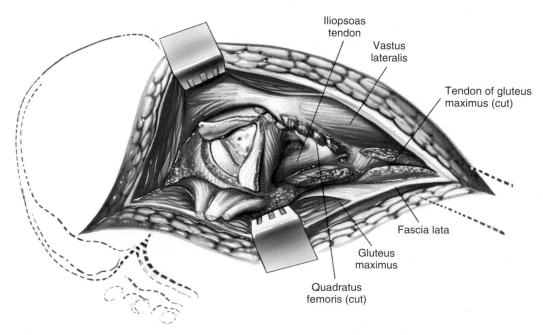

**Figure 8-72**   To gain additional exposure, cut the quadratus femoris and the tendinous insertion of the gluteus maximus.

ply is useful both when the muscle is transposed and in treatment of some cases of nonunion of femoral neck fractures (Fig. 8-72).

4. Detach the insertion of the gluteus maximus tendon from the femur to increase the exposure of the femoral neck and shaft. This maneuver is particularly useful during total joint replacement,

especially revision joint replacement. If you detach the tendon, position acetabular retractors on the rim of the acetabulum as you would in the anterolateral approach. As long as the retractors are firmly on bone and do not crush soft tissues against the acetabular rim, no vital structures will be damaged (see Fig. 8-72).

# Posterior Approach to the Acetabulum

The posterior approach gives access to the posterior wall of the acetabulum and its posterior column (Fig. 8-73). It is by far the easiest of all acetabular approaches, and extensive blood loss is not usually encountered. The approach does not allow access to the anterior column. Its uses include reduction and fixation of:

1. Fractures of the posterior lip of the acetabulum
2. Fractures of the posterior column
3. Fractures of the posterior lip and posterior column
4. Simple transverse fractures

## Position of the Patient

Two positions are possible. If the approach is to be used for fractures of the posterior lip and/or posterior column, place the patient in the **lateral position.** Skeletal traction can be used in this position to aid retraction of the femoral head. In this case, place a skeletal pin transversely through the lower end of the femur. If you are using skeletal traction, ensure that the knee is placed in full flexion to reduce the risk of a traction injury to the sciatic nerve.

Alternatively, if the approach is to be used for transverse fractures, place the patient in the prone position (Fig. 8-74). Place a skeletal pin transversely through the lower end of the femur with the knee flexed to reduce the risk of a traction injury to the sciatic nerve.

With the patient in the lateral position, there is a natural tendency for the femoral head to move medially in cases of transverse acetabular fracture. Operating in the lateral position therefore makes reduction of these fractures more difficult. Reduction of the fracture in this position can only be obtained by an assistant lifting the femoral head out of the acetabulum. The use of the prone position facilitates reduction of transverse fractures.

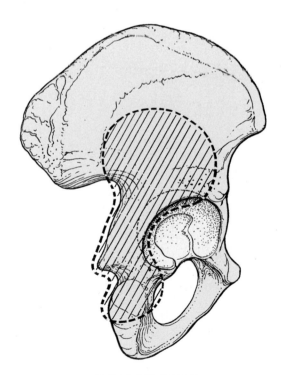

Lateral view of pelvis

External surface

**Figure 8-73**   The posterior approach to the acetabulum allows access to the posterior column, posterior lip and dome segment of the acetabulum.

## Landmarks and Incision

### Landmarks

Palpate the greater trochanter on the outer aspect of the thigh. Note that the posterior edge is easier to palpate than the anterior one.

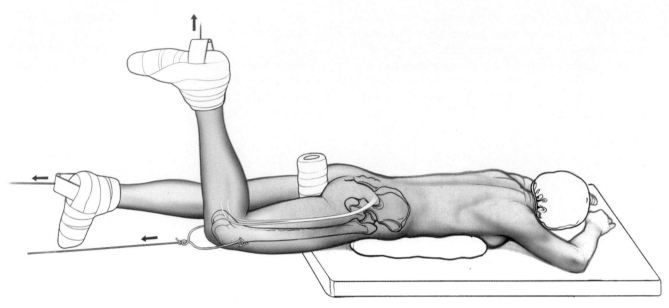

**Figure 8-74**   Position of the patient for posterior approach to the acetabulum. Note the flexed position of the knee to prevent stretching of the sciatic nerve.

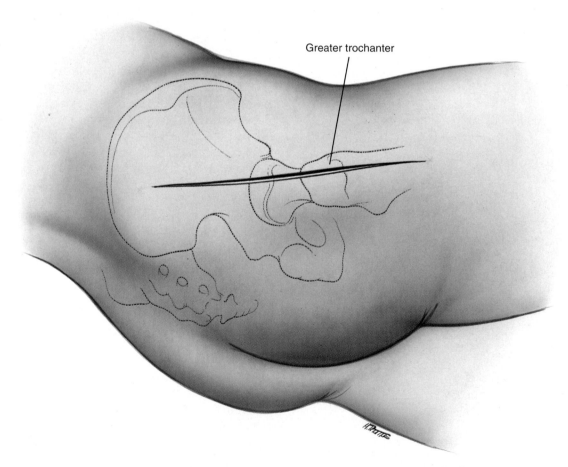

Greater trochanter

**Figure 8-75**   Make a longitudinal incision centered on the greater trochanter extending from just below the iliac crest to 10 cm below the greater trochanter.

## Incision

Make a longitudinal incision centered on the greater trochanter extending from just below the iliac crest to 10 cm below the tip of the greater trochanter (Fig. 8-75).

## Internervous Plane

There is no true internervous plane in this approach. However, the gluteus maximus that is split in the line of its fibers is not significantly denervated because it receives its nerve supply well proximal to the split.

## Superficial Surgical Dissection

Deepen the incision through subcutaneous fat. Incise the fascia lata in the line of the skin incision in the lower half of the wound, and extend this incision superiorly along the anterior border of the gluteus maximus muscles (Fig. 8-76). Retract the split edges

of the fascia to reveal the piriformis muscle and the short external rotators of the hip (Fig. 8-77).

Internally rotate the leg to put the short external rotators and the piriformis on the stretch and detach these muscles as they insert into the femur (Fig. 8-78). The posterior capsule of the hip joint is now revealed. This usually will be torn or detached in cases of trauma.

## Deep Surgical Dissection

Posterior lip fractures of the acetabulum can be adequately visualized and fixed at this stage. If you require more extensive exposure of the posterior column, perform an osteotomy of the greater trochanter. Divide the greater trochanter from posterior to anterior, removing a piece of bone 5 mm in size. This bone will have the gluteal muscles attached to it superiorly and the vastus lateralis attached to it inferiorly. Displace this piece of bone, with its attached muscles, anterior to the femur to increase exposure of the posterior column

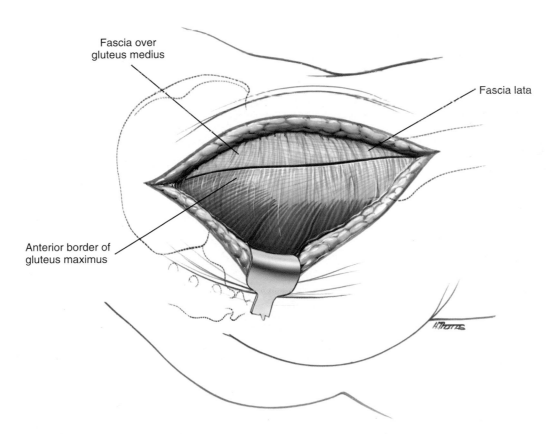

Fascia over gluteus medius

Fascia lata

Anterior border of gluteus maximus

**Figure 8-76**  Incise the fascia lata in line with the skin incision. Extend the incision superiorly along the anterior border of the gluteus maximus muscle.

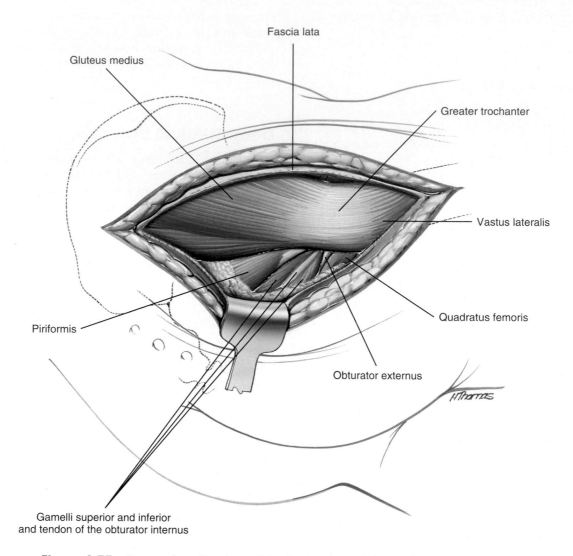

Fascia lata

Gluteus medius

Greater trochanter

Vastus lateralis

Quadratus femoris

Obturator externus

Piriformis

Gamelli superior and inferior
and tendon of the obturator internus

**Figure 8-77**   Retract the split edges of the fascia to reveal the piriformis muscle and the short external rotators of the hip.

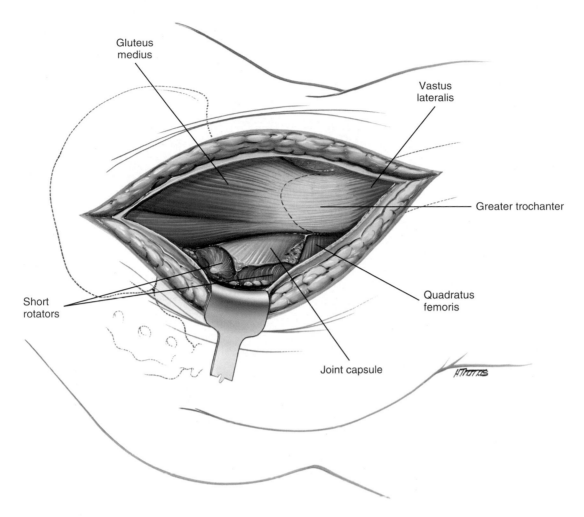

**Figure 8-78**   Divide the short external rotator muscles and the piriformis as they insert into the femur.

(Fig. 8-79). This trochanteric fragment can be reattached easily with screws during closure. Note that trochanteric osteotomies are associated with heterotopic bone formation in acetabular surgery.

## Dangers

### Nerves

The **sciatic nerve** is often contused by the original trauma. Great care must be taken throughout the operation that the nerve is not forcibly retracted. The divided external rotators will protect the nerve from direct trauma, but the nerve may still be injured by indirect forces transmitted through the retractor. The nerve is in most danger if a fracture table with continuous traction is used. You must be certain that the knee is flexed to avoid stretching the nerve.

### Vessels

The **inferior gluteal artery** leaves the pelvis beneath the piriformis. This vessel may be damaged by the original fracture or the artery may be injured during the surgical dissection. If the artery is transected, it will retract into the pelvis and bleeding will be brisk. To control the bleeding apply direct pressure, then turn the patient over into the supine position. If the artery has retracted into the pelvis, vascular control can only be achieved by tying off the external iliac artery via a retroperitoneal approach.

The **superior gluteal artery and nerve** leaves the pelvis above the piriformis and enters the deep surface of the gluteus medius. This attachment tethers the muscle, limiting the amount of upward retraction of the muscle and prevents you from reaching the iliac crest.

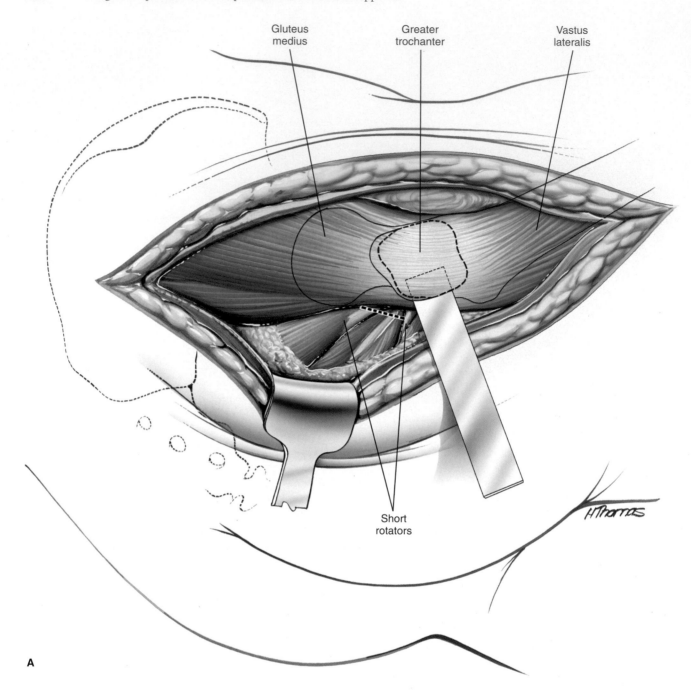

Gluteus medius

Greater trochanter

Vastus lateralis

Short rotators

A

**Figure 8-79** **(A)** Elevate a small sliver of bone from the greater trochanter, leaving the attachments of the gluteus medius and this vastus lateralis intact.

## How to Enlarge the Approach

### Local Measures
Visualization of the inside of the acetabulum is always difficult because of the presence of an intact femoral head. In addition to using longitudinal femoral traction, specialized femoral head retractors are available that allow the head to be partially dislocated, thereby facilitating clear visualization of the dome of the acetabulum. It is critically important to obtain good visualization of the inside of the joint, because the screws used for internal fixation may penetrate the joint.

### Extensile Measures
The skin incision can be extended distally down to the level of the knee. Either split the vastus lateralis or elevate it from the lateral intermuscular septum to allow exposure of the lateral surface of the entire shaft of the femur.

The exposure cannot be usefully extended proximally.

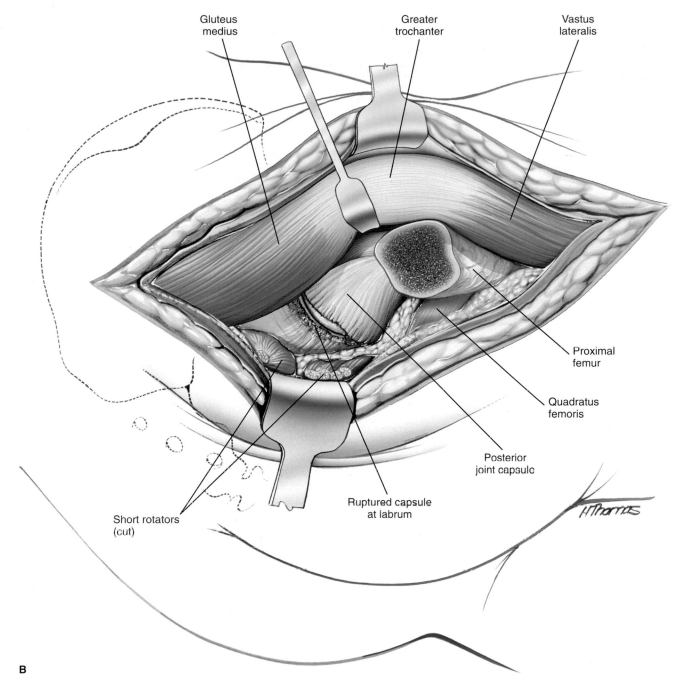

**Figure 8-79 (continued)**  **(B)** Retract the bone sliver anteriorly on its muscular attachments.

# Applied Surgical Anatomy of the Posterior Approaches to the Hip and Acetabulum

## Overview

The muscles covering the posterior aspect of the hip joint form two sheaths or layers. The outer layer consists of the gluteus maximus. The inner layer consists of the short external rotators of the hip, the piriformis, the superior gemellus, the obturator internus, the inferior gemellus, and the quadratus femoris. The sciatic nerve runs vertically between the two lay-

ers, down through the operative field (Figs. 8-80 and 8-81).

The gluteus maximus sits on the other structures in the buttock like the front cover of a book. It inserts partly into the iliotibial band and partly into the gluteal tuberosity of the femur. Also inserting into the band, but further anteriorly, is the tensor fasciae latae. Together, the gluteus maximus, the fascia lata (which covers the gluteus medius), and the tensor

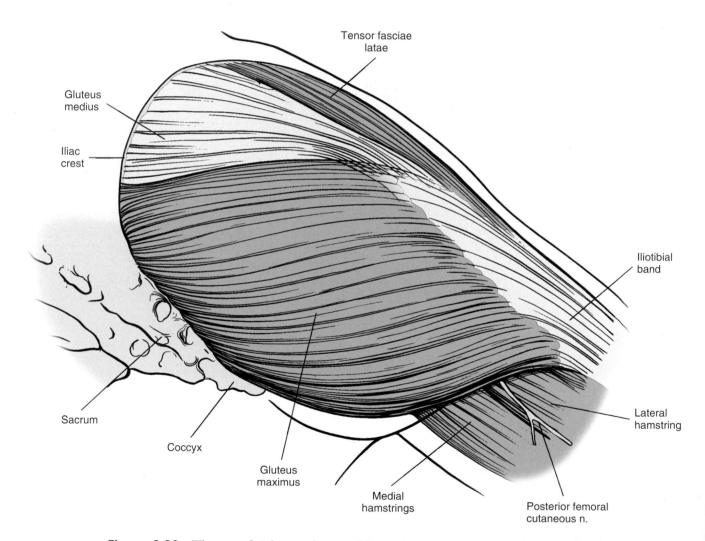

**Figure 8-80**   The superficial musculature of the posterior approach of the hip joint. The gluteus maximus predominates.

**Gluteus Maximus.** *Origin.* From posterior gluteal line of ilium and that portion of the bone immediately above and behind it; from posterior surface of lower part of sacrum and from side of coccyx; and from fascia covering gluteus medius. *Insertion.* Into iliotibial band of fascia lata and into gluteal tuberosity. *Action.* Extends and laterally rotates thigh. *Nerve supply.* Interior gluteal nerve.

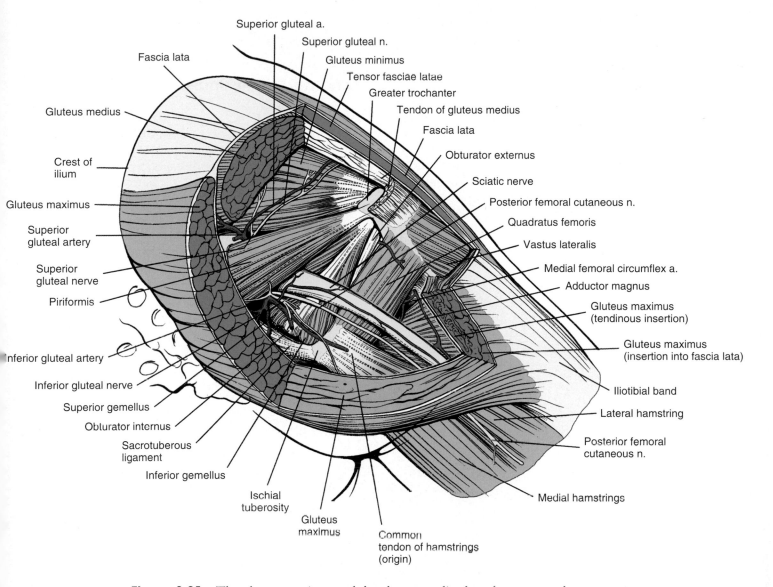

**Figure 8-81** The gluteus maximus and the gluteus medius have been resected to reveal the gluteus minimus, the piriformis, and the short rotator muscles. Note the relationship of the neurovascular structures to the piriformis.

**Gluteus Minimus.** *Origin.* From outer surface of ilium between anterior and inferior gluteal lines. *Insertion.* Into impression on anterior border of greater trochanter via tendon that gives expansion to joint capsule. *Action.* Rotates thigh medially and abducts it. *Nerve supply.* Superior gluteal nerve.

**Piriformis.** *Origin.* From front of sacrum via fleshy digitations from second, third, and fourth portions of sacrum. *Insertion.* Into upper border of greater trochanter via round tendon. *Action.* Rotates thigh laterally and abducts it. *Nerve supply.* Branches from first and second sacral nerves.

**Obturator Internus.** *Origin.* From inner surface of anterolateral wall of pelvis and from surfaces of greater part of obturator foramen. *Insertion.* Onto medial surface of greater trochanter above trochanteric fossa. *Action.* Rotates thigh laterally. *Nerve supply.* Any nerve from sacral plexus.

**Quadratus Femoris.** *Origin.* From upper part of external border of tuberosity of ischium. *Insertion.* Into upper part of linea quadrata, the line that extends vertically downward from intertrochanteric crest. *Action.* Rotates thigh laterally. *Nerve supply.* Branch from sacral plexus.

fasciae latae form a continuous fibromuscular sheath, the outer layer of the hip musculature (see Fig. 8-80). As Henry[18] noted, the layer can be viewed as the "pelvic deltoid": it covers the hip much as the deltoid muscle covers the shoulder.

The outer layer can be breached at different points, each of which changes the posterior approach. The most natural separation, the Marcy-Fletcher approach,[19] lies at the anterior border of the gluteus maximus, between the gluteus maximus (inferior gluteal nerve) and the gluteus medius. This approach uses a true internervous plane.

Other more posterior approaches (like the Moore approach[13] and the Osborne approach[20]) involve splitting the fibers of the gluteus maximus. They are more popular than the Marcy-Fletcher approach even though they do not operate in an internervous plane, mainly because they offer excellent exposure of the hip joint.

## Landmarks and Incision

### Landmarks

The *greater trochanter*, over which the skin incision is centered, is the easiest bony prominence to palpate around the hip. Its posterior aspect is relatively free of muscles; its anterior and lateral aspects are covered by the tensor fasciae latae and the gluteus medius and minimus muscles and are much less accessible.

The greater trochanter arises from the junction of the neck and the shaft of the femur. From there, it projects both upward and backward (Fig. 8-83). The following five muscles insert into it:

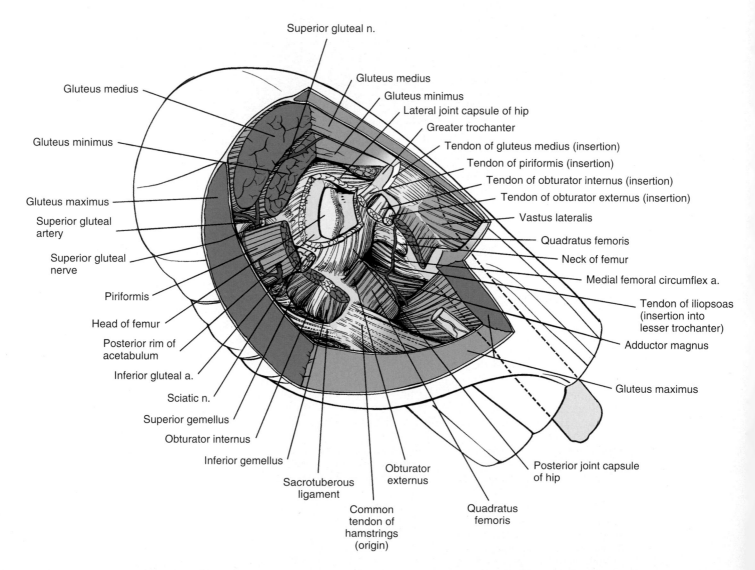

**Figure 8-82**   The gluteus minimus, piriformis, and short rotators have been resected to uncover the posterior aspect of the hip joint.

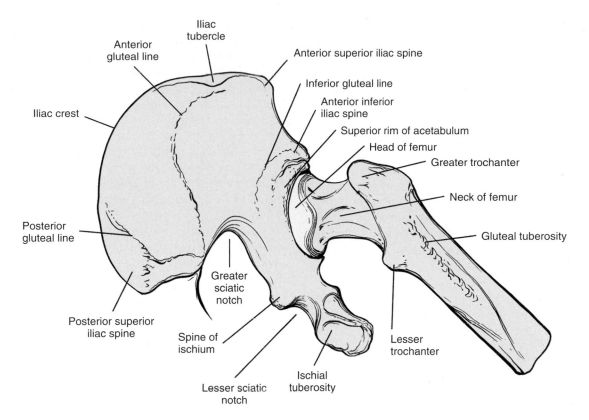

**Figure 8-83**  Osteology of the posterior aspect of the hip and pelvis.

`1. The *gluteus medius* attaches by a broad insertion into its lateral aspect. Below this insertion, the bone is covered by the beginnings of the iliotibial tract. A bursa, occasionally a site of inflammation, lies between the tract and the bone over the relatively bare portion of the trochanter. The bursa can be the site of bacterial infection (historically, most frequently tuberculosis).

2. The *gluteus minimus* is attached to the anterior aspect of the trochanter, where its tendon is divided in the anterolateral approach (see Fig. 8-81).

3. The *piriformis* inserts via a tendon into the middle of the upper border of the greater trochanter. Its insertion forms a surgical landmark for the insertion of certain types of intramedullary rods into the femur. The bone is perforated just medial to it, the easiest route into the medulla of the femoral shaft (see Fig. 8-81).

4. *Obturator externus tendon.* Immediately below the insertion of the piriformis lies the trochanteric fossa, a deep pit that marks the attachment of the obturator externus tendon (see Fig. 8-81).

5. The *obturator internus* tendon inserts with the two gemelli into the upper border of the trochanter, posterior to the insertion of the piriformis (see Fig. 8-81).

### Incision

The upper part of the incision crosses the lines of cleavage of the skin at almost 90°, but the resulting scar is always hidden by clothing. Most patients who undergo this approach are elderly and tend not to form exuberant scar tissue, and they heal with a fine line scar.

## Superficial Surgical Dissection and its Dangers

Superficial dissection consists of cutting through the outer muscle layer by splitting the fibers of the gluteus maximus, the single largest muscle in the body. The fibers of the gluteus maximus are extremely coarse; they run obliquely downward and laterally across the buttock. The muscle's innervation, the inferior gluteal nerve, emerges from the pelvis beneath the inferior border of the piriformis and almost immediately enters the muscle's deep surface close to its medial border, its origin. From there, the nerve's branches spread throughout the muscle. Splitting the gluteus maximus close to its lateral insertion does not denervate significant portions of the muscle, because its main nerve supply passes well medial to the most medial point of splitting (see Fig. 8-80).

The gluteus maximus is quiet during normal walking or standing still; it comes into play during stair climbing or standing up from a sitting position. (During normal walking, hip extension is primarily a function of the hamstrings rather than the gluteus maximus.)

## Deep Surgical Dissection and its Dangers

Deep dissection consists of incising some portion of the inner muscular layer (the short external rotators of the hip) to expose the posterior hip joint capsule (see Fig. 8-82). Five muscles form the inner layer: the piriformis, the superior gemellus, the tendon of the obturator internus, the inferior gemellus, and the quadratus femoris.

Recognizing the relationship of the piriformis to passing structures is the key to understanding the neurovascular anatomy of the area (see Fig. 8-81). All neurovascular structures that enter the buttock from the pelvis pass through the greater sciatic notch, either superior or inferior to the piriformis, which itself passes from the pelvis to the buttock through the notch.

The 10 critical neurovascular structures are as follows:

1. Superior gluteal nerve    } Above the
2. Superior gluteal artery    } piriformis

(These are the only structures to pass above the piriformis, hence, their name "superior.")

3. Inferior gluteal nerve
4. Inferior gluteal artery
5. Pudendal nerve
6. Internal pudendal artery    } Below the
7. Nerve to obturator internus    } piriformis
8. Sciatic nerve
9. Posterior femoral cutaneous nerve
10. Nerve to quadratus femoris

The *superior gluteal nerve* emerges from the pelvis above the piriformis. It crosses behind the posterior border of the gluteus medius and runs in the space between the gluteus medius and the gluteus minimus, supplying both before sending fibers to the tensor fasciae latae.

The *superior gluteal artery*, the largest branch of the internal iliac artery, enters the pelvis above the upper border of the piriformis and runs with its nerve, supplying the gluteus medius and gluteus minimus and sending a nutrient vessel to the ilium on the gluteal line. The nutrient vessel may bleed when a larger posterior iliac bone graft is taken. The superior gluteal artery also sends branches to the overlying gluteus maximus, forming part of the muscle's dual arterial supply.

The superior gluteal artery can be damaged in pelvic fractures, especially in those involving the greater sciatic notch. If it retracts into the pelvis, its bleeding must be controlled by an extraperitoneal approach to the pelvis so that its feeding vessel, the internal iliac artery, can be ligated. In pelvic fractures, selective angiography may aid in the diagnosis of a ruptured superior gluteal artery. During the angiography, the artery may be embolized through the diagnostic cannula, avoiding a pelvic exploration.[21] If you are using the anterior or posterior approaches to the acetabulum using a trochanteric osteotomy, the superior gluteal vessels must be intact in order to avoid muscle necrosis of the gluteus medius and minimus. This is because the origin and insertion of the muscles is detached in these approaches. If the acetabular fracture involves a displaced fracture of the greater sciatic notch, preoperative angiography is advised to ensure that the neurovascular pedicle to these structures is intact.

The *inferior gluteal nerve* reaches the buttock beneath the lower border of the piriformis. It enters the deep surface of the gluteus maximus almost immediately.

The *inferior gluteal artery*, which follows the inferior gluteal nerve, supplies the gluteus maximus. The branch it sends along the sciatic nerve was the original axial artery of the limb. In rare cases, this artery can serve as one guide to the sciatic nerve during surgery. The inferior gluteal artery may also be torn in pelvic fractures, but not as frequently as the superior gluteal artery.

The *pudendal nerve* is not encountered during the posterior approach to the hip because its course in the buttock is very short. It turns around the sacrospinous ligament before entering the perineum.

The *internal pudendal artery* runs with the pudendal nerve. The artery is usually well clear of the operative field during posterior approaches, but damage to it has been reported. Local pressure against the ischial spine usually controls bleeding; if not, or if the artery has retracted, an extraperitoneal approach through the space of Retzius[22] may be needed to ligate the parent trunk.

The *nerve to the obturator internus* enters its muscle almost as soon as it emerges from behind the inferior border of the piriformis. The nerve also supplies the superior gemellus.

The massive *sciatic nerve*, which is formed by roots from the lumbosacral plexus (L4, L5, S1, S2, S3), appears in the buttock from beneath the lower border of the piriformis, just lateral to the inferior gluteal and pudendal nerves and vessels. It is usually surrounded by fat and is often easier to feel than to see. It passes vertically down the buttock together with its artery, lying on the short external rotator muscles of the inner muscular sleeve, the obturator internus, the two gemelli, and the quadratus femoris. Farther distally, it passes deep (anterior) to the biceps femoris and disappears from view, lying on the adductor magnus.

The sciatic nerve is safe during posterior approaches as long as you are aware of its position. It can be injured if it is trapped in the posterior blade of the self-retaining retractor that holds the fascial edge. It also can be damaged if it is not protected during reduction of the prosthetic head into the acetabulum.

The tibial portion of the sciatic nerve supplies all the hamstring muscles except the short head of the biceps femoris and the extensor portion of the adductor magnus in the thigh. All its branches arise from the medial side of the nerve. Dissections around the sciatic nerve in the thigh therefore should remain on the lateral (safe) side, since the only branch coming off that side runs to the short head of the biceps, a muscle that causes few clinical problems if its nerve supply is damaged (see Fig. 8-81).

The *common peroneal and tibial nerves*, the terminal branches of the sciatic nerve, supply all the muscles below the knee. In addition, they (and other sciatic branches) supply skin over the sole of the foot, the dorsum of the foot (except for its medial side), and the calf and lateral side of the lower leg. Damage to the sciatic nerve at the level of the hip joint injures both tibial and common peroneal elements, resulting in a balanced flaccid paralysis below the knee, together with paralysis of the hamstring muscles. Complete sciatic nerve lesions are relatively rare; more often, the damage seems to affect either the tibial or the common peroneal components. Hence, neurologic findings may vary regardless of the level of the lesion.

Common peroneal nerve palsies do occur after posterior approaches to the hip. The question then arises as to whether the nerve was damaged at the operative site or whether it was compressed as it turns around the fibular head, usually during postoperative care. The differential diagnosis can be made by doing an electromyogram (EMG) of the short head of the biceps, the only muscle of the thigh that is supplied by the common peroneal division of the sciatic nerve. Lesions in the pelvis or at the level of the hip joint denervate this muscle. Lesions at the level of the fibular head leave it unaffected.

Only 20% of the cross section of the sciatic nerve at the hip joint is formed by nerve fibers. The remaining 80% is made up of connective tissue. Nerve repairs in this area are often unsuccessful, because bundle-to-bundle contact is difficult to achieve.

The *posterior femoral cutaneous nerve (posterior cutaneous nerve of the thigh)* supplies a large area of skin on the back of the thigh. The nerve actually lies on the sciatic nerve until the sciatic passes deep to the biceps femoris. Then the posterior femoral cutaneous nerve continues superficial to the hamstring muscles but deep to the fascia lata, sending out several cutaneous branches.

The *nerve to the quadratus femoris* emerges from the pelvis behind the sciatic nerve and runs with it on its deep surface as it crosses the tendon of the obturator internus and the two gemelli. The nerve then passes deep to the quadratus femoris before entering its anterior surface. It also gives off muscular branches to the inferior gemellus.

## Obturator Internus

The obturator internus is one of the few muscles that make a right-angled turn; it curves round the lesser sciatic notch of the ischium. The muscle has a tricipital tendon that is reinforced at its insertion by the superior and inferior gemelli.

## Quadratus Femoris

The quadratus femoris is quadrate, that is, four-sided. Its transversely running fibers form a clear surgical landmark. The muscle has an excellent blood supply. At the lower border of its insertion lies the cruciate anastomosis, consisting of the ascending branch of the first perforating artery, the descending branch of the inferior gluteal artery, and transverse branches of the medial and lateral femoral circumflex arteries (see Fig. 8-81).

The muscle's blood supply can be used to revascularize an avascular femoral head and neck.[17] In this maneuver, the quadrate tubercle of the femur is detached, leaving the muscular insertion of the quadratus femoris intact. The resultant muscle-bone pedicle can be swung upward, and the bone can be inserted across the fracture site.

## Medial Approach to the Hip

The medial approach, attributed to Ludloff,[23] was originally designed for surgery on flexed, abducted, and externally rotated hips, the kinds of deformities caused by certain types of congenital dislocation of the hip.

The uses of the medial approach include the following:

1. Open reduction of congenital dislocation of the hip. The approach gives an excellent exposure of the psoas tendon, which can block reduction of the hip.[24]
2. Biopsy and treatment of tumors of the inferior portion of the femoral neck and medial aspect of proximal shaft
3. Psoas release
4. Obturator neurectomy

The upper part of the approach can be used for an obturator neurectomy. If a neurectomy is combined with an adductor release, the approach can be performed through a short transverse incision or a short longitudinal incision in the groin that permits division of the adductors close to their pelvic origin, an area where there is less bleeding.

### Position of the Patient

Place the patient supine on the operating table with the affected hip flexed, abducted, and externally rotated. This may not be possible in cases with fixed deformity, when the position is often determined for you. The sole of the foot on the affected side should lie along the medial side of the contralateral knee (Fig. 8-84).

### Landmarks and Incision

#### Landmarks
Palpate the *adductor longus* from the medial side of the thigh and follow it up to its origin at the pubis, in

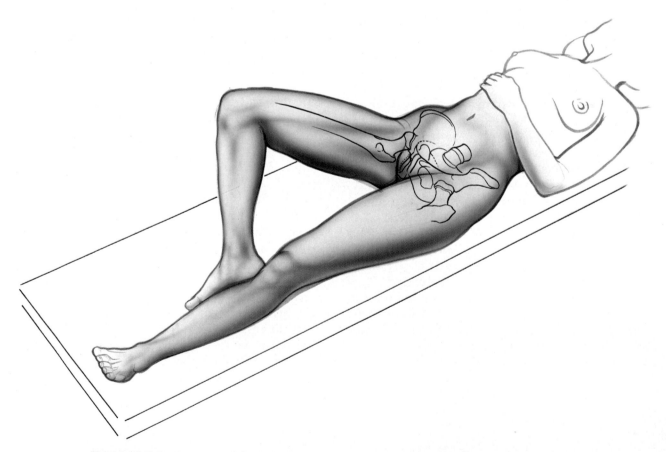

**Figure 8-84**    Position of the patient on the operating table for the medial approach to the hip.

the angle between the pubic crest and the symphysis. The adductor longus is the only muscle of the adductor group that is easy to palpate.

With your finger anchored on the greater trochanter, move your thumb along the inguinal creases medially and obliquely downward until you can feel the *pubic tubercle*. They are at the same level as the top of the greater trochanter.

### Incision

Make a longitudinal incision on the medial side of the thigh, starting at a point 3 cm below the pubic tubercle. The incision runs down over the adductor longus. Its length is determined by the amount of femur that must be exposed (Fig. 8-85).

### Internervous Plane

The superficial dissection does not exploit an internervous plane, since both the adductor longus and the gracilis are innervated by the anterior division of the obturator nerve. The plane is nevertheless safe for dissection; both muscles receive their nerve supplies proximal to the dissection (Fig. 8-86).

More deeply, the plane of dissection lies between the adductor brevis and the adductor magnus. The adductor brevis is supplied by the anterior division of the obturator nerve. The adductor magnus has two nerve supplies: Its adductor portion is supplied by the posterior division of the obturator nerve, and its ischial portion is supplied by the tibial part of the sciatic nerve. The two muscles, therefore, form the boundaries of an internervous plane (see Fig. 8-89).

### Superficial Surgical Dissection

Begin the superficial dissection by developing a plane between the gracilis and the adductor longus. Like other intermuscular planes in the adductor group, this plane can be developed with your gloved finger (Fig. 8-87*A*).

### Deep Surgical Dissection

Continue the dissection in the interval between the adductor brevis and the adductor magnus until you feel the lesser trochanter on the floor of the wound. Try to protect the posterior division of the obturator

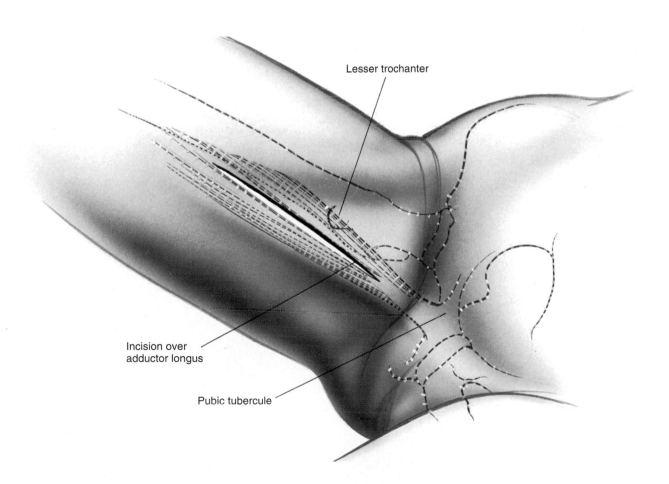

Lesser trochanter

Incision over adductor longus

Pubic tubercule

**Figure 8-85**    Incision for the medial approach to the hip.

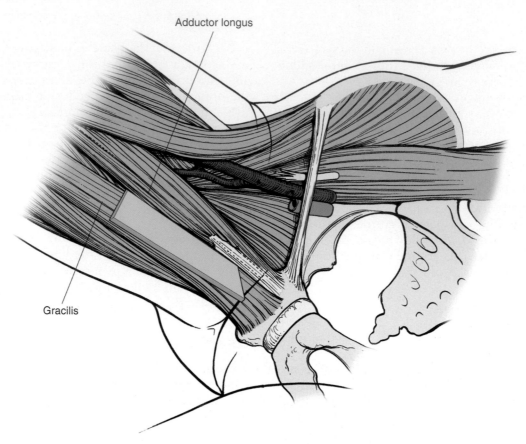

**Figure 8-86** The intermuscular interval between the adductor longus and the gracilis is not an internervous plane, since both muscles are innervated by the anterior division of the obturator nerve. The plane is safe, however, since the muscles receive their nerve supplies proximal to the dissection.

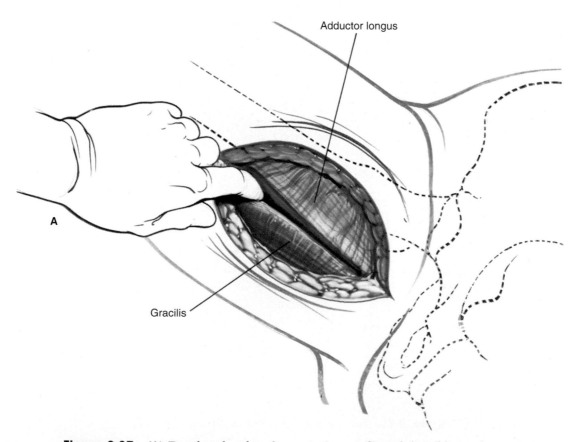

**Figure 8-87** (A) Develop the plane between the gracilis and the adductor longus.

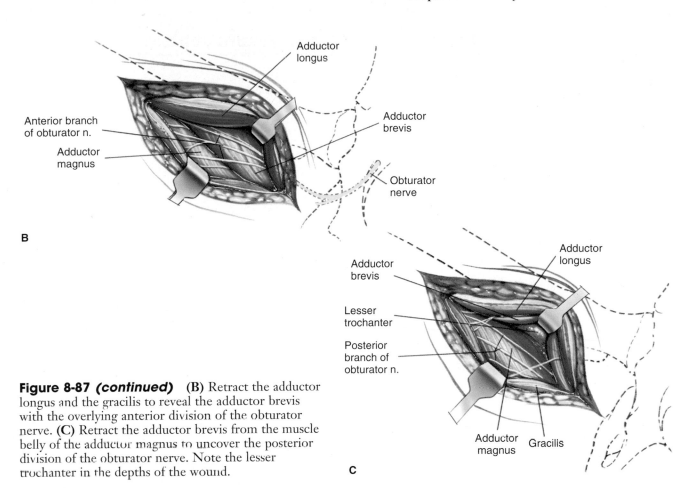

**Figure 8-87 (continued)** **(B)** Retract the adductor longus and the gracilis to reveal the adductor brevis with the overlying anterior division of the obturator nerve. **(C)** Retract the adductor brevis from the muscle belly of the adductor magnus to uncover the posterior division of the obturator nerve. Note the lesser trochanter in the depths of the wound.

nerve, the innervation to the muscle's adductor portion, to preserve the hip extensor function of the adductor magnus (see Dangers below). Place a narrow retractor (such as a bone spike) above and below the lesser trochanter to isolate the psoas tendon.

## Dangers

### Nerves
The **anterior division of the obturator nerve** lies on top of the obturator externus and runs down the medial side of the thigh between the adductor longus and the adductor brevis, to which it is bound by a thin tissue. It supplies the adductor longus, the adductor brevis, and the gracilis in the thigh (Fig. 8-87*B*).

The **posterior division of the obturator nerve** lies in the substance of the obturator externus, which it supplies before it leaves the pelvis. The nerve then runs down the thigh on the adductor magnus and under the adductor brevis; it supplies the adductor portion of the adductor magnus (Fig. 8-87*C*).

Most of the time, the approach is designed specifically to cut these nerves to relieve muscular spastic-ity. If you are not using it for that purpose, avoid transecting them.

### Vessels
The **medial femoral circumflex artery** (see Applied Surgical Anatomy of the Thigh in Chapter 9) passes around the medial side of the distal part of the psoas tendon. It is in danger, especially in children, if you try to detach the psoas without isolating the tendon and cutting it under direct vision (Fig. 8-89).

## How to Enlarge the Approach

### Local Measures
After reaching the femur and detaching the insertions of the psoas and iliacus, you can expose some 5 cm of femoral shaft distal to the lesser trochanter by blunt dissection.

### Extensile Measures
This exposure is almost never enlarged by extensile measures.

# Applied Surgical Anatomy of the Medial Approach

## Overview

The anatomy of this approach is the anatomy of the adductor compartment of the thigh. The adductors do not cover the hip joint, since they all originate below the level of the joint itself.

The adductor compartment of the thigh consists of three layers of muscles, with the two divisions of the obturator nerve running between each pair of layers. The superficial layer consists of the adductor longus and the gracilis; the middle layer, the adductor brevis; and the deep layer, the adductor magnus.

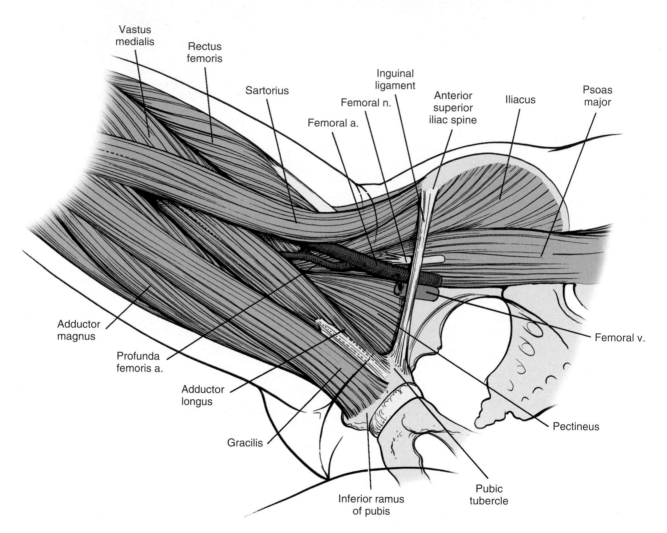

**Figure 8-88**   Anatomy of the medial approach to the hip. The thigh is abducted, slightly flexed, and externally rotated. The plane of the superficial dissection runs between the adductor longus and the gracilis.

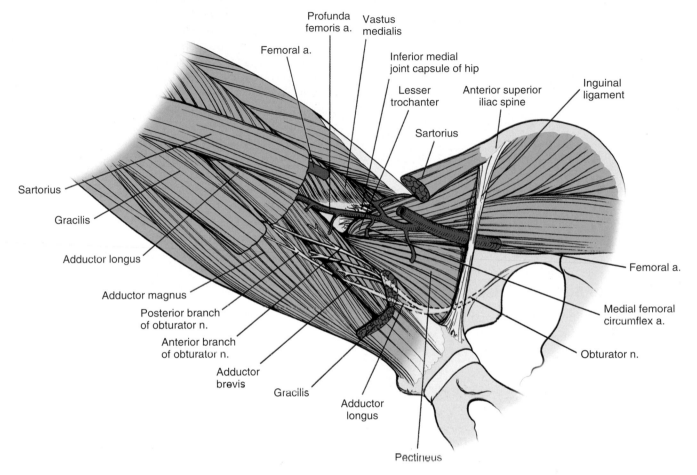

Profunda femoris a.
Vastus medialis
Femoral a.
Inferior medial joint capsule of hip
Lesser trochanter
Anterior superior iliac spine
Inguinal ligament
Sartorius
Sartorius
Gracilis
Femoral a.
Adductor longus
Adductor magnus
Medial femoral circumflex a.
Posterior branch of obturator n.
Anterior branch of obturator n.
Obturator n.
Adductor brevis
Gracilis
Adductor longus
Pectineus

**Figure 8-89** The muscular layer of the medial approach to the hip. The dissection lies between the adductor brevis and the adductor magnus. The gracilis, adductor longus, and sartorius have been resected to reveal the deeper structures of the medial aspect of the thigh. Note the relationships of the anterior and posterior divisions of the obturator nerve to the adductor longus and adductor brevis. Note the proximity of the medial femoral circumflex artery to the insertion of the psoas tendon.

**Psoas Major.** *Origin.* Anterior surface of transverse processes and bodies of the lumbar vertebrae and corresponding intervertebral disks. *Insertion.* Lesser trochanter of femur. *Action.* Flexor of hip and flexor of lumbar spine when leg is fixed. *Nerve supply.* Segmental nerves from second and third lumbar roots.

**Iliacus.** *Origin.* Upper two thirds of iliac fossa, inner lip of iliac crest, anterior aspect of sacroiliac joint, and from the lumbosacral and iliolumbar ligaments. *Insertion.* Lesser trochanter of femur by common tendon with psoas. *Action.* Flexor of hip. Tilts pelvis forward when leg is fixed. *Nerve supply.* Femoral nerve (L2-L4).

## Landmarks and Incision

### Landmarks

The *adductor longus* is the only muscle of the adductor group that is easily palpable at its tendinous origin. Its structure is considered in detail in the superficial surgical dissection.

The *pubic tubercle* is the most lateral part of the body of the pubis. Easily palpable, it marks the medial attachment of the inguinal ligament (Fig. 8-90).

### Incisions

A longitudinal incision crosses the lines of cleavage obliquely, since they run down and medially cross the front of the thigh. A transverse insertion made in the groin, used for release of the adductors, is parallel with the lines and should heal with minimal scar formation. Meticulous closure of the deep fascia minimizes ugly depressed scars.

## Superficial Surgical Dissection

The approach runs between the adductor longus and the gracilis. Both muscles are supplied by the anterior division of the obturator nerve, but the nerves enter them close to their pubic origins, leaving the intermuscular plane available for surgical use (see Fig. 8-88).

The *gracilis* is extremely long and thin, with long parallel-running fibers. Its aponeurotic origin, a thin sheet of tendinous fibers arising from the pubis, lies in an anteroposterior plane.

The *adductor longus* arises by a strong tendon, which accounts for its involvement in the relatively high incidence of avulsion fractures. The origin may ossify in those who, like horseback riders, use their hip adductors excessively. This ossification is known as rider's bone. Calcification and ossification are also seen in soccer players in whom the lesion may give rise to chronic pain and loss of function.

Given the size and relative "weakness" of these two muscles, it is difficult to understand why they were once given the name of *custodes virginitatis.*[25]

The *obturator nerve* is derived from anterior divisions of the L2-L4 nerve roots. The nerve divides in the obturator notch into *anterior* and *posterior* divisions. The anterior division passes over the upper border of the obturator externus and descends on the medial side of the thigh behind the adductor longus, on the anterior surface of the adductor brevis. It supplies sensory fibers to the hip joint.

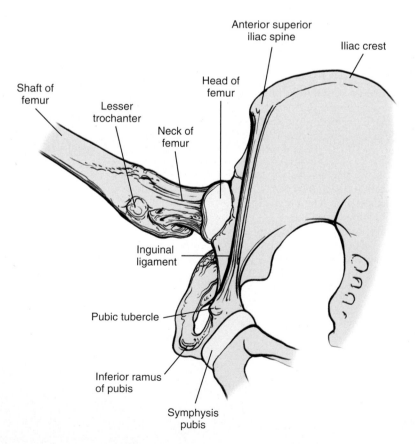

**Figure 8-90**  Osteology of the medial approach to the hip.

The nerve is commonly transected in cases of adduction contractures of the hip caused by spasticity of the adductor muscles. To find it, define the interval between the adductor longus and the adductor brevis, the point at which the nerve is available for section. The nerve lies on the anterior surface of the adductor brevis, bound to it by a thin areolar covering. There, it may divide into three or even four bundles. Therefore, when performing an anterior obturator neurectomy, dissect the nerve bundles proximally as far as possible to avoid overlooking branches coming off higher up.

The anterior branch gives cutaneous distribution to the medial side of the knee, perhaps the reason hip pain is often referred to the knee, especially in cases of slipped upper femoral epiphysis. (A second pain commonly referred to the inside of the knee, originating in the ovary, is thought to be due to direct irritation of the obturator nerve by ovarian pathology, because the nerve runs adjacent to the ovary in the pelvis.)

## Deep Surgical Dissection

The intermuscular interval used in deep surgical dissection lies between the adductor brevis and the adductor magnus (see Fig. 8-90).

The *adductor brevis* runs down the thigh, sandwiched between the anterior and posterior divisions of the obturator nerve.

In certain animals, the *adductor magnus* inserts into the tibia. In humans, the superficial medial ligament of the knee is thought to have arisen as the degenerative tendon of the adductor magnus and is sometimes referred to as the fourth hamstring muscle.

The *posterior division of the obturator nerve* runs distally on the surface of the adductor magnus, supplying it.

## REFERENCES

1. LETOURNEL E: Acetabular fractures: classification and management. Clin Orthop Relatres 151:81, 1980
2. TILE M: Fractures of the pelvis and acetabulum. Baltimore, Williams and Wilkins, 1984
3. JUDET R, JUDET T, LETOURNEL E: Fractures of the acetabulum classification and surgical approaches: open reduction. J Bone Joint Surg 46-A:1615, 1964
4. SENEGAS J, LIOUR Z, YATES M: Complex acetabular fractures: a transtrochanteric lateral surgical approach. Clin Orthop Related Research 151:107,1980
5. SMITH-PETERSEN MN: A new supra-articular subperiosteal approach to the hip joint. Am J Orthop Surg 15:592, 1917
6. SMITH-PETERSEN MN: Approach to and exposure of the hip joint for mold arthroplasty. J Bone Joint Surg (Am) 31:40, 1949
7. HONORTH MB: Congenital dislocation of the hip: technique of open reduction. Ann Surg 135:508, 1952
8. CHARNLEY J: Low friction arthroplasty of the hip: theory and practice. New York, Springer-Verlag, 1979
9. HARRIS WH: A new lateral approach to the hip joint. J Bone Joint Surg (Am) 49:891, 1967
10. MÜLLER ME: Total hip prosthesis. Clin Orthop 72:46, 1970
11. CHARNLEY J: Arthroplasty of the hip: a new operation. Lancet 2:129, 1961
12. EVANS P: The postural function of the iliotibial tract. Ann R Coll Surg Engl 61:271, 1979
13. MOORE AT: The Moore self-locking vitallium prosthesis in fresh femoral neck fractures: a new low posterior approach (the southern exposure). In American Academy of Orthopaedic Surgeons: Instructional Course Lectures, Vol. 16. St. Louis, CV Mosby, 1959
14. MOORE AT: The self-locking metal hip prosthesis. J Bone Joint Surg (Am) 39:811, 1957
15. THOMPSON FR: Vitallium intramedullary hip prosthesis: preliminary report. N Y State J Med 52:3011, 1958
16. CHARNLEY J: Anchorage of the femoral head prosthesis to the shaft of the femur. J Bone Joint Surg (Br) 42:28, 1960
17. MYERS MH, HARVEY JP, MOORE TM: Treatment of displaced subcapital and transcervical fractures of the femoral neck by muscle pedicle—bone graft and internal fixation. J Bone Joint Surg (Am) 55:257, 1973
18. HENRY AK: Extensile exposure, 3rd ed. Edinburgh, Churchill Livingstone, 1972
19. MARCY GH, FLETCHER RS: Modification of the posterolateral approach to the hip for insertion of femoral head prosthesis. J Bone Joint Surg (Am) 36:142, 1954
20. OSBORNE RP: The approach to the hip joint: a critical review and a suggested new route. Br J Surg 18:49, 1930-1931
21. NACHBUR B, MEYER RP, VRKKALA K ET AL: The mechanisms of severe arterial injury in surgery of the hip joint. Clin Orthop 141:122 (June) 1979
22. RETZIUS AA: Ueber das Ligamentjm Pelvioprostaticum Oper Den Apparat, durch Welchen die Harnblane, die Prostata Uno der Untern Becken Öffnung Befestgt Sind. Arch Anat Physiol 188–189, 1841
23. LUDLOFF K: Zur Blutigen Einrenkung DerAngeborenen Huftluxation. Z Orthop Chir 22:272, 1908
24. FERGUSON AB JR: Primary open reduction of congenital dislocation of the hip using a median adductor approach. J Bone Joint Surg (Am) 55:671, 1973
25. LAST RJ: Anatomy regional and applied. New York, Churchill Livingstone, 1978

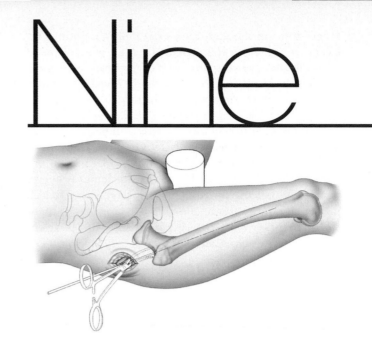

# The Femur

Operations on the femur are extremely common. The lateral approach to the proximal femur, which is used to treat the growing number of patients who have intertrochanteric hip fractures, is the most frequently used approach in orthopaedic surgery.

The four basic approaches, the *lateral, posterolateral, anterolateral*, and *anteromedial*, all penetrate elements of the quadriceps muscle. Only the posterolateral approach uses an internervous plane, but all are relatively straightforward because the femoral nerve, which supplies the quadriceps femoris muscle, divides proximally in the thigh, allowing the more distal muscle elements to be separated without denervation. (The posterior approach is reserved for exploration of the sciatic nerve and for patients who cannot undergo more anterior approaches because of skin problems.)

Femoral shaft fractures are now most commonly treated with intramedullary nails inserted using a closed technique. A minimal access approach to the proximal femur for the insertion of intramedullary nails is described.

Because the key vascular structures spiral down the thigh, passing in an anterior to posterior direction, the anatomy of the thigh is discussed in a separate section in this chapter following the descriptions of the surgical approaches. Within this section, the unique anatomic features of each approach are discussed individually.

## Lateral Approach

The lateral approach is the incision used most often for gaining access to the upper third of the femur. It also can be extended inferiorly to expose virtually the whole length of the bone. Although it is an extremely quick and easy approach, it involves splitting the vastus lateralis muscle. The subsequent blood loss that results from the rupture of vessels during this procedure may make surgery awkward, but rarely is life-threatening.

The uses of the lateral approach include the following:

1. Open reduction and internal fixation of intertrochanteric fractures (this is by far the most common use of the approach)
2. Insertion of internal fixation in the treatment of subcapital fractures or slipped upper femoral epiphysis
3. Subtrochanteric or intertrochanteric osteotomy
4. Open reduction and internal fixation of femoral shaft fractures and supracondylar fractures of the femur
5. Extraarticular arthrodesis of the hip joint
6. Treatment of chronic osteomyelitis of the femur
7. Biopsy and treatment of bone tumors

### Position of the Patient

Patients with trochanteric or subtrochanteric fractures should be placed on an orthopaedic table in the supine position so that their fractures can be manipulated or controlled during surgery. Use an orthopaedic table for any procedure that involves the use of an image intensifier (Fig. 9-1). Internally rotate the leg 15° to overcome the natural anteversion of the femoral neck and to bring the lateral surface of the bone into a true lateral position.

For surgery on the shaft of the femur, use a lateral position. Place the patient on his or her side, with the affected limb uppermost. Take care to pad the bony prominences of the bottom limb to avoid pressure necrosis of the skin. Place other pillows between the two limbs to pad the medial surface of the knee and the medial malleolus of the side that is being operated on.

### Landmarks and Incision

#### Landmarks

The posterior edge of the *greater trochanter* is relatively uncovered. Palpate it, moving the fingers anteriorly and proximally to identify its tip.

The *shaft of the femur* is palpable as a line of resistance on the lateral side of the thigh.

#### Incision

Make a longitudinal incision, beginning over the middle of the greater trochanter and extending down the lateral side of the thigh over the lateral aspect of the femur. The length of the incision will vary with the requirements of the surgery (Fig. 9-2).

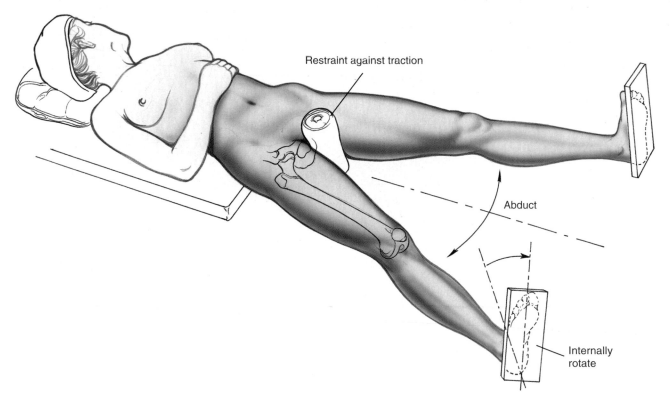

**Figure 9-1**  Position of the patient on the operating table for the lateral approach to the proximal femur.

## Internervous Plane

There is no internervous or intermuscular plane, because the dissection splits the vastus lateralis muscle, which is supplied by the femoral nerve. The muscle receives its nerve supply high in the thigh, however, so splitting the muscle distally does not denervate it.

## Superficial Surgical Dissection

Incise the fascia lata of the thigh in line with the skin incision. At the upper end of the wound, the distal portion of the tensor fasciae latae may have to be split in line with its fibers to expose the vastus lateralis (Fig. 9-3). This split is needed in about one third of patients, those who have tensor fasciae latae

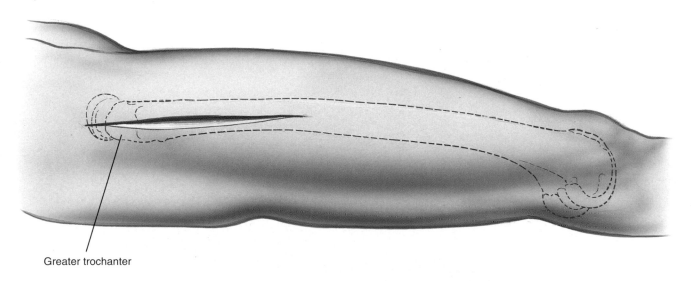

**Figure 9-2**  Incision for the lateral approach to the proximal femur.

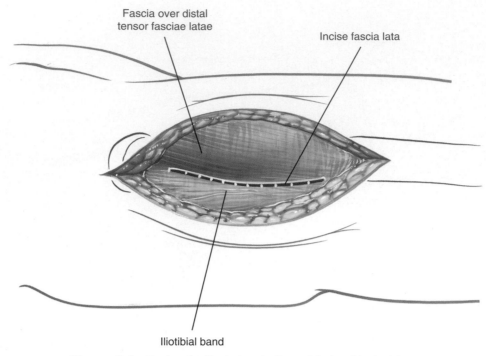

**Figure 9-3** Incise the fascia lata in line with the skin incision.

fibers extending distally beyond the greater trochanter.

## Deep Surgical Dissection

Carefully incise the fascial covering of the vastus lateralis muscle (Fig. 9-4). Insert a Homan or Bennett retractor through the muscle, running the tip of the retractor over the anterior aspect of the femoral shaft. Then, insert a second retractor through the same gap and down to the femoral shaft. Manipulate the second retractor so that it moves underneath the femur, and pull the two retractors apart to split the vastus lateralis in the line of its fibers (Fig. 9-5).

Continue splitting by blunt dissection. As dissection proceeds, several vessels that cross the field will be exposed. Coagulate them, if possible, before they are avulsed by the blunt dissection.

Splitting the vastus lateralis reveals the underlying lateral surface of the femur.

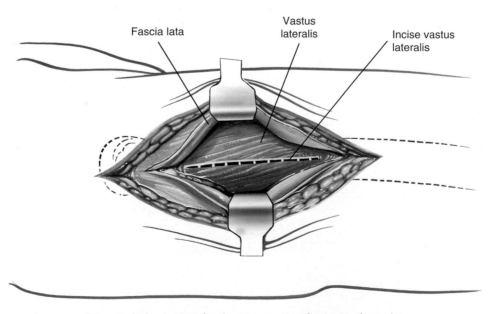

**Figure 9-4** Incise the fascia covering the vastus lateralis.

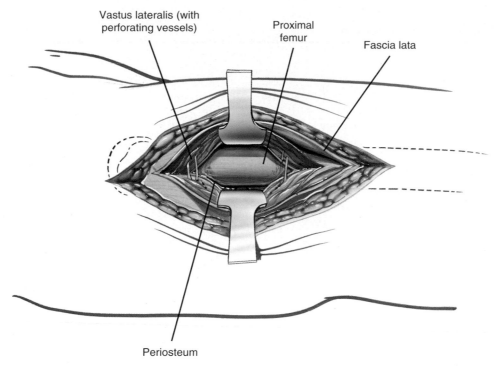

**Figure 9-5** Split the fibers of the vastus lateralis. To develop a subperiosteal plane, squeeze two Homan retractors down to the femoral shaft and separate them to split the vastus lateralis further.

## Dangers

### Vessels

Numerous **perforating branches of the profunda femoris artery** traverse the vastus lateralis muscle (see Fig. 9-31). They are damaged during the approach and should be ligated or coagulated. These arterial branches can be identified more easily if the muscle is split gently with a blunt instrument rather than cut straight through with a knife.

## How to Enlarge the Approach

### Extensile Measures

The approach is most useful for exposing the proximal third of the bone for internal fixation of a hip fracture. It can be extended to the knee joint, however, to allow full exposure of the lateral aspect of the femoral shaft for reduction and fixation of all types of femoral fractures (Fig. 9-6; see Figs. 9-34 and 9-35).

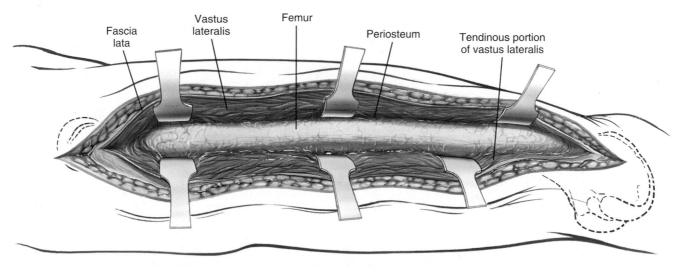

**Figure 9-6** The incision may be extended distally to expose the entire shaft of the femur.

# Posterolateral Approach

The posterolateral approach[1] can expose the entire length of the femur. Because it follows the lateral intermuscular septum, it does not interfere with the quadriceps muscle. Although other lateral approaches involve splitting the vastus lateralis or vastus intermedius muscles, the functional results of the posterolateral approach do not differ significantly from those of other approaches, probably because the vastus lateralis originates partly from the lateral intermuscular septum. As a result, surgery still involves detaching a part of the muscle's origin and does not use a true intermuscular plane.

The lateral intramuscular septum lies posterior to the femoral shaft at its proximal end. This septum overlies the middle of the shaft at its distal end. The posterolateral approach is therefore ideal for exposure of the distal one third of the femur. The more proximal the approach, the greater the bulk of the vastus lateralis that will need to be retracted anteriorly and the more difficult the approach will be.

The uses of the posterolateral approach include the following:

1. Open reduction and plating of femoral fractures, especially supracondylar fractures
2. Open intramedullary rod placement for femoral shaft fractures
3. Treatment of nonunion of femoral fractures
4. Femoral osteotomy (which is performed rarely in the region of the femoral shaft)
5. Treatment of chronic or acute osteomyelitis
6. Biopsy and treatment of bone tumors

## Position of the Patient

Place the patient supine on the operating table with a sandbag beneath the buttock on the affected side to

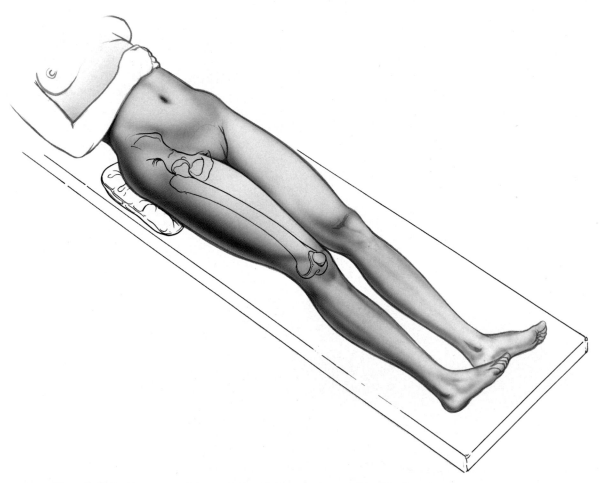

**Figure 9-7**   Position of the patient on the operating table for the posterolateral approach to the femur.

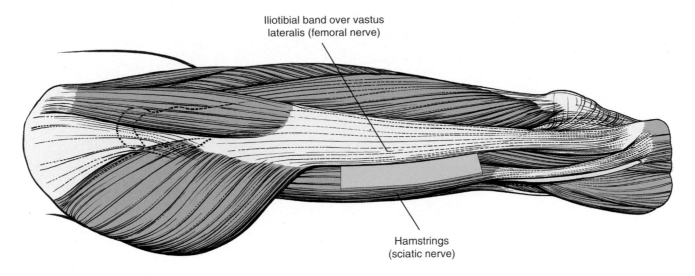

Iliotibial band over vastus
lateralis (femoral nerve)

Hamstrings
(sciatic nerve)

**Figure 9-8**   The internervous plane lies between the vastus lateralis (which is supplied
by the femoral nerve) and the hamstring muscles (which are supplied by the sciatic
nerve).

elevate the buttock and to rotate the leg internally, bringing the posterolateral surface of the thigh clear of the table (Fig. 9-7).

## Landmarks and Incision

### Landmarks
Palpate the *lateral femoral epicondyle* on the lateral surface of the knee joint. The epicondyle actually is a

flare of the condyle. Moving superiorly, note that the femur cannot be palpated above the epicondyle.

### Incision
Make a longitudinal incision on the posterolateral aspect of the thigh. Base the distal part of the incision on the lateral femoral epicondyle and continue proximally along the posterior part of the femoral shaft. The exact length of the incision depends on the surgery to be performed (Fig. 9-9).

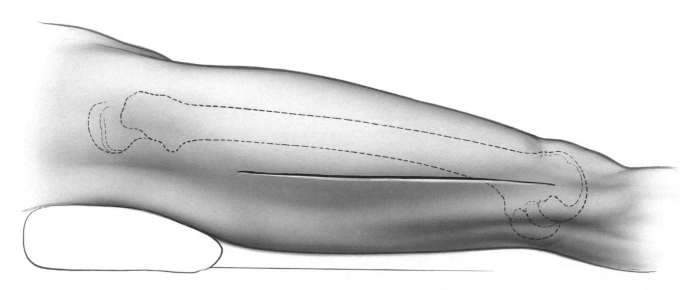

**Figure 9-9**   Incision for the posterolateral approach to the thigh.

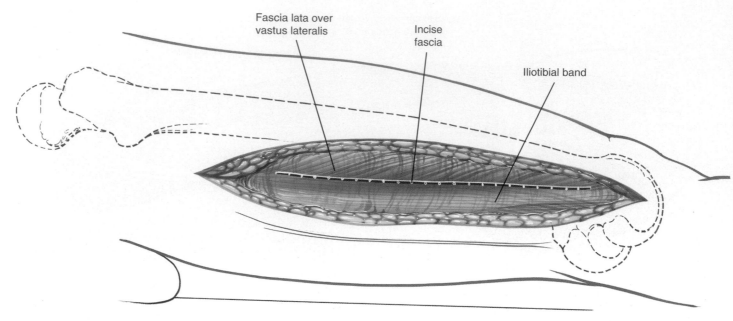

**Figure 9-10**    Incise the fascia of the thigh in line with its fibers and the skin incision.

## Internervous Plane

The approach exploits the plane between the *vastus lateralis* muscle (which is supplied by the femoral nerve) and the *lateral intermuscular septum*, which covers the *hamstring muscles* (which are supplied by the sciatic nerve; Fig. 9-8).

## Superficial Surgical Dissection

Incise the deep fascia of the thigh in line with its fibers and the skin incision (Fig. 9-10).

## Deep Surgical Dissection

Identify the vastus lateralis under the fascia lata (Fig. 9-11). Follow the muscle posteriorly to the lateral intermuscular septum. Then, reflect the muscle anteriorly, dissecting between muscle and septum. Numerous branches of the perforating arteries cross this septum to supply the muscle; they must be ligated or coagulated (Fig. 9-12).

Continue the dissection, following the plane between the lateral intermuscular septum and the vastus lateralis muscle, detaching those parts of the

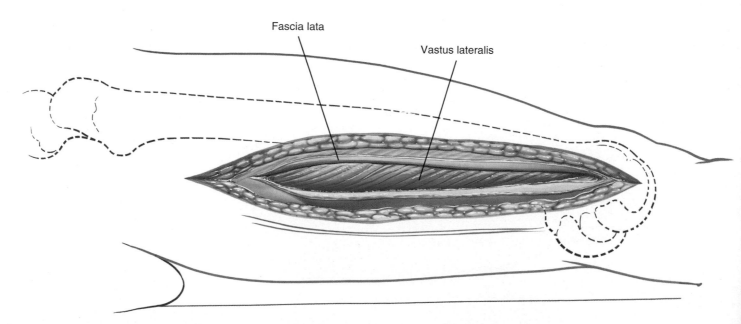

**Figure 9-11**    Identify the vastus lateralis under the incised fascia lata.

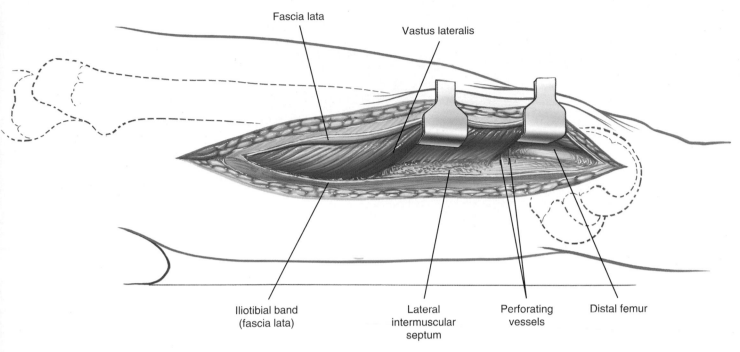

**Figure 9-12**   Elevate the vastus lateralis anteriorly, separating the muscle from the septum.

vastus lateralis that arise from the septum until the femur is reached at the linea aspera (Fig. 9-13). Incise the periosteum longitudinally at this point and strip off the muscles that cover the femur, using subperiosteal dissection. Detaching muscles from the linea aspera itself usually has to be done by sharp dissection (Fig. 9-14).

It is very easy to open up the plane between the vastus lateralis muscle and the lateral intermuscular septum in the distal third of the femur. Moving prox-

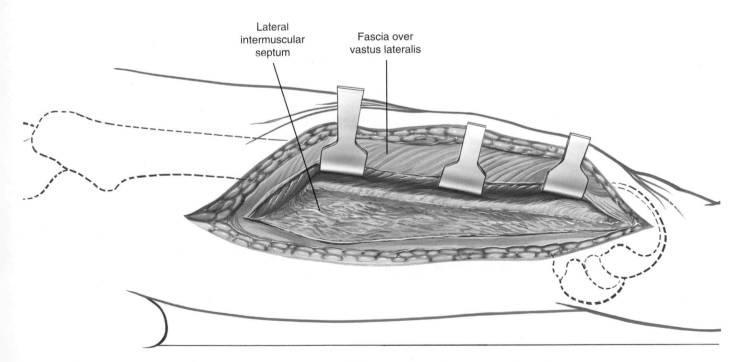

**Figure 9-13**   Detach those portions of the vastus lateralis that arise from the septum until the femur and linea aspera are reached. Then, incise the periosteum longitudinally.

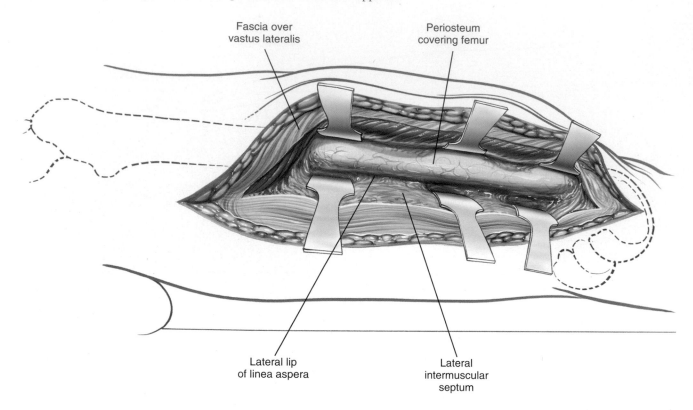

**Figure 9-14** Expose the shaft of the femur.

imally, the muscle becomes thicker, and it becomes more difficult to lift the muscle bulk anteriorly to reveal the femoral shaft. To aid in this process, place a Homan or Bennett retractor over the anterior aspect of the femoral shaft, lifting the vastus lateralis forward. A retractor placed on the lateral intermuscular septum will help open up the gap and facilitate proximal dissection.

## Dangers

### Vessels
The **perforating arteries** (which are branches of the profunda femoris artery) pierce the lateral intermuscular septum to supply the vastus lateralis muscle. They must be ligated or coagulated one by one as the dissection progresses. If they are torn flush with the lateral intermuscular septum, they may begin to bleed out of control as they retract behind it (see Fig. 9-35).

The **superior lateral geniculate artery and vein** cross over the lateral surface of the femur at the top of the femoral condyles. These vessels will need to be ligated for exposure to the bone.

## How to Enlarge the Approach

### Extensile Measures
The major value of this incision lies in its exposure of the distal two thirds of the femur. It can be extended superiorly, however, up to the greater trochanter, to expose virtually the entire femoral shaft. Note that, superiorly, the tendon of the gluteus maximus muscle lies behind the lateral intermuscular septum.

The approach can be extended easily into a lateral parapatellar approach to the knee joint. This allows accurate visualization of the entire distal end of the femur. This extension is used to allow reduction and fixation of intraarticular fractures of the distal femur.

# Anteromedial Approach to the Distal Two Thirds of the Femur

The anteromedial approach provides an excellent view of the lower two thirds of the femur and the knee joint. Its uses include the following:

1. Open reduction and internal fixation of fractures of the distal femur, particularly those that extend into the knee joint (its major use)
2. Open reduction and internal fixation of femoral shaft fractures
3. Treatment of chronic osteomyelitis
4. Biopsy and treatment of bone tumors
5. Quadricepsplasty

## Position of the Patient

Place the patient supine on the operating table, and drape the extremity so that it can move freely (Fig. 9-15).

## Landmark and Incision

### Landmark

The *vastus medialis* muscle is a distinct bulge supero-medial to the upper pole of the patella. Only the inferior portion can be seen and palpated distinctly. The vastus medialis atrophies rapidly in many patients with knee pathology; therefore, it may be difficult to find.

### Incision

Make a 10- to 15-cm longitudinal incision on the anteromedial aspect of the thigh over the interval between the rectus femoris and vastus medialis muscles. (There are no specific landmarks for this interval other than the contour of the vastus medialis.) Extend the incision distally along the medial edge of

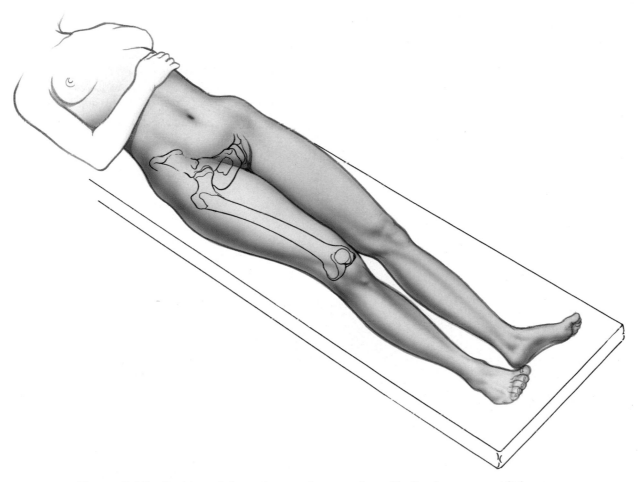

**Figure 9-15** Position of the patient on the operating table for the anteromedial approach to the femur.

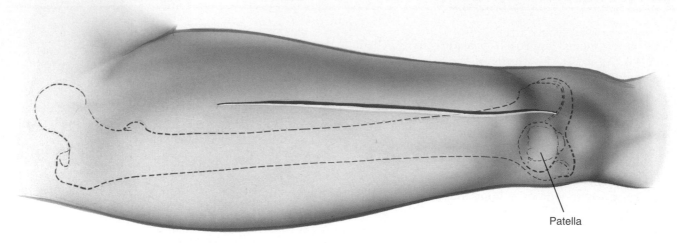

Patella

**Figure 9-16**    Incision for the anteromedial approach to the thigh.

the patella to the joint line of the knee, if the knee joint must be opened. The exact length of the incision depends on the pathology being treated (Fig. 9-16).

## Internervous Plane

There is no internervous plane; the dissection descends between the vastus medialis and rectus femoris muscles, both of which are supplied by the femoral nerve. The intermuscular plane can be used safely to expose the distal two thirds of the femur, however, because both muscles receive their nerve supplies well up in the thigh.

## Superficial Surgical Dissection

Incise the fascia lata (deep fascia) in line with the skin incision, and identify the interval between the vastus medialis and rectus femoris muscles (Fig. 9-17). Develop this plane by retracting the rectus femoris laterally (Fig. 9-18).

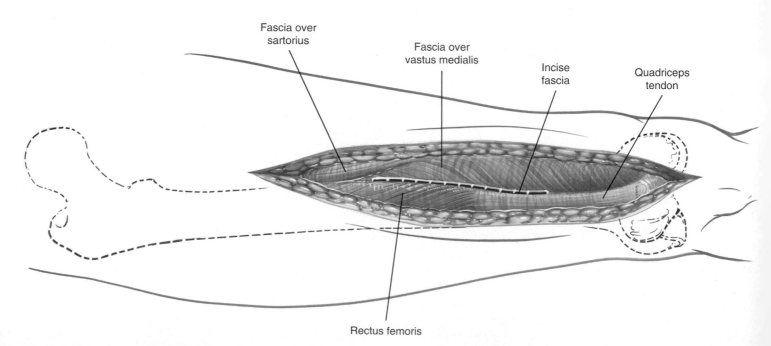

Fascia over
sartorius

Fascia over
vastus medialis

Incise
fascia

Quadriceps
tendon

Rectus femoris

**Figure 9-17**    Incise the fascia lata in line with the skin incision, and identify the interval between the vastus medialis and the rectus femoris.

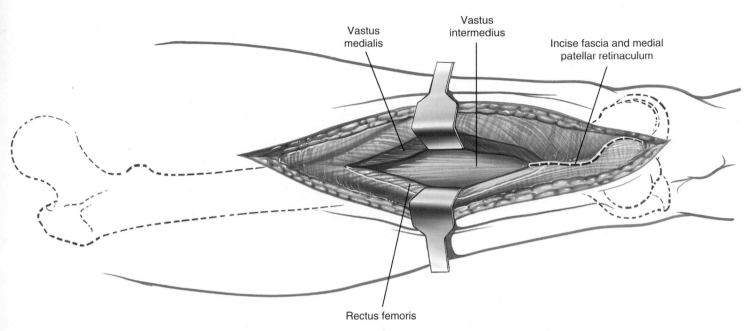

Vastus medialis

Vastus intermedius

Incise fascia and medial patellar retinaculum

Rectus femoris

**Figure 9-18**   Develop the plane between the vastus medialis and the rectus femoris, retracting the rectus femoris laterally. Begin the parapatellar incision into the joint capsule.

## Deep Surgical Dissection

Begin distally, opening the capsule of the knee joint in line with the skin incision by cutting through the medial patellar retinaculum (see Fig. 9-18). Continue proximally, splitting the quadriceps tendon almost on its medial border. Open up the plane by sharp dissection, staying within the substance of the quadriceps tendon and leaving a small cuff of the tendon with the vastus medialis attached to it. This preserves the insertion of these fibers and allows easy closure. If the vas-tus medialis is stripped off the quadriceps tendon, it is very difficult to reinsert, and muscle function will be compromised. Next, continue to develop the interval between the vastus medialis and rectus femoris muscles proximally to reveal the vastus intermedius muscle. Split the vastus intermedius in line with its fibers; directly below lies the femoral shaft, covered with periosteum. Incise the periosteum longitudinally, and continue the dissection in the subperiosteal plane to get to the bone (Figs. 9-19 and 9-20).

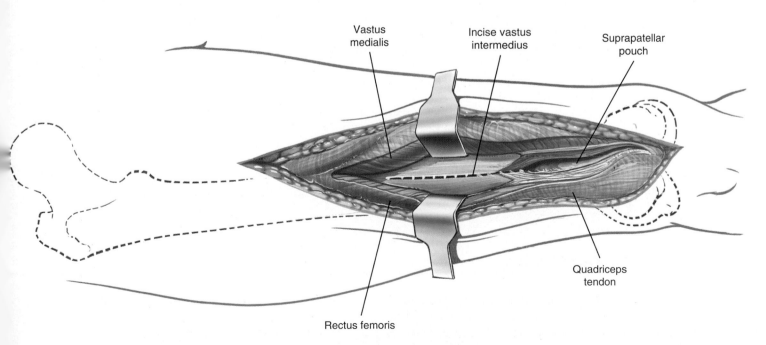

Vastus medialis

Incise vastus intermedius

Suprapatellar pouch

Rectus femoris

Quadriceps tendon

**Figure 9-19**   Continue the parapatellar incision proximally, opening the joint capsule and suprapatellar region. Carry the incision into the substance of the vastus intermedius.

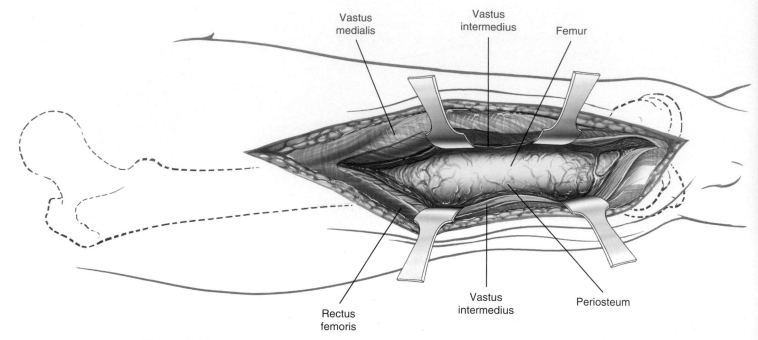

**Figure 9-20**    Incise the periosteum of the femur longitudinally, and expose the distal femur by subperiosteal dissection.

## Dangers

### Vessels

The **medial superior genicular artery** crosses the operative field just above the knee, winding around the lower end of the femur. Although it looks small, it must be ligated or coagulated to avoid hematoma formation (see Fig. 10-43).

### Muscles and Ligaments

The lowest fibers of the **vastus medialis** muscle insert directly onto the medial border of the patella. Their main job is to stabilize the patella and prevent lateral subluxation (see Fig. 9-32). The fiber attachments of the muscle inevitably are disrupted during this approach, unless a small cuff of quadriceps tendon is taken with the muscle. Make sure to repair the incision meticulously during closure to prevent subsequent lateral subluxation of the patella.

## How to Enlarge the Approach

### Extensile Measures

*Superior Extension.* The approach can be extended along the same interval between the rectus femoris and vastus medialis muscles. To extend the deep dissection, continue to split the vastus intermedius muscle. The extension offers excellent exposure of the lower two thirds of the femur. Higher up, however, the femoral artery, vein, and nerve intrude into the dissection; the upper third of the femur is explored best by a lateral approach.

*Inferior Extension.* Continue the skin incision downward, and curve it laterally so that it ends just below the tibial tubercle. Incise the medial retinaculum in line with the skin incision, making the patella more mobile and subject to lateral subluxation for full exposure of the knee joint. Take care not to avulse the quadriceps tendon from its insertion during the maneuver (see Medial Parapatellar Approach in Chapter 10).

## Posterior Approach

The posterior approach[4] is useful in patients who cannot undergo more anterior approaches because of local skin problems. It provides access to the middle three fifths of the bone, as well as to the sciatic nerve. Although it is performed rarely, its uses include the following:

1. Treatment of infected cases of nonunion of the femur
2. Treatment of chronic osteomyelitis
3. Biopsy and treatment of bone tumors
4. Exploration of the sciatic nerve

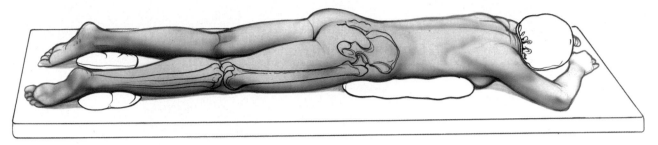

**Figure 9-21**   Position of the patient on the operating table for the posterior approach to the femur.

The approach is unusual in that surgery remains lateral to the biceps muscle in its proximal half, but proceeds medial to it in its distal half. This is because of the relationship of the posterior aspect of the femur to the sciatic nerve.

## Position of the Patient

Place the patient prone on the operating table, supporting the pelvis and chest on longitudinally placed pillows or thick foam pads to allow the abdomen and chest to move freely, ensuring adequate ventilation (Fig. 9-21).

## Landmark and Incision

### Landmark
The *gluteal folds* are visible clearly on the buttock.

### Incision
Make a straight longitudinal incision about 20 cm long down the midline of the posterior aspect of the thigh. The incision should end proximally at the inferior margin of the gluteal fold, and its length will vary with surgical need (Fig. 9-23).

## Internervous Plane

The plane of dissection lies between the *lateral intermuscular septum*, which covers the *vastus lateralis* muscle (which is supplied by the femoral nerve), and the *biceps femoris* muscle (which is supplied by the sciatic nerve; Fig. 9-22).

## Superficial Surgical Dissection

Incise the deep fascia of the thigh in line with the skin incision, or lateral to it, taking care not to damage the posterior femoral cutaneous nerve, which runs longitudinally under the deep fascia (and roughly in line with the fascial incision), in the groove between the biceps and semitendinosus muscles (Fig. 9-24). Identify the lateral border of the biceps femoris in the proximal end of the wound by

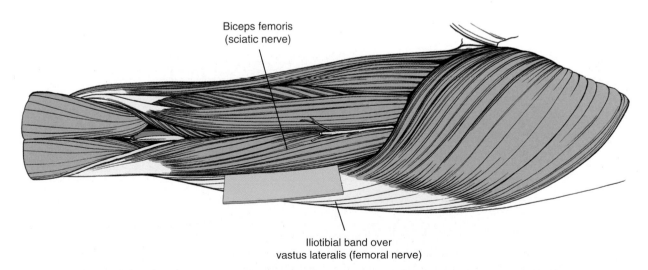

Biceps femoris
(sciatic nerve)

Iliotibial band over
vastus lateralis (femoral nerve)

**Figure 9-22**   The internervous plane lies between the vastus lateralis (which is supplied by the femoral nerve) and the biceps femoris (which is supplied by the sciatic nerve).

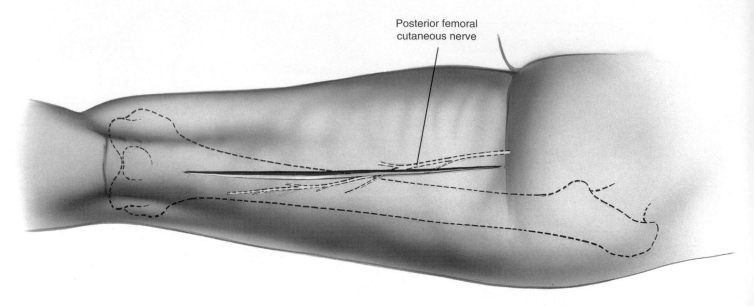

**Figure 9-23** Make a straight longitudinal incision in the midline of the posterior aspect of the thigh.

palpating it. Then, develop the plane between the biceps femoris and vastus lateralis muscles, which are covered by the lateral intermuscular septum (Fig. 9-25).

## Deep Surgical Dissection

Begin proximally. Retract the long head of the biceps femoris muscle medially and the lateral intermuscu-

lar septum laterally, developing the plane with a finger (see Fig. 9-25). Identify the short head of the biceps as it arises from the lateral lip of the linea aspera. Detach its origin from the femur by sharp dissection, and reflect it medially to expose the posterior aspect of the femur (Fig. 9-26).

In the distal half of the wound, retract the long head of the biceps laterally to expose the sciatic nerve (Fig. 9-27). Gently retract the sciatic nerve laterally

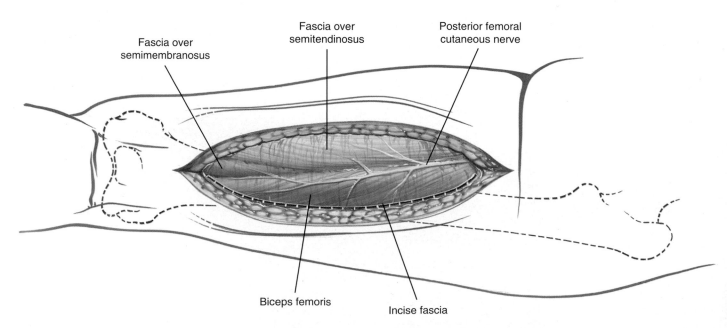

Fascia over semimembranosus

Fascia over semitendinosus

Posterior femoral cutaneous nerve

Biceps femoris

Incise fascia

**Figure 9-24** Incise the deep fascia of the thigh in line with the skin incision or just lateral to it, taking care not to damage the posterior femoral cutaneous nerve.

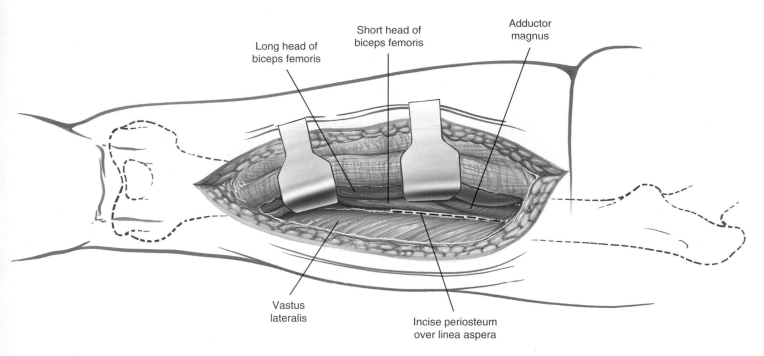

**Figure 9-25** Identify the lateral border of the biceps femoris; develop the plane between the biceps femoris and the vastus lateralis.

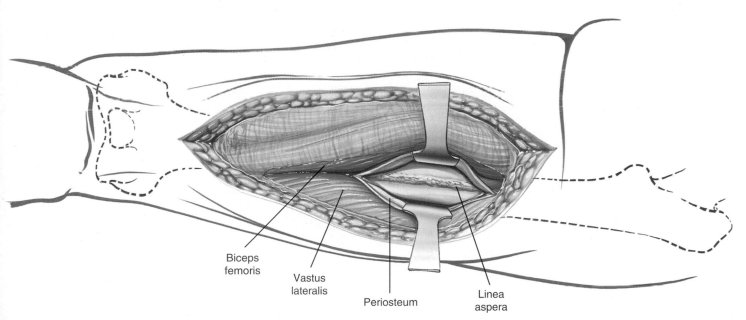

**Figure 9-26** Detach the origin of the short head of the biceps from the femur by sharp dissection, and reflect it medially to expose the posterior aspect of the femur.

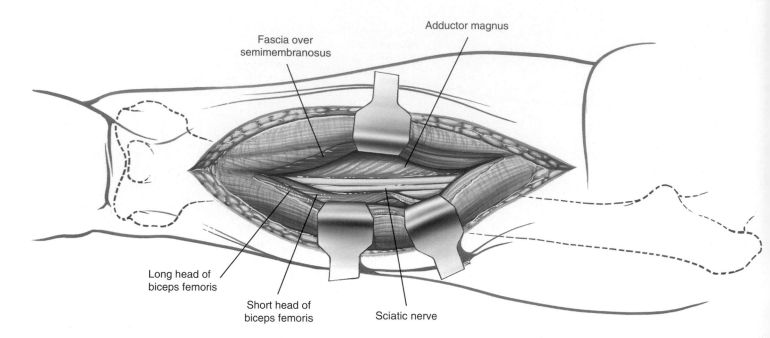

**Figure 9-27** Retract the long head of the biceps laterally to expose the sciatic nerve.

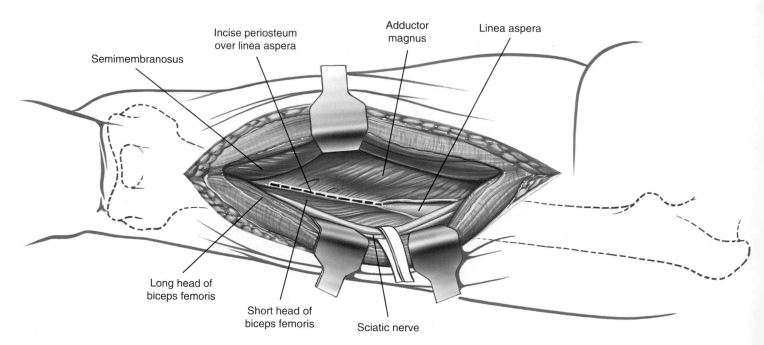

**Figure 9-28** Retract the sciatic nerve laterally to expose the posterior aspect of the femur. Incise the periosteum.

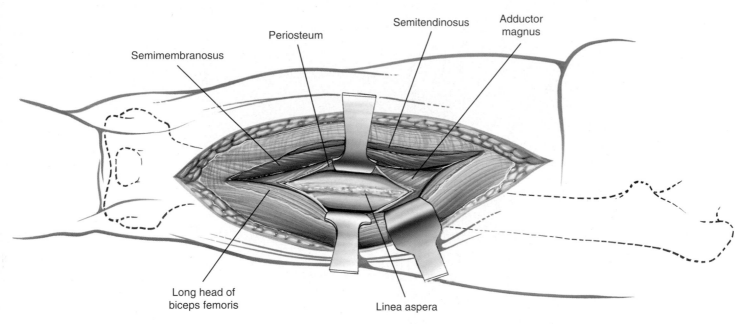

Semimembranosus  Periosteum   Semitendinosus   Adductor magnus

Long head of biceps femoris   Linea aspera

**Figure 9-29**   Develop the subperiosteal plane to expose the posterior aspect of the femur.

to reveal the posterior aspect of the femur, which is covered with periosteum (Fig. 9-28). Incise the periosteum longitudinally (Fig. 9-29; see Fig. 9-28).

## Dangers

### Nerves

The **sciatic nerve** courses down the back of the thigh in the posterior compartment. Because it lies medial to the biceps muscle in the upper part of the incision, it is protected from damage during the proximal part of the approach as long as the correct intermuscular plane is maintained. Distally, the nerve

must be identified and care taken not to retract it overzealously (see Fig. 9-36).

The **nerve to the biceps femoris** branches from the sciatic nerve and enters the biceps from its medial side well up in the thigh. Because the dissection is on the safe lateral side, the nerve cannot be damaged proximally.

## How to Enlarge the Approach

The approach cannot be extended usefully either superiorly or inferiorly. It is valuable solely for its exposure of the middle three fifths of the shaft of the femur.

# Applied Surgical Anatomy of the Thigh

## Overview

### Muscle Groups

There are three major muscle groups in the thigh (Figs. 9-30 through 9-32):

1. The adductors of the hip are supplied by the obturator nerve and occupy the medial segment of the thigh. The adductor magnus both adducts and extends the hip, and it has a dual nerve supply, the obturator and sciatic nerves.
2. The extensors of the knee are supplied by the femoral nerve and occupy the anterior segment of the thigh.

3. The flexors of the knee (which also extend the hip) are supplied by the sciatic nerve and lie in the posterior segment of the thigh.

The knee extensors are separated from the hip adductors by the thin medial intermuscular septum and from the knee flexors by the tough lateral intermuscular septum. The adductors and flexors are not separated by an intermuscular septum.

### Nerves

Three major nerves run down the thigh. The *obturator nerve*, which arises from the lumbar plexus (L2-4), runs in the adductor group, supplying all these muscles.

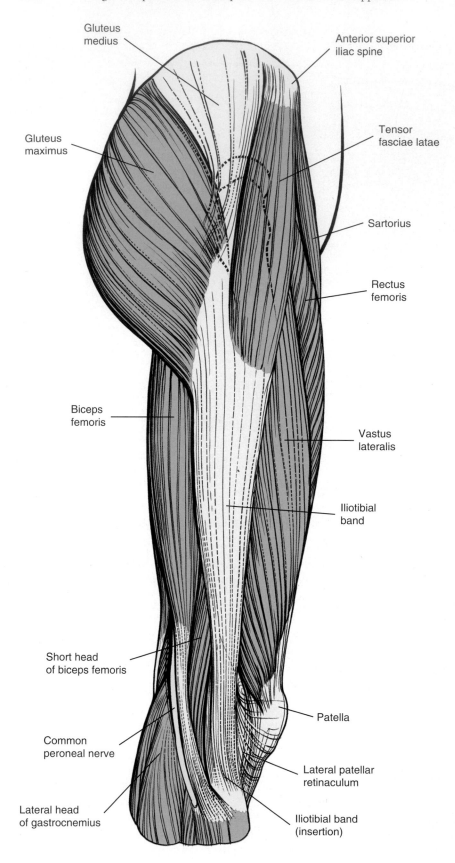

**Figure 9-30**   The superficial musculature of the lateral aspect of the thigh. The iliotibial band (tract) overlies the vastus lateralis proximally.

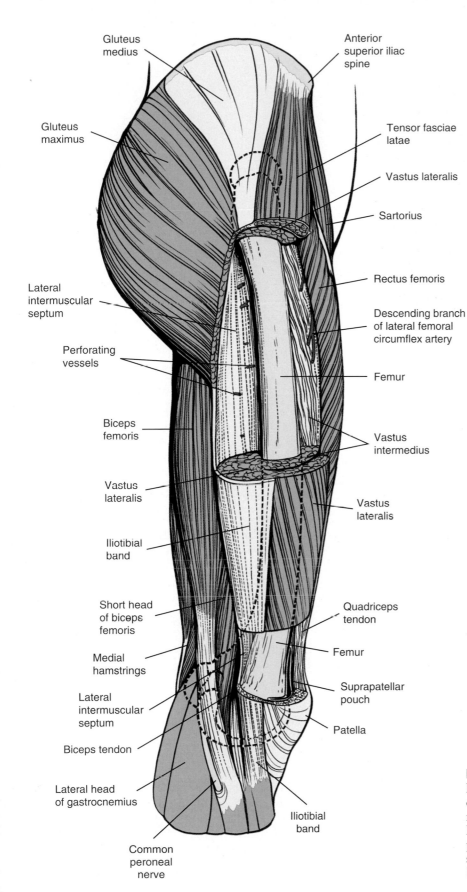

Gluteus medius

Gluteus maximus

Lateral intermuscular septum

Perforating vessels

Biceps femoris

Vastus lateralis

Iliotibial band

Short head of biceps femoris

Medial hamstrings

Lateral intermuscular septum

Biceps tendon

Lateral head of gastrocnemius

Common peroneal nerve

Anterior superior iliac spine

Tensor fasciae latae

Vastus lateralis

Sartorius

Rectus femoris

Descending branch of lateral femoral circumflex artery

Femur

Vastus intermedius

Vastus lateralis

Quadriceps tendon

Femur

Suprapatellar pouch

Patella

Iliotibial band

**Figure 9-31** The tensor fasciae latae, the vastus lateralis, and a portion of the vastus intermedius have been resected to reveal the femur and the lateral intermuscular septum. Note the perforating vessels as they pierce the septum. Note that the vastus lateralis bulges posteriorly.

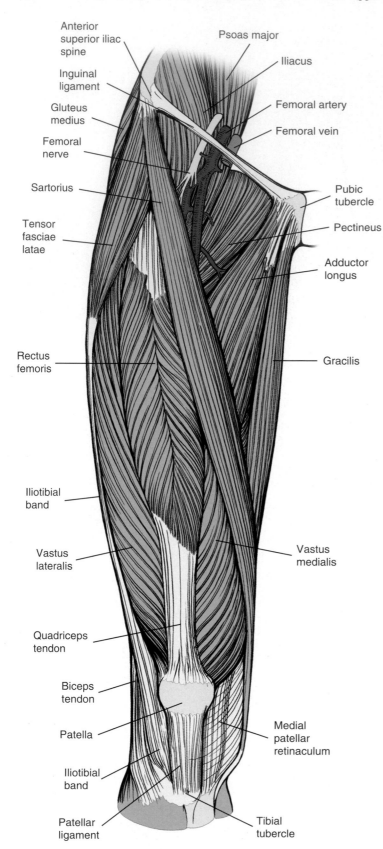

Anterior superior iliac spine

Inguinal ligament

Gluteus medius

Femoral nerve

Sartorius

Tensor fasciae latae

Rectus femoris

Iliotibial band

Vastus lateralis

Quadriceps tendon

Biceps tendon

Patella

Iliotibial band

Patellar ligament

Psoas major

Iliacus

Femoral artery

Femoral vein

Pubic tubercle

Pectineus

Adductor longus

Gracilis

Vastus medialis

Medial patellar retinaculum

Tibial tubercle

**Figure 9-32**   The superficial musculature of the anterior aspect of the thigh.

**Rectus Femoris.** *Origin.* Reflected head from just above acetabulum and anterior capsule of hip joint; straight head from anterior inferior iliac spine. *Insertion.* Upper border of patella, tibial tubercle. *Action.* Powerful extensor of knee and weak flexor of hip. *Nerve supply.* Femoral nerve (L2-L4).

The *sciatic nerve*, which arises from the lumbosacral plexus (L4-5, S1-3), lies in the posterior segment of the thigh, supplying the hamstrings and the extensor portion of the adductor magnus. Running deep to the long head of the biceps and lying on the adductor magnus, it ends up medial to the biceps as the muscle crosses from the ischial tuberosity toward the head of the fibula (see Fig. 9-36).

The *femoral nerve*, which is a branch of the lumbar plexus (L2-4), divides into its branches soon after entering the thigh and supplies all the extensors of the knee (Fig. 9-33).

## Vessels

The *femoral artery* is the artery of transit through the thigh. Its major branch, the profunda femoris artery, is the main blood supply of the thigh musculature. After the femoral artery gives off the profunda femoris artery in the femoral triangle, it gives off no other major branches of importance in the thigh (Fig. 9-34).

The femoral artery actually enters the thigh under the inguinal ligament at the midinguinal point, directly over the head of the femur. That is why the femoral pulse is the surface marking of the femoral head. The artery then travels distally on the iliopsoas muscle and disappears at the bottom of the femoral triangle beneath the sartorius muscle, running on the adductor longus muscle. There, the artery lies in a depression known as the subsartorial canal of Hunter. The canal runs between the extensor and adductor compartments of the thigh and is roofed by a thick fascial layer and the sartorius muscle. The posterior wall is formed by the adductor muscles (the adductor longus superiorly and the adductor magnus inferiorly), and the anterior wall is formed by the vastus medialis muscle. Running with the artery in the canal is the saphenous nerve (a cutaneous nerve that is derived from the femoral nerve), the femoral vein, and, in the upper half, the nerve to the vastus medialis muscle.

The femoral artery ultimately pierces the adductor magnus muscle one handbreadth above the knee to join the sciatic nerve in the popliteal fossa before entering the posterior compartments of the thigh. There, it lies deep and medial to the sciatic nerve (see Fig. 9-36).

The femoral artery is lateral to the femoral vein in the femoral triangle, but medial to it in the popliteal fossa, perhaps as a result of the rotation of the limb that occurs during fetal development.

The artery also changes position in relation to the femur; it is anterior to it at its upper end, medial to it in its middle portion, and behind it at its lower end. These changes influence not only the planning of approaches, but also the insertion of skeletal pins for traction and the application of external fixative devices.

The *profunda femoris artery* supplies the thigh musculature. It arises from the femoral artery in the femoral triangle, coming off its lateral side before passing behind it quickly. The two arteries then leave the femoral triangle. The profunda femoris artery passes behind the adductor longus muscle, whereas the femoral artery passes anterior to it. Thus, the muscle is sandwiched between the two arteries (Fig. 9-35; see Fig. 9-34).

Four of the perforating branches of the profunda femoris artery pass posteriorly through the medial compartment of the thigh. They wind around the femur just as the medial femoral circumflex artery does and enter the anterior compartment again by piercing the lateral intermuscular septum. They must be ligated at that point in the posterolateral approach to the femur (see Fig. 9-34).

The *medial femoral circumflex artery* passes between the iliopsoas and pectineus muscles to lie on the upper border of the adductor longus muscle. From there, it winds around the interval between the quadratus femoris and adductor magnus muscles, where it divides. The ascending branch runs along the superior border of the quadratus femoris, where it may be cut in posterior approaches to the hip, causing troublesome bleeding. The horizontal branch passes between the quadratus femoris and the adductor magnus to form one limb of the cruciate anastomosis (see Fig. 9-34).

The *lateral femoral circumflex artery* passes lateral to the rectus femoris muscle, where it appears in the upper part of the anterolateral approach. There, it divides into three branches:

1. The ascending branch runs upward toward the anterior superior iliac spine in the intermuscular interval between the sartorius and tensor fasciae latae muscles. There, it requires ligation in the anterior approach to the hip.
2. The transverse branch continues to wind around the femur and joins the transverse branch of the medial femoral circumflex, contributing to the cruciate anastomosis.
3. The descending branch passes along the interval between the vastus intermedius and vastus lateralis muscles, where it is encountered in the anterolateral approach to the femur (see Fig. 9-34).

The *saphenous vein* arises on the dorsum of the ankle at the medial end of the dorsal venous arch. Passing anterior to the medial malleolus (where it can be found during cutdown for the insertion of intravenous lines), it passes behind the knee before spiraling forward on the medial side of the thigh into

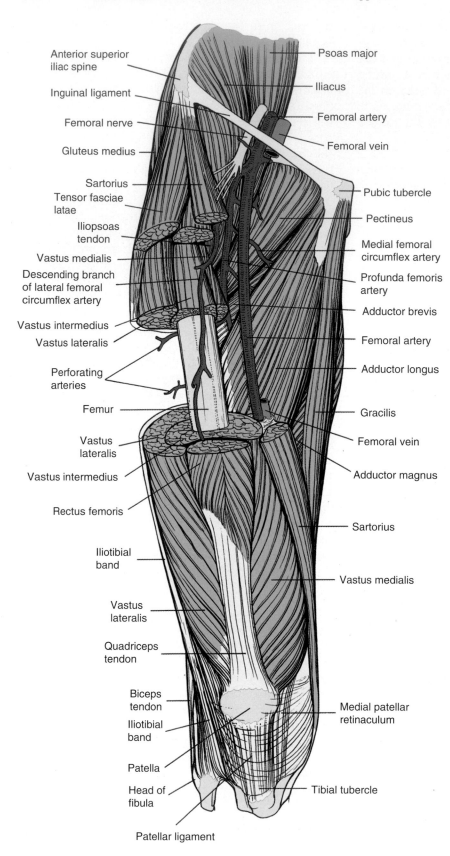

Anterior superior iliac spine

Inguinal ligament

Femoral nerve

Gluteus medius

Sartorius

Tensor fasciae latae

Iliopsoas tendon

Vastus medialis

Descending branch of lateral femoral circumflex artery

Vastus intermedius

Vastus lateralis

Perforating arteries

Femur

Vastus lateralis

Vastus intermedius

Rectus femoris

Iliotibial band

Vastus lateralis

Quadriceps tendon

Biceps tendon

Iliotibial band

Patella

Head of fibula

Patellar ligament

Psoas major

Iliacus

Femoral artery

Femoral vein

Pubic tubercle

Pectineus

Medial femoral circumflex artery

Profunda femoris artery

Adductor brevis

Femoral artery

Adductor longus

Gracilis

Femoral vein

Adductor magnus

Sartorius

Vastus medialis

Medial patellar retinaculum

Tibial tubercle

**Figure 9-33**   The sartorius, the rectus femoris, the tensor fasciae latae, the vastus lateralis, and the vastus intermedius have been resected to reveal the course of the femoral and profunda femoris arteries; note the relationship of the arteries to the quadriceps and the adductor muscles.

**Vastus Lateralis.** *Origin.* Upper half of intertrochanteric line. Vastus lateralis ridge, lateral lip of linea aspera, and upper two thirds of lateral supracondylar line of femur. Also from lateral intermuscular septum. *Insertion.* Lateral border of patella and tibial tubercle. *Action.* Extensor of knee. *Nerve supply.* Femoral nerve (L2-L4).
**Vastus Intermedius.** *Origin.* Anterior and lateral aspect of upper two thirds of femoral shaft. *Insertion.* Tibial tubercle. *Action.* Extensor of knee. *Nerve supply.* Femoral nerve (L2-L4).
**Vastus Medialis.** *Origin.* Medial lip of linea aspera and spiral line of femur. *Insertion.* Tibial tubercle and medial border of patella. *Action.* Extensor of knee. *Nerve supply.* Femoral nerve (L2-L4).

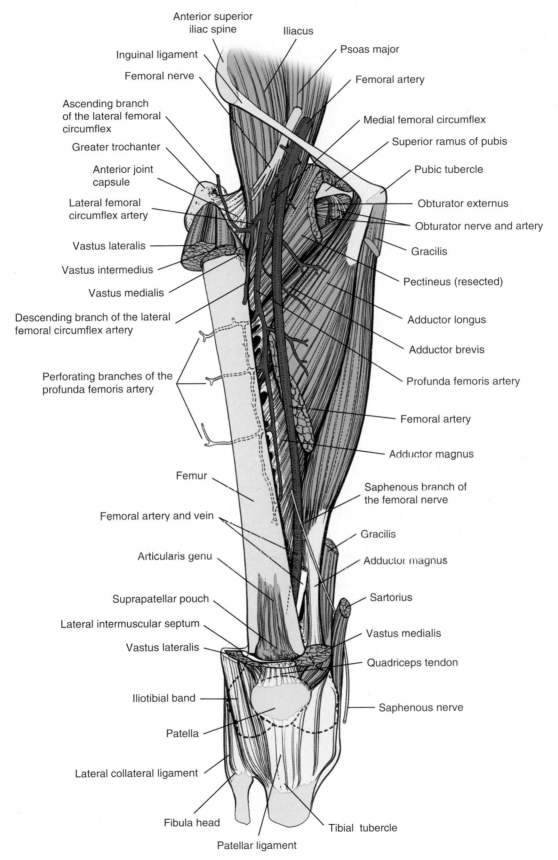

**Figure 9-34** The complete course of the femoral artery and profunda femoris artery. Note the perforating branches of the profunda femoris artery. Note that the adductor longus muscle has been resected to show the course of the profunda femoris artery, which runs posterior to it.

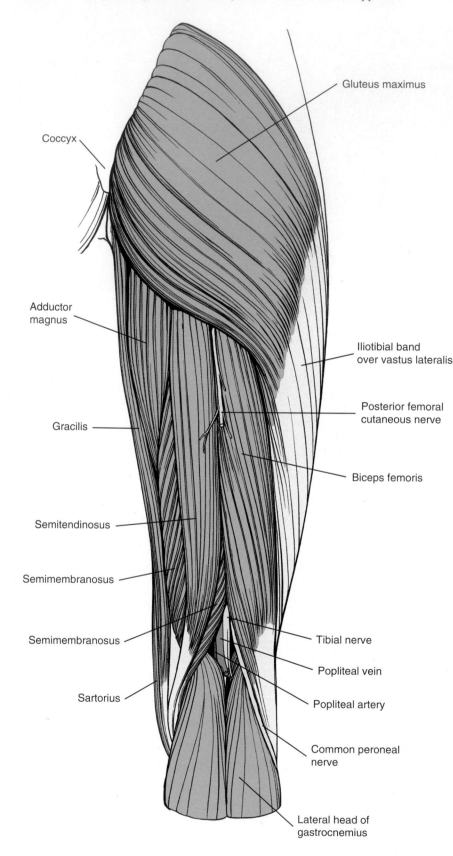

Coccyx

Adductor magnus

Gracilis

Semitendinosus

Semimembranosus

Semimembranosus

Sartorius

Gluteus maximus

Iliotibial band over vastus lateralis

Posterior femoral cutaneous nerve

Biceps femoris

Tibial nerve

Popliteal vein

Popliteal artery

Common peroneal nerve

Lateral head of gastrocnemius

**Figure 9-35**  The superficial musculature of the posterior aspect of the thigh. Note the central course of the posterior femoral cutaneous nerve.

**Biceps Femoris.** *Origin.* Long head from ischial tuberosity. Short head from linea aspera and lateral supracondylar line of femur. *Insertion.* Head of fibula. *Action.* Flexor of knee, extensor of hip, and lateral rotator of leg. *Nerve supply.* Long head: sciatic nerve (tibial division) (L5, S1, S2). Short head: sciatic nerve (common peroneal division (S1-S2).

**Semimembranosus.** *Origin.* Ischial tuberosity. *Insertion.* Medial condyle of tibia. *Action.* Weak extensor of hip, flexor of knee, and medial rotator of leg. *Nerve supply.* Tibial nerve (L5, S1, S2).

**Semitendinosus.** *Origin.* Ischial tuberosity (common origin with biceps femoris). *Insertion.* Subcutaneous surface of tibia. *Action.* Flexor of knee, extensor of hip, and medial rotator of leg. *Nerve supply.* Tibial nerve (L5, S1, S2).

the femoral vein. The saphenous vein is the major superficial vein of the thigh, but although it frequently is the object of general surgical procedures, it has little importance for the orthopaedic surgeon.

## Landmark and Incisions

### Landmark

Most of the *femur* is cloaked deeply in muscle; only the greater trochanter and the femoral condyles are easily palpable. The femur has a natural anterior bow, which is important for the design of intramedullary rods.

The angle between the femoral shaft and the femoral neck varies, but usually is about 130°. The femoral neck is displaced about 15° in anteversion on the femoral shaft. These angles should be borne in mind when pins or nails are inserted up the femoral neck.

### Incisions

Longitudinal incisions in the thigh parallel the lines of cleavage of the skin; the resultant scars usually are cosmetically acceptable.

## Superficial and Deep Surgical Dissection

Four of the approaches to the femur penetrate the knee extensor compartment. (The posterior approach penetrates the hamstring compartment and is considered separately.)

The knee extensor compartment consists of a single muscle that arises from four heads and inserts through the extensor apparatus of the knee into the tibial tubercle. This muscle, the quadriceps femoris, is the largest muscle in the body. It is supplied by the femoral nerve (Fig. 9-36; see Figs. 9-32 through 9-34).

Different muscle elements in the quadriceps group contract differently. Because the gliding that occurs between muscle elements is so vital to function, any incision that penetrates the muscle may endanger its efficacy. The distal third of the quadriceps is free to glide over the anterior aspect of the femur, because no part of the muscle is attached to that part of the bone.

The four heads of the quadratus femoris are as follows:

1. *Rectus femoris.* The rectus femoris is bipinnate in structure, like the feathers of an arrow. It is the only part of the quadriceps that crosses two joints, the hip and knee, as it descends the thigh over the vastus intermedius. Its ability to slide over the vastus intermedius during movement of the knee is the result of the presence of a thick fascial layer on its underside. Because its origins are so close to the hip joint, both heads of the rectus femoris must be detached to allow access to the anterior aspect of the hip and to the inner and outer walls of the pelvis at the upper margin of the acetabulum.

2. *Vastus lateralis.* The plane between the lateral intermuscular septum and the vastus lateralis is difficult to define, and dissection is bloody, mainly because the muscle arises in part from the septum itself. Following the plane between the lateral intermuscular septum and the muscle leads to the posterior aspect of the femur at the linea aspera (the origin of the muscle) and not onto the lateral aspect of the bone. The plane is defined most easily and is most useful in the distal third of the femur.

   The vastus lateralis glides on the vastus intermedius during movement. As is true for the rectus femoris, its deep surface is covered with a thick fascial attachment.

3. *Vastus intermedius.* The vastus intermedius cloaks the anterior and lateral aspects of the upper two thirds of the femoral shaft and forms the innermost layer of the quadriceps. This muscle is split during most approaches to the femur.

4. *Vastus medialis.* The nerve supply of the vastus medialis is the largest branch of the femoral nerve, a branch that contains a large number of proprioceptive fibers. When trauma affects the knee, fibers of the vastus medialis that attach to the patella tend to lose tone quickly, possibly because of a neuromuscular reflex mediated via the nerve to the vastus medialis. Wasting of these muscle fibers produces a subjective sense of instability that persists until the muscle bulk returns to normal. Therefore, rehabilitating the vastus medialis is vital in the treatment of any knee injury.

The lowest fibers of the vastus medialis insert into the patella, pulling it medially. They are crucial in preventing lateral subluxation of the patella during flexion of the knee.

## Posterior Approach to the Femur

The posterior approach involves dissection of the posterior compartment of the thigh (see Figs. 8-39 and 8-40). The key to the approach lies in understanding the anatomy of the sciatic nerve and its relationship to the biceps femoris muscle.[5]

The sciatic nerve runs vertically down the thigh more or less in a straight line. The biceps femoris muscle angles across the posterior aspect of the thigh

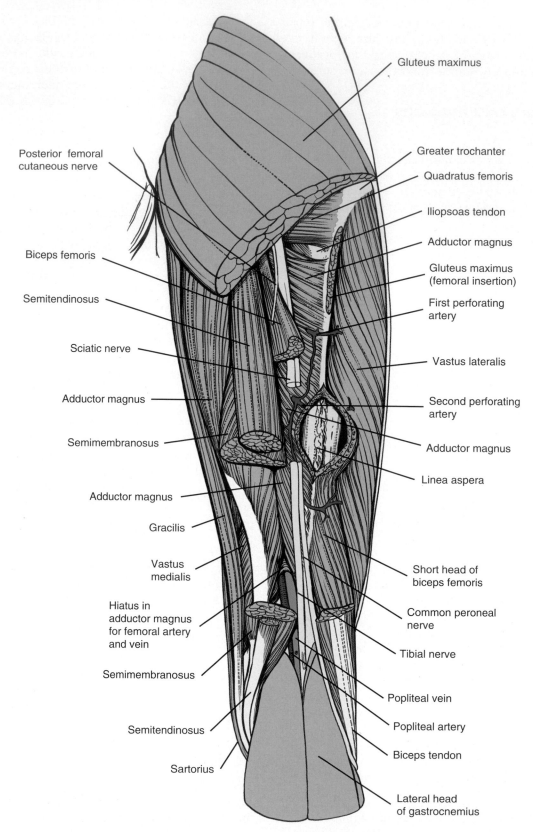

**Figure 9-36**   The course of the sciatic nerve and the anatomic location of the linea aspera. The gluteus maximus and hamstring muscles are resected.

in a medial to lateral direction, forming a bridge under which the sciatic nerve runs. The nerve, therefore, lies underneath the biceps femoris in the proximal thigh and lateral to it in the distal thigh. Hence, during exposure of the proximal half of the posterior aspect of the bone, the biceps should be retracted medially, taking with it and protecting the sciatic nerve. For more distal exposures, the biceps requires retraction laterally, and the nerve must be retracted with it. If a wide exposure of the whole length of this piece of the bone is required, the long head of the biceps should be divided; the proximal half of the muscle, together with the short head, should be retracted medially with the sciatic nerve.

The three hamstring muscles arise from the ischium and run down the posterior compartment of the thigh. All cross two joints, the hip and the knee, and all act as hip extensors and knee flexors. The hamstring muscles are supplied by branches of the sciatic nerve.

### Semimembranosus Muscle

The insertions of the semimembranosus muscle greatly reinforce the posterior and posteromedial joint capsule of the knee (see Applied Surgical Anatomy of the Medial Side of the Knee in Chapter 10). The muscle may be transferred to the anterior surface of the lateral femoral condyle, together with the semitendinosus tendon, to correct internal rotation deformity of the hip in patients with a variety of neurologic lesions, a technique that is used only rarely.[6]

### Semitendinosus Muscle

As its name implies, the semitendinosus muscle has an extremely long tendon in relation to the size of its muscle belly. The tendon is at least 13 cm long and can be used in a variety of surgical procedures. It may be left attached to the tibia, even as it is attached via a drill hole to the patella, to hold that bone medially in cases of recurrent dislocation.[7] It also may be used for posterior[8] and anterior[9] cruciate reconstruction; in that procedure, the tendon is separated from the muscle at the musculotendinous junction and is threaded through the femur so that it mimics the function of the missing cruciate ligaments. In addition, it may be used to reinforce a torn medial collateral knee ligament.

## Minimal Access Approach to the Proximal Femur

The minimal access approach to the proximal femur is used for the insertion of intramedullary nails for the treatment of the following:

1. Acute femoral shaft fractures
2. Pathological femoral shaft fractures
3. Delayed union and nonunion of femoral shaft fractures

The entry point for the insertion of an intramedullary nail into the femur is determined radiographically. It depends on the design of the nail and the anatomy of the proximal femur in the individual patient. The majority of intramedullary nails are straight when viewed in the anterior-posterior plane. The nail should be inserted so that its entry point into the bone is exactly in line with the intramedullary canal on both anterior-posterior and lateral radiographs. The use of preoperative templates overlying radiographs allows for a precise calculation of the entry point. The nearest anatomical landmark to this entry point is the piriform fossa, but it cannot be used reliably in all patients because it does not always line up with the intramedullary canal in both planes. In addition, the fossa cannot be palpated because of overlying musculature.

For nails that are straight when viewed in the anterior-posterior plane, the skin incision, the entry point of the nail in the bone, and the medullary canal of the femur should all be in a straight line.

Some nails are angled at their upper end and require insertion via the tip of the greater trochanter. These nails require a skin incision directly over the tip of the greater trochanter.

### Position of the Patient

Two positions are available for the insertion of femoral nails. The supine position allows easier control of fracture reduction and distal locking of the nail (Fig. 9-37). The lateral position allows easier access to the entry point in the proximal end of the femur.

#### Supine Position

Place the patient supine on a traction table. Employ traction using a supracondylar femoral pin or a trac-

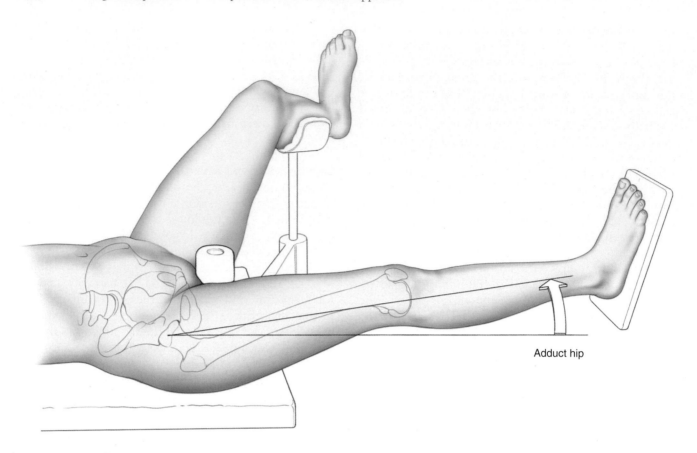

**Figure 9-37**   Place the patient supine on the traction table. Reduce the fracture by traction and manipulation. Adduct the leg as much as possible around the traction pole. Abduct and flex the opposite hip to allow c-arm access to the whole of the femur.

tion boot. Adduct the leg as much as possible around the traction post to make it anatomically possible to enter the upper end of the femur via the skin on the lateral aspect of the buttock. Laterally flex the trunk of the patient away from the operative side. Flex and abduct the opposite hip and flex the knee, placing the leg in a support (see Figs. 9-37 and 9-38*A*). Ensure that adequate anterior-posterior and lateral radiographs of the entry point of the nail and the fracture site can be obtained. Be sure that the fracture is reduced or reducible before commencing surgery. Although this may be time-consuming, it is important to obtain good-quality radiographs before commencing surgery, or you will struggle to obtain quality imaging during the case. Five minutes of preoperative time may shorten your operating time by 2 hours.

In proximal femoral shaft fractures, the proximal fragment will flex and abduct due to the unopposed pull of the psoas and the abductor muscles. Displaced proximal femoral fractures cannot be reduced by traction alone. Control of the proximal fragment frequently requires percutaneous insertion of a Stein-

mann pin into the proximal fragment, allowing its manipulation.

Inserting a nail in a very obese patient cannot be done successfully in the supine position (Fig. 9-38).

**Lateral Position**

Place the patient in a lateral position on a traction table with the affected limb uppermost. Apply traction to the femur through a distal supracondylar pin or a plaster boot. Adduct the leg over the traction pole. Place the contralateral limb in a flexed position at both hip and knee. Take care to pad the bony prominences of the bottom leg to prevent skin breakdown due to pressure. Ensure that adequate anterior-posterior and lateral radiographs of the entry point and the fracture site can be obtained. The fracture must be reduced or reducible before commencing surgery. Proximal femoral fractures will require ancillary modes of reduction (Steinmann pins) (see Supine Position above).

The lateral position allows easier access to the proximal femur than the supine position because it allows more adduction, which is particularly useful in

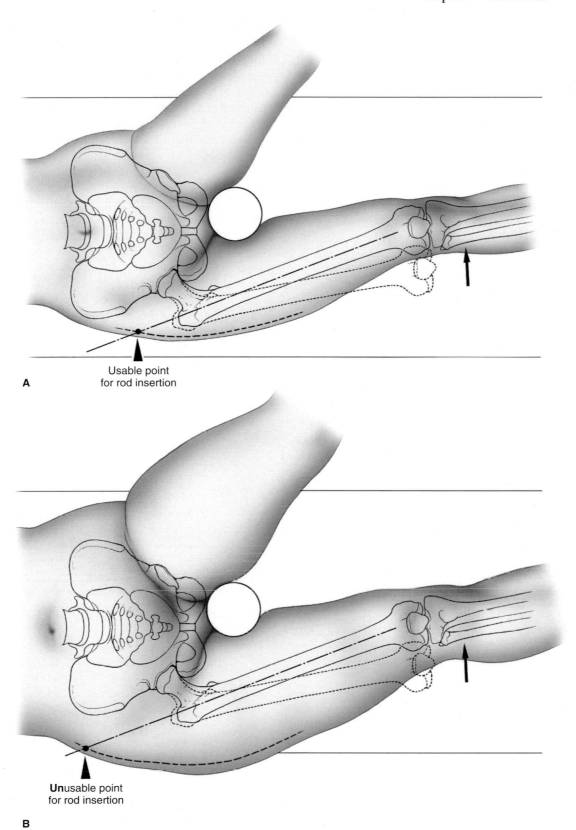

**A**

Usable point
for rod insertion

**B**

Unusable point
for rod insertion

**Figure 9-38** **(A)** Adducting the leg moves the skin incision distally. **(B)** In obese patients, nailing in this supine position is impossible. Note that even with maximal adduction, the ideal incision lies above the iliac crest.

obese patients. In cases of extreme obesity, even this position may not permit successful intramedullary nailing; such patients are probably best treated by a retrograde nailing technique with an entry point into the bone in the intercondylar notch.

## Landmarks and Incision

### Landmarks

The *greater trochanter* is a large mass of bone that projects upward and backward from the junction of the shaft of the femur and its neck (see Fig. 8-40).

The *anterior superior iliac spine* can be felt as the anterior margin of the iliac crest (see Fig. 8-40).

The *shaft of the femur* can be felt as resistance through the massive vastus lateralis muscle on the lateral side of the thigh.

### Incision

There are two techniques for planning the correct placement of the incision.

*Radiographic Technique.* Palpate the shaft of the femur on the lateral aspect of the thigh through the bulk of the vastus lateralis muscle. With a marker pen, draw a line on the skin, marking the lateral aspect of the shaft of the femur (Fig. 9-39). This line is curved because the femur is bowed anteriorly when viewed in the lateral plane. Extend this gently curving line proximal to the tip of the greater trochanter, up to the level of the iliac crest (Fig. 9-40).

Place a long guidewire, such as a reaming guidewire, on the anterior aspect of the thigh. Using radiographic control, ensure that the guidewire is overlying the center of the medullary canal when viewed in the anterior-posterior plane (Fig. 9-41).

Take a long artery forceps and move it proximally along the line you have drawn on the skin. Screen this instrument using an image intensifier in the anterior-posterior planes (see Fig. 9-41). When the image of the tip of the forceps coincides with the guidewire radiographically, mark the skin (see Fig. 9-41). This skin mark will be the center of the skin

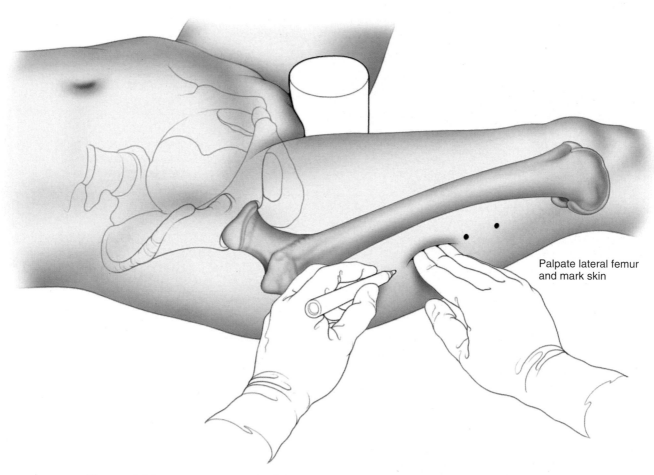

Palpate lateral femur and mark skin

**Figure 9-39**   Palpate the shaft of the femur through the vastus lateralis muscle. Draw a line on the skin, marking the line of the shaft of the femur. Note that this line is curved.

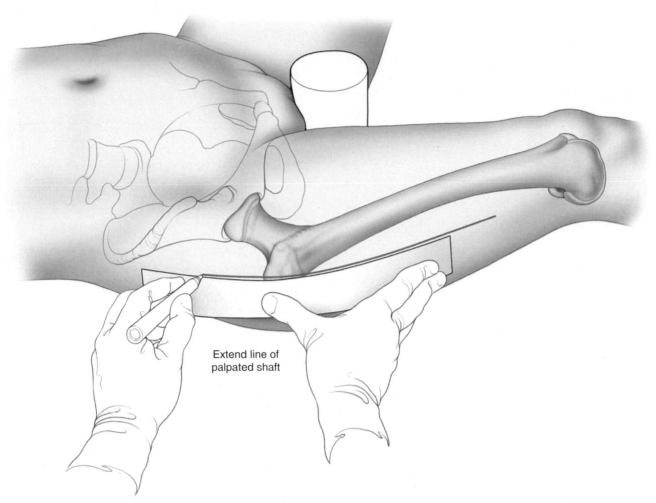

Extend line of
palpated shaft

**Figure 9-40**   Extend the drawn line above the tip of the greater trochanter to the level of the anterior superior iliac spine.

incision. A wire inserted through this incision and through the correct entry point in the bone will pass perfectly down the center of the medullary canal of the femur in both anterior-posterior and lateral planes.

If the patient is obese and/or you are unable to adduct the leg, then this entry point will be above the level of the iliac crest (see Fig. 9-38*B*). Such an entry point is clearly not usable. If this is the case, then alternative techniques using curved instrumentation will need to be used through a more proximally based incision.

*Landmark Technique.* Palpate the shaft of the femur through the bulk of the vastus lateralis muscle. With a marker pen, draw a curved line on the skin of the lateral aspect of the thigh, marking the shaft of the femur (see Fig. 9-39). Extend this line proximally beyond the tip of the greater trochanter, curving it slightly posteriorly.

Palpate the anterior superior iliac spine. Draw a line perpendicularly downward from the iliac spine toward the buttock. The incision should be centered at the point where these two lines cross (Fig. 9-42).

### Incision

Make a longitudinal incision centered on the skin mark. The size of the incision depends on the type of nail to be used. Nails that have proximal interlocking jigs that are considerably offset from the nail can be inserted through a 3-cm incision. Nails whose proximal jigs attach close to the nail require a longer skin incision (up to 7 cm).

### Internervous Plane

There is no internervous plane or intramuscular plane. The dissection splits fibers of the gluteus maximus and gluteus medius but does not denervate either muscle.

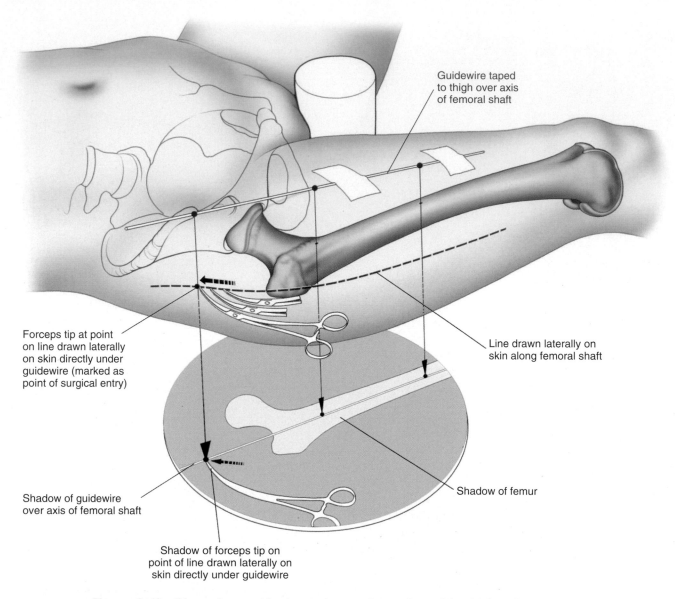

Guidewire taped
to thigh over axis
of femoral shaft

Forceps tip at point
on line drawn laterally
on skin directly under
guidewire (marked as
point of surgical entry)

Line drawn laterally on
skin along femoral shaft

Shadow of femur

Shadow of guidewire
over axis of femoral shaft

Shadow of forceps tip on
point of line drawn laterally on
skin directly under guidewire

**Figure 9-41**    Place a long guidewire on the anterior surface of the thigh and position it under image intensifier control so that its image overlies the center of the medullary canal of the femur. Take a long artery forceps and move it proximally along the drawn line on the lateral aspect of the thigh. When the image of the forceps coincides with the image of the guidewire radiographically, mark the skin.

## Superficial Surgical Dissection

Incise the subcutaneous fat and the fascia overlying the gluteus maximus in line with the incision. Split the fibers of gluteus maximus for 3 cm in the line of its fibers using a curved clamp.

## Deep Surgical Dissection

Continue the dissection distally using a long curved clamp to split the fibers of the gluteus medius muscle

to gain access to the proximal femur. Careful use of a finger as a blunt dissector to identify the medial aspect of the greater trochanter is often helpful as well. Insert a marker wire (or rod) through the completed dissection onto the proximal end of the femur, and adjust the position of the wire using X-ray control in both anterior-posterior and lateral planes until the wire is at the correct entry point into the bone. The wire must line up with the intramedullary canal on both anterior-posterior and lateral planes (Figs. 9-43 and 9-44).

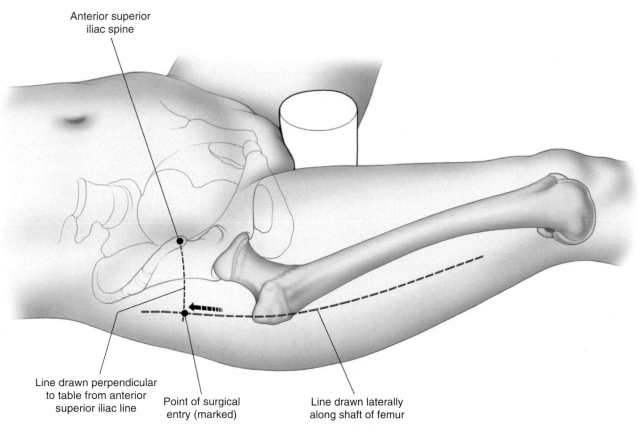

Anterior superior
iliac spine

Line drawn perpendicular
to table from anterior
superior iliac line

Point of surgical
entry (marked)

Line drawn laterally
along shaft of femur

**Figure 9-42**   Landmark technique. Draw a line perpendicularly downwards from the anterior superior iliac spine. Where this line crosses the previously drawn line on the lateral aspect of the thigh, mark the skin.

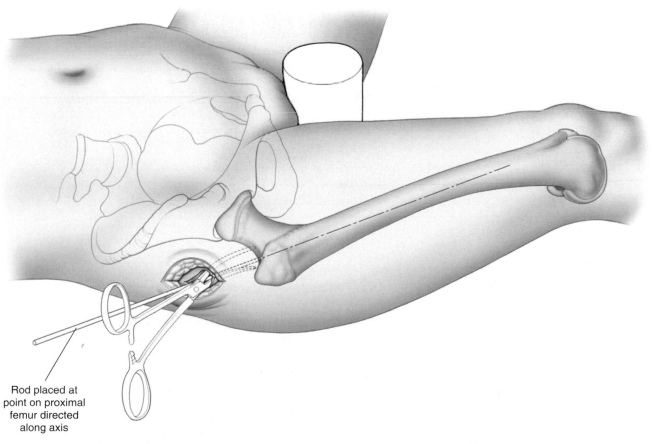

Rod placed at
point on proximal
femur directed
along axis

**Figure 9-43**   Split the fibers of the gluteus maximus in line with the skin incision. Deepen the incision down to the femur by splitting the fibers of the gluteus medius.

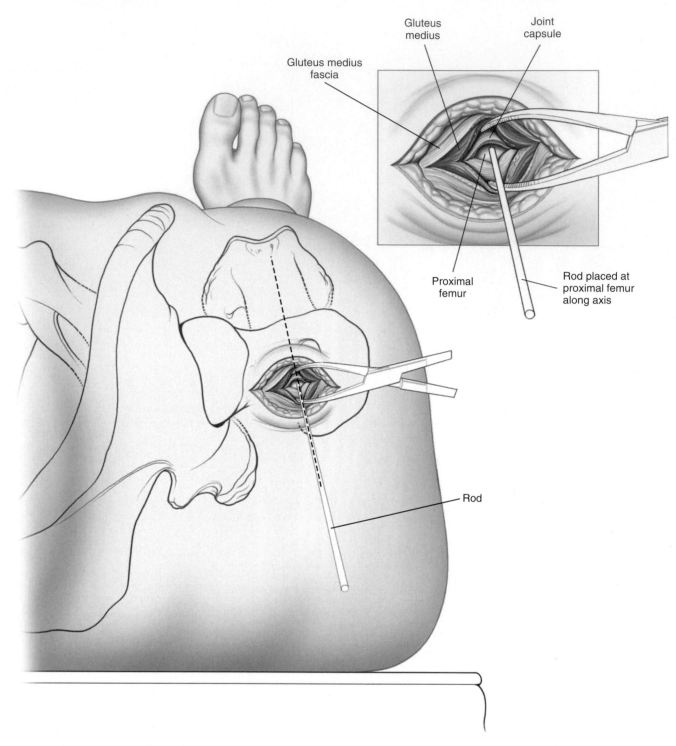

**Figure 9-44**    Insert a guidewire (or rod) into proximal femur, checking its position in both A-P and lateral planes using a c-arm.

The exact techniques for entering the proximal femur vary from nail to nail. You must consult the appropriate literature to ensure that the instrumentation is used correctly.

## Dangers

### Bone Deformity

The presence of an incorrect entry point is potentially hazardous in intramedullary nailing of the femur.

An entry point that is too far lateral commonly occurs. This will create a *varus deformity* at the fracture site if the nail used is rigid. Lateral entry points may also create an iatrogenic fracture of the medial femoral cortex during nail insertion.

An entry point that is too far medial may create an iatrogenic fracture of the femoral neck, usually a vertical basicervical fracture. On occasion, medial entry points may also damage the blood supply to the femoral head, creating avascular necrosis.

### Nerves

The *superior gluteal nerve* runs posteriorly to anteriorly through the substance of the gluteus medius muscle 3 to 5 cm above the tip of the greater trochanter. If the femur is adducted, the nerve will not be damaged during insertion of a nail. If, however, a retrograde nailing technique is used when the femur is not necessarily abducted, then damage to the nerve may occur.

## How to Enlarge the Approach

This approach cannot be usefully enlarged proximally or distally because it does not utilize an internervous plane.

## REFERENCES

1. MARCY GH: The posterolateral approach to the femur. J Bone Joint Surg 29:676, 1947
2. THOMPSON JE: Anatomical methods of approach in operations on the long bones of the extremities. Ann Surg 68:309, 1918
3. HENRY AK: Exposure of the humerus and femoral shaft. Br J Surg 12:84, 1924
4. BOSWORTH DM: Posterior approach to the femur. J Bone Joint Surg 26:687, 1944
5. GRAY H: Anatomy of the human body, 27th ed. Goss CM, ed. Philadelphia, Lea & Febiger, 1959:1049
6. SUTHERLAND DH ET AL: Clinical and electromyographic study of seven spastic children with internal rotation gait. J Bone Joint Surg [Am] 51:1070, 1969
7. GALBAZZI R: Nuove applicazion del trapianto muscolare e tendineo (XII Congress Societa Italiana di Ortopedia). In: Archivo di Ortopedia, 1922:38
8. KENNEDY JC, GRAINGER RW: The posterior cruciate ligament. J Trauma 7:357, 1967
9. CITO KO: Reconstruction of the anterior cruciate ligament by semitendinosus tenodesis. J Bone Joint Surg [Am] 57:605, 1975

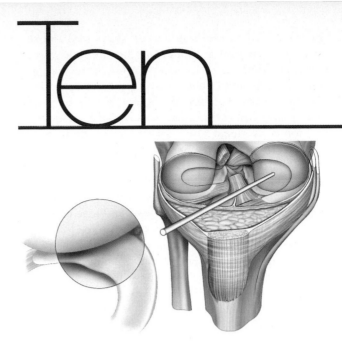

# Ten

# The Knee

The knee is a synovial hinge joint, supported and stabilized by powerful muscular and ligamentous forces. It is superficial on three sides (anterior, medial, and lateral), and approaches to it are comparatively straightforward. Because the knee joint is only covered by skin and retinaculae on three of its four sides, the joint is ideal for arthroscopic approaches. Arthroscopy of the knee is also facilitated by the large size of the joint cavity. Arthroscopic approaches have largely replaced open surgical approaches for the treatment of meniscal pathology, anterior cruciate ligament reconstruction, and removal of loose bodies.

Two *arthroscopic approaches* are described that allow complete exploration of the knee joint.

Seven open approaches to the knee are described. These approaches are useful where arthroscopic equipment is not available. They are also of great importance when dealing with trauma of the knee joint associated with open wounds. Because the major neurovascular structures of the leg all pass posterior to the joint, the posterior approach is used mainly for exploration of these structures.

The *medial parapatellar approach*, the most common knee incision, can be used for a variety of procedures. The length of the incision depends on the pathology to be treated; when it is used fully, this approach gives an unrivaled exposure of the whole joint. It is suitable for total joint replacement.

The *approach for medial meniscectomy* is much more restricted. The introduction of the operative arthroscope has limited its use.

The *medial approach to the knee joint* affords easier access to the medial supporting structures of the knee. Because of its slightly more posterior placement and the curving nature of the approach, a flap can be developed that allows better visualization of the posteromedial corner of the joint.

The anatomy of the medial side of the knee is considered in a separate section after these approaches are described.

The *approach for lateral meniscectomy* provides adequate exposure, but its use is limited. The *lateral approach* is used for ligamentous reconstruction of the knee's lateral supporting structures. The anatomy of the knee's lateral side is considered after these two approaches are outlined.

The *lateral approach to the distal femur*, an adjunct to the medial parapatellar incision, is used for repairs of ruptured anterior cruciate ligaments. The approach enters the intercondylar notch from behind, allowing reattachment of the distal stump of a torn anterior cruciate ligament or the insertion of a graft. It usually is used in conjunction with an anteromedial approach to the knee.

The *posterior approach* to the knee is performed rarely, and then usually for the repair of neurovascular structures. Its anatomy is considered after this approach is described.

## General Principles of Arthroscopy

See Chapter 1, General Principles of Arthroscopy, Figs. 1-60 through 1-62.

## Arthroscopic Approaches to the Knee

The knee is a large unconstrained hinge joint that is often described as subcutaneous. Its anteromedial and anterolateral coverings consist largely of fibrous tissue—the patellar retinaculum and joint capsule (see Figs. 10-40, 10-54). Incisions through these coverings can be safely made without endangering any vital structures.

Arthroscopy of the knee has largely replaced open procedures for the following:

1. Meniscal resection or repair
2. Removal of loose bodies
3. Anterior cruciate ligament reconstruction
4. Synovial biopsy

5. Synovectomy
6. Debridement of early osteoarthritic knees, including microfracture
7. Treatment of osteochondritis dissecans

Numerous arthroscopic portals have been described in knee arthroscopy surgery.[1,2]

The anterolateral portal is the one most commonly used for diagnostic purposes; it is nearly always used in conjunction with the anteromedial portal. The combination of these approaches allows the use of the arthroscope along with arthroscopic instrumentation. Usually the arthroscope is inserted via the anterolateral portal and instruments are inserted via the anteromedial portal. However, either portal can be used for either purpose. These two approaches are described in this section.

## Position of the Patient

Place the patient supine on the operating table. Apply a well-padded tourniquet to the mid-thigh. Exsanguinate the limb and inflate the tourniquet. Remove the end of the table (Fig. 10-1; see Figs. 10-9 and 10-41). Prep and drape the limb so that you

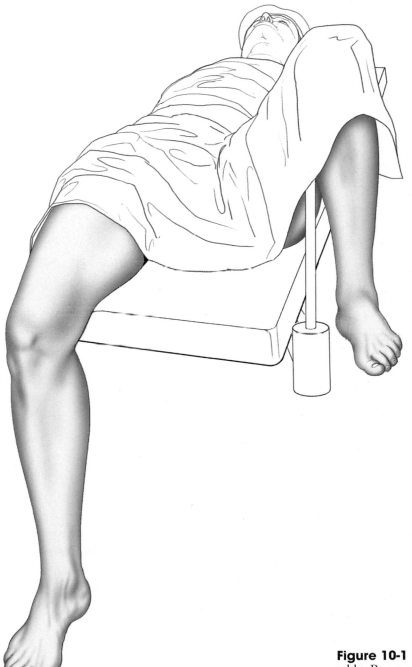

**Figure 10-1** Place the patient supine on the operating table. Remove the end of the table so that you are able to manipulate the knee during surgery.

are able to manipulate the knee during surgery. The use of an arthroscopic clamp placed around the tourniquet allows the surgeon to apply a valgus and external rotation force to the knee, facilitating access to the medial compartment. The use of a clamp, however, makes it more difficult to place the knee in the figure-of-eight position (placing the lateral malleolus of the involved extremity on the opposite thigh; see Figs. 10-8, *inset*, and 10-42) to allow access to the lateral compartment of the knee. If a surgical

assistant is available to provide the appropriate forces, the use of a clamp is not indicated.

## Landmarks and Incision

### Lateral

Flex and extend the knee and use your thumb to palpate the *lateral joint lines*. Move your thumb toward the midline. You will feel the resistance of the lateral edge of the *patellar tendon*. Flex the knee to 90°. Place your

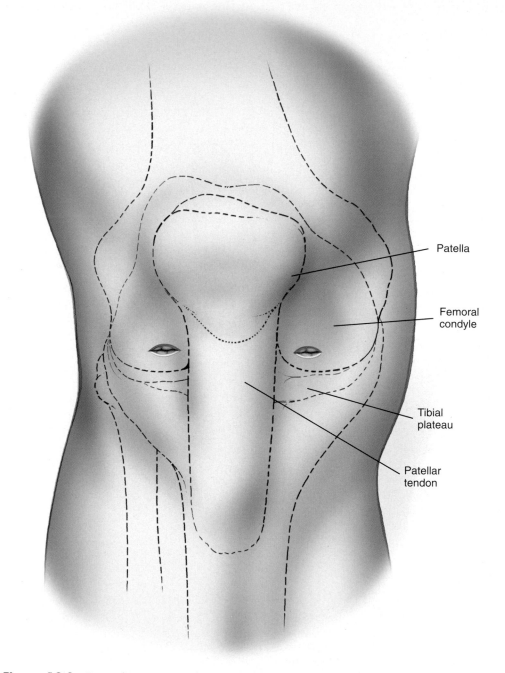

Patella

Femoral condyle

Tibial plateau

Patellar tendon

**Figure 10-2**    Lateral incision: make a small 8-mm transverse stab incision 1½ cm above the lateral joint line. Medial incision: make an 8-mm stab incision 1½ cm above the medial joint line.

forefinger in the recess created by the lateral border of the patellar tendon and the lateral joint space. This is the so-called soft spot. Make an 8-mm transverse stab incision approximately 5 mm proximal to your finger, 1 cm to 1½ cm above the joint line (Fig. 10-2).

### Medial

Move your finger to palpate the *medial joint line* and the medial edge of the *patellar tendon*. Place your finger in the medial soft spot, and make an 8-mm stab incision some 1½ cm above the joint line. Note that because the lateral tibial plateau is slightly lower than the medial plateau, the lateral incision will be slightly lower than the medial one (see Fig. 10-2).

## Internervous Plane

There is no internervous plane in these surgical approaches, which consist of incisions made in the medial and lateral patellar retinacula and joint capsule. No major nerves are present in these areas.

## Surgical Dissection

With the knee flexed to 90°, deepen the anterolateral skin incision using a sharp-ended blade. As you incise the retinaculum, you will suddenly feel a decrease in resistance. Withdraw the blade and insert the arthroscopic sheath and blunt trochar. Push the sheath and trochar into the anterolateral portion of the knee, taking care not to hit the underlying femur; then carefully extend the knee while advancing the arthroscopic sheath up into the suprapatellar pouch. Remove the trochar. Insert the 30° arthroscopic telescope. Switch on the irrigation fluid before switching on the light source to avoid thermal damage to the synovium.

# Arthroscopic Exploration of the Knee

Although the use of a preoperative MRI facilitates the discovery of pathology within the knee, it is important to ensure that each arthroscopic exploration examines all portions of the knee and not merely the site of the presumed pathology.

## Order of Scoping

Begin with placing a 30° arthroscope in the suprapatellar pouch (Fig. 10-3, *view 1*). The arthroscope should be easily mobile, allowing you to examine all portions of the suprapatellar pouch, noting especially the synovium and checking for the presence of any loose bodies.

Keeping the knee fully extended, withdraw the arthroscope into the patellofemoral joint, rotating the telescope to allow examination of both the femoral and patellar aspects of the joint (see Fig. 10-3, *view 2*). Manipulating the patella medially and laterally facilitates this procedure.

Keeping the leg extended, slide the tip of the arthroscope into the lateral recess or gutter of the knee, passing the scope between the lateral aspect of the femur and the lateral capsule of the joint (see Fig. 10-3, *view 3*). Observe the lateral surface of the femur, and ensure that you can see the insertion of the popliteus muscle (see Fig. 10-3, *view 4*). The popliteal hiatus is a common recess for the presence of loose bodies.

Keeping the knee in full extension, sweep the arthroscope into the lateral portion of the knee, observing the anterior part of the lateral meniscus (Fig. 10-4, *view 5*). Pass the arthroscope medially, and rotate the scope so that you are looking posteriorly. This will allow you visualization of the medial femoral recess or gutter (see Fig. 10-4, *view 6*).

Withdraw the arthroscope into the center of the knee and gently flex to 90°, allowing the tip of the arthroscope to enter the medial compartment of the knee. Observe the articular cartilage of the medial femoral condyle and medial tibial plateau. Also observe the medial meniscus and meniscal rim (Fig. 10-5, *view 7*). Apply a valgus and external rotation force to the knee, and rotate the scope so that it is looking laterally, to allow examination of the posterior horn of the medial meniscus (Fig. 10-6, *view 8*).

Withdraw the arthroscope into the intercondylar notch, observing the anterior and posterior cruciate ligaments (Fig. 10-7, *view 9*).

With the arthroscope in the area of the intercondylar notch, flex the knee to just over 90°, abduct the hip, and place the lateral malleolus of the operative side on the anterior aspect of the contralateral knee (see Fig. 10-42). This is known as the figure-of-eight position and allows arthroscopic inspection of the entire lateral compartment (Fig. 10-8, *inset*). Observe the articular surfaces of the lateral femoral condyle and lateral tibial plateau. Examine the lateral meniscus in its entirety (see Fig. 10-8, *view 10*).

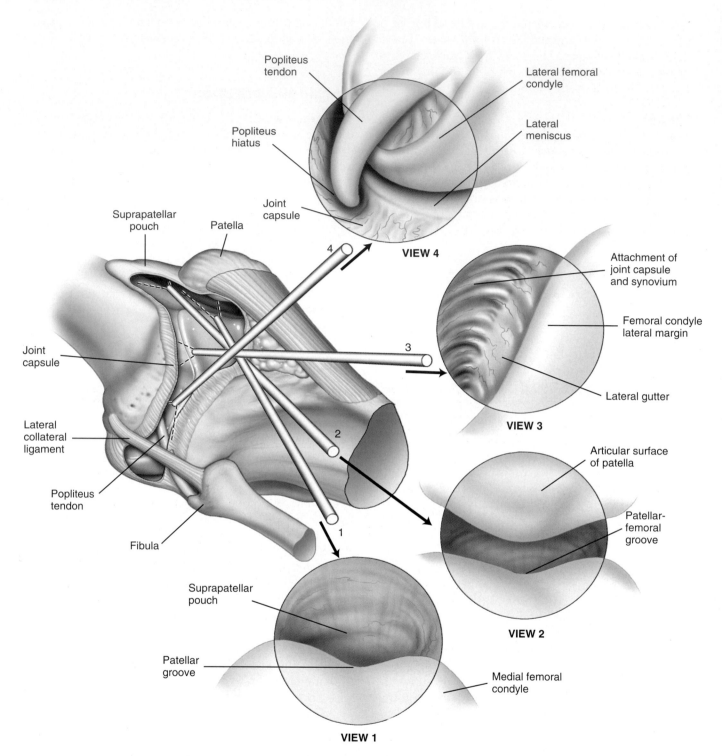

**Figure 10-3**   **(View 1)** Begin with the arthroscope in the suprapatellar pouch and observe the synovium, checking for the presence of loose bodies. **(View 2)** Withdraw the arthroscope into the patellofemoral joint. To observe the full extent of the joint, rotate the scope in both directions and move the patella medially and laterally. **(View 3)** Slide the scope into the lateral recess of the knee and observe the lateral aspect of the lateral femoral condyle. **(View 4)** Advance the arthroscope into the lateral gutter to view the insertion of the popliteal muscle.

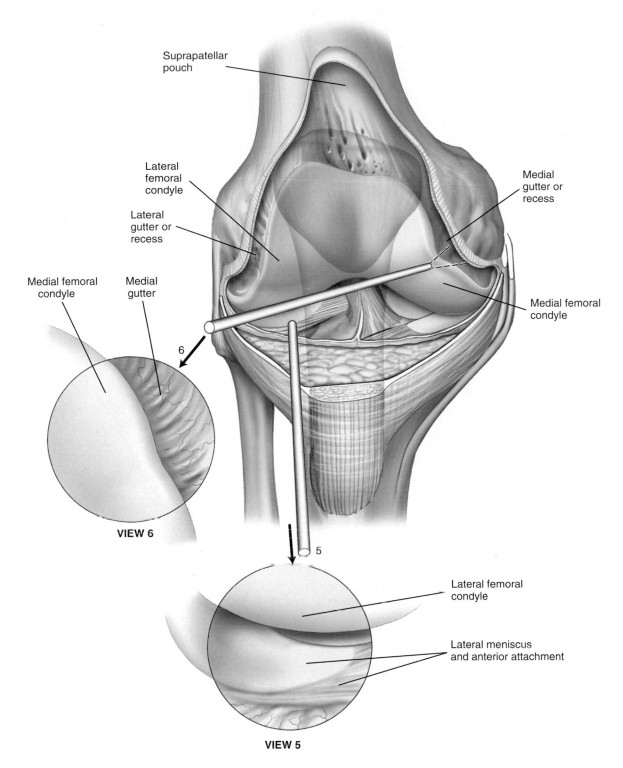

Suprapatellar pouch

Lateral femoral condyle

Lateral gutter or recess

Medial gutter or recess

Medial femoral condyle

Medial femoral condyle

Medial gutter

VIEW 6

6

5

VIEW 5

Lateral femoral condyle

Lateral meniscus and anterior attachment

**Figure 10-4**   **(View 5)** With the knee in full extension, sweep the arthroscope into the lateral portion of the knee and observe the anterior horn of the lateral meniscus and the anterior part of the lateral femoral condyle. **(View 6)** Advance the arthroscope medially and rotate it to look posteriorly. Observe the medial femoral recess.

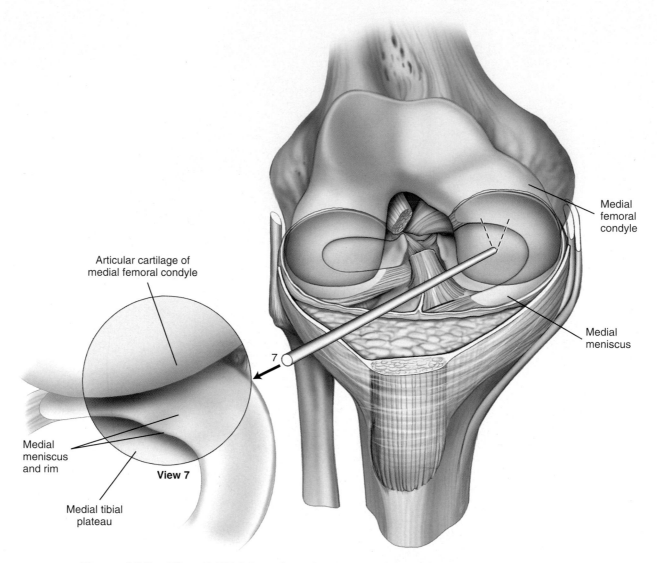

Articular cartilage of
medial femoral condyle

Medial
meniscus
and rim

**View 7**

Medial tibial
plateau

Medial
femoral
condyle

Medial
meniscus

**Figure 10-5**    **(View 7)** Withdraw the arthroscope into the center of the joint, and then
flex the knee to allow the arthroscope to enter the medial compartment. Observe the rim
of the medial meniscus, the medial femoral condyle, and the medial tibial plateau.

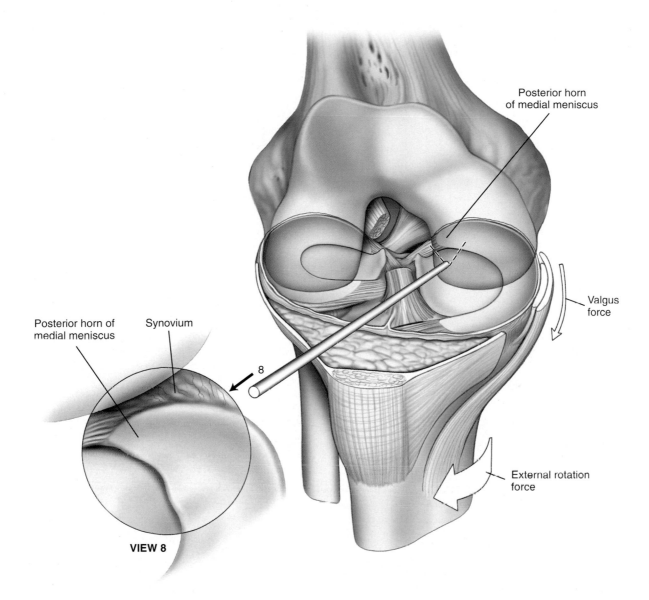

**Figure 10-6** **(View 8)** Apply a valgus/external rotation force to the knee, and rotate the arthroscope so that it is looking laterally. Observe the posterior horn of the medial meniscus.

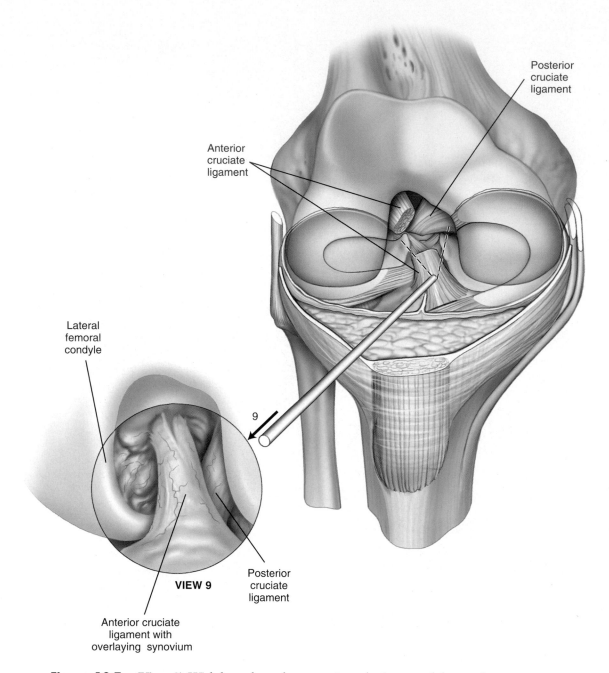

**Figure 10-7**   **(View 9)** Withdraw the arthroscope into the intercondylar notch to observe the cruciate ligaments.

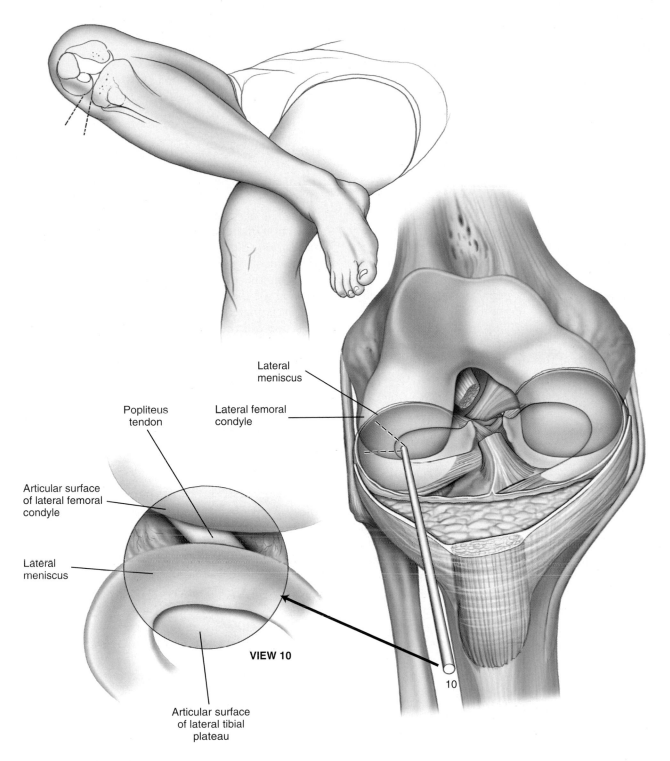

Lateral
meniscus

Lateral femoral
condyle

Popliteus
tendon

Articular surface
of lateral femoral
condyle

Lateral
meniscus

**VIEW 10**

Articular surface
of lateral tibial
plateau

10

**Figure 10-8**   **(Inset)** Flex the knee 90° above the hip, and place the lateral malleolus of the operative side on the anterior aspect of the contralateral knee (figure-of-eight position). **(View 10)** Advance the arthroscope into the lateral compartment of the knee to observe the lateral meniscus in its entirety.

To allow inspection of the undersurface of the menisci and to assess the integrity of the cruciate ligaments, insert the arthroscopic hook through the anteromedial portal and use it under direct vision of the arthroscope to palpate these structures.

## Dangers

### Articular Cartilage

The *articular cartilage* of the knee may be damaged at two stages during arthroscopy: by the incision or by the forceful insertion of an arthroscope. If the incision is made carefully, this problem should not occur. Remember that if you meet with resistance when manipulating the arthroscope within the knee, then it is certain that you are damaging the articular cartilage. More posteriorly based incisions on the medial side may easily damage the articular surface of the medial femoral condyle if performed blind. Therefore, it is recommended that more posterior medial or lateral incisions, if needed, should be made under direct arthroscopic control. Ten seconds of careless use of an arthroscope within the knee may create the equivalent of 10 years of wear in that joint.

### Meniscus

The *meniscus* may be damaged by the scalpel or the arthroscope if the incisions are made too close to the joint line.

## How to Enlarge the Approach

### Local Measures

Manipulation of the knee is the key to success in visualizing all portions of the joint. To allow complete inspection of the knee, apply a valgus external rotation force to assess the posterior aspect of the medial compartment of the knee. You will also need to apply a varus internal rotation stress to examine the lateral portions of the knee. Remember that the telescope you use is angled at 30°. Changing the direction of the telescope will therefore significantly change the view that you obtain (see Figs. 1-60 through 1-62). This is most important when examining the posterior third of the medial compartment of the knee.

# Medial Parapatellar Approach

The medial parapatellar approach[3] is the workhorse approach to the knee. Extended to its full length, it allows excellent access to most structures. Portions of the incision can be used to gain access to the suprapatellar pouch, the patella, and the medial side of the joint. When a straight, midline, longitudinal skin incision is used in conjunction with a medial parapatellar capsular approach, the incision offers an exposure large enough for total knee arthroplasty.

The uses of the medial parapatellar approach include the following:

1. Synovectomy[4,5]
2. Medial meniscectomy
3. Removal of loose bodies[6]
4. Ligamentous reconstructions
5. Patellectomy
6. Drainage of the knee joint in cases of sepsis
7. Total knee replacement[7–14]
8. Repair of the anterior cruciate ligament (see the section regarding the lateral approach to the distal femur)
9. Open reduction and internal fixation of distal femoral fractures when a medial plate is to be used

## Position of the Patient

Place the patient in a supine position on the operating table. The approach can be made with or without the use of a tourniquet. Operating without a tourniquet slows the surgical approach, but bleeding points are easy to pick up in the superficial surgical dissection. If you are using a tourniquet, it will need to be removed prior to closure of the wound to allow you to obtain hemostasis of the wound. If you are using a tourniquet, exsanguinate the leg by applying a compressive bandage or by elevating the limb for five minutes; then, inflate a tourniquet (Fig. 10-9).

Place a sandbag on the table in such a position that it supports the heel when the knee is flexed to 90°. This sandbag will help maintain the knee in a flexed position during joint replacement surgery. Position a table support on the outer aspect of the upper thigh to prevent the leg from falling into abduction when the knee is flexed.

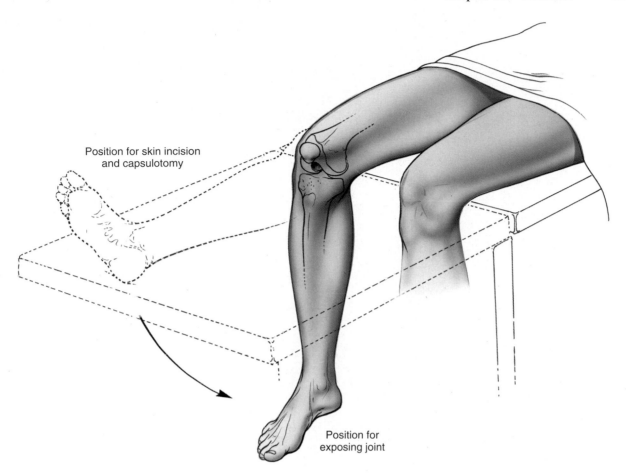

Position for skin incision
and capsulotomy

Position for
exposing joint

**Figure 10-9**   Position of the patient for the medial parapatellar approach. Begin with the straight leg position, and then flex the knee for the deeper dissection.

## Landmarks and Incision

### Landmarks
Palpate the patella. Run fingers down to the *patellar ligament* (ligamenta patellae), which runs from the inferior border of the patella and is palpable to its insertion into the tibial tubercle.

### Incision
Make a longitudinal straight midline incision, extending from a point 5 cm above the superior pole of the patella to below the level of the tibial tubercle (see Fig. 10-10).

## Internervous Plane

There is no internervous plane in this approach, even when the incision is extended superiorly into the intermuscular plane between the vastus medialis and rectus femoris muscles. Both of these muscles are supplied by the femoral nerve well proximal to this dissection, leaving the plane safe for knee surgery.

## Superficial Surgical Dissection

Divide the subcutaneous tissues in the line of the skin incision, ensuring hemostasis. Develop a medial skin flap to expose the quadriceps tendon, the medial border of the patella, and the medial border of the patellar tendon. Enter the joint by cutting through the joint capsule. Begin on the medial side of the patella, taking care to leave a cuff of capsular tissue medial to the patella and lateral to the quadriceps muscle to facilitate closure. Divide the quadriceps tendon in the midline to enter the suprapatellar pouch. Finally, complete the capsule incision by dividing the fibrous tissue on the medial aspect of the patellar tendon. The capsular incision will almost certainly also cut through the synovium, since the capsule and synovium are intimately related.

Retract the fat pad, or excise it, as dictated by the exposure requirements. As the joint line is approached, care should be taken not to damage the anterior insertion of the medial meniscus unless the approach is being used for joint replacement surgery (Figs. 10-10 through 10-12).

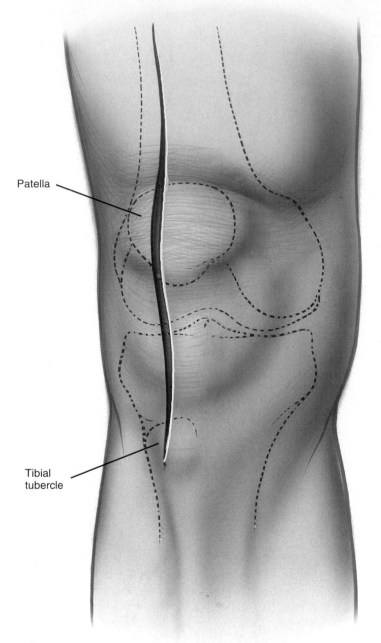

Patella

Tibial
tubercle

**Figure 10-10** Make a longitudinal, straight, midline incision.

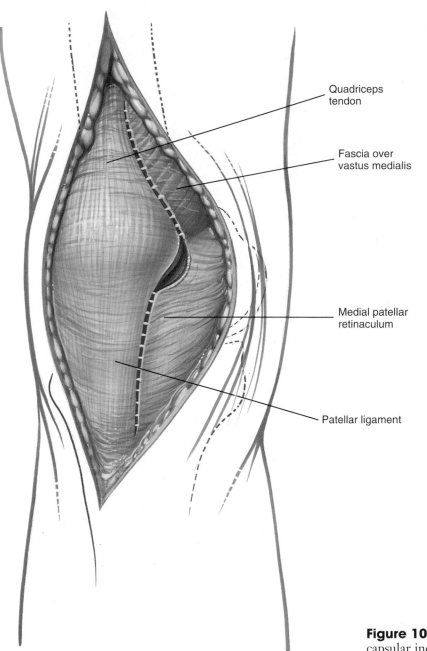

Quadriceps
tendon

Fascia over
vastus medialis

Medial patellar
retinaculum

Patellar ligament

**Figure 10-11** Make a medial parapatellar
capsular incision.

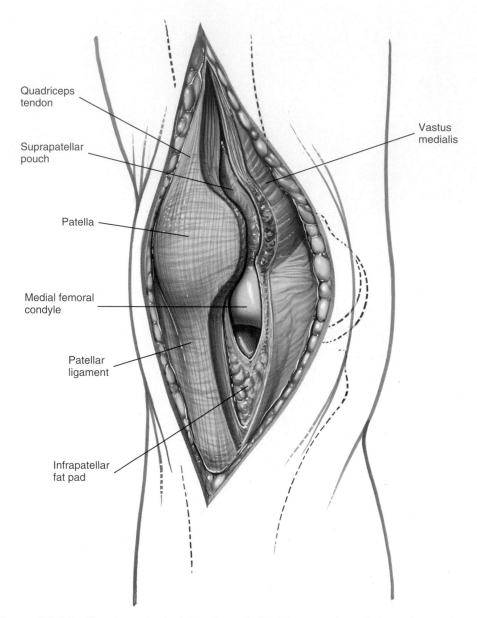

Quadriceps
tendon

Suprapatellar
pouch

Patella

Medial femoral
condyle

Patellar
ligament

Infrapatellar
fat pad

Vastus
medialis

**Figure 10-12**     Continue the incision through the joint capsule and along the patellar ligament and quadriceps tendon to gain access to the joint.

## Deep Surgical Dissection

Dislocate the patella laterally and rotate it 180°; then, flex the knee to 90° (Fig. 10-13; see Fig. 10-9). Try to avoid avulsion of the patellar ligament from its insertion on the tibia as the patella is dislocated, because reattaching the tendon to the bone is difficult. If the patella does not dislocate easily, it can be given added mobility by extending the skin incision superiorly over the interval between the rectus femoris and vastus medialis muscles. Continue the dissection deeper, splitting the quadriceps tendon farther just lateral to its medial border (see Fig. 10-13).

In those rare cases in which the patella still does not dislocate, carefully remove the patellar ligament attachment with an underlying block of bone. The bone makes subsequent reattachment easier (Fig. 10-14). Be aware that the tibial components of many knee replacements incorporate a central peg that makes reattachment of a bone block impossible if a screw is to be used. In such cases, a staple fixation may be indicated.

When the patella is dislocated and the knee is flexed fully, this incision provides the widest possible exposure of the entire knee joint.

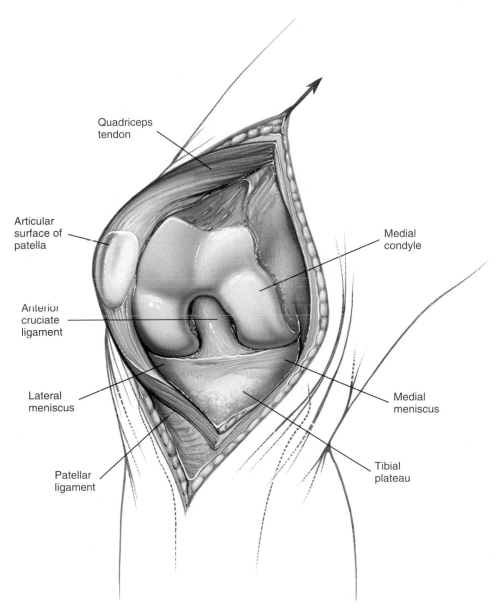

**Figure 10-13**   Dislocate the patella laterally, and flex the knee to 90°.

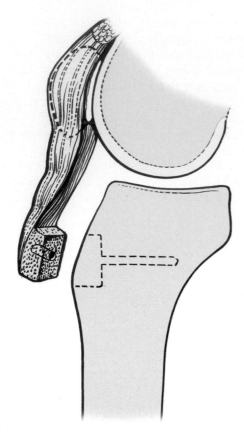

**Figure 10-14**   Detach the patellar ligament attachment with an underlying block of bone.

## Dangers

### Nerves

The **infrapatellar branch of the saphenous nerve** often is cut during this approach. The major danger

in cutting the nerve is the development of a postoperative neuroma. Because the area of anesthesia produced usually is not troublesome, do not repair the nerve if it is cut. Instead, resect it and bury its end in fat to decrease the chances that a painful neuroma will form (see Figs. 10-32 and 10-35).

### Muscles and Ligaments

If the patellar ligament becomes avulsed from its insertion on the tibia, it is difficult to reattach.

## How to Enlarge the Approach

### Local Measures

*Superior Extension.* Extend the approach proximally between the rectus femoris and vastus medialis muscles. Then, split the underlying vastus intermedius muscle to expose the distal two thirds of the femur. Stay in the distal third of the thigh; more proximally, the branches of the femoral nerve may become involved, resulting in partial denervation (see Anteromedial Approach to the Distal Two Thirds of the Femur in Chapter 9).

*Inferior Extension.* Mobilize the upper part of the attachment of the patellar ligament to the tibia or remove the patellar ligament with an underlying block of bone. This extension may be useful in dealing with complex intraarticular fractures of the knee joint. (See the section detailing the lateral approach to the distal femur for combined use in repair of the cruciate ligament.)

## Approach for Medial Meniscectomy

The approach for medial meniscectomy[15] is a common formal incision for the knee. It is quite flexible, with several acceptable locations for incision and many different ways to position the patient. Some surgeons advocate a transverse skin incision over the joint line; although this limits the view of the knee, it provides better access to the meniscus itself. Others prefer longitudinal or oblique incisions, which offer a better view of such other intraarticular structures as the cruciate ligaments. Although operative arthroscopy has reduced dra-

matically the need for this approach, it remains a useful one.

The uses of the anteromedial approach include the following:

1. Medial meniscectomy
2. Partial meniscectomy
3. Removal of loose bodies
4. Removal of foreign bodies
5. Treatment of osteochondritis of the medial femoral condyle[6]

## Position of the Patient

Arrange the patient in a supine position on the operating table. Place a sandbag under the affected thigh, taking care that it is not directly beneath the popliteal fossa, where it will compress the popliteal artery and posterior joint capsule against the back of the femur and tibia, increasing the risk of accidental injury during excision of the posterior third of the meniscus (Fig. 10-15). Remove the end of the table so that the knee can be flexed beyond a right angle.

This position requires good lighting so that the meniscus can be seen during surgery. The light must be adjusted continually to keep it shining directly into the depths of the wound. A headlamp is the best light source.

Exsanguinate the limb by elevating it for 2 to 5 minutes or by applying a soft rubber bandage. Then, apply a tourniquet.

## Landmarks and Incision

### Landmarks

The *medial joint line* must be identified, because incisions easily can be made too high. Flexion and extension of the knee allows the line to be palpated with certainty.

Locate the *inferomedial corner of the patella.*

### Incision

Begin the incision at the inferomedial corner of the patella. Angle it inferiorly and posteriorly, ending

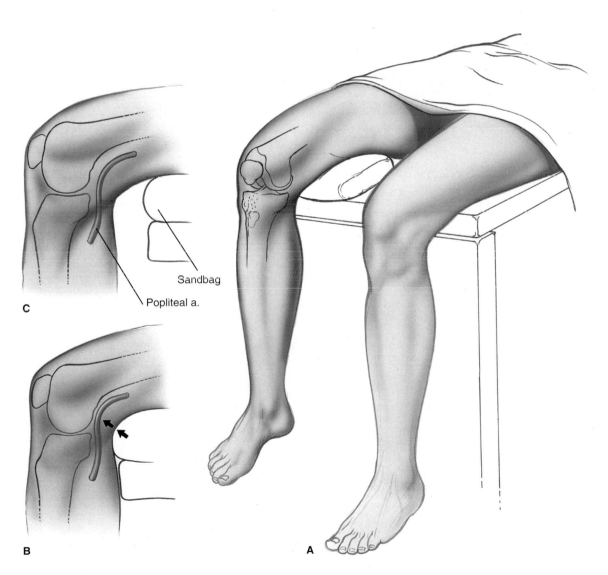

Sandbag

Popliteal a.

**Figure 10-15**   **(A)** Position of the patient for medial meniscectomy. **(B)** Improper placement of the sandbag pushes the popliteal artery against the posterior joint capsule. **(C)** Proper placement of the sandbag under the affected thigh.

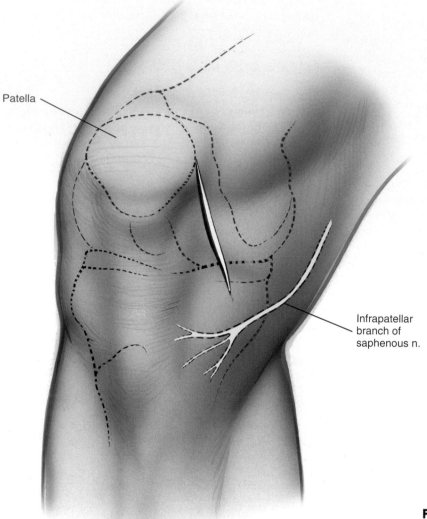

Patella

Infrapatellar branch of saphenous n.

**Figure 10-16** Incision for anteromedial approach for medial meniscectomy.

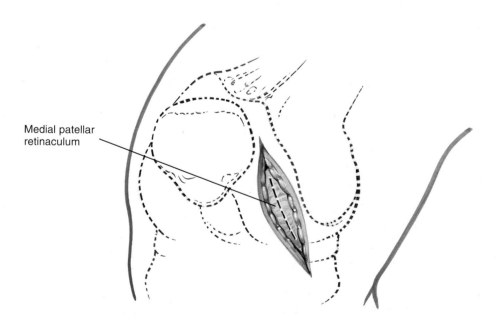

Medial patellar retinaculum

**Figure 10-17** Incise down to the anteromedial aspect of the joint capsule.

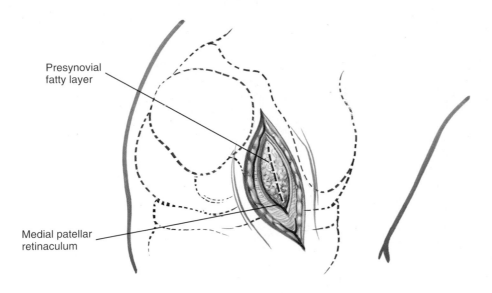

**Figure 10-18**   Incise the joint capsule in line with the incision to reveal the extrasynovial fat.

about 1 cm below the joint line. Incisions continued farther inferiorly can cut the infrapatellar branch of the saphenous nerve as it traverses the upper leg (Fig. 10-16).

## Internervous Plane

There is no internervous plane in this approach because the deep incision is made through the medial patellar retinaculum and joint capsule.

## Superficial Surgical Dissection

Deepen the wound in line with the skin incision down to the anteromedial aspect of the joint cap-

sule, the true joint capsule, which is reinforced by the medial retinaculum of the patella (Fig. 10-17). Incise the capsule in line with the skin incision, which also is in line with the capsular fibers (Fig. 10-18).

## Deep Surgical Dissection

Open the synovium, together with the extrasynovial fat, well above the joint line to gain access to the anteromedial portion of the joint (Fig. 10-19). Opening the joint above the joint line avoids damage to the intrasynovial fat pad, medial meniscus, and coronary ligament (Figs. 10-20 and 10-21).

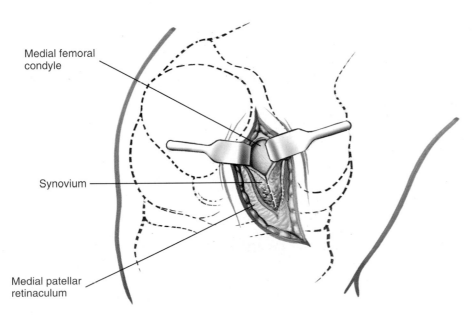

**Figure 10-19**   Incise the synovium to gain access to the joint.

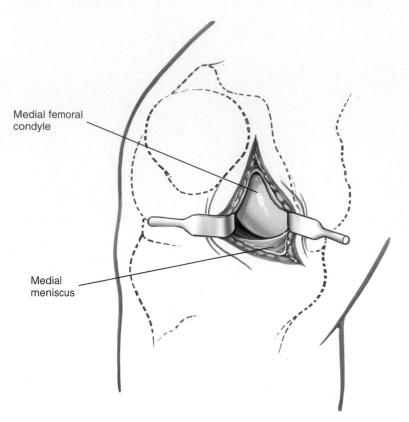

Medial femoral
condyle

Medial
meniscus

**Figure 10-20**   Open the joint capsule and synovium to the joint line to prevent damage to the meniscus and synovial fat pad.

## Dangers

### Nerves

The **infrapatellar branch of the saphenous nerve** may be cut if the incision is extended farther inferiorly than 1 cm below the joint line (see Fig. 10-16).

### Vessels

Because the **popliteal artery** is immediately behind the posterior joint capsule, any injury to the posterior joint capsule may damage the artery. If the knee is flexed, the posterior joint capsule falls away from the tibia and femur, taking the artery with it. A sandbag placed directly under the popliteal fossa prevents the capsule from moving posteriorly and must be avoided at all costs (see Fig. 10-15*B,C*).

### Muscles and Ligaments

The **coronary ligament** (the meniscotibial element of the deep medial ligament) connects the periphery of the meniscus with the joint capsule and tibia, and may be damaged if the incision through the syn-

ovium is made at the joint line (see Figs. 10-33 and 10-34).

Incisions made too far posteriorly may cut the **superficial medial ligament** (the tibial collateral ligament) as it runs from the medial epicondyle of the femur to its insertion on the tibia under cover of the pes anserinus (see Figs. 10-27 and 10-28).

### Special Structures

The **fat pad** occupies varying amounts of the anterior portion of the knee joint and should not be damaged. Damage may produce adhesions within the joint and, in theory, can interfere with the blood supply to the patella (see Fig. 10-12).

The **medial meniscus** may be incised accidentally during the opening of the synovium unless the knee joint is entered well above the joint line.

## How to Enlarge the Approach

### Local Measures

Three factors may improve the exposure offered by this approach:

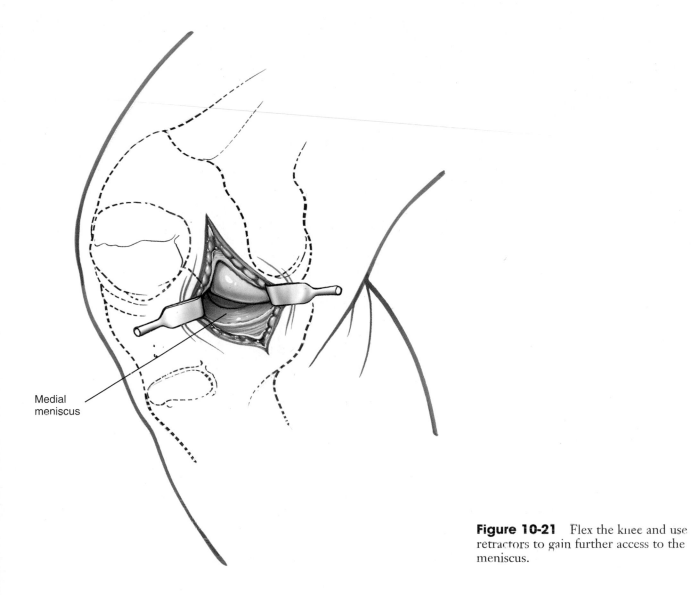

Medial
meniscus

**Figure 10-21**   Flex the knee and use retractors to gain further access to the meniscus.

1. *Retraction.* Retractors must be positioned and repositioned carefully to ensure the best possible view of the intraarticular structures.
2. *Position of light.* Light should shine directly into the wound, usually from over the surgeon's shoulder. Constant readjustment is necessary, and the use of a headlamp is invaluable.
3. An outward stress will open up the medial side of the joint. Flexion of the knee allows better access to the back of the medial side of the joint. If the posterior horn of the medial meniscus must be seen, however, a better view is obtained by putting the leg into full extension and applying distraction and outward force.

**Extensile Measures**

*Posterior Extension.* The dissection is limited posteriorly by the superficial medial ligament, which crosses the joint just in front of the midpoint of the femur. For better access to the posterior half of the joint, a second incision must be made behind this ligament.

Insert a blunt instrument into the joint and push it slowly backward, running along the inside of the medial joint capsule at the level of the joint itself. As the instrument is pushed, the superficial medial ligament will be sensed; from inside the knee, it feels like a firm structure beneath the tip of the instrument. As

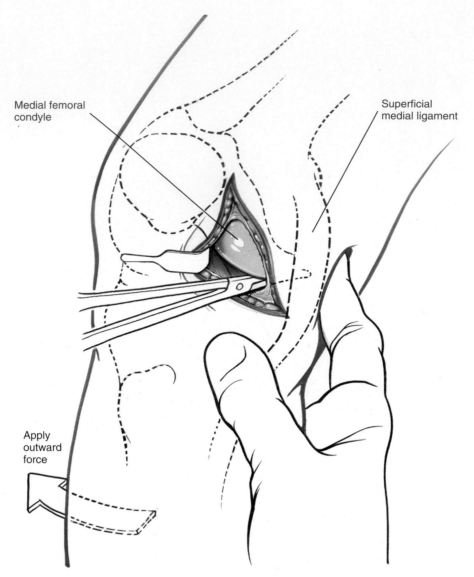

Medial femoral
condyle

Superficial
medial ligament

Apply
outward
force

**Figure 10-22**    Insert a blunt instrument into the joint, and push it backward along the inside of the medial joint capsule. Palpate posteriorly until the instrument can be felt beneath the skin.

the instrument is passed posteriorly, there will be a give in the resistance corresponding to a point just posterior to the superficial medial ligament (Fig. 10-22). At that point, make a second longitudinal posterior incision through the skin and knee joint capsule (Fig. 10-23).

***Superior Extension.*** To extend the incision superiorly, continue incising the skin along the medial border of the patella. Then, incise the medial patellar retinaculum and the underlying joint capsule in the

same line to reach the back of the patella. Further superior extension exposes the suprapatellar pouch, which is a frequent site of loose bodies in the knee.

The incision may be extended still farther proximally in the muscular plane between the vastus medialis and rectus femoris muscles, exposing the distal two thirds of the femur.

***Inferior Extension.*** Inferior extension can cut the infrapatellar branch of the saphenous nerve and is not recommended.

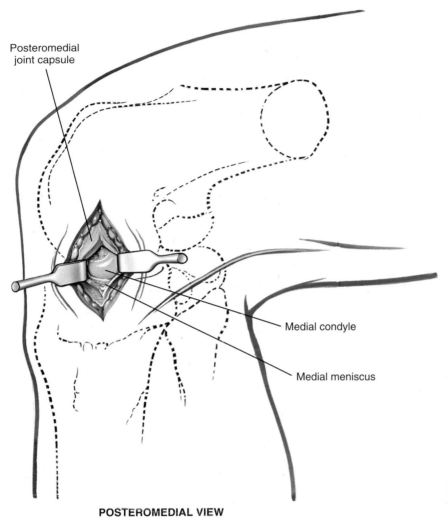

Posteromedial
joint capsule

Medial condyle

Medial meniscus

**POSTEROMEDIAL VIEW**

**Figure 10-23**   Make a second
longitudinal posterior incision to enter
the posteromedial aspect of the joint.

# Medial Approach to the Knee and Its Supporting Structures

The medial approach[16] provides the widest possible exposure of the ligamentous structures on the medial side of the knee. Although it is used mainly for the exploration and treatment of damage to the superficial medial (collateral) ligament and medial joint capsule, the approach also can be used for a medial meniscectomy in conjunction with ligamentous repair and for the repair of a torn anterior cruciate ligament. (See the section regarding the lateral approach to the distal femur.)

## Position of the Patient

Place the patient supine on the operating table. Flex the affected knee to about 60°. Abduct and externally rotate the hip on that side, placing the foot on the opposite shin. Then, use a tourniquet after exsanguinating the limb. Various thigh rests have been designed to make it easier to maintain this position (Fig. 10-24).

## Landmark and Incision

### Landmark
Palpate the *adductor tubercle* on the medial surface of the medial femoral condyle. It lies on the posterior part of the condyle in the distal end of the natural depression between the vastus medialis and hamstring muscles.

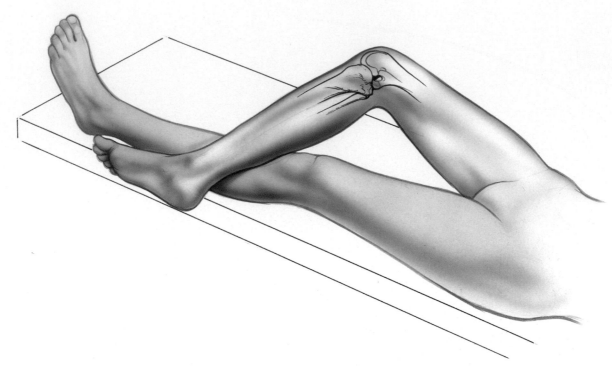

**Figure 10-24**  Position for the medial approach to the knee.

### Incision

Make a long, curved incision, beginning at a point 2 cm proximal to the adductor tubercle of the femur. Curve it anteroinferiorly to a point 6 cm below the joint line on the anteromedial aspect of the tibia. The middle of this incision runs parallel to the medial border of the patella about 3 cm medial to it (Fig. 10-25).

### Internervous Plane

There is no true internervous plane in this approach. Because the nerves at the level of the knee pass posterior to the approach in the popliteal fossa, dissection is quite safe. The only cutaneous nerve that may be damaged is the saphenous nerve and its branches.

### Superficial Surgical Dissection

Raise the skin flaps to expose the fascia. The exposure should extend from the midline anteriorly to the posteromedial corner of the knee posteriorly (Fig. 10-26).

The infrapatellar branch of the saphenous nerve crosses the operative field transversely and is sacrificed; however, the saphenous nerve itself, which emerges from between the gracilis and sartorius muscles, must be preserved, must the long saphenous vein in the posteromedial aspect of the dissection. (The infrapatellar branch of the saphenous nerve should be cut and the end buried in fat to diminish the chances of the formation of a painful neuroma.)

### Deep Surgical Dissection

Exposing the deep structures within the knee involves incising the layers that cover them, either in front of or behind the superficial medial ligament (the medial collateral ligament). These separate incisions provide access to the anterior and posterior parts of the medial side of the joint, respectively.

#### Anterior to the Superficial Medial Ligament

Use the anterior approach to expose the superficial medial ligament, the anterior part of the medial meniscus, and the cruciate ligament.

Incise the fascia along the anterior border of the sartorius muscle in line with the muscle's fibers, starting from its attachment to the subcutaneous surface of the tibia and extending proximally to a point 5 cm above the joint line (see Fig. 10-26). The anterior

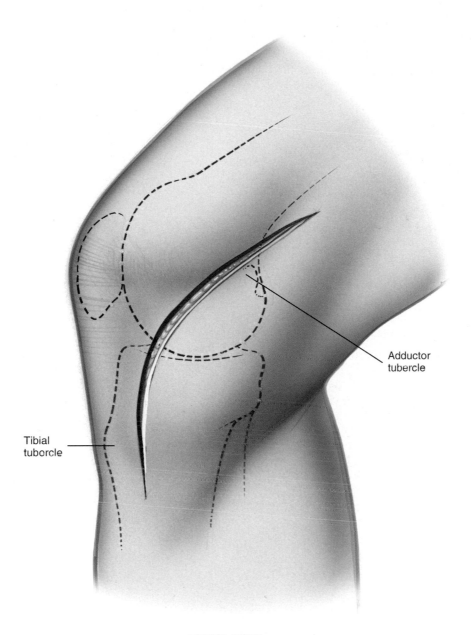

Adductor
tubercle

Tibial
tuborcle

**MEDIAL VIEW**

**Figure 10-25** Make a long, curved incision. The middle of this incision runs parallel
and about 3 cm medial to the medial border of the patella.

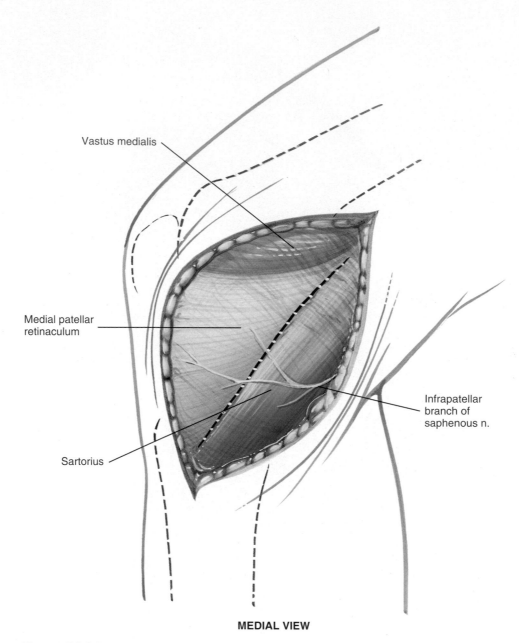

Vastus medialis

Medial patellar
retinaculum

Sartorius

Infrapatellar
branch of
saphenous n.

**MEDIAL VIEW**

**Figure 10-26**    Retract the skin flaps to expose the fascia of the knee. Note that the infrapatellar branch of the saphenous nerve crosses the operative field transversely. Incise the fascia along the anterior border of the sartorius.

border of the sartorius is hard to define at the level of the knee joint, so it should be sought either at the muscle's tibial insertion or at the proximal end of the wound. Now, flex the knee further to allow the sartorius muscle to retract posteriorly, uncovering the other two components of the pes anserinus, the semitendinosus and gracilis muscles, which lie beneath and behind the sartorius (Fig. 10-27).

Retract all three muscles posteriorly to expose the tibial insertion of the superficial medial ligament, which lies deep and distal to the anterior edge of the sartorius. Note that the ligament inserts some 6 to 7 cm below the joint line, not close to it (Fig. 10-28). Apply gentle traction to the superficial medial ligament to reveal its point of injury. Alternatively, apply a strong outward force to the knee,

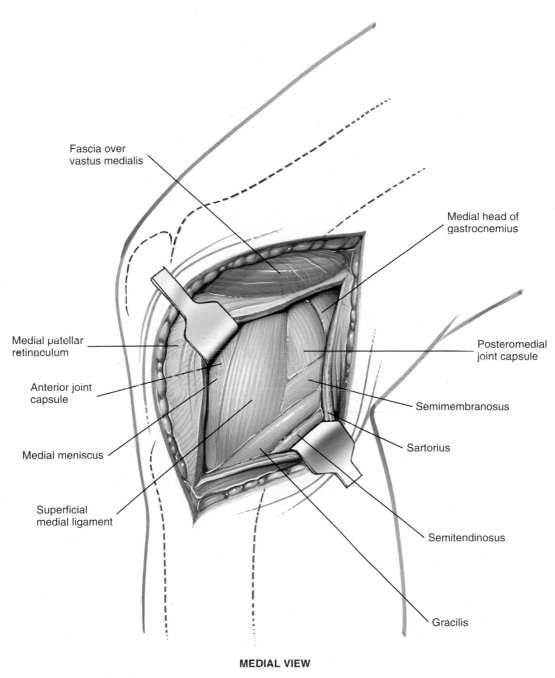

Fascia over vastus medialis

Medial head of gastrocnemius

Medial patellar retinaculum

Posteromedial joint capsule

Anterior joint capsule

Semimembranosus

Medial meniscus

Sartorius

Superficial medial ligament

Semitendinosus

Gracilis

**MEDIAL VIEW**

**Figure 10-27**   Flex the knee and retract the sartorius posteriorly to uncover the remaining components to the pes anserinus.

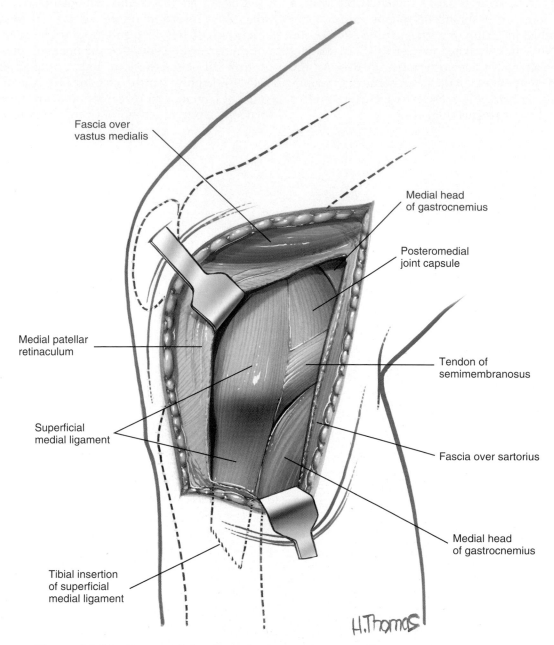

**Figure 10-28**   Retract all three muscles (sartorius, semitendinosus, and gracilis) posteriorly to expose the tibial insertion of the superficial medial ligament.

which will make obvious the site of the ligamentous disruption.

Make a longitudinal medial parapatellar incision to gain access to the inside of the front of the joint. To avoid damage to the underlying medial meniscus, begin the incision well above the joint line and cut down carefully (Fig. 10-29).

## Posterior to the Superficial Medial Ligament

The posterior approach exposes the posterior third of the meniscus and the posteromedial corner of the knee.

Incise the fascia along the anterior border of the sartorius muscle in the same way as for the anterior approach (see Fig. 10-26). Retract the muscle poste-

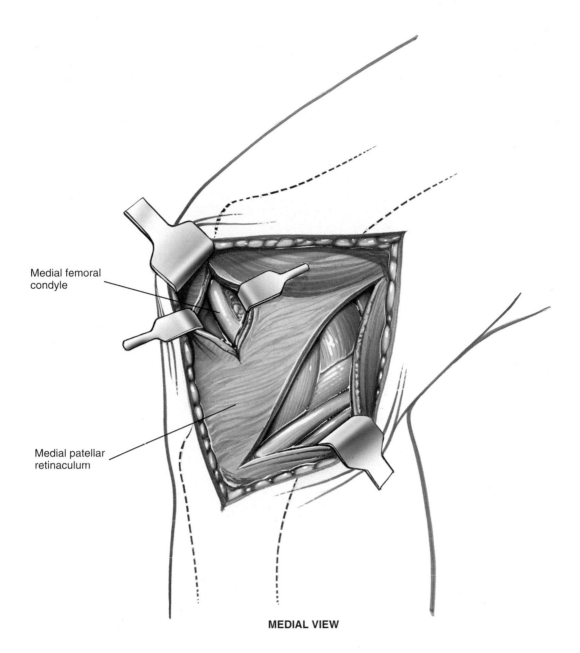

Medial femoral condyle

Medial patellar retinaculum

**MEDIAL VIEW**

**Figure 10-29**   Make a longitudinal medial parapatellar incision to gain access to the inside of the front of the knee joint.

riorly, together with the semitendinosus and gracilis muscles (Fig. 10-30). In cases of damage to the posteromedial joint capsule, the back of the medial femoral condyle usually will be seen, with its underlying meniscus visible through the torn posteromedial joint capsule. If the capsule is intact, expose the posteromedial corner of the joint by separating the medial head of the gastrocnemius muscle from the semimembranosus muscle. Although both muscles

are supplied by the tibial nerve, this intermuscular plane is a safe area for dissection, because the semimembranosus receives its nerve supply well proximal to the approach and the gastrocnemius receives it well distal.

Finally, separate the medial head of the gastrocnemius muscle from the posterior capsule of the knee joint almost to the midline by blunt dissection (Fig. 10-31). Full exposure allows the posteromedial cor-

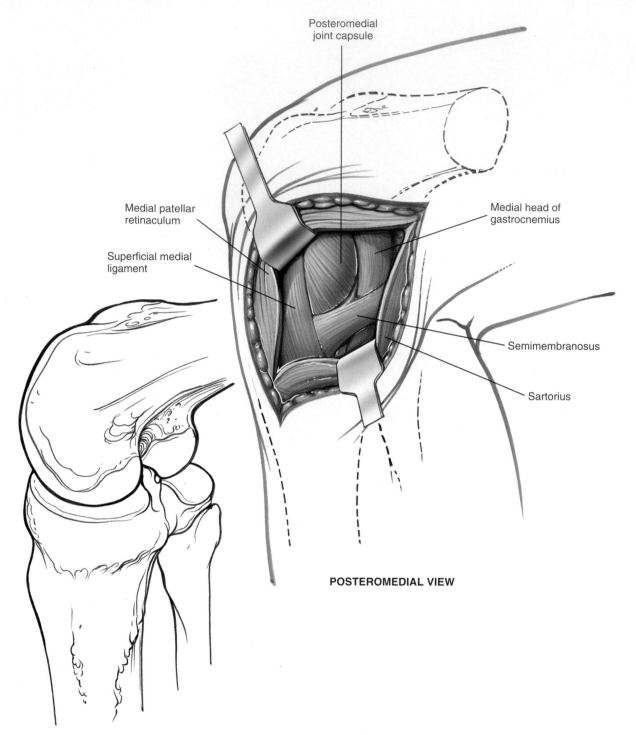

**Figure 10-30** Retract the sartorius, semitendinosus, and gracilis posteriorly to expose the posteromedial corner of the joint. Orientation of the knee *(inset)*.

ner of the capsule to be inspected for damage. A second arthrotomy posterior to the superficial medial ligament (the tibial collateral ligament) permits inspection or treatment of posterior intraarticular or periarticular pathology (see Fig. 10-31). Repair of the posteromedial corner of the joint also is possible.

## Dangers

### Nerves
The cut end of the **infrapatellar branch of the saphenous nerve** should be buried in fat to prevent the formation of a postoperative neuroma.

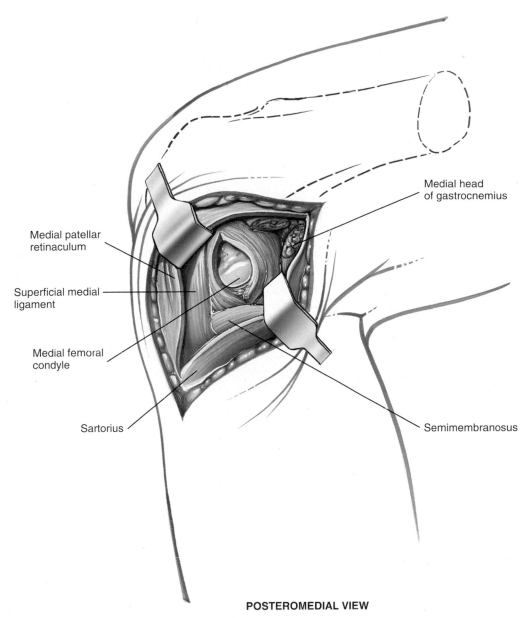

Medial head
of gastrocnemius

Medial patellar
retinaculum

Superficial medial
ligament

Medial femoral
condyle

Sartorius

Semimembranosus

**POSTEROMEDIAL VIEW**

**Figure 10-31**   Expose the posteromedial corner of the knee joint by first separating the gastrocnemius muscle and the posterior capsule of the joint, and then performing a capsulotomy posterior to the tibial collateral ligament.

The saphenous nerve emerges from between the gracilis and sartorius muscles, and runs with the long saphenous vein. It provides sensation for some of the non–weight-bearing portions of the foot and should be preserved (Fig. 10-32; see Fig. 10-35).

## Vessels

The **saphenous vein** appears in the posterior corner of the superficial dissection. Because it may be required for future vascular procedures, it should be preserved (see Fig. 10-35).

The **medial inferior genicular artery** curves around the upper end of the tibia. It may be damaged when the medial belly of the gastrocnemius muscle is lifted off the posterior capsule: the damage may go unnoticed until the wound is closed and the tourniquet is released (see Figs. 10-38 and 10-39).

The **popliteal artery** lies against the posterior joint capsule in the midline and is adjacent to the medial head of the gastrocnemius muscle. Take care to avoid injuring the vessel during separation of the

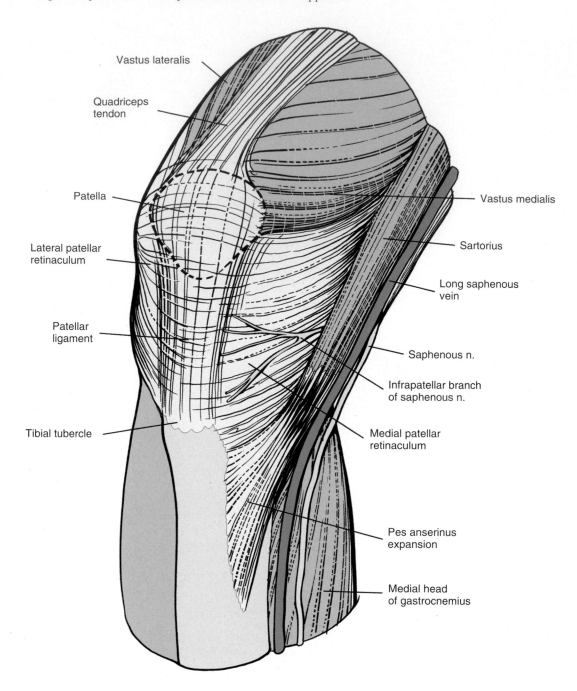

**Figure 10-32**    The outer layer of the anteromedial aspect of the knee joint.

gastrocnemius from the joint capsule (see Figs. 10-58 and 10-61).

## Special Problems

Hematomas under the skin flap that develop postoperatively can cause skin necrosis. Therefore, the large skin flaps that are created in this approach should be drained well.

## How to Enlarge the Approach

The incision already is extensive, providing exposure to all the medial structures of the knee, and cannot be extended usefully in either direction. (For repair of the anterior cruciate ligament, see the section describing the lateral approach to the distal femur.)

# Applied Surgical Anatomy of the Medial Side of the Knee

## Overview

As Warren and Marshall pointed out, the ligaments on the medial side of the knee are merely "condensations within tissue planes."[17] They blend with each other at various points, making definition of each layer difficult, especially in cases of trauma, when bleeding and edema can complicate the problem further. For this reason, it is important to have an understanding of the normal anatomy and supporting structures on the medial side of the knee.

The anatomy of the medial side is understood readily when it is described in three separate layers.[17] Approaches to the knee enter the joint by incising these layers sequentially, from outside to inside.

## Outer Layer

The outer layer consists of the proximal continuation of the deep fascia of the thigh. It encloses the sartorius muscle, whose fibers blend with the fascial layer before they insert into the tibia.

Anteriorly, the outer layer blends with fibrous tissue derived from the vastus medialis muscle to form the medial patellar retinaculum. Posteriorly, the layer is continuous with the deep fascia, which covers the gastrocnemius muscle and the roof of the popliteal fossa (Fig. 10-35; see Fig. 10-32).

## Middle Layer

The middle layer consists of the superficial medial ligament (the tibial or medial collateral ligament), which is attached superiorly just below the adductor tubercle of the femur. The ligament, which is quadrangular, fans out as it travels down to insert into the subcutaneous border of the tibia some 6 to 7 cm below the knee joint. It lies behind the axis of rotation of the knee (Figs. 10-33 and 10-34).

Above the superficial medial ligament, fibrous tissue from the middle layer passes to the medial side of the patella, forming the medial patellofemoral ligament (see Fig. 10-34).

Posterior to the superficial medial ligament, the fibrous tissue of the middle layer merges with that of the true joint capsule (deep layer) and the tendon of the semimembranosus muscle (Fig. 10-36).

The semimembranosus muscle runs down across the popliteal fossa before it inserts into the back of the medial condyle of the tibia. Three expansions of fibrous tissue come from the muscle's tendon to reinforce the supporting structures of the knee. The tough *oblique popliteal ligament*, one of the expansions, crosses the popliteal fossa, extending upward and laterally before attaching to the lateral femoral condyle (Fig. 10-38). Another expansion of the tendon of the semimembranosus muscle passes forward along the medial surface of the tibial plateau and under the superficial medial ligament before attaching to bone (Fig. 10-39). The expansion lies below the inferior attachment of the joint capsule (in the deep layer). A third, thin expansion passes over the popliteus muscle (see Fig. 10-38). These muscular insertions are thought to be very important for the dynamic stabilization of the knee. In cases of damage to the posteromedial corner of the knee, they should be reattached in their anatomic position, if possible.

The *semitendinosus* and *gracilis* muscles run between the superficial and middle layers of the supporting structures of the knee. They insert into the tibia under the tendon of the sartorius muscle (in the outer layer), where they become part of the outer layer (see Figs. 10-34 and 10-36).

## Deep Layer

The deep layer consists of the joint capsule itself as it attaches just above and below the margins of the articular surfaces of the tibia and femur. Anteriorly, the true capsule lies over the fat pad; it is not part of the medial retinaculum that covers it.

The deep layer is thickened in only one place on the medial side of the knee: by the deep medial ligament, which extends from the medial epicondyle of the femur to the medial meniscus. The deep medial ligament is deep to and separate from the superficial medial ligament. In addition, the deep layer anchors the meniscus to the tibia (the coronary ligament). This results in the limitation of meniscal motion, which may be a factor in the genesis of meniscal tears (see Figs. 10-34 and 10-39).

## Incision

The lines of cleavage of the skin run roughly transversely across the knee joint. Therefore, the more transverse the incision, the more cosmetic the resulting scar. Longitudinal incisions, such as those that are used for the medial parapatellar approaches, often leave broad, obvious scars, which are distressing, especially in young women.

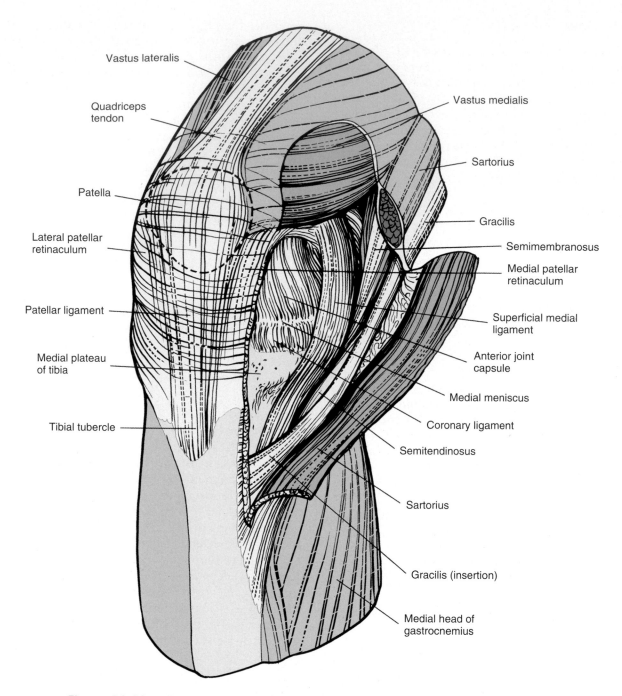

Vastus lateralis

Quadriceps tendon

Patella

Lateral patellar retinaculum

Patellar ligament

Medial plateau of tibia

Tibial tubercle

Vastus medialis

Sartorius

Gracilis

Semimembranosus

Medial patellar retinaculum

Superficial medial ligament

Anterior joint capsule

Medial meniscus

Coronary ligament

Semitendinosus

Sartorius

Gracilis (insertion)

Medial head of gastrocnemius

**Figure 10-33**   The sartorius and the medial patellar retinaculum (outer layer) have been resected to reveal the superficial medial ligament of the middle layer. The true joint capsule (deep layer) also is exposed.

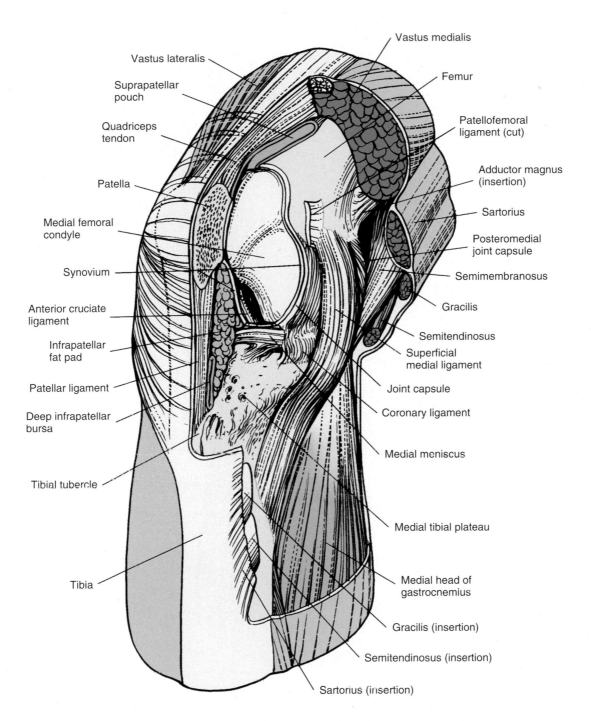

**Figure 10-34**   The joint cavity of the knee, with all the more superficial structures removed.

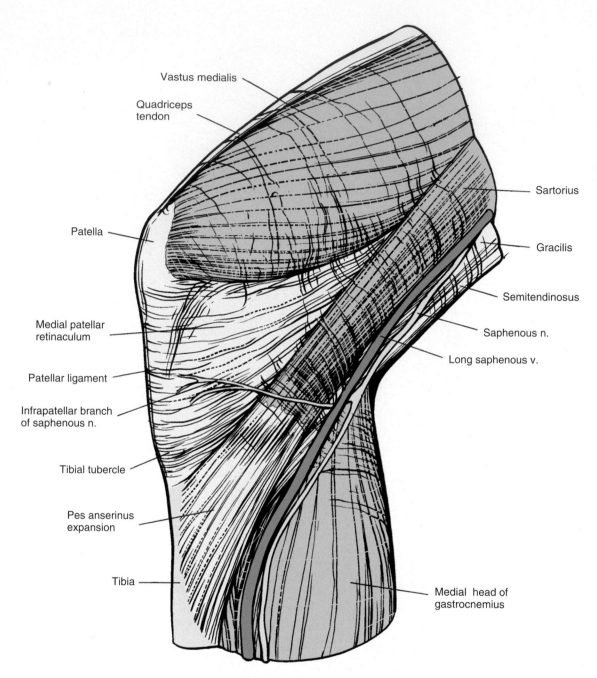

**Figure 10-35**    The outer layer of the medial aspect of the knee joint consists of the sartorius, the fascia of the thigh, and the medial patellar retinaculum.

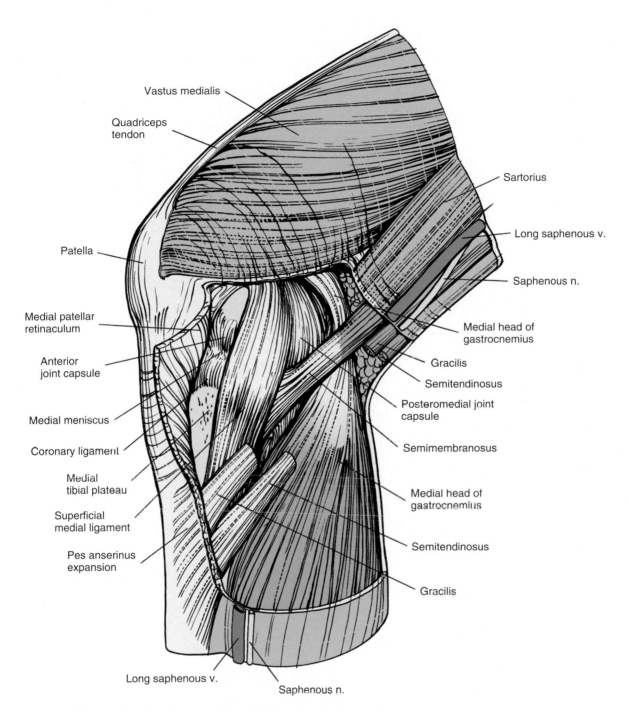

**Figure 10-36** The outer layer has been resected to reveal the intermediate layer, consisting of the superficial medial ligament. Between the superficial and medial layers run the semitendinosus and gracilis muscles. The deep medial ligament (meniscofemoral ligament) of the deep layer is visible. The true joint capsule anterior to the superficial medial ligament also is visible.

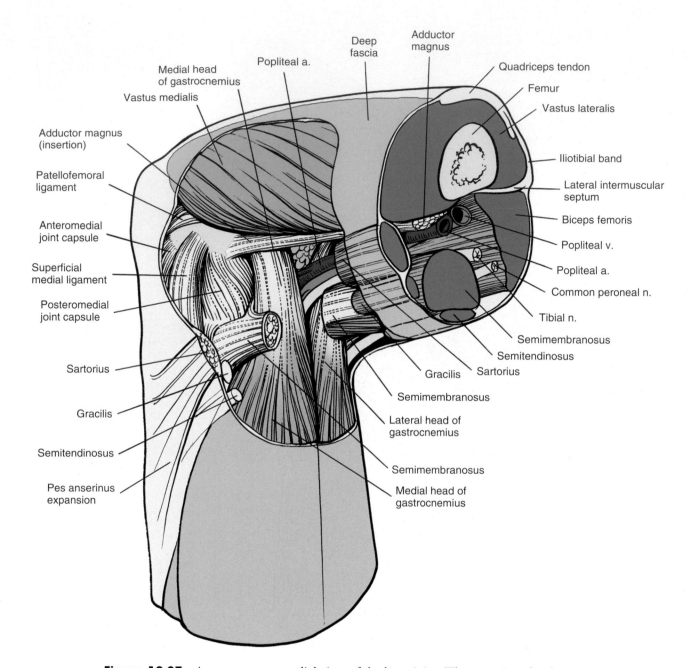

**Figure 10-37**   A more posteromedial view of the knee joint. The sartorius, the deep fascia of the outer layer, the gracilis, the semitendinosus, and the semimembranosus have been resected to reveal the superficial medial ligament (middle layer), the posteromedial joint capsule (deep layer), and the medial head of the gastrocnemius.

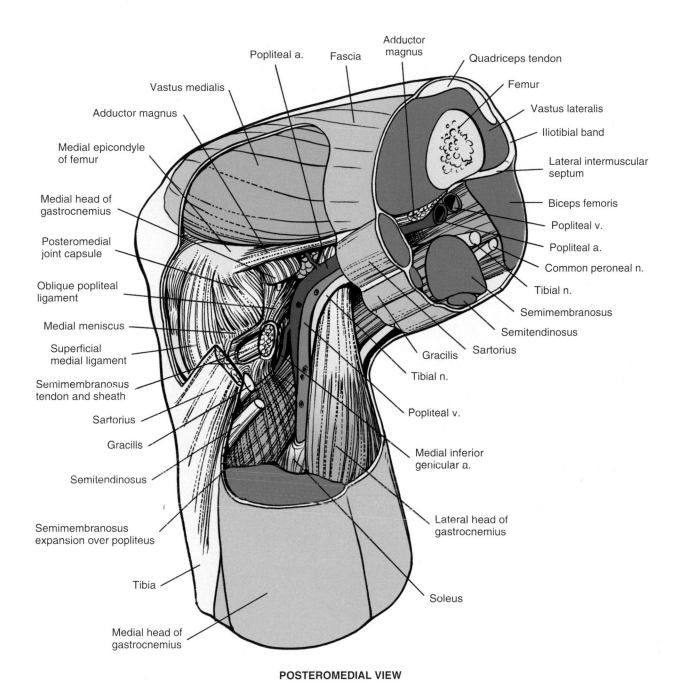

Popliteal a.   Fascia   Adductor magnus   Quadriceps tendon

Vastus medialis

Adductor magnus

Medial epicondyle of femur

Medial head of gastrocnemius

Posteromedial joint capsule

Oblique popliteal ligament

Medial meniscus

Superficial medial ligament

Semimembranosus tendon and sheath

Sartorius

Gracills

Semitendinosus

Semimembranosus expansion over popliteus

Tibia

Medial head of gastrocnemius

Femur

Vastus lateralis

Iliotibial band

Lateral intermuscular septum

Biceps femoris

Popliteal v.

Popliteal a.

Common peroneal n.

Tibial n.

Semimembranosus

Semitendinosus

Sartorius

Gracilis   Tibial n.

Popliteal v.

Medial inferior genicular a.

Lateral head of gastrocnemius

Soleus

**POSTEROMEDIAL VIEW**

**Figure 10-38**   The medial head of the gastrocnemius has been resected to reveal the three expansions of the semimembranosus.

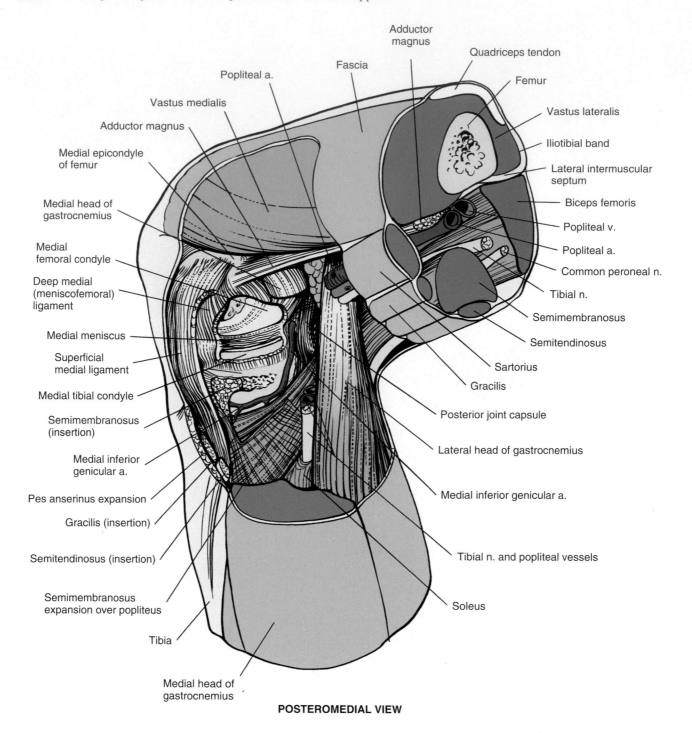

**POSTEROMEDIAL VIEW**

**Figure 10-39** The posterior aspect of the superficial medial ligament (middle layer) has been excised to reveal the true joint capsule and its thickening, the deep medial ligament (the meniscofemoral ligament and the coronary ligaments). The posteromedial joint capsule has been excised to reveal the corner of the joint. The insertion of the semimembranosus and a portion of its expansion are visible.

## Superficial and Deep Surgical Dissections

The three-layer pattern offers a step-by-step approach to the medial exposure of the knee that is consistent with the anatomy.

I. *Medial exposure of the knee and its supporting structures*

A. With anterior arthrotomy

1. The *outer layer* is incised in front of the sartorius muscle for exposure of the middle and deep layers (see Fig. 10-35).
2. Retraction of the sartorius muscle posteriorly uncovers the two structures lying between the superficial and middle layers: the semitendinosus and gracilis muscles (see Fig. 10-36).
3. Retraction of all three muscles of the pes anserinus reveals the *middle layer*, the superficial medial ligament (see Fig. 10-36).
4. Vertical incision through the medial patellar retinaculum exposes the thin underlying capsule, the *deep layer* (see Fig. 10-36).
5. Incision of this capsule makes accessible the intraarticular structures of the anterior half of the joint (see Fig. 10-34).

B. With posterior arthrotomy

1. Incision of the *outer layer* anterior to the sartorius muscle (and posterior retraction of this muscle, the semitendinosus muscle, and the gracilis muscle) reveals the superficial medial ligament (see Fig. 10-37).
2. Further posterior retraction brings the posteromedial corner of the joint into view. The cover consists of fibrous tissue derived from the semimembranosus muscle (the *middle layer*), which has fused with the true joint capsule (the *deep layer*; see Fig. 10-38).
3. Covering the medial side of the posterior joint capsule is the medial head of the gastrocnemius muscle. This head can be reflected backward off the capsule to extend the exposure posteriorly (see Figs. 10-37 and 10-39).
4. Arthrotomy posterior to the superficial medial ligament consists of incising the deep and middle layers together, exposing the intraarticular structures in the posterior half of the joint (Fig. 10-40; see Fig. 10-39).

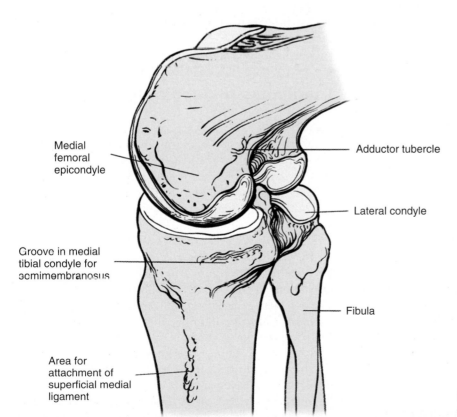

Medial femoral epicondyle

Adductor tubercle

Groove in medial tibial condyle for semimembranosus

Lateral condyle

Fibula

Area for attachment of superficial medial ligament

**Figure 10-40** Osteology of the posteromedial aspect of the knee joint.

II. *Approach for medial meniscectomy*
  A. Incising the medial patellar retinaculum exposes the true capsule of the joint, which is very thin at this point.
  B. The true capsule of the joint, incised with the synovium, allows access to the anteromedial portion of the joint (see Figs. 10-33 and 10-34).
III. *Medial parapatellar approach to the knee*
  A. The joint is dissected through the same fascial layers as in the approach for the medial meniscus.

## Special Anatomic Points

Three muscles, the sartorius, semitendinosus, and gracilis, insert into the upper part of the subcutaneous surface of the tibia. Each muscle has a different nerve supply: the sartorius is innervated by the femoral nerve, the semitendinosus by the sciatic nerve, and the gracilis by the obturator nerve. In addition, each muscle crosses both the hip and the knee.

The actions of the three muscles are duplicated by other, more powerful, muscles. At their pelvic origins, the three attach to three points on the bony pelvis that are separated as widely as the pelvis allows: the anterior superior iliac spine (sartorius), the ischial tuberosity (semitendinosus), and the inferior pubic ramus (gracilis). With these origins and insertions, the muscles are arranged ideally to stabilize the pelvis on the leg.

The sartorius, semitendinosus, and gracilis insert into the subcutaneous surface of the tibia at a point called the *pes anserinus* (goose foot). Acting together, they not only flex the knee, but also internally rotate the tibia.

# Approach for Lateral Meniscectomy

A lateral meniscectomy can be performed through several types of incisions. Longitudinal and oblique incisions provide better access to other structures within the joint, whereas a transverse incision provides limited access to the knee, but excellent exposure of the meniscus itself. All incisions enter the lateral compartment of the knee anterior to the superficial lateral ligament.

The approach is used for the following:

1. Lateral meniscectomy, total and partial[18]
2. Removal of loose bodies
3. Removal of foreign bodies
4. Treatment of osteochondritis of the lateral femoral condyle

## Position of the Patient

### Table-Bent Position
The table-bent position is identical to that used for medial meniscectomy. Two points are critical:

1. The sandbag must be placed under the thigh, not under the knee, to keep the popliteal artery and the posterior capsule from being compressed against the back of the femur and tibia.
2. The knee should be free to flex more than 90° to allow the best possible access to the back of the joint (Fig. 10-41).

### Crossed-Leg Position
Place the patient supine on the operating table. Drop the end of the table so the knees can flex. Then, place the calf of the affected side over the opposite thigh to flex the affected knee and abduct and externally rotate the hip. Now, place the table in 45° of Trendelenburg to bring the lateral side of the knee up to eye level. Finally, flex the head of the table up so that the patient does not slide backward (Fig. 10-42).

For both positions, exsanguinate the limb either by elevating it for 2 minutes or by applying a soft rubber bandage. Next, inflate a tourniquet.

## Landmarks and Incision

### Landmarks
The *lateral femoral condyle* is palpable along its smooth surface as far as the joint line.

The *head of the fibula* is situated at about the same level as the tibial tubercle. From the lateral femoral epicondyle, move a thumb inferiorly and posteriorly across the joint line to find it.

Palpate the *lateral border of the patella*.

To find the *lateral joint line*, flex and extend the knee; palpate the hinge area with a thumb to feel the movement of the femur and the tibia.

To palpate the *superficial lateral ligament (fibular collateral ligament*, lateral collateral ligament), cross the patient's leg so that his or her ankle rests on the opposite knee. When the knee is flexed to 90° and the hip is abducted and externally rotated, the iliotibial tract relaxes and makes the superficial lateral ligament easier to isolate. The ligament stands away from the joint itself, stretching from the fibular head to the lateral femoral condyle.

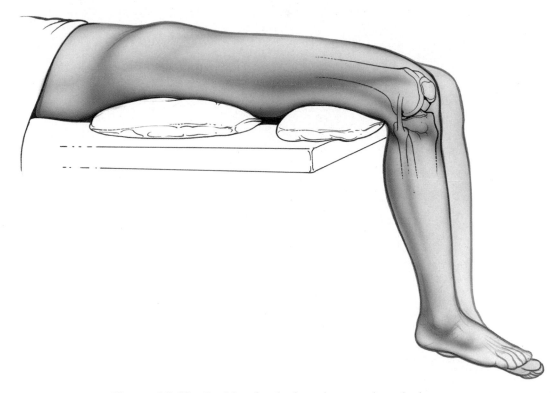

**Figure 10-41**   Position for the lateral approach to the knee.

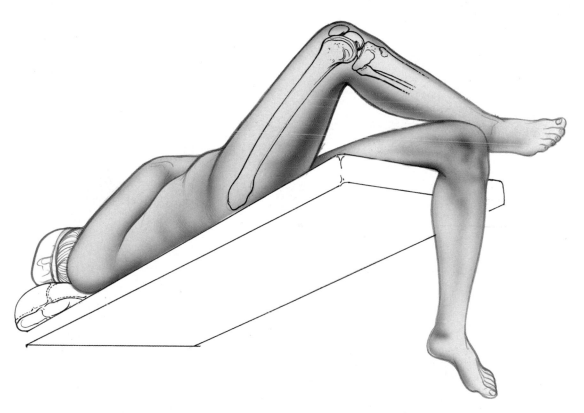

**Figure 10-42**   With the patient supine on the operating table, drop the end of the table so the knee can flex. The crossed-leg position allows a direct approach to the lateral aspect of the knee.

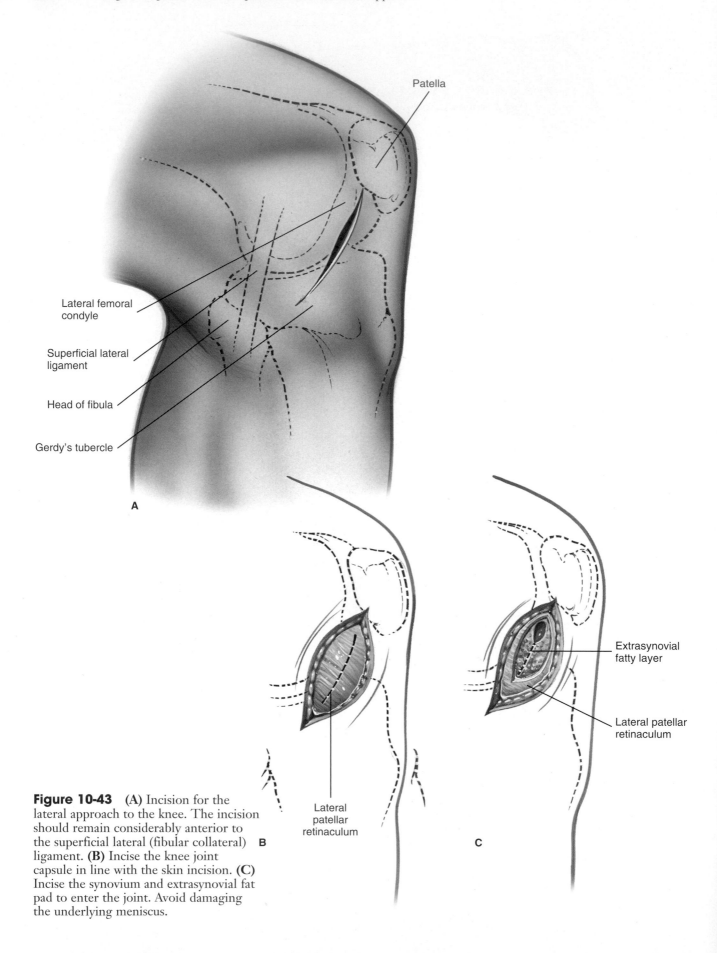

Patella

Lateral femoral
condyle

Superficial lateral
ligament

Head of fibula

Gerdy's tubercle

**A**

Extrasynovial
fatty layer

Lateral patellar
retinaculum

Lateral
patellar
retinaculum

**B**

**C**

**Figure 10-43** **(A)** Incision for the
lateral approach to the knee. The incision
should remain considerably anterior to
the superficial lateral (fibular collateral)
ligament. **(B)** Incise the knee joint
capsule in line with the skin incision. **(C)**
Incise the synovium and extrasynovial fat
pad to enter the joint. Avoid damaging
the underlying meniscus.

### Incision

Of all the skin incisions made around the knee, the oblique incision offers the most leeway, both for meniscectomy and for other intraarticular procedures, should they prove necessary. To make the incision, start at the inferolateral corner of the patella and continue downward and backward for about 5 cm. The cut should remain considerably anterior to the superficial lateral ligament, which lies under a line drawn vertically up from the head of the fibula to the lateral femoral condyle (Fig. 10-43*A*).

### Internervous Plane

There is no internervous plane in this approach, which consists mainly of incisions of the lateral patellar retinaculum and the joint capsule. No major nerves are located in or near the area.

### Superficial Surgical Dissection

Open the anterolateral aspect of the knee capsule in line with the incision (see Fig. 10-43*B*).

### Deep Surgical Dissection

Incise the synovium and extrasynovial fat of the knee joint in line with the incision to open the anterolateral portion of the joint. To avoid damaging the underlying meniscus, begin the incision well above the joint line and cut down carefully (Fig. 10-44; see Fig. 10-43*C*).

### Dangers

#### Vessels

The *lateral inferior genicular artery* runs around the upper part of the tibia. The artery lies next to the peripheral attachment of the lateral meniscus; it may be damaged if the meniscus is detached along with a portion of the capsule during meniscectomy, leading to massive postoperative hemarthrosis. It is not in danger during the approach (see Fig. 10-50).

#### Muscles and Ligaments

The **superficial lateral ligament** (fibular collateral ligament) limits posterior extension at the incision. If it is cut and not repaired, it may affect lateral stability. Its position may be estimated by a line drawn from the head of the fibula to the lateral femoral condyle (see Fig. 10-50).

### Special Problems

The lateral meniscus may be damaged if the synovium is incised too close to the joint line.

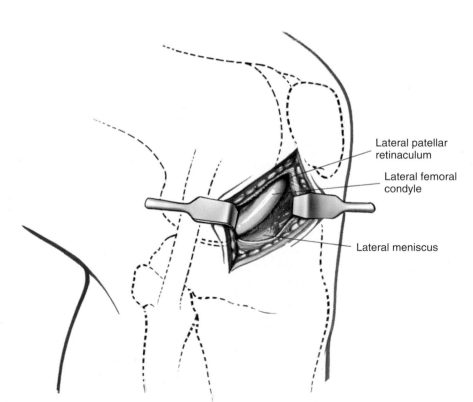

Lateral patellar retinaculum

Lateral femoral condyle

Lateral meniscus

**Figure 10-44**  Expose the meniscus. Place retractors to allow maximum exposure of the joint.

## How to Enlarge the Approach

This particular approach restricts the view of the inside of the joint because of the relative immobility of the structures that are incised and the difficulty in retracting them. The exposure may be improved in three ways without extending the incision:

1. *Retraction.* Retractors should be readjusted frequently to allow the best possible view.
2. *Position* of *the joint.* An inward stress opens up the lateral side of the joint (one advantage of the crossed-leg position), which automatically puts an inward stress on the knee. Flexion of the knee allows better access to the back of the lateral side of the joint. If the very back of the joint must be seen, however, the best view may be obtained by putting the knee into extension and applying distraction and inward force.
3. *Lights.* The direction of the light should be adjusted frequently so that it shines into the depths of the wound. A headlamp can be used to advantage for lateral meniscectomy.

### Extensile Measures

***Posterior Extension.*** The incision cannot be extended posteriorly because of the presence of the superficial lateral ligament.

***Superior Extension.*** To extend the incision superiorly, incise the skin and lateral patellar retinaculum along the lateral border of the patella, increasing access to the back of the patella. To widen the exposure still further, extend the incision superiorly and open the plane between the posterior border of the vastus lateralis muscle and the lateral intramuscular septum. Extending this approach into a posterolateral approach to the femur offers the theoretic possibility of extending the exposure as far as the greater trochanter (see Posterolateral Approach in Chapter 9). This extended exposure is very useful in the treatment of supracondylar fractures of the femur with intraarticular components.

***Inferior Extension.*** To extend the incision inferiorly, incise the skin vertically downward, staying lateral to the tibial tubercle and running vertically down the leg about 1 cm from the subcutaneous border of the tibia. Incise the lateral patellar retinaculum, then carefully detach part of the origin of the tibialis anterior muscle from the lateral border of the tibia. This will allow access to the upper third of the tibia and good visualization of the inside of the joint. This extension can be used for the internal fixation of lateral tibial plateau fractures. In these fractures, it is critically important to achieve good visualization of the articular surface of the lateral tibial condyle to allow anatomic reconstruction of this surface.

# Lateral Approach to the Knee and Its Supporting Structures

The lateral approach provides access to all the supporting structures on the lateral side of the knee. It may be extended for intraarticular exploration of the knee's anterior and posterior structures as well.

Normally, only part of the exposure is needed for any single surgical procedure. Its major use is in the assessment of ligamentous damage, a type of pathology that is more common on the medial side because outward stress is more common than inward stress.

## Position of the Patient

Place the patient supine on the operating table with a sandbag under the buttock of the affected side. This position rotates the leg medially to expose better the lateral aspect of the knee. Flex the knee to 90°. Exsanguinate the limb either by elevating it for 3 to 5 minutes or by applying a soft rubber bandage, then inflate a tourniquet (see Fig. 10-41).

## Landmarks and Incision

### Landmarks
Locate the *lateral border of the patella* and the *lateral joint line.*

*Gerdy's tubercle* (the lateral tubercle of the tibia), a smooth, circular facet on the anterior surface of the lateral condyle of the tibia, marks the inferior attachment of the iliotibial band. Palpate it just lateral to the patellar ligament.

## Incision

A long, curved incision is needed for adequate exposure of all the lateral structures of the knee. Begin the incision at the level of the middle of the patella and 3 cm lateral to it. With the knee still flexed, extend the cut downward, over Gerdy's tubercle on the tibia and 4 to 5 cm distal to the joint line. Complete the incision by curving its upper end to follow the line of the femur (Fig. 10-45).

## Internervous Plane

The dissection exploits the plane between the *iliotibial band* and the *biceps femoris* muscle. The iliotibial band is the fascial aponeurosis of two muscles, the gluteus maximus and the tensor fasciae latae, both of which are supplied by the superior gluteal nerve. The biceps femoris is supplied by the sciatic nerve. Although the iliotibial band itself has no nerve sup-

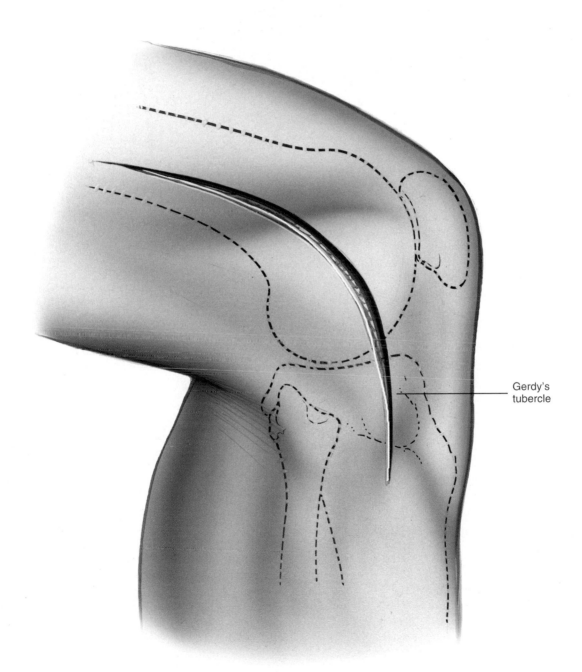

Gerdy's tubercle

**Figure 10-45** Incision for the lateral approach to the knee joint. The incision should be made with the knee flexed.

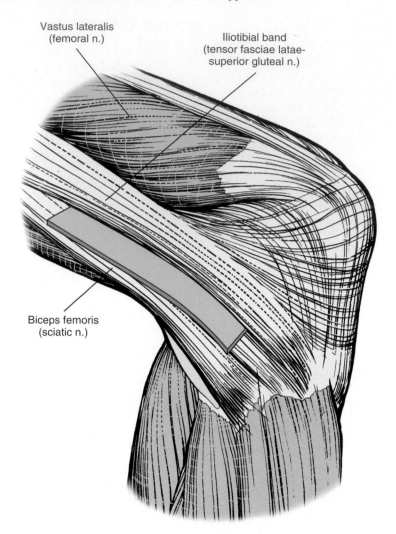

**Figure 10-46**   Internervous plane between the *iliotibial band* (which is supplied by the superior gluteal nerve) and the *biceps femoris* (which is supplied by the sciatic nerve).

ply, the plane between it and the biceps femoris can be considered an internervous one because of the band's muscular origin (Fig. 10-46).

## Superficial Surgical Dissection

Mobilize the skin flaps widely. Underneath are two major structures: the iliotibial band, sweeping down to attach to the anterolateral border of the tibia and Gerdy's tubercle, and the biceps femoris muscle, passing downward and forward to attach to the head of the fibula. Both these structures may be avulsed

from their insertions during severe inward stress to the knee.

Incise the fascia in the interval between the iliotibial band and the biceps femoris muscle, avoiding the common peroneal nerve on the posterior border of the biceps tendon (Fig. 10-47). Retract the iliotibial band anteriorly and the biceps femoris muscle (with the peroneal nerve) posteriorly, uncovering the superficial lateral ligament (fibular collateral ligament) as it runs from the lateral epicondyle of the femur to the head of the fibula. The posterolateral corner of the knee capsule also is visible (Fig. 10-48).

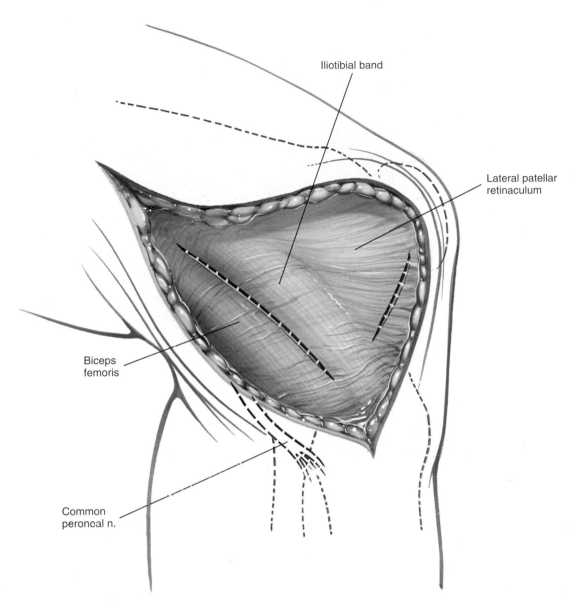

**Figure 10-47**   Incise the fascia in the interval between the iliotibial band and the biceps femoris to uncover the superficial lateral (fibular collateral) ligament and the posterior joint complex. Make a separate fascial incision anteriorly to create a lateral parapatellar approach.

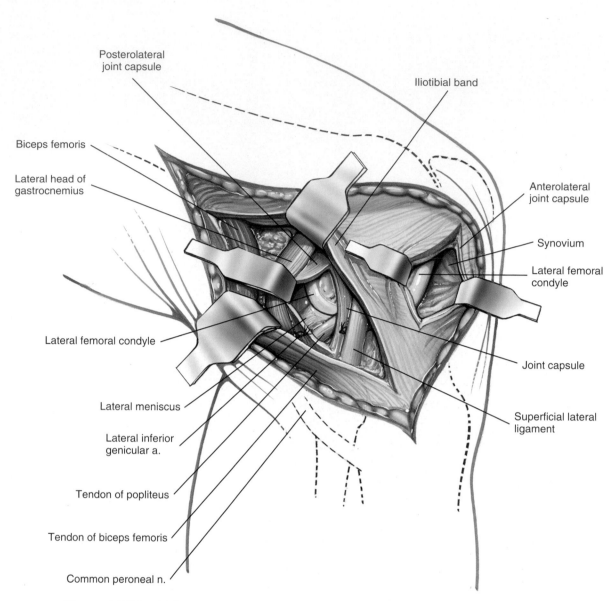

Posterolateral
joint capsule

Iliotibial band

Biceps femoris

Lateral head of
gastrocnemius

Anterolateral
joint capsule

Synovium

Lateral femoral
condyle

Lateral femoral condyle

Joint capsule

Lateral meniscus

Lateral inferior
genicular a.

Superficial lateral
ligament

Tendon of popliteus

Tendon of biceps femoris

Common peroneal n.

**Figure 10-48** Make an incision into the joint capsule anterior to the superficial lateral ligament for a standard anterolateral approach. To enter the posterior portion of the joint, retract the iliotibial band anteriorly and the biceps femoris posteriorly, revealing the superficial lateral ligament and the posterolateral aspect of the joint. Incise the joint capsule posterior to the ligament to reveal the contents of the joint.

## Deep Surgical Dissection

Enter the joint either in front of or behind the superficial lateral ligament (see Fig. 10-48).

### Anterior Arthrotomy

To inspect the entire lateral meniscus, incise the capsule in front of the ligament. Make a separate fascial incision to create a lateral parapatellar approach. To avoid incising the meniscus, begin the arthrotomy 2 cm above the joint line (see Fig. 10-47).

## Posterior Arthrotomy

To inspect the posterior horn of the lateral meniscus, find the lateral head of the gastrocnemius muscle at its origin at the back of the lateral condyle of the femur. Dissect between it and the posterolateral corner of the joint capsule. The lateral superior genicular arteries are in this area; they must be ligated or coagulated.

Note that the popliteus muscle inserts into the femur by way of a tendon that lies inside the joint capsule; the posterolateral corner of the knee may be hidden by the popliteus and its tendon. In cases of trauma, the dissection in this area already may have been done.

Make a longitudinal incision in the capsule, starting the arthrotomy well above the joint line to avoid damaging the meniscus or the tendon of the popliteus. An arthrotomy of the posterior half of the joint capsule must be performed carefully to avoid damaging the popliteus tendon, which lies outside the meniscus. The arthrotomy allows inspection of the posterior half of the lateral compartment behind the superficial lateral ligament (see Fig. 10-48).

## Dangers

### Nerves

The **common peroneal nerve** is the structure most at risk during this approach. It lies on the posterior border of the biceps tendon and must be found early in the approach, as the supporting structures of the lateral side of the knee are being dissected; thereafter, it must be protected, because it is easy to damage. The nerve should be identified proximal to any damage and traced from a normal area into an abnormal one (Fig. 10-49).

### Vessels

The **lateral superior genicular artery** runs between the lateral head of the gastrocnemius muscle and the posterolateral capsule, and requires ligation for full exposure of that corner of the joint (Fig. 10-51). Because this vessel may cause a significant postoperative hematoma if it is not ligated adequately, it is advisable to remove the tourniquet before closing the incision.

### Muscles and Ligaments

The **popliteus tendon** is at risk as it travels within the joint before it attaches to the posterior aspect of the meniscus and the femur. Take care when opening the posterior half of the knee joint capsule to avoid cutting the tendon (see Fig. 10-51).

## Special Problems

The **lateral meniscus** or its **coronary ligament** may be incised accidentally if arthrotomy is performed too close to the joint line.

## How to Enlarge the Approach

### Local Measures

The approach as described gives a complete view of the lateral structures of the knee and cannot be improved usefully.

### Extensile Measures

The exposure cannot be extended usefully.

# Applied Surgical Anatomy of the Lateral Side of the Knee

## Overview

The supporting structures on the lateral side of the knee fall into three layers. Because the anatomy can be distorted in pathologic states, a clear understanding of the normal anatomy is required before explorations[19] are carried out.

## Outer Layer

The outer layer is continuous with the deep fascia of the thigh (see Fig. 10-49). The *iliotibial band*, the aponeurotic tendon of the tensor fasciae latae and gluteus maximus muscles, is a thickening in the deep fascia of the thigh. Its fibers run longitudinally.

The band inserts into a smooth facet on the anterior surface of the lateral condyle of the tibia that is known as Gerdy's tubercle. It also sends fibers into the deep fascia of the leg and reinforces the lateral patellar retinaculum. In injuries to the knee involving severe inward stress, its insertion may be avulsed. When the knee is in extension, the iliotibial band is anterior to the axis of rotation and maintains extension. With the knee flexed to 90°, it moves behind the axis of rotation and can act as a flexor. This variable relationship to the axis of rotation may be a feature in the genesis of the pivot shift test for a torn anterior cruciate ligament.[20]

The *biceps femoris* muscle, a part of the outer layer, is enclosed by the deep fascia, as is the sartorius muscle on the medial side.

The *lateral patellar retinaculum* is a tough structure derived largely from the fascia covering the vastus lateralis muscle.

## Middle Layer

The superficial lateral ligament (fibular collateral ligament) runs from the lateral epicondyle of the femur to the head of the fibula. The lateral inferior genicular vessels run between the ligament and the joint capsule itself. Because the ligament is attached to the femoral

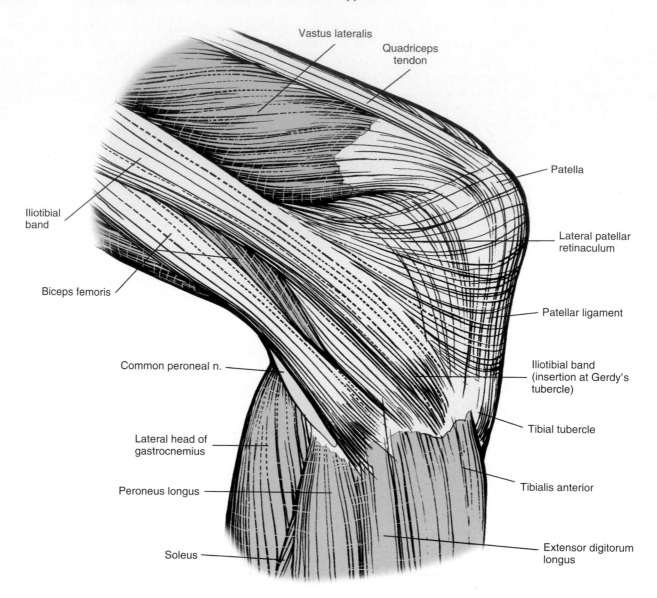

**Figure 10-49**  A slightly anterolateral view of the outer layer of the knee. The lateral patellar retinaculum, the biceps femoris, and the iliotibial band constitute the outer layer.

condyle behind the axis of rotation, it is tight in extension. When the ligament is damaged, subsequent functional problems are minimized by the existence of other supporting structures on the lateral side of the knee, especially the iliotibial band (see Fig. 10-50).

### Deep Layer
The deep layer consists of the true capsule of the knee joint, the fibrous tissue attached just above and

below the articular surfaces of the knee. Two other structures run with the capsule:

1. The *popliteus* muscle originates from the popliteal surface of the tibia above the soleal line. Its tendon, which lies within the joint capsule, attaches to the lateral condyle of the femur and the posterior aspect of the lateral meniscus.

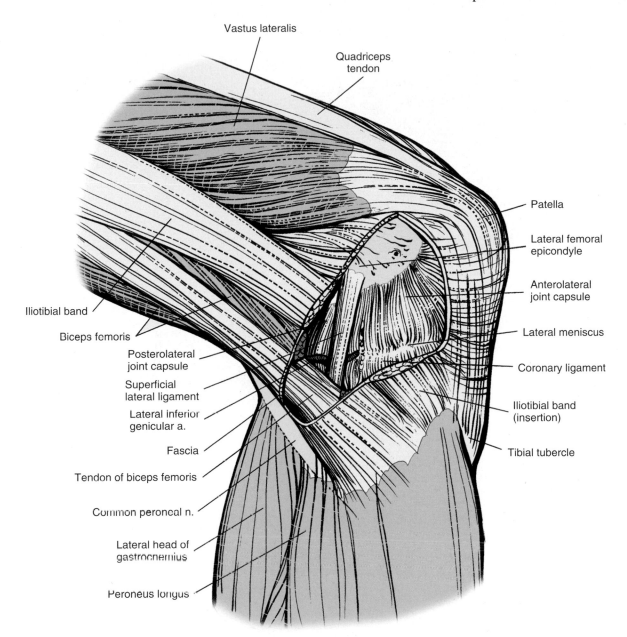

**Figure 10-50**   The lateral patellar retinaculum, the iliotibial band, and the deep fascia (outer layer) have been excised to reveal the superficial lateral ligament (middle layer) and the joint capsule (deep layer). Note that the lateral inferior genicular artery runs along the joint line between the middle and deep layers.

2. The *short lateral ligament* (deep lateral ligament) is a thickening in the true capsule of the knee. The ligament is developed poorly; it runs underneath the superficial lateral ligament (fibular collateral ligament), from the lateral femoral condyle to the head of the fibula. Unlike the medial ligament, the lateral ligament does not attach to the meniscus. That is why the lateral meniscus can move far more freely than can its medial counterpart (see Fig. 10-51).

## Landmarks and Incision

Oblique or longitudinal skin incisions cross the lines of cleavage almost perpendicularly and may result in broad scars.

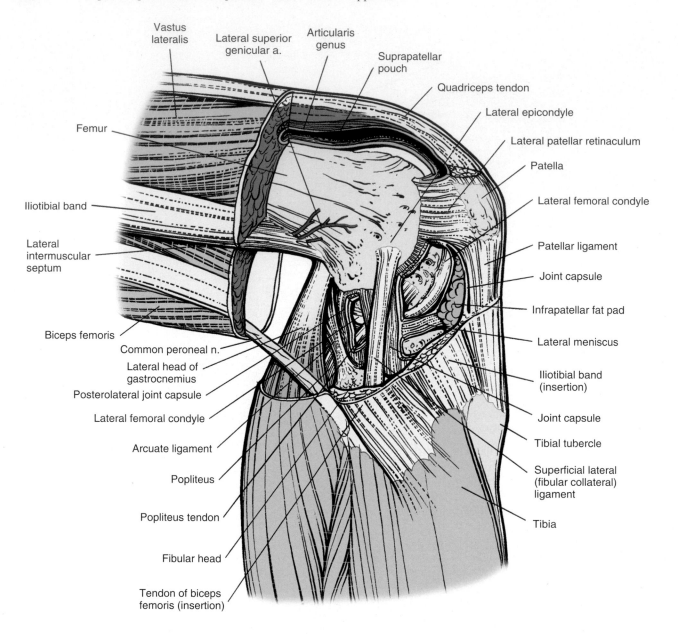

**Figure 10-51**   A true lateral view of the knee joint. The biceps femoris, iliotibial band, and vastus lateralis have been excised to reveal the deeper layers. The joint capsule has been excised anterior and posterior to the superficial lateral ligament (fibular collateral ligament) to expose the intraarticular structures, notably the popliteus tendon and the lateral meniscus.

## Superficial and Deep Dissections

I. *Approach for lateral meniscectomy*
   A. Incise the *superficial* and *deep layers*, cutting the lateral patellar retinaculum (see Fig. 10-50).
   B. The true capsule of the joint is very thin at this point. Incise it with its synovium to gain access to the joint surface.

II. *Lateral exposure of the knee and its supporting structures*
   A. Open the *superficial layer* in the plane between the biceps femoris muscle and the iliotibial band (see Fig. 10-50).
   B. Incise the joint either in front of or behind the superficial lateral ligament, the *middle layer* of the lateral side (see Fig. 10-51).
   C. Incise the capsule of the joint (the *deep layer*) in front of or behind the superficial lateral ligament. Do not damage the tendon of the popliteus muscle, which lies between the outer border of the lateral meniscus and the capsule of the joint (see Fig. 10-51).

# Posterior Approach to the Knee

The posterior approach[3,21] is primarily a neurovascular approach. Orthopaedically, it rarely is needed because the medial and lateral approaches each provide good access to half the posterior capsule. Its uses include the following:

1. Repair of the neurovascular structures that run behind the knee in cases of trauma
2. Repair of avulsion fractures of the site of attachment of the posterior cruciate ligament to the tibia
3. Recession of gastrocnemius muscle heads in cases of contracture
4. Lengthening of hamstring tendons
5. Excision of Baker's cyst and other popliteal cysts
6. Access to the posterior capsule of the knee

## Position of the Patient

Place the patient prone on the operating table. Use a tourniquet for all procedures except vascular repairs (Fig. 10-52).

## Landmarks and Incision

### Landmarks

Palpate the two heads of the *gastrocnemius muscle* at their origin on the posterior femoral surface just above the medial and lateral condyles. They are not as easy to feel as are the hamstring tendons just above them.

Palpate the *semimembranosus* and *semitendinosus muscles* on the medial border of the popliteal fossa.

The semitendinosus feels round; the semimembranosus is deeper and remains muscular to its insertion.

### Incision

Use a gently curved incision. Start laterally over the biceps femoris muscle, and bring the incision obliquely across the popliteal fossa. Turn downward over the medial head of the gastrocnemius muscle, and run the incision inferiorly into the calf (Fig. 10-53).

## Internervous Plane

There is no true internervous plane in this dissection, which exposes the contents of the popliteal fossa by incising the deep fascia over it and pulling apart the three muscles that form its boundaries.

## Superficial Surgical Dissection

Reflect the skin flaps with the underlying subcutaneous fat. The vein is easier to identify if the leg is not exsanguinated fully before the tourniquet is applied. Running on the lateral side of the vein is the medial sural cutaneous nerve. The small saphenous vein can be used as a guide to the nerve, and the nerve can be used as a guide to dissecting the popliteal fossa. The nerve, which continues beneath the deep fascia of the calf, is a branch of the tibial nerve (Fig. 10-54; see Fig. 10-57).

Incise the fascia of the popliteal fossa just medial to the small saphenous vein. Trace the medial sural cutaneous nerve proximally back to its source, the

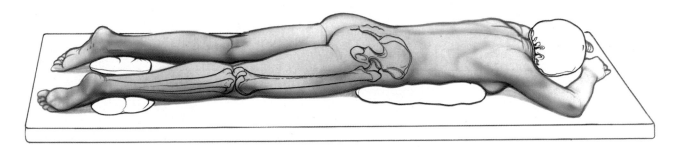

**Figure 10-52**   Position of the patient on the operating table for the posterior approach to the knee.

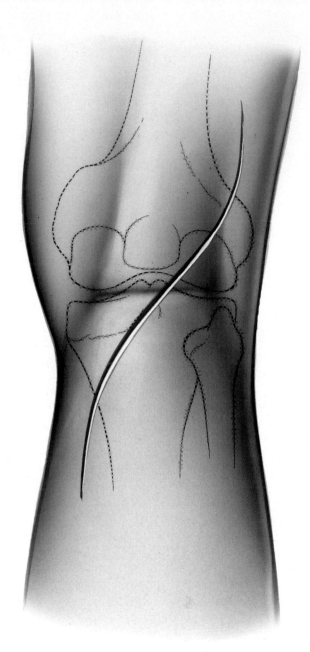

**Figure 10-53** Make a curved incision over the popliteal fossa. Start laterally over the biceps femoris, and bring the incision obliquely across the popliteal fossa. Turn the incision downward over the medial head of the gastrocnemius.

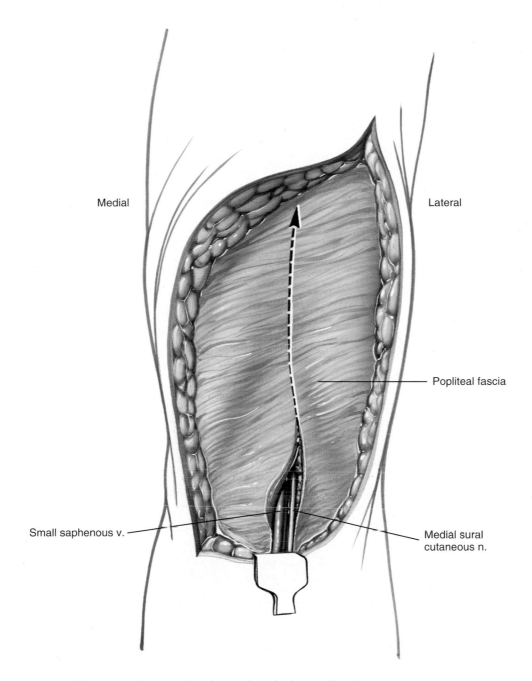

Medial

Lateral

Popliteal fascia

Small saphenous v.

Medial sural
cutaneous n.

**Figure 10-54**  Reflect the skin flaps. Identify the small saphenous vein as it passes upward in the midline of the calf. On the lateral side of the vein is the medial sural cutaneous nerve. Incise the fascia of the fossa just lateral to the small saphenous vein.

tibial nerve. Dissect up to the apex of the popliteal fossa, following the tibial nerve (Fig. 10-55).

The apex of the popliteal fossa is formed by the semimembranosus muscle on the medial side and the biceps femoris muscle on the lateral side. Roughly at the apex, the common peroneal nerve separates from the tibial nerve. Dissect out the common peroneal nerve in a proximal to distal direction as it runs along the posterior border of the biceps femoris muscle (Fig. 10-56; see Fig. 10-59).

Now, turn to the popliteal artery and vein, which lie deep and medial to the tibial nerve (Fig. 10-57).

The artery has five branches around the knee: two superior, two inferior, and one middle genicular artery. One or more of these branches may have to be ligated if the artery needs to be mobilized (see Fig. 10-60).

The popliteal vein lies medial to the artery as it enters the popliteal fossa from below. Then it curves, lying directly posterior to the artery while in the fossa. Above the knee joint, it moves to the postero-lateral side of the artery. Be very careful in mobilizing this structure. Intimal damage may cause thrombosis.

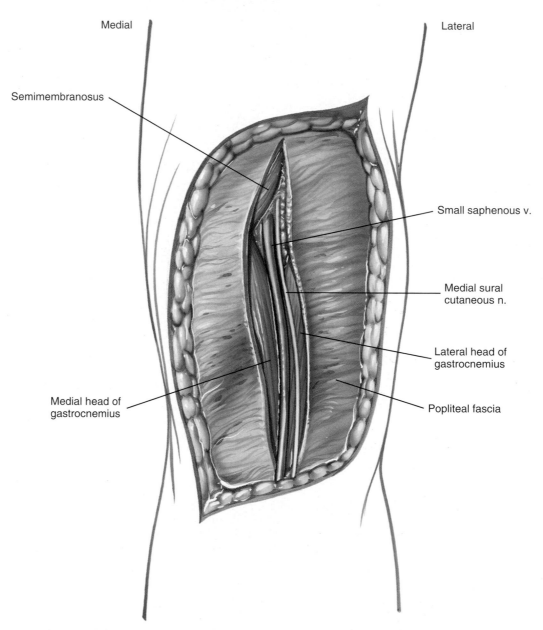

**Figure 10-55**   Incise the fascia of the popliteal fossa. Trace the medial sural cutaneous nerve proximally, back to its source, the tibial nerve.

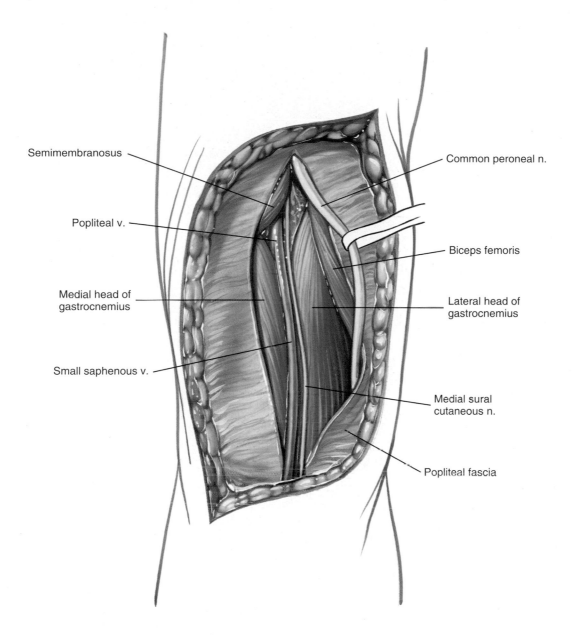

Semimembranosus

Popliteal v.

Medial head of
gastrocnemius

Small saphenous v.

Common peroneal n.

Biceps femoris

Lateral head of
gastrocnemius

Medial sural
cutaneous n.

Popliteal fascia

**Figure 10-56** Dissect out the common peroneal nerve in a proximal to distal direction as it runs along the posterior border of the biceps femoris muscle.

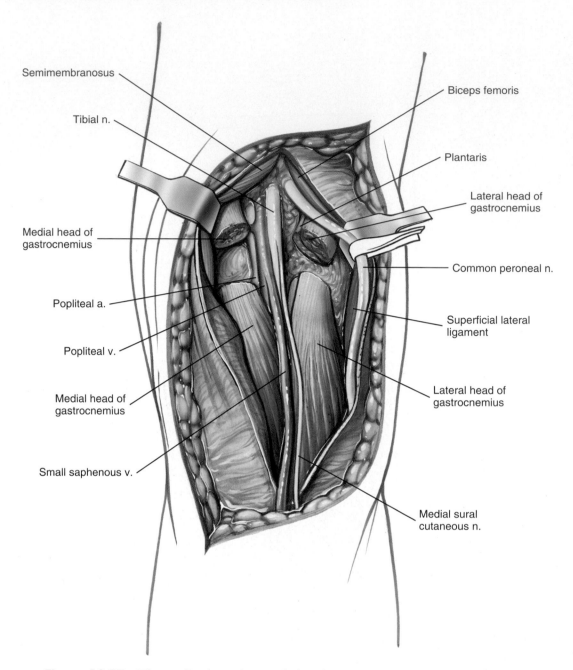

**Figure 10-57**   The popliteal vein lies medial to the artery as it enters the popliteal fossa from below. Then it curves, lying directly posterior to the artery while in the fossa.

## Deep Surgical Dissection

Retracting the muscles that form the boundaries of the popliteal fossa exposes various parts of the posterior joint capsule. There are two ways to gain greater access to the joint if this is necessary:

1. Posteromedial joint capsule. Detach the tendinous origin of the medial head of the gastrocnemius muscle from the back of the femur. Retract

the head laterally and inferiorly, pulling the nerves and vessels out of the way to reach the posteromedial corner of the joint. The exposure now is the same as that achieved by posterior extension of the medial approach to the knee (Fig. 10-58; see Fig. 10-57).

2. Posterolateral corner of the joint. Detach the origin of the lateral head of the gastrocnemius muscle from the lateral femoral condyle. Develop the

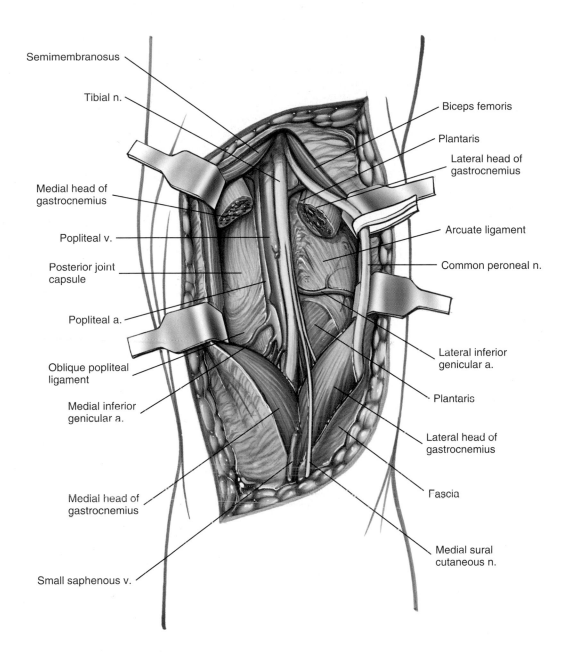

**Figure 10-58** Retract the muscles that form the boundaries of the popliteal fossa, exposing the various parts of the posterior joint capsule. Detach the tendinous origin of the medial head of the gastrocnemius in the back of the femur to expose the posteromedial portion of the joint capsule. Detach the origin of the lateral head of the gastrocnemius from the lateral femoral condyle to expose the posterolateral corner of the joint capsule.

interval between it and the biceps femoris muscle, creating the same exposure as in the lateral approach to the knee (see Figs. 10-57 and 10-58).

Note that the posterior approach is no better than the lateral and medial approaches in dealing with pathology of the posteromedial and posterolateral corners of the knee joint. It should be used mainly for exploring structures within the popliteal fossa and for reattaching the avulsed tibial insertion of the posterior cruciate ligament.

## Dangers

### Nerves
The **medial sural cutaneous nerve,** which lies lateral to the **small saphenous vein,** may be damaged as it travels beneath the deep fascia of the calf. Incising the deep fascia of the calf **medial** to the vein, therefore, will preserve the nerve. Cutting the medial sural cutaneous nerve may produce a painful neuroma, but the resulting anesthesia usually is not significant (Fig. 10-59; see Fig. 10-54).

The **tibial nerve** may be damaged in the popliteal fossa. Damage to the nerve at this level produces paralysis of all the flexors of the toes and feet (Fig. 10-60; see Fig. 10-58).

The **common peroneal nerve** also is susceptible to damage in the popliteal fossa. Damage to the nerve at this level produces paralysis of the extensors and the evertors of the foot (see Figs. 10-58 and 10-59).

### Vessels
The *small saphenous vein* may need to be ligated; this is an uncomplicated procedure.

The *popliteal vessels* can be damaged during deep dissection, producing ischemia of the calf and foot (see Fig. 10-58).

## How to Enlarge the Approach

### Local Measures
The exposure described gives an adequate view of the contents of the popliteal fossa. Retracting the muscles of the fossa improves the view. To expose the knee capsule itself, detach one or both of the heads of the gastrocnemius muscle.

Extend the approach inferiorly to expose the trifurcation of the popliteal artery. At that point, the anterior tibial artery passes forward above the upper border of the interosseous membrane into the extensor compartment of the leg. This pattern makes it difficult to mobilize the artery; anastomoses in these areas are quite challenging.

# Applied Surgical Anatomy of the Posterior Approach to the Knee

## Overview

The anatomy of the posterior approach to the knee is the anatomy of the popliteal fossa.

The popliteal fossa is diamond shaped in cadavers. In live patients, the lower "V" of the diamond (the gap between the two heads of the gastrocnemius muscle) is nonexistent until the heads are retracted from one another.

The fossa is bounded on its superior border by the semimembranosus and semitendinosus muscles medially and by the biceps femoris muscle laterally. Its inferior boundaries are the two heads of the gastrocnemius muscle. The roof of the fossa is the popliteal fascia, which is formed by the outer layer of the knee's supporting structures. The floor is the posterior aspect of the distal end of the femur, the posterior capsule of the joint, and the popliteus muscle, which overlies the proximal tibia (see Fig. 10-59).

## Incision

The lines of cleavage in the skin run almost transversely across the back of the knee joint. The curved incision described, therefore, has a variable relation to these lines. The resultant scar usually is cosmetically acceptable.

The incision crosses a major flexor crease at the back of the knee, but because the incision is almost parallel to the skin crease at this level, a flexion contracture of the knee does not occur when the wound heals.

## Superficial Surgical Dissection

Superficial surgical dissection involves incising the roof of the popliteal fossa, using the small (short) saphenous vein and the medial sural cutaneous nerve of the calf as guides.

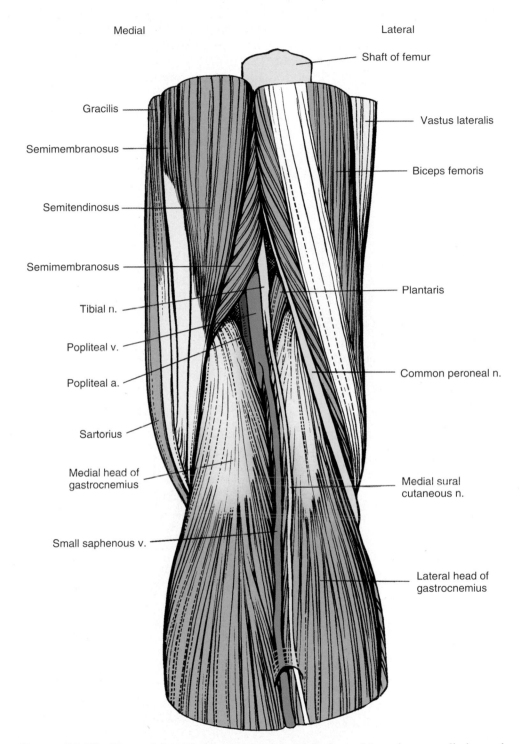

**Figure 10-59**   View of the superficial structures of the knee. Note the centrally located small (short) saphenous vein and medial sural cutaneous nerve.

The *roof* of the popliteal fossa consists of the popliteal fascia, a continuation of the deep fascia of the thigh, and part of the outer layer of the knee. Two key structures pierce it to form the basis for the dissection of the fossa itself:

1. The *small (short) saphenous vein* arises in the foot and runs behind the lateral malleolus into the

back of the calf. It travels roughly along the midline of the calf and penetrates the popliteal fascia before joining the popliteal vein.

2. The *medial sural cutaneous nerve* also runs in the midline of the calf beneath the deep fascia, just lateral to the small saphenous vein. This nerve, which is a branch of the tibial nerve, supplies varying amounts of skin on the back of the calf.

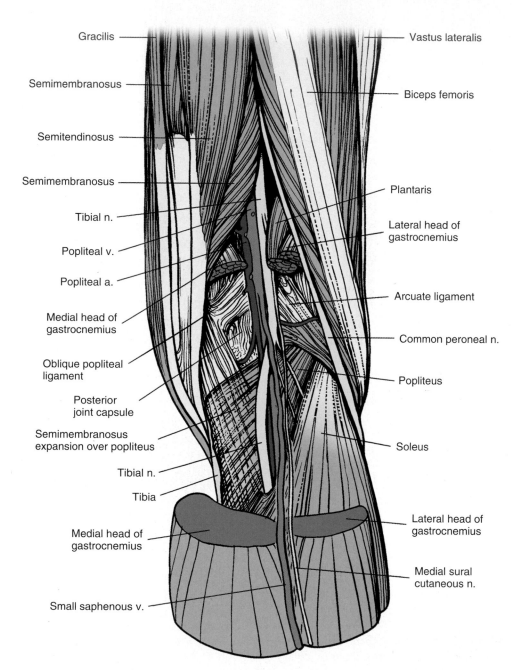

**Figure 10-60**   The gastrocnemius and the plantaris have been resected to reveal the neurovascular bundle in the popliteal fossa.

Knowing the location of these two structures makes it easier to find the tibial nerve (see Fig. 10-59).

The *tibial nerve*, a continuation of the sciatic nerve, is lateral to the popliteal artery as it enters the popliteal fossa. Then, at the midpoint of the fossa, it crosses the artery and lies medial to it as they leave the fossa together. The tibial nerve passes vertically downward in the fossa, giving branches to the plantaris, gastrocnemius, soleus, and popliteus muscles. Its sole cutaneous branch, the sural nerve, is of surgical interest in nerve grafting. The tibial nerve leaves the fossa between the two heads of the gastrocnemius muscle. Tibial nerve palsy affects the plantar flexors of the toes and ankle (see Fig. 10-60).

The *common peroneal nerve* slopes downward across the fossa, running laterally toward the medial side of the tendon of the biceps muscle. It disappears into the peroneus longus muscle, usually under a fibrous arch, where it may be entrapped before it winds around the fibula. Because patients naturally lie with their legs externally rotated, the head of the fibula often is in contact with the bed and compression palsy of the nerve can occur. For this reason, it is critically important to pad the head of the fibula when the patient is placed on the operating table in such a position that the head of this bone may come in contact with the operating table surface. Its division into deep and superficial peroneal nerves occurs within the substance of the peroneus longus muscle. Common peroneal nerve palsy affects all the extensors and evertors of the foot (see Figs. 10-23, 10-25, and 10-60).

The vascular structures lie more deeply in the fossa. The popliteal artery runs obliquely through the fossa after entering on the medial side of the femur. It lies directly behind the posterior capsule of the knee joint, dividing into its terminal branches, the posterior tibial, anterior tibial, and peroneal arteries, behind the gastrocnemius muscle. In the fossa, it gives off five branches:

The *two superior genicular arteries* encircle the lower end of the femur. The lateral artery requires ligation in the posterolateral approach to the knee. The medial artery requires ligation if the medial head of the gastrocnemius muscle has to be detached from the femur to expose the posteromedial corner of the knee.

The *middle genicular artery* passes forward in the knee and supplies the cruciate ligaments. Traumatic rupture of the cruciate ligaments, therefore, is associated with brisk intraarticular bleeding that usually manifests as an immediate posttraumatic effusion. The artery holds its parent trunk firmly to the posterior capsule of the joint. For this reason, it can be damaged easily in dislocations of the knee during trauma or surgery. It also may be damaged as the posterior structures in the knee are dissected out from medial or lateral approaches. To avoid endangering the artery, flex the knee to allow the joint capsule to fall away from the back of the femur and tibia.

The *two inferior genicular arteries* (medial and lateral) encircle the upper end of the tibia, passing deep to the medial and lateral superficial ligaments. The lateral artery is the most commonly damaged structure during lateral meniscectomy; it runs right at the level of the joint line and, therefore, is vulnerable in cases in which the meniscus is detached too far laterally (see Fig. 10-60).

The *popliteal vein* lies between the popliteal artery and the tibial nerve. The small saphenous vein pierces the popliteal fascia to enter the popliteal vein within the fossa.

## Deep Surgical Dissection and Its Dangers

Deep surgical dissection consists of retracting and, sometimes, mobilizing the boundaries of the popliteal fossa. These boundaries are formed by the semimembranosus and semitendinosus muscles superomedially, by the biceps femoris muscle superolaterally, by the medial head of the gastrocnemius muscle inferomedially, and by the lateral head of the gastrocnemius muscle inferolaterally (see Fig. 10-60). For more information on these muscles, see Applied Surgical Anatomy of the Thigh in Chapter 9 and Posterolateral Approach to the Tibia in Chapter 11.

The floor of the popliteal fossa is formed by the *popliteus*, one of the few muscles in the body whose origin is distal to its insertion. The tendon enters the joint by passing through a gap in the posterolateral capsule, beneath the arcuate ligament (Figs. 10-61 and 10-62).

The popliteus muscle unlocks the knee from its fully extended (screw home) position. It also draws the lateral femoral condyle backward on the tibia and pulls the lateral meniscus back, preventing it from being trapped between the tibia and femur. The convex rounded posterior aspect of the lateral tibial plateau allows this movement to take place.

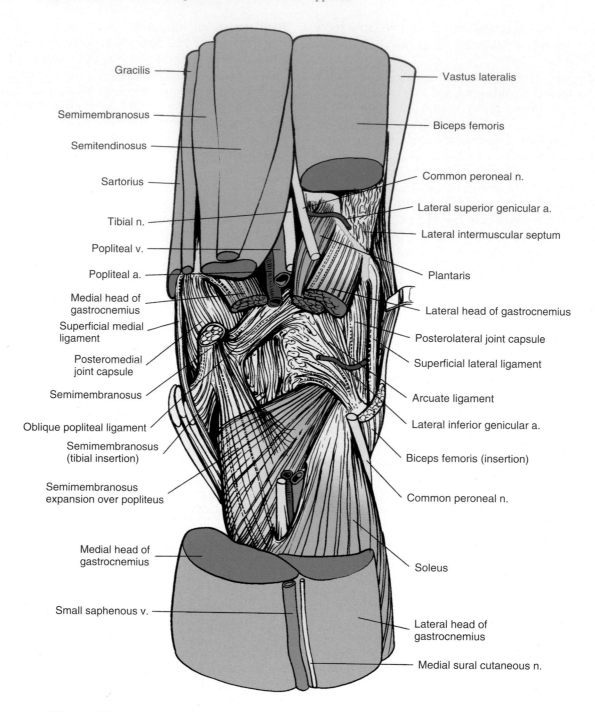

**Figure 10-61** The medial and lateral hamstrings and the neurovascular bundle have been resected to reveal the posterior joint capsule of the knee. Note the three expansions of the semimembranosus sheath.

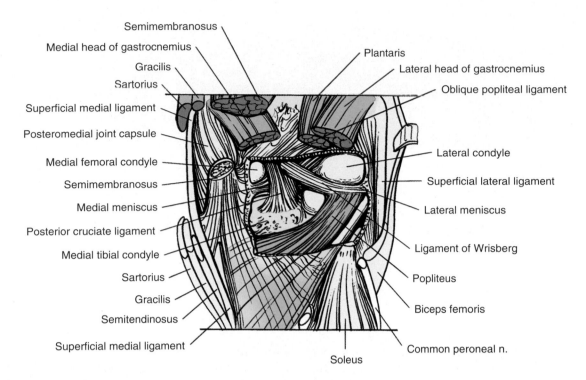

**Figure 10-62**  The posterior joint capsule of the knee has been resected to reveal the intraarticular structures of the posterior aspect of the knee, most notably the posterior cruciate ligament and the popliteus.

**Popliteus.** *Origin.* Popliteal surface of tibia above soleal line. *Insertion.* Lateral epicondyle of femur and posterior aspect of lateral meniscus. *Action.* Rotates femur laterally on tibia. *Nerve supply.* Tibial nerve.

# Lateral Approach to the Distal Femur

The lateral approach to the distal femur, known as the "over-the-top" approach, is used in conjunction with the medial parapatellar approach for repair or reconstruction of the anterior cruciate ligament (see the section regarding the medial parapatellar approach). Therefore, it is not used as an isolated incision. The approach exposes the posterior aspect of the intercondylar notch by passing over the top of the posterior aspect of the lateral femoral condyle.

The lateral approach to the distal femur also provides access to the lateral aspect of the lateral femoral condyle so that drill holes can be made in the condyle

(if they are needed) for reattachment of the femoral end of the anterior cruciate ligament or attachment of the femoral end of an anterior cruciate substitute.

## Position of the Patient

Place the patient supine on the table with a bolster under the thigh so that the knee rests in 30° of flexion. Place a tourniquet high on the patient's thigh and exsanguinate the leg using a compression bandage or prolonged elevation before the tourniquet is inflated (Fig. 10-63).

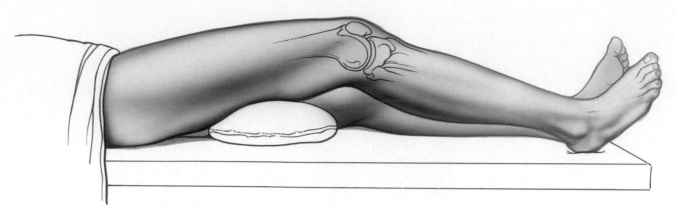

**Figure 10-63**    Position for the lateral approach to the distal femur.

## Landmarks and Incision

### Landmarks

Palpate the posterior lateral margin of the *lateral femoral condyle* as it flares out from the shaft of the femur.

Note the intersection between the *iliotibial band* and the *biceps femoris* muscle.

### Incision

Make a 10-cm incision parallel to and over the indentation between the biceps femoris muscle and

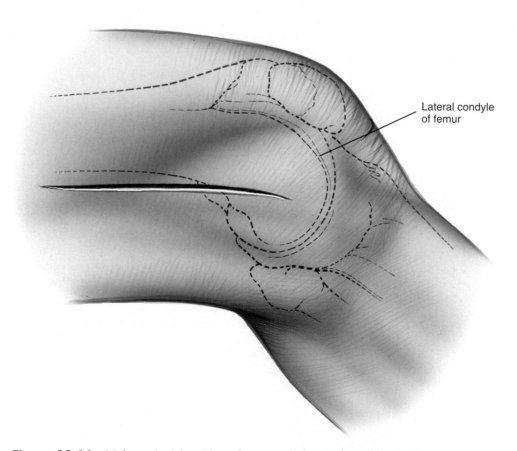

Lateral condyle of femur

**Figure 10-64**    Make an incision 10 cm long parallel to and over the indentation between the biceps femoris and the iliotibial band.

the iliotibial band. Distally, the incision ends at the flare of the femoral condyle (Fig. 10-64).

## Internervous Plane

The dissection exploits the internervous plane between the *vastus lateralis muscle* (which is supplied by the femoral nerve) and the *biceps femoris* muscle (which is supplied by the sciatic nerve; see Fig. 10-51).

## Superficial Surgical Dissection

Incise the iliotibial band just anterior to the lateral intermuscular septum, in line with the skin incision. The incision is slightly anterior to the skin incision itself (Fig. 10-65).

## Deep Surgical Dissection

Identify the vastus lateralis muscle anterior to the intermuscular septum, and retract it anteriorly and medially. Below the muscle lies the lateral superior genicular artery; it must be ligated (Figs. 10-66 and 10-67). Using cautery, incise the periosteum at the junction of the shaft and flare of the femur. Pass a small clamp or a small Cobb elevator behind the posterolateral flare of the lateral femoral condyle, staying in a subperiosteal plane. Carefully carry the dissection distally and medially over the top of the lateral femoral condyle until the instrument can be felt to enter the intercondylar notch (Fig. 10-68). Sticking to bone, pass the tip of the instrument anteriorly until it is visible in the knee, as viewed from the anteromedial incision (medial parapatellar) (Fig. 10-69).

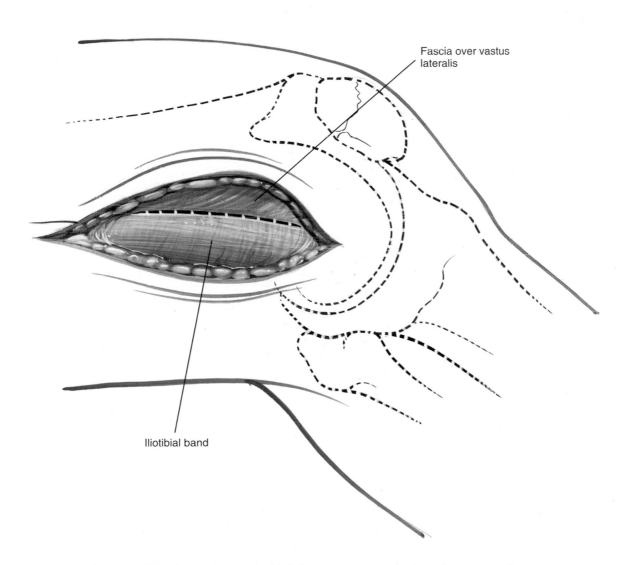

Fascia over vastus lateralis

Iliotibial band

**Figure 10-65** Incise the iliotibial band just anterior to the lateral intermuscular septum, in line with the skin incision.

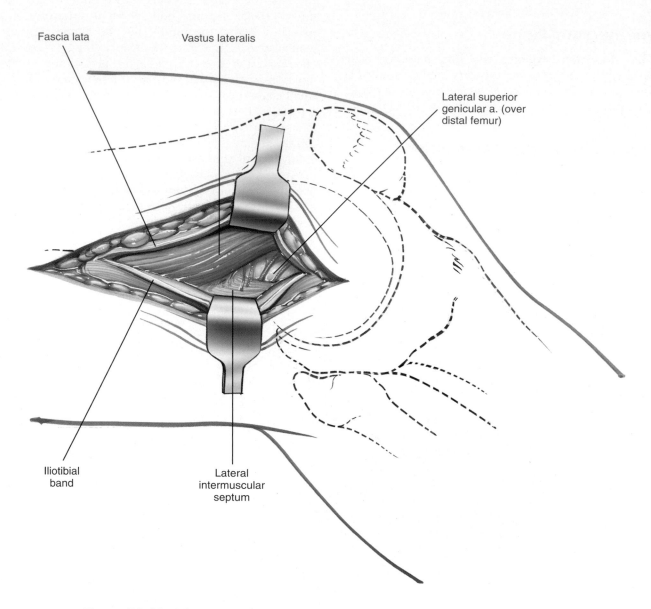

Fascia lata

Vastus lateralis

Lateral superior
genicular a. (over
distal femur)

Iliotibial
band

Lateral
intermuscular
septum

**Figure 10-66**   The vastus lateralis anterior to the intermuscular septum is retracted anteriorly and medially. Identify the lateral superior genicular artery.

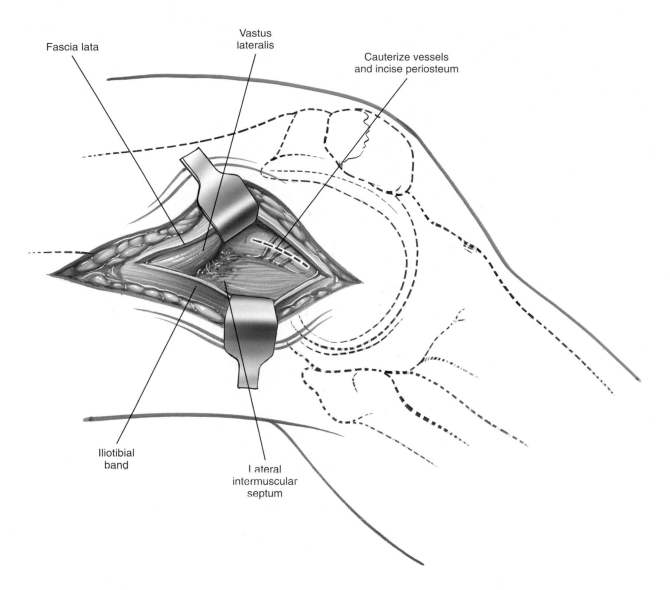

Fascia lata

Vastus
lateralis

Cauterize vessels
and incise periosteum

Iliotibial
band

Lateral
intermuscular
septum

**Figure 10-67**   Retract the muscles further, ligate the lateral superior genicular artery, and incise the periosteum at the junction of the shaft and the flare of the femur.

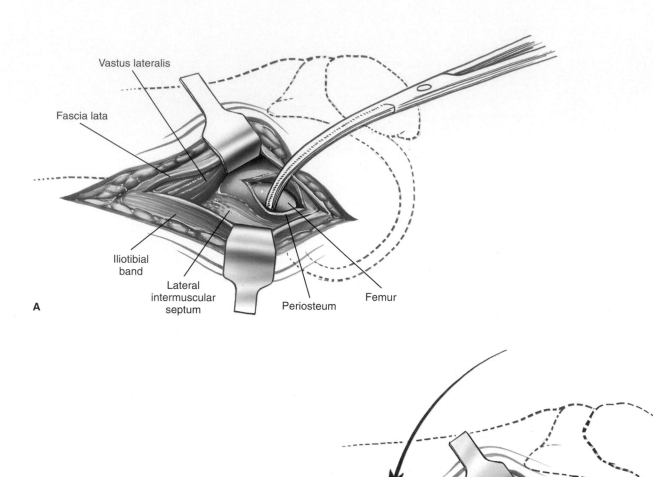

**Vastus lateralis**

**Fascia lata**

**Iliotibial band**

**Lateral intermuscular septum**

**Periosteum**

**Femur**

**A**

**B**

**Figure 10-68**   **(A)** Pass a small instrument behind the posterolateral flare of the lateral femoral condyle deep to the periosteum. **(B)** Continue passing the instrument distally and medially over the top of the lateral femoral condyle until it can be felt entering the intercondylar notch.

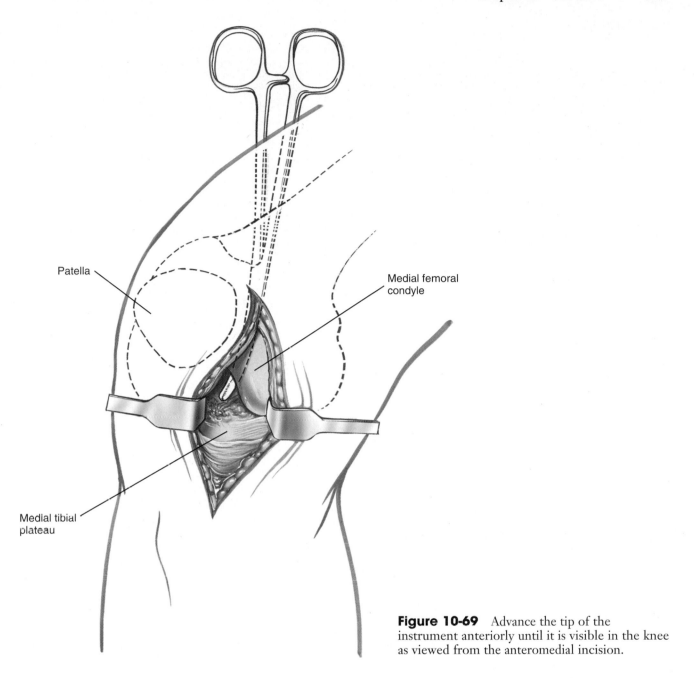

Patella

Medial femoral
condyle

Medial tibial
plateau

**Figure 10-69**  Advance the tip of the
instrument anteriorly until it is visible in the knee
as viewed from the anteromedial incision.

## Dangers

### Nerves and Vessels

The **peroneal nerve** can be injured if the surgical
plane is strayed out of to the posterior side of the
biceps femoris muscle.

The **lateral superior genicular artery** must be
ligated. Otherwise, it can cause a large postoperative
hematoma.

The **popliteal artery** may be injured if the surgical
plane does not remain subperiosteal. As the intercondylar notch is felt, bend the knee to 90° to allow the
popliteal artery to fall posteriorly with the joint capsule.

## How to Enlarge the Approach

### Local Measures

Retract the vastus lateralis muscle vigorously toward
the midline of the knee with a right-angled retractor.

### Extensile Measures

This incision is very extensile. It can be extended as
far proximally and distally as it has to be (see Lateral
Approach in Chapter 9). In addition, the incision can
be used in its more proximal extensions for an ili-
otibial-fascial graft.

## REFERENCES

1. SCOTT WN, INSALL JN, KELLY MA: Arthroscopy and meniscectomy; surgical approaches, anatomy and techniques
2. INSALL JN, ED: Surgery of the knee, 2nd ed. New York, Churchill Livingstone, 1993
3. ABBOTT LC, CARPENTER WF: Surgical approaches to the knee joint. J Bone Joint Surg 27:277, 1945
4. CONATY JP: Surgery of the hip and knee in patients with rheumatoid arthritis. J Bone Joint Surg [Am] 55:301, 1973
5. McMASTER M: Synovectomy of the knee in juvenile rheumatoid arthritis. J Bone Joint Surg [Br] 54:263, 1972
6. AICHROTH P: Osteochondritis dissecans of the knee: a clinical survey. J Bone Joint Surg [Br] 53:440, 1971
7. COVENTRY MB ET AL: Geometric total knee arthroplasty, 1: conception, design, indications, and surgical technic. Clin Orthop 94:171, 1973
8. FREEMAN MAR: Total replacement of the knee. Orthop Rev 3:21, 1974
9. FREEMAN MAR, TODD RC, BAMERT P ET AL: ICLH arthroplasty of the knee, 1968–1977. J Bone Joint Surg [Br] 60:339, 1978
10. GUNSTON FH, MacKENZIE RI: Complications of polycentric knee arthroplasty. J Bone Joint Surg [Br] 59:506, 1977
11. HABERMAN ET, DEUTSCH SD, ROVERE GD: Knee arthroplasty with the use of the Waldius total knee prosthesis. Clin Orthop 94:72, 1973
12. INSALL IN, SCOTT WN, RANAWAT CS: The total condylar knee: a report of 220 cases. J Bone Joint Surg [Am] 61:173, 1979
13. LASKIN RS: Modular total knee replacement arthroplasty: a review of 89 patients. J Bone Joint Surg [Am] 58:766, 1978
14. SHEEHAN JM: Arthroplasty of the knee. J Bone Joint Surg [Br] 60:333,1978
15. SMILLIE IS: Injuries of the knee joint, 4th ed. Baltimore, Williams & Wilkins, 1971
16. HUGHSTON JC: A surgical approach to the medial and posterior ligaments of the knee. J Bone Joint Surg [Am] 55:923, 1973
17. WARREN LF, MARSHALL JL: The supporting structure and layers on the medial side of the knee. J Bone Joint Surg [Am] 61:56, 1979
18. POGRUND H: A practical approach for lateral meniscectomy. J Trauma 16:365, 1976
19. KAPLAN EB: Surgical approach to the lateral [peroneal] side of the knee joint. Surg Gynecol Obstet 104:346, 1957
20. SLOCUM DB, JAMES SL, LARSEN RL ET AL: Late reconstruction of ligament injuries to the medial compartment of the knee. Clin Orthop 118:63, 1976
21. BRACKETT EG, OSGOOD RB: The popliteal incision for the removal of "joint mick" in the posterior capsule of the knee joint: a report of cases. Boston J Med Surg 165:975, 1911

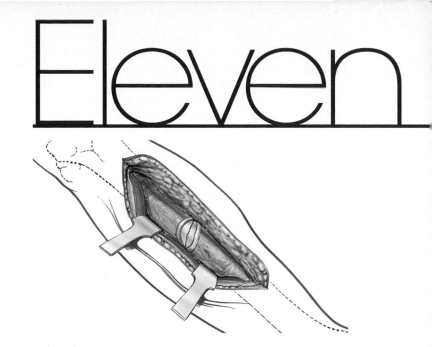

# Eleven

# The Tibia and Fibula

The tibia and fibula are approximately equal in length, but are different in structure and function. The tibia is large, transmits most of the stress of walking, and has a broad, accessible subcutaneous surface. The fibula is slender and plays an important role in ankle stability; it is surrounded by muscles, except at its ends. Surgical approaches to the fibula are more complex than are those to the tibia, because of both the depth of the bone and the presence of the common peroneal nerve, which winds around its upper third.

There are three main tibial approaches. The *anterior approach* is used most often because it affords easy access to the subcutaneous surface of the bone. The *anterolateral* and *posterolateral approaches* are used rarely, but can save the limb when skin breakdown has made anterior approaches impossible during bone grafting for nonunited fractures.

The majority of tibial shaft fractures treated operatively are treated by the insertion of intramedullary nails. The *minimal access approach* to the proximal tibia is used for this technique.

The *approach to the fibula* is classically extensile, using the internervous plane between muscles supplied by the superficial peroneal nerve (the peroneal muscles) and those supplied by the tibial nerve (the flexor muscles). Although this approach can expose the whole bone, the full approach rarely is required.

Because the surgical anatomy of the approaches overlap, the anatomy of the area is considered as a whole.

# Anterior Approach to the Tibia

The anterior approach offers safe, easy access to the medial (subcutaneous) and lateral (extensor) surfaces of the tibia. It is used for the following:

1. Open reduction and internal fixation of tibial fractures[1]
2. Bone grafting for delayed union or nonunion of fractures[2]
3. Implantation of electrical stimulators[3]
4. Excision of sequestra or saucerization in patients with osteomyelitis
5. Excision and biopsy of tumors
6. Osteotomy

Plates applied to the subcutaneous surface of the tibia are placed correctly biomechanically on the medial (tensile) side of the bone; they also are easier to contour there. Some surgeons prefer to use the lateral surface for plating, however, to avoid the problems of subcutaneous placement.

The anterior approach is the preferred approach to the tibia except when the skin is scarred or has draining sinuses in it.

## Position of the Patient

Place the patient supine on the operating table. The use of a tourniquet is optional. Tourniquets should not be used if this approach is to be used in conjunction with the exploration of an open wound. If you wish to use a tourniquet, exsanguinate the limb by elevating it for 3 to 5 minutes, then inflate a tourniquet (Fig. 11-1).

## Landmarks and Incision

### Landmarks
The *shaft of the tibia* is roughly triangular when viewed in cross section. It has three borders, one anterior, one medial, and one interosseous (posterolateral). These borders define three distinct surfaces: (1) a medial subcutaneous surface between the anterior and medial borders, (2) a lateral (extensor) surface between the anterior and interosseous borders, and (3) a posterior (flexor) surface between the medial and interosseous (posterolateral) borders. The anterior and medial borders and the subcutaneous surface are easily palpable.

### Incision
Make a longitudinal incision on the anterior surface of the leg parallel to the anterior border of the tibia and about 1 cm lateral to it. The length of the incision depends on the requirements of the procedure because of the poor vascularity of the skin. It is safer to make a longer incision than to retract skin edges forcibly to obtain access. The tibia can be exposed along its entire length (Fig. 11-2).

## Internervous Plane

There is no internervous plane in this approach. The dissection essentially is subperiosteal and does not disturb the nerve supply to the extensor compartment.

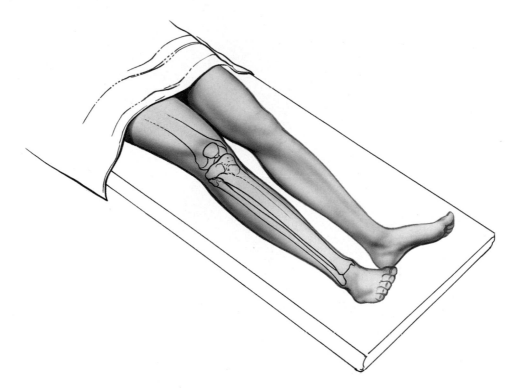

**Figure 11-1**   Position for the anterior approach to the tibia.

## Superficial Surgical Dissection

Elevate the skin flaps to expose the subcutaneous surface of the tibia. The long saphenous vein is on the medial side of the calf and must be protected when the medial skin flap is reflected (Fig. 11-3).

## Deep Surgical Dissection

Two surfaces of the tibia can be approached through this incision.

### Subcutaneous (Medial) Surface

The periosteum of the tibia provides a small but vital blood supply to the bone in fractures that interfere with its main blood supply. For this reason, periosteal stripping must be kept to an absolute minimum. In particular, never strip the periosteum off an isolated fragment of bone, or the bone will become totally avascular.

To expose the bone, incise the periosteum longitudinally in the middle of the subcutaneous surface of the tibia. Reflect it anteriorly and posteriorly to uncover only as much bone as is absolutely necessary (Fig. 11-4). Note the superior insertion of the pes anserinus into the subcutaneous surface of the tibia.

Detach it if that portion of the bone needs to be exposed, but this rarely is necessary.

### Lateral (Extensor) Surface

Incise the periosteum longitudinally over the anterior border of the tibia. Reflect the tibialis anterior muscle subperiosteally, and retract it laterally to expose the lateral surface of the bone. The tibialis anterior is the only muscle to take origin from the lateral surface of the tibia; detaching the muscle completely exposes that surface (see Figs. 11-4 and 11-21).

## Dangers

### Vessels

The **long saphenous vein,** which runs up the medial side of the calf, is vulnerable during superficial surgical dissection and should be preserved for future vascular procedures, if at all possible (see Fig. 11-21).

## Special Surgical Points

Skin flaps must be closed meticulously after surgery to avoid infection of the tibia. Although longitudinal incisions over the tibia heal well, transverse incisions

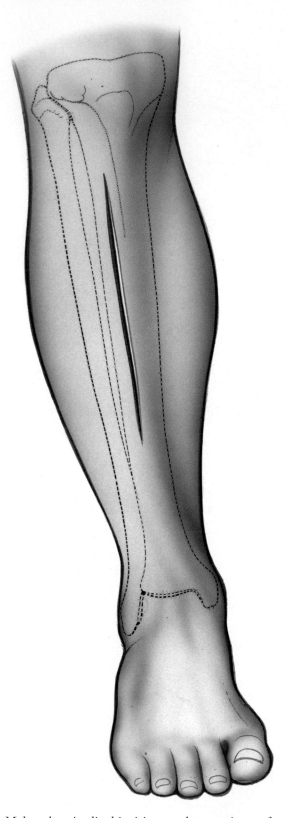

**Figure 11-2**    Make a longitudinal incision on the anterior surface of the leg.

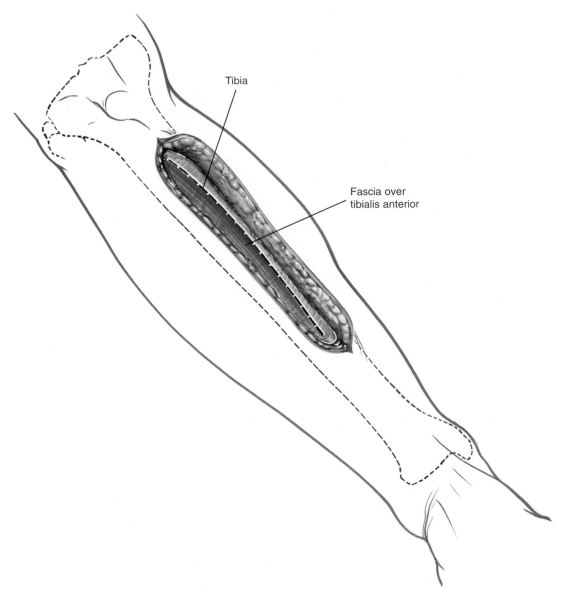

**Figure 11-3**   Elevate the skin flaps over the medial portion of the tibialis anterior and the subcutaneous medial surface of the tibia. To expose the lateral surface of the tibia, incise the deep fascia over the medial border of the tibialis anterior.

Tibia

Fascia over
tibialis anterior

and irregular wounds may heal poorly, especially in elderly individuals. The skin over the lower third of the tibia is very thin; wounds in that area heal badly, especially in patients with chronic venous insufficiency.

It is important to minimize the amount of soft tissue that is stripped from bone in this approach when it is used for fracture work. Devascularized bone, no matter how well it is reduced and fixed, will not unite. Using care and appropriate reduction forceps, it usually is possible to preserve soft-tissue attachments of all but the smallest fragments of bone.

## How to Enlarge the Approach

### Local Measures
The extent of the exposure is determined by the size of the skin incision; the whole subcutaneous surface of the tibia may be exposed, if necessary.

To reach the posterior surface of the tibia from an anterior approach, continue the subperiosteal dissection posteriorly around the medial border. Proximally, lift the flexor digitorum longus muscle off the posterior surface of the tibia subperiosteally. Distally, lift off the tibialis posterior muscle. This

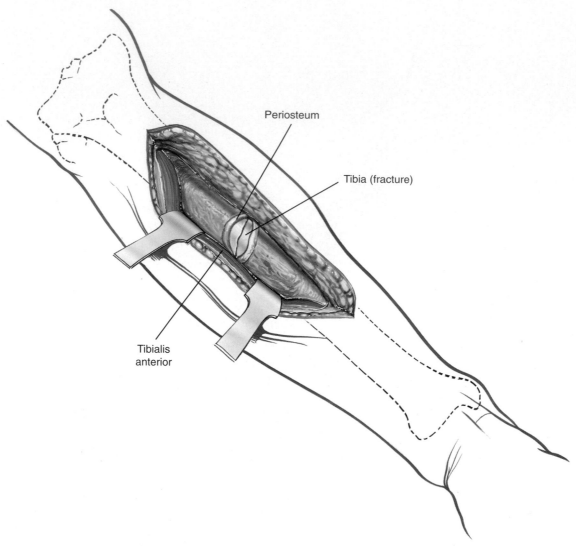

**Figure 11-4**   Elevate the tibialis anterior from the lateral surface of the tibia. Incise the periosteum; elevate it only as necessary.

procedure exposes the posterior surface of the bone, but does not offer as full an exposure as does the posterolateral approach. It probably is useful only for the insertion of bone graft as part of an internal fixation carried out through this anterior route.

### Extensile Measures

***Proximal Extension.*** To extend the approach proximally, continue the skin incision along the medial side of the patella. Deepen the incision through the medial patellar retinaculum to gain access to the knee joint and the patella. (For details, see Medial Para-

patellar Approach in Chapter 10.) Alternatively, extend the wound proximally along the lateral side of the patella. Deepen that wound through the lateral patellar retinaculum to gain access to the lateral compartment of the knee.

***Distal Extension.*** To extend the approach distally, curve the incision over the medial side of the hind part of the foot. Deepening the wound provides access to all the structures that pass behind the medial malleolus. Continue the incision onto the middle and front parts of the foot. (For details, see Anterior and Posterior Approaches to the Medial Malleolus in Chapter 12.)

# Anterolateral Approach to the Tibia

The anterolateral approach is used to expose the middle two thirds of the tibia when the skin over the subcutaneous surface of the bone is unsuitable for a direct anterior approach. It is of most use in the treatment of infected nonunion of the tibia. Its uses include:

1. Anterolateral bone grafting of the tibia
2. Tibia profibula grafting (cross-tibiofibular grafting).[11]

This approach is technically simple. Because it only provides limited exposure of the tibia, it usually is inadequate for the internal fixation of fractures.

## Position of the Patient

Place the patient on his or her side with the affected limb on top. Protect the bony prominences of the bottom leg to avoid the development of pressure sores. Exsanguinate the limb either by elevating it for 5 minutes or by applying a compression bandage and then inflating a tourniquet.

## Landmarks and Incision

### Landmarks
Palpate the subcutaneous surface of the fibula in the distal third of the limb. Also palpate the fibula head proximally.

### Incision
Make a longitudinal incision that overlies the shaft of the fibula, centering it at the level of the tibial pathol-

ogy. The length of the incision depends on the length of the tibia that must be exposed. Note that the length of tibia exposed will be considerably shorter than the length of the fibula incision (Fig. 11-5).

## Internervous Plane

Superficially, the internervous plane lies between the peroneus brevis muscle (which is supplied by the superficial peroneal nerve) and the extensor digitorum longus muscle (which is supplied by the deep peroneal nerve).

Deeply, the internervous plane lies between the tibialis posterior muscle (which is supplied by the tibial nerve) and the extensor muscles of the ankle and foot (which are supplied by the deep peroneal nerve). These muscles are separated by the interosseous membrane.

## Superficial Surgical Dissection

Deepen the incision, taking care not to damage the short saphenous vein that may appear in the posterior aspect of the wound. Incise the fascia in the line of the skin incision, and identify the underlying peroneal muscles (Fig. 11-6). Develop a plane between the anterior aspect of the peroneus brevis muscle and the extensor digitorum longus muscle to come down onto the anterolateral aspect of the fibula (Fig. 11-7). Protect the superficial peroneal nerve, which can be seen lying on the peroneus brevis muscle.

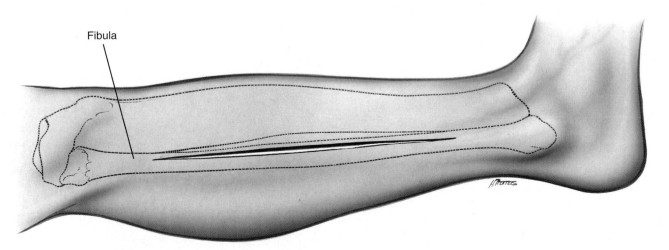

Fibula

**Figure 11-5**   Make a longitudinal incision centered over the site of the fracture.

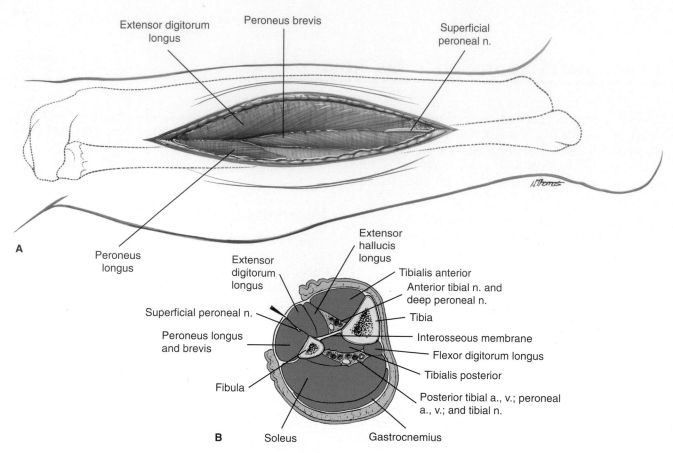

**Figure 11-6** **(A)** Identify the peroneal muscles and the short saphenous vein. **(B)** Identify the plane between the peroneus brevis and the extensor digitorum longus.

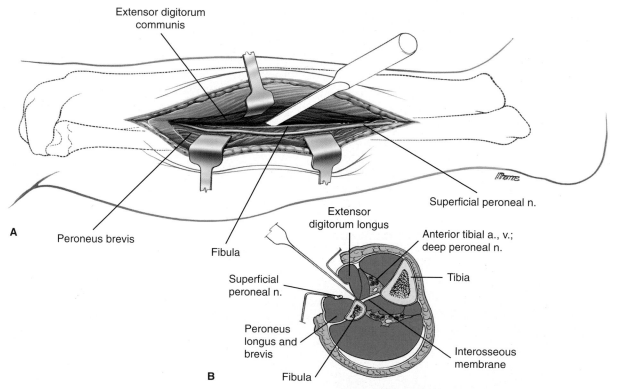

**Figure 11-7** **(A)** Develop a plane in a distal to proximal direction between the peroneus brevis and the extensor digitorum longus. **(B)** Note the superficial peroneal nerve lying on the peroneus brevis muscle.

## Deep Surgical Dissection

Gently detach the extensor musculature from the anterior aspect of the interosseous membrane using blunt instruments. Follow the anterior aspect of this membrane onto the lateral border of the tibia (Fig. 11-8). Because this approach almost always is used in cases of trauma, the plane often is difficult to develop. Make sure to stay firmly on the interosseous membrane; straying anteriorly may cause damage to the anterior neurovascular bundle. Expose the posterolateral corner of the tibia. Gently strip off as much tissue as necessary from the lateral aspect of the tibia, elevating some of the origin of the tibialis anterior muscle in the process. As in all approaches to the tibia, only the minimum amount of soft tissue that is required to gain adequate access should be dissected to avoid devascularization of bone.

## Dangers

### Vessels and Nerves

The small saphenous vein may be damaged in the posterior skin flap (see Fig. 11-6A).

The superficial peroneal nerve runs down the leg in the peroneal or lateral compartment. It gives off all its motor branches in the upper third of the leg. Hence, it is sensory only at the level of this approach. Identify and preserve the nerve to avoid numbness on the dorsum of the foot (see Fig. 11-7B).

The anterior tibial artery and the deep peroneal nerve run down the leg in the anterior compartment, which is anterior to the interosseous membrane. Therefore, as long as the plane of operation remains on the interosseous membrane and does not wander off anteriorly, no damage will result until the periosteum of the tibia is reached.

## How to Enlarge the Approach

### Local Measures

The longer the incision, the less retraction that is required for adequate visualization.

### Extensile Measures

This approach cannot be extended easily proximally or distally.

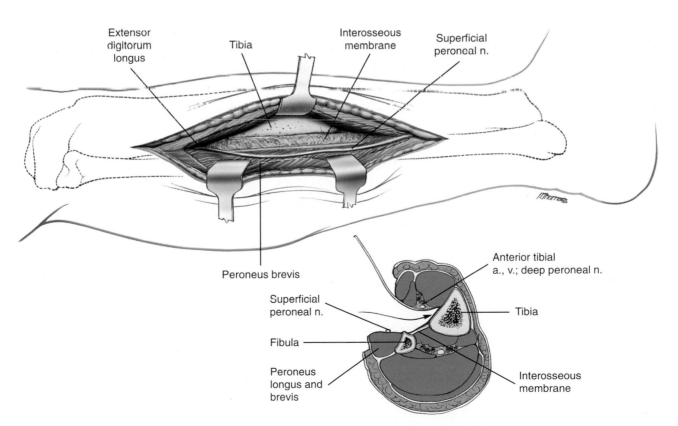

**Figure 11-8** Develop a plane by detaching the extensor musculature from the anterior aspect of the interosseous membrane to expose the posterolateral corner of the tibia.

# Posterolateral Approach to the Tibia

The posterolateral approach[4] is used to expose the middle two thirds of the tibia when the skin over the subcutaneous surface is badly scarred or infected. It is a technically demanding operation. The approach is suitable for the following uses:

1. Internal fixation of fractures
2. Treatment of delayed union or nonunion [5] of fractures, including bone grafting

The approach also permits exposure of the middle of the posterior aspect of the fibula.

## Position of the Patient

Place the patient on his or her side, with the affected leg uppermost. Protect the bony prominences of the bottom leg to avoid the development of pressure sores. Exsanguinate the limb by elevating it for 5 minutes, then apply a tourniquet (Fig. 11-9).

## Landmark and Incision

### Landmark
The lateral border of the *gastrocnemius muscle* is easy to palpate in the calf.

### Incision
Make a longitudinal incision over the lateral border of the gastrocnemius muscle. The length of the incision depends on the length of bone that must be exposed (Fig. 11-10).

## Internervous Plane

The internervous plane lies between the *gastrocnemius, soleus, and flexor hallucis longus muscles* (all of which are supplied by the tibial nerve), and the *peroneal muscles* (which are supplied by the superficial peroneal nerve)—between the posterior and lateral muscular compartments (Fig. 11-11).

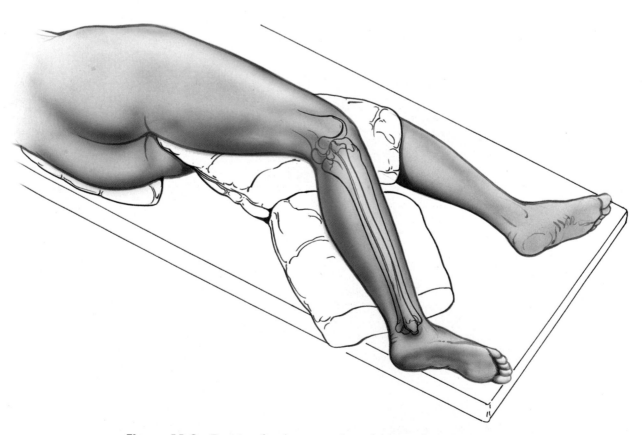

**Figure 11-9**    Position for the posterolateral approach to the tibia.

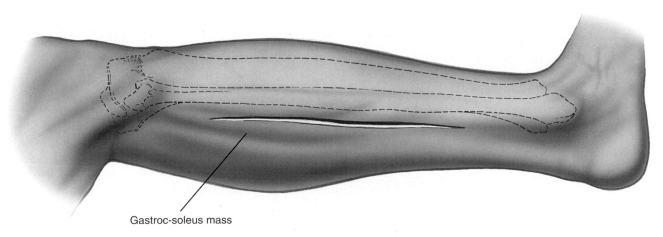

Gastroc-soleus mass

**Figure 11-10** Incision of the lateral border of the gastrocnemius.

## Superficial Surgical Dissection

Reflect the skin flaps, taking care not to damage the short saphenous vein, which runs up the posterolateral aspect of the leg from behind the lateral malleolus. Incise the fascia in line with the incision and find the plane between the lateral head of the gastrocnemius and soleus muscles posteriorly, and the peroneus brevis and longus muscles anteriorly. Muscular branches of the peroneal artery lie with the peroneus brevis in the proximal part of the incision and may have to be ligated (Fig. 11-12).

Find the lateral border of the soleus and retract it with the gastrocnemius medially and posteriorly; underneath, arising from the posterior surface of the fibula, is the flexor hallucis longus (Fig. 11-13).

## Deep Surgical Dissection

Detach the lower part of the origin of the soleus muscle from the fibula and retract it posteriorly and medially. Detach the flexor hallucis longus muscle from its origin on the fibula and retract it

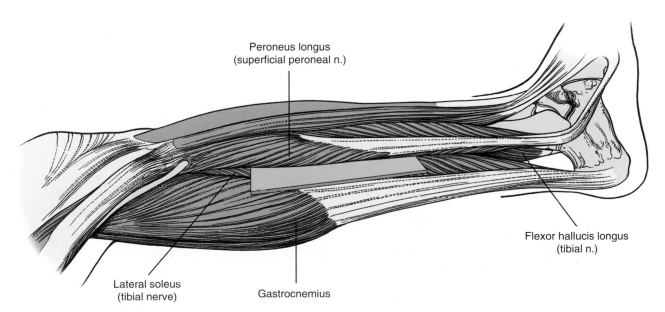

Peroneus longus
(superficial peroneal n.)

Flexor hallucis longus
(tibial n.)

Lateral soleus
(tibial nerve)

Gastrocnemius

**Figure 11-11** The internervous plane lies between the *gastrocnemius, soleus,* and *flexor hallucis longus muscles* (which are supplied by the tibial nerve) and the *peroneal muscles* (which are supplied by the superficial peroneal nerve).

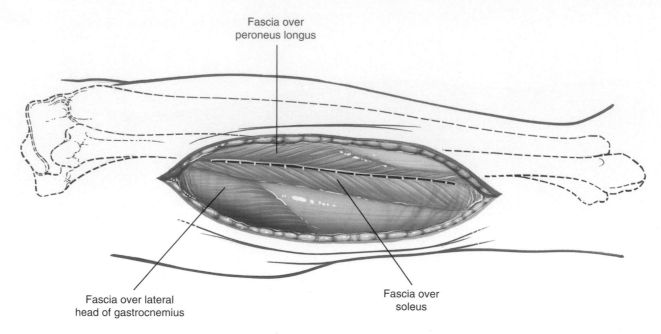

Fascia over
peroneus longus

Fascia over lateral
head of gastrocnemius

Fascia over
soleus

**Figure 11-12** Reflect the skin flaps. Incise the fascia in line with the incision. Find the plane between the lateral head of the gastrocnemius and soleus posteriorly, and the peroneus brevis and longus anteriorly.

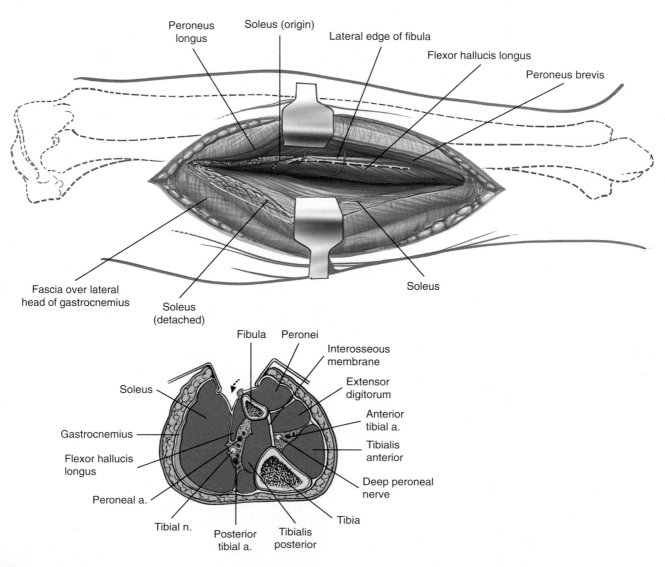

Peroneus
longus

Soleus (origin)

Lateral edge of fibula

Flexor hallucis longus

Peroneus brevis

Fascia over lateral
head of gastrocnemius

Soleus
(detached)

Soleus

Fibula    Peronei

Interosseous
membrane

Soleus

Extensor
digitorum

Gastrocnemius

Anterior
tibial a.

Flexor hallucis
longus

Tibialis
anterior

Peroneal a.

Deep peroneal
nerve

Tibial n.

Posterior
tibial a.

Tibialis
posterior

Tibia

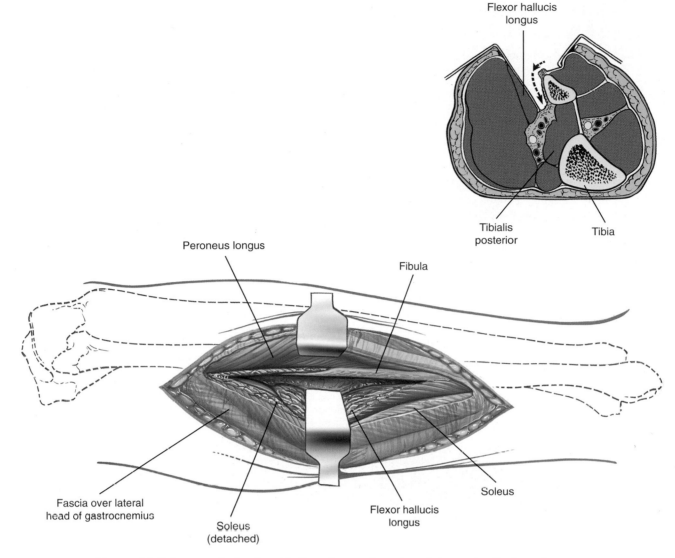

**Figure 11-14** Detach the flexor hallucis longus from its origin on the fibula and retract it posteriorly and medially. Continue dissecting posteriorly, staying on the posterior surface of the fibula. Detach the flexor hallucis longus from its origin on the fibula, staying close to the bone *(cross section)*. Retract the muscle medially.

posteriorly and medially (Fig. 11-14; see Fig. 11-13). Continue dissecting medially across the interosseous membrane, detaching those fibers of the tibialis posterior muscle that arise from it. The posterior tibial artery and tibial nerve are posterior to the dissection, separated from it by the bulk of

the tibialis posterior and flexor hallucis longus muscles (Fig. 11-15). Follow the interosseous membrane to the lateral border of the tibia, detaching the muscles that arise from its posterior surface subperiosteally, and expose its posterior surface (Fig. 11-16).

**Figure 11-13** Detach the origin of the soleus from the fibula, and retract it posteriorly and medially along with the gastrocnemius. Retract the peroneal muscles anteriorly. Detach the flexor hallucis longus from its origin on the fibula. Develop the plane between the gastrocnemius-soleus group posteriorly and the peroneal muscles anteriorly *(cross section)*. Note the flexor hallucis longus on the posterior surface of the fibula.

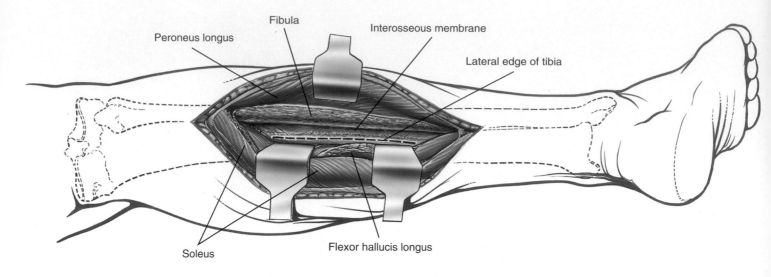

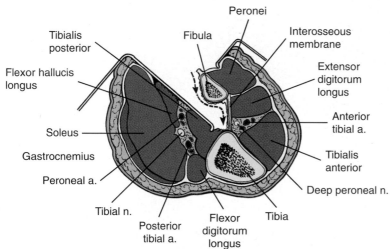

**Figure 11-15** Continue dissecting medially across the interosseous membrane, detaching those fibers of the tibialis posterior that arise from it. Continue dissecting across the membrane until the posterior aspect of the tibia can be seen. Incise the periosteum on the lateral border of the tibia. Continue the dissection posteriorly across the fibula and the interosseous membrane until the lateral border of the tibia is reached *(cross section)*. Note that the neurovascular structures are protected by the bulk of the tibialis posterior.

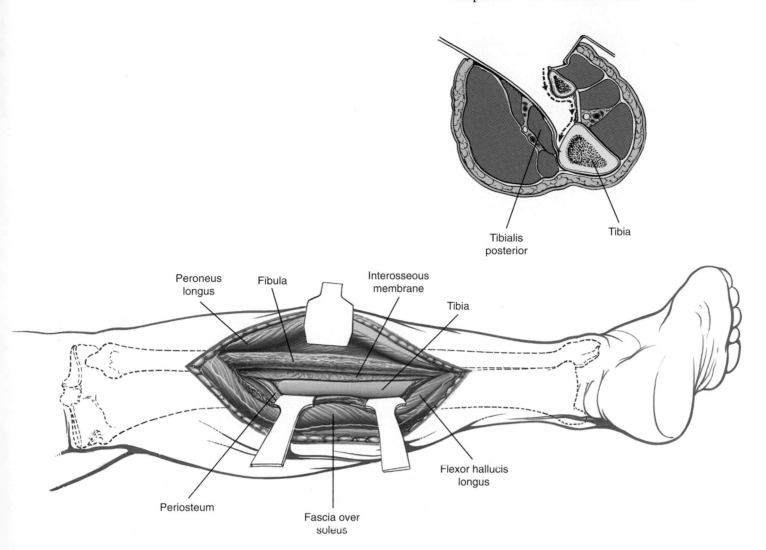

**Figure 11-16** Detach the muscles that arise from the posterior surface of the tibia subperiosteally. Expose the posterior border of the tibia subperiosteally *(cross section)*. The detached tibialis posterior muscle protects the neurovascular structures.

## Dangers

### Vessels

The **small (short) saphenous vein** may be damaged when the skin flaps are mobilized. Although the vein should be preserved if possible, it may be ligated, if necessary, without impairing venous return from the leg.

Branches of the **peroneal artery** cross the intermuscular plane between the gastrocnemius and peroneus brevis muscles. They should be ligated or coagulated to reduce postoperative bleeding (see Fig. 11-27).

The **posterior tibial artery** and tibial nerve are safe as long as the surgical plane of operation remains on the interosseous membrane and does not wander into a plane posterior to the flexor hallucis longus and tibialis posterior muscles (see Fig. 11-27).

## How to Enlarge the Approach

### Extensile Measures

*Proximal Extension.* The approach cannot be extended into the proximal fourth of the tibia.

There, the back of the tibia is covered by the popliteus muscle and the more superficial posterior tibial artery and tibial nerve, making safe dissection impossible.

*Distal Extension.* The approach can be made continuous with the posterior approach to the ankle if the skin incision is extended distally between the posterior aspect of the lateral malleolus and the Achilles tendon.

# Approach to the Fibula

The approach to the fibula employs a classic extensile exposure[6] and offers access to all parts of the fibula. Its uses include the following:

1. Partial resection of the fibula during tibial osteotomy[7] or as part of the treatment of tibial nonunion[8,9]
2. Resection of the fibula for decompression of all four compartments of the leg[10]
3. Resection of tumors
4. Resection for osteomyelitis
5. Open reduction and internal fixation of fractures of the fibula
6. Removal of bone grafts

Although the bone can be exposed completely, only a part of the approach usually is required for any one procedure.

## Position of the Patient

Place the patient on his or her side on the operating table with the affected side uppermost. Pad the bony prominences of the other leg to prevent the development of pressure sores. Exsanguinate the limb by elevating it for 3 to 5 minutes, then apply a tourniquet (see Fig. 11-9). Alternatively, if this approach is used in conjunction with a surgical approach to the tibia, place the patient supine on the operating table. A sandbag placed underneath the affected buttock will rotate the leg internally, allowing adequate exposure of the lateral aspect of the leg for the approach to the fibula. Subsequently, if the sandbag is removed, the leg naturally will rotate externally, providing access to the tibia.

## Landmarks and Incision

### Landmarks

The *head of the fibula* is easily palpable about 2 to 3 cm below the lateral femoral condyle.

The common peroneal nerve can be rolled underneath the fingers as it winds around the fibular neck.

The lower *fourth of the fibula* is subcutaneous.

### Incision

Make a linear incision just posterior to the fibula, beginning behind the lateral malleolus and extending to the level of the fibular head. Continue the incision up and back, a handbreadth above the head of the fibula and in line with the biceps femoris tendon. Watch out for the common peroneal nerve, which runs subcutaneously over the neck of the fibula and can be cut if the skin incision is too bold. The length of the incision depends on the amount of exposure needed (Fig. 11-17).

## Internervous Plane

The internervous plane lies between the *peroneal muscles*, supplied by the superficial peroneal nerve, and the *flexor muscles*, supplied by the tibial nerve (see Fig. 11-11).

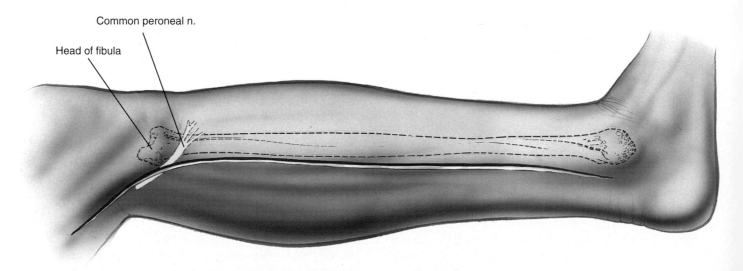

Common peroneal n.

Head of fibula

**Figure 11-17** Make a long linear incision just posterior to the fibula.

## Superficial Surgical Dissection

To expose the fibular head and neck, begin proximally by incising the deep fascia in line with the incision, taking great care not to cut the underlying common peroneal nerve. Find the posterior border of the biceps femoris tendon as it sweeps down past the knee before inserting into the head of the fibula. Identify and isolate the common peroneal nerve in its course behind the biceps tendon; trace it as it winds around the fibular neck (Fig. 11-18). Mobilize the nerve from the groove on the back of the neck by cutting the fibers of the peroneus longus that cover the nerve and gently pulling the nerve forward over the fibular head with a strip of corrugated rubber drain. Identify and preserve all branches of the nerve (Fig. 11-19).

Develop a plane between the peroneal and the soleus; with the common peroneal nerve retracted anteriorly, incise the periosteum of the fibula longi-

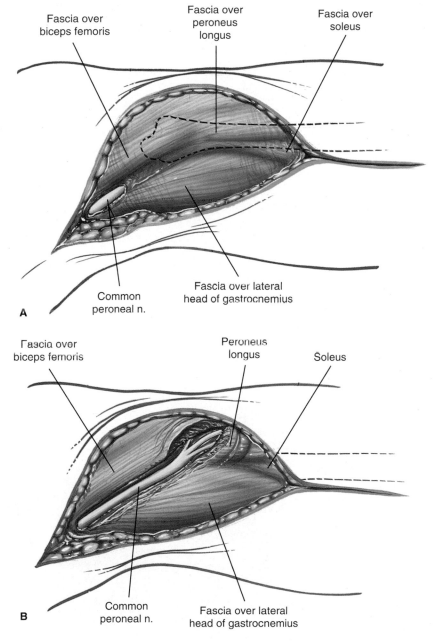

**Figure 11-18**   **(A)** Expose the common peroneal nerve in the proximal end of the incision along the posterior border of the biceps. **(B)** Continue exposing the common peroneal nerve distally as it winds around the neck of the fibula in the substance of the peroneus longus.

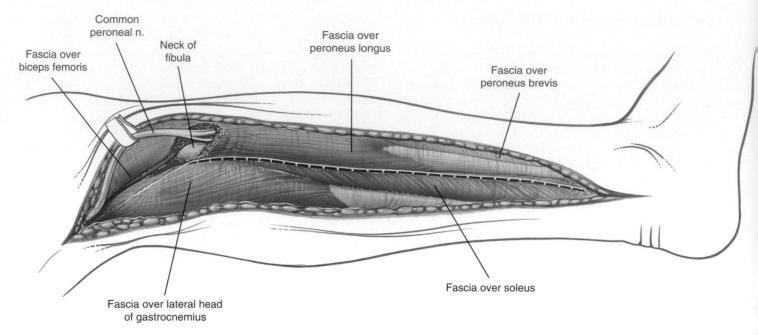

**Figure 11-19**   Retract the peroneal nerve anteriorly, and incise the fascia between the peroneal muscles and the soleus muscle.

tudinally in the line with this plane of cleavage. Continue the incision down to bone (Fig. 11-20).

## Deep Surgical Dissection

Strip the muscle off the fibula by dissection. All muscles that originate from the fibula have fibers that run distally toward the foot and ankle. Therefore, to strip them off cleanly, you must elevate them from distal to proximal. Most muscles originate from periosteum or fascia; they can be stripped. Muscles attached directly to bone are difficult to strip; they usually must be cut (Fig. 11-21, and *cross-section*).

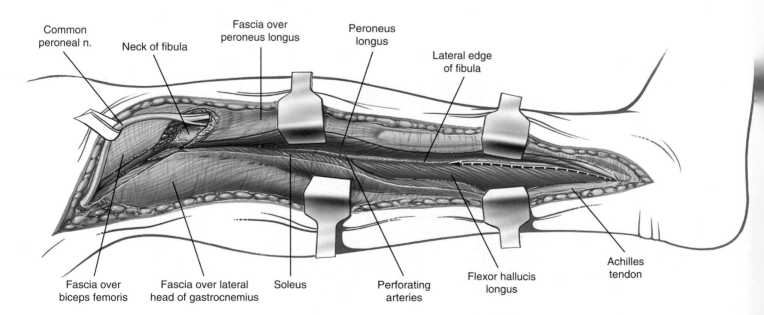

**Figure 11-20**   Develop the intermuscular plane between the peroneal muscles and the soleus muscle down the lateral edge of the fibula. Strip the flexor muscles from the posterior aspect of the fibula in a distal to proximal direction.

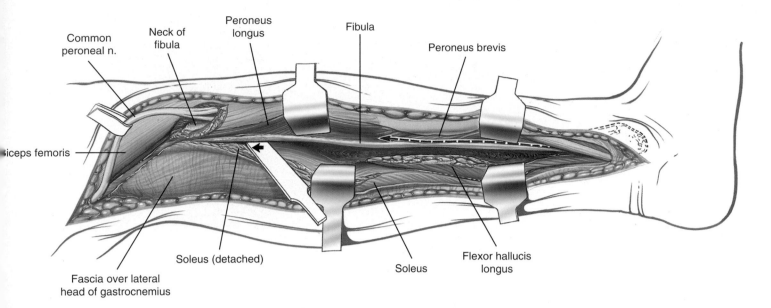

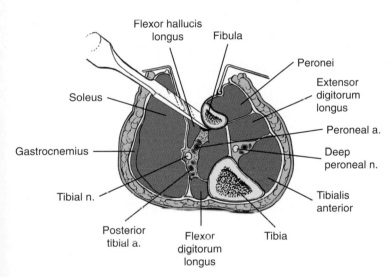

**Figure 11-21**  Strip the flexor hallucis longus and the soleus from the posterior aspect of the fibula, and strip the peroneal muscles from the anterior surface of the fibula in a distal to proximal direction. Strip the flexor muscles from the posterior aspect of the fibula *(cross section)*. Avoid neurovascular structures by staying close to the bone.

The other structure attached to the fibula, the interosseous membrane, has fibers that run obliquely upward. To complete the dissection, strip the interosseous membrane subperiosteally from proximal to distal (Fig. 11-22, and *cross-section*).

## Dangers

### Nerves

The **common peroneal nerve** is vulnerable as it winds around the neck of the fibula. The key to pre-serving the nerve is to identify it proximally as it lies on the posterior border of the biceps femoris. It then can be safely traced through the peroneal muscle mass and retracted. The dorsal cutaneous branch of the superficial peroneal nerve is susceptible to injury at the junction of the distal and middle thirds of the fibula; if it is damaged, it causes numbness on the dorsum of the foot (see Fig. 11-30).

### Vessels

Terminal branches of the **peroneal artery** lie close to the deep surface of the lateral malleolus. To avoid

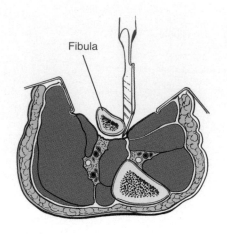

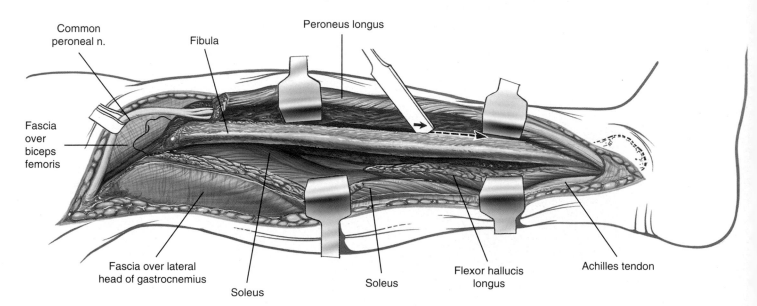

**Figure 11-22**   Retract the peroneal muscles anteriorly. Strip the interosseous membrane from the anterior border of the fibula in a proximal to distal direction. Strip the muscles from the anterior surface of the fibula, and strip the interosseous membrane from its fibular attachment in a proximal to distal direction *(cross section)*.

damaging them, you must keep the dissection subperiosteal (see Fig. 11-27).

The **small (short) saphenous vein** may be damaged; you may ligate it if necessary.

## How to Enlarge the Approach

### Local Measures
The exposure described allows exposure of the entire bone.

### Extensile Measures

*Distal Extension.* Extend the skin incision distally by curving it over the lateral side of the tarsus. To gain access to the sinus tarsi and the talocalcaneal, talonavicular, and calcaneocuboid joints, reflect the underlying extensor digitorum brevis muscle. This extension is used frequently for lateral operations on the leg and foot (see Lateral Approach to the Hindpart of the Foot in Chapter 12).

# Applied Surgical Anatomy of the Leg

## Overview

The tibia and fibula are very different bones. The tibia has a large subcutaneous surface that allows access to the bone along its entire length; the fibula is enclosed almost completely in muscle. Only at its proximal end and in the lower third of the bone does the fibula develop a subcutaneous surface, which terminates in the lateral malleolus. For this reason, operations on most of the fibula almost always involve extensive stripping of muscle off bone. In addition, the tibia has no major neurovascular structures running directly on it

other than its nutrient artery; the fibula has close ties to the common peroneal nerve and its branches.

The deep fascia of the leg is a tough, fibrous, unyielding structure that encloses the calf muscles. Where the bones become subcutaneous, the fascia usually is attached to the border of the bone.

Two intermuscular septa, one anterior and one posterior, pass from the deep surface of the encircling fascia to the fibula and enclose the peroneal or lateral compartment of the leg.

Three separate muscular compartments exist in the lower leg (Fig. 11-23).

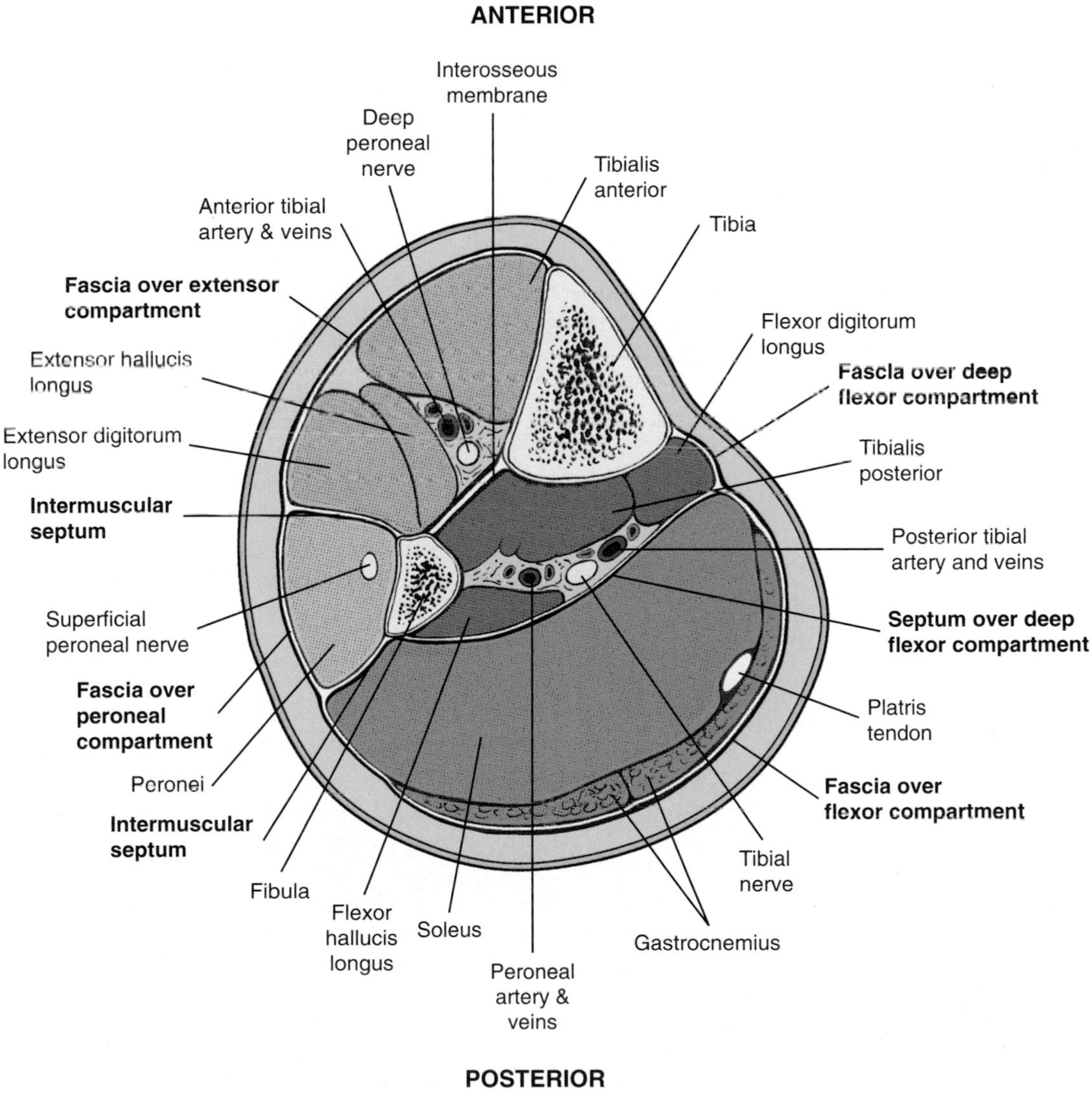

**Figure 11-23**   The fibro-osseous compartments of the leg.

### Anterior (Extensor) Compartment

The anterior compartment contains the extensor muscles of the foot and ankle. Its medial boundary is the lateral (extensor) surface of the tibia, and its lateral boundary is the extensor surface of the fibula and anterior intermuscular septum. The anterior compartment is enclosed by the deep fascia of the leg and all its muscles are supplied by the deep peroneal nerve. The compartment's artery is the anterior tibial artery.

### Lateral (Peroneal) Compartment

The peroneal compartment is bounded by the anterior intermuscular septum in front, by the posterior intermuscular septum behind, and by the fibula medially. It contains the peroneal muscles, which evert the foot. The superficial peroneal nerve supplies all the muscles in the compartment. No artery runs in it; its muscles receive their supply from several branches of the peroneal artery.

### Posterior (Flexor) Compartment

The flexor compartment contains the flexors of the foot and ankle. This compartment is separated from the other compartments by a fibro-osseous complex: laterally, from the peroneal compartment, by the posterior intermuscular septum and the posterior medial surface of the fibula; and anteriorly, from the extensor compartment, by the interosseous membrane and the posterior (flexor) surface of the tibia. The tibial nerve innervates all the muscles in the compartment, and the posterior tibial artery supplies them with blood. The peroneal artery also runs in this compartment and forms part of the blood supply of the muscles.

The flexor compartment consists of two groups of muscles, superficial (gastrocnemius, soleus, plantaris) and deep (tibialis posterior, flexor digitorum longus, flexor hallucis longus), which are separated by a fascial layer.

## Anterior Approach to the Tibia

### Landmark and Incision

#### Landmark

For the surgeon, the *subcutaneous surface of the tibia* is the most accessible bit of bone in the body. Unfortunately, this ease of access makes the bone attractive as a source of grafts. This procedure weakens the bone, something that is reflected in the high incidence of subsequent fractures.

#### Incision

The longitudinal incision roughly parallels the lines of cleavage in the skin. The resultant scar is not unduly prominent, but often is visible in women because of its position.

### Superficial Surgical Dissection

The *periosteum of the tibia* is a thick fibrous membrane that can be peeled off the bone easily, especially in children. Only 10% of the blood supply of the bone comes from the periosteum; the remaining 90% comes from medullary vessels. Therefore, the periosteum can be elevated off a normal bone without significant impairment of its blood supply. In cases of fracture, however, soft-tissue attachments may form the only remaining blood supply to isolated bone fragments and must be preserved.

The *long saphenous vein* is the longest superficial vein in the body. It originates just distal and anterior to the medial malleolus and continues proximally on the medial side of the leg superficial to the fascia. It may be ligated if necessary.

### Deep Surgical Dissection

The *tibialis anterior* is the only muscle to arise from the tibia in the anterior compartment (Fig. 11-24). The muscle may be avulsed partially from the tibia in joggers and other athletes, and is one of the causes of shin splints. The pathology of this particular complaint, however, is unclear. Some believe that it results from stress fractures of the tibia itself; others contend that it represents a compartment syndrome.[10]

The *common peroneal nerve* runs over the neck of the fibula in the substance of the peroneus longus muscle and divides into deep and superficial branches (Fig. 11-25).

The *deep peroneal nerve* continues to wind around the fibular neck deep to the extensor digitorum longus muscle before reaching the anterior surface of the interosseous membrane. It runs down the leg on the interosseous membrane between the tibialis anterior and extensor hallucis longus muscles, supplying all the muscles of the extensor portion of the leg (see Fig. 11-25). The nerve to extensor hallucis longus may split off the deep peroneal nerve up to 15 cm below the fibula neck.[11] This means that lateral approaches to the fibula may produce a neuropraxia

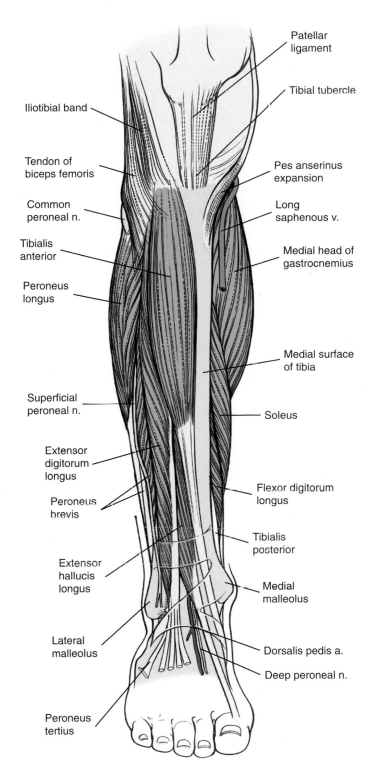

Patellar
ligament

Tibial tubercle

Iliotibial band

Tendon of
biceps femoris

Pes anserinus
expansion

Common
peroneal n.

Long
saphenous v.

Tibialis
anterior

Medial head of
gastrocnemius

Peroneus
longus

Medial surface
of tibia

Superficial
peroneal n.

Soleus

Extensor
digitorum
longus

Flexor digitorum
longus

Peroneus
brevis

Tibialis
posterior

Extensor
hallucis
longus

Medial
malleolus

Lateral
malleolus

Dorsalis pedis a.

Deep peroneal n.

Peroneus
tertius

**Figure 11-24** The superficial structures of the anterior compartment of the leg.

**Tibialis Anterior.** *Origin.* Lateral condyle of tibia, upper two thirds of lateral surface of tibia, interosseous membrane, deep fascia, lateral intermuscular septum. *Insertion.* Medial cuneiform and base of first metatarsal. *Action.* Dorsiflexor and invertor of foot. *Nerve supply.* Deep peroneal nerve.
**Extensor Hallucis Longus.** *Origin.* Middle half of anterior surface of fibula and interosseous membrane. *Insertion.* Base of distal phalanx of hallux. *Action.* Extensor of hallux and ankle. *Nerve supply.* Deep peroneal nerve.
**Extensor Digitorum Longus.** *Origin.* Upper three fourths of anterior surface of fibula, small area of tibia adjacent to superior tibiofibular joint, and interosseous membrane. *Insertion.* Via extensor hoods to middle and distal phalanges of lateral four toes. *Action.* Extensor of toes and of ankle. *Nerve supply.* Deep peroneal nerve.
**Peroneus Tertius.** *Origin.* Lower third of anterior surface of fibula. *Insertion.* Base of fifth metatarsal. *Action.* Evertor and dorsiflexor of foot. *Nerve supply.* Deep peroneal nerve.

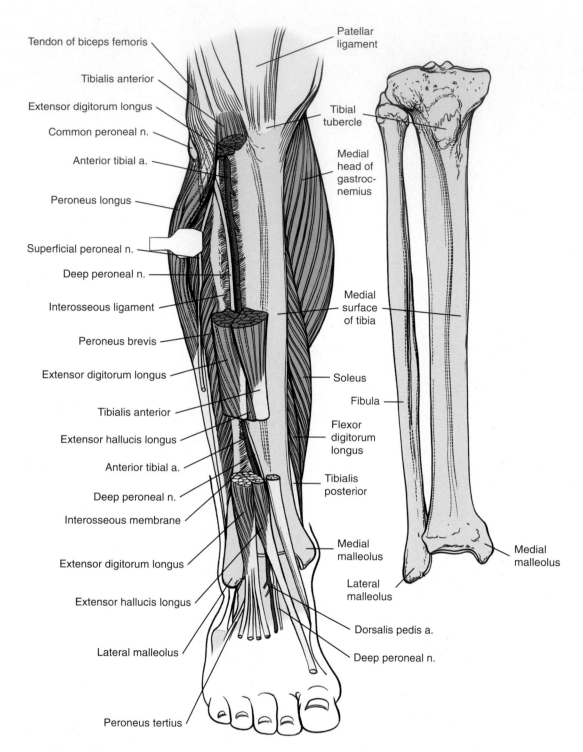

**Figure 11-25**  Muscles of the anterior compartment have been resected to reveal the anterior surface of the tibia, the neurovascular structures, the interosseous membrane, and the anterior surface of the fibula.

of this nerve even if they are carried out well below the level of the fibula neck.

The *superficial peroneal nerve* runs down the peroneal compartment of the leg, supplying the peroneus longus and brevis muscles. Its dorsal cutaneous branch supplies the skin on the dorsum of the foot (see Fig. 11-25).

The *anterior tibial artery* is a branch of the popliteal artery. It reaches the anterior portion of the leg by passing above the interosseous membrane. It lies so close to the fibula that its venae comitantes often leave a notch in the bone large enough to be visible on radiographs, a relationship that must be respected when the fibular head is excised. The artery runs with the deep peroneal nerve on the interosseous membrane; it continues in the foot as the dorsalis pedis artery (see Fig. 11-25).

Three other muscles, the extensor hallucis longus, extensor digitorum longus, and peroneus tertius, also occupy the anterior compartment of the leg. They are not involved in the anterior approach to the tibia, but are part of the approach to the anterior compartment and may be seen during the exploration of wounds caused by open tibial fractures. Together with the tibialis anterior muscle, they are implicated in the anterior compartment syndrome (see Fig. 11-25).

# Posterolateral Approach to the Tibia

## Incision

The longitudinal incision almost parallels the lines of cleavage in the skin, and the resultant scar is not unduly broad. Cosmesis rarely is a problem with this exposure; it is reserved largely for cases in which the skin on the anterior aspect of the tibia is unsuitable for surgery.

## Superficial Surgical Dissection

Superficial surgical dissection consists of finding the plane that separates the gastrocnemius and soleus muscles from the peroneus brevis muscle (see Fig. 11-29).

The fibers of the *gastrocnemius* are arranged generally longitudinally, giving the muscle the ability to contract a considerable distance at the expense of muscle strength. The gastrocnemius crosses two joints. During quiet walking, plantar flexion of the ankle is carried out largely by the powerful soleus muscle, which crosses only one joint. The gastrocnemius is capable of acting as a fast plantar flexor of the ankle, but only if the soleus provides power to overcome the inertia of the body weight. The gastrocnemius, therefore, comes into play mainly during running and jumping.

The major surgical importance of the soleus muscle lies in the numerous plexuses of small veins that it contains. This multipinnate muscle is one of the major pumps involved in venous return from the limb; lack of muscular action (i.e., after surgery or fractures) may lead to venous stasis and thrombosis.

The *peroneus brevis* tendon, which grooves the back of the lateral malleolus, is useful in reconstruction of the lateral side of the ankle. On occasion, the peroneus brevis may avulse the styloid process of the fifth metatarsal in association with inversion injuries of the ankle (Fig. 11-26; see Fig. 11-29).

## Deep Surgical Dissection

Deep surgical dissection consists of detaching the flexor hallucis longus muscle from the fibula and the tibialis posterior muscle from the interosseous membrane. Some fibers of the flexor digitorum longus muscle also must be reflected off the posterior surface of the tibia to permit access to that bone.

Generally, the dissection is carried out subperiosteally. Nevertheless, at those points where muscle actually originates from bone, it must be detached by sharp dissection, because a subperiosteal plane cannot be developed (Figs. 11-27 and 11-28).

The *flexor hallucis longus* muscle helps support the longitudinal arch of the foot. In the sole of the foot, it sends slips to the flexors of the second and third toes. It is muscular down to the level of the ankle joint, a characteristic that makes it identifiable at that level.

## Dangers

### Nerves and Vessels

The posterior tibial artery and the tibial nerve lie superficial (posterior) to the plane of dissection; they may be damaged if the appropriate surgical plane is not adhered to.

The **tibial nerve,** the medial portion of the sciatic nerve, enters the calf deep under the fibrous arch of the soleus muscle. It sends branches to all the muscles of the flexor compartment. Passing behind the medial malleolus, it divides into three branches: a calcaneal branch, a small lateral plantar nerve, and, finally, a larger medial plantar nerve (see Fig. 11-27).

The **posterior tibial artery,** a branch of the popliteal artery, runs under the fibrous arch of the soleus muscle. Its major branch in the calf is the peroneal artery.

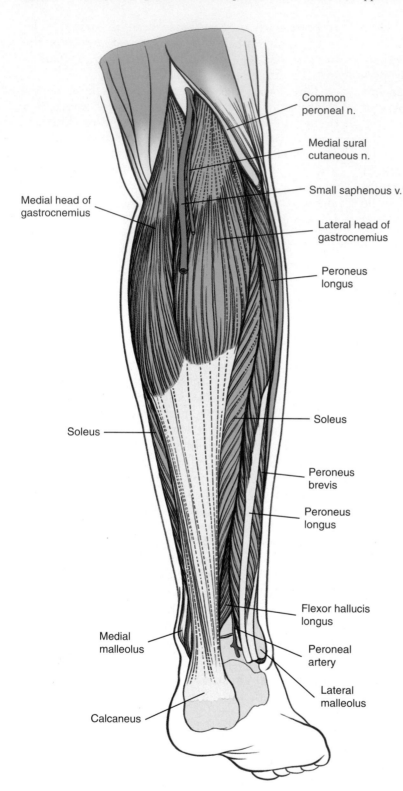

Common peroneal n.

Medial sural cutaneous n.

Small saphenous v.

Medial head of gastrocnemius

Lateral head of gastrocnemius

Peroneus longus

Soleus

Soleus

Peroneus brevis

Peroneus longus

Flexor hallucis longus

Medial malleolus

Peroneal artery

Lateral malleolus

Calcaneus

**Figure 11-26**   The superficial structures of the posterolateral aspect of the leg.

**Gastrocnemius.** *Origin.* Medial head from medial condyle and popliteal surface of femur. Lateral head from lateral surface of lateral femoral condyle. Middle third of posterior aspect. *Insertion.* Calcaneus. Into Achilles tendon with soleus and plantaris muscles. Achilles tendon then inserts into calcaneus. *Action.* Plantar flexor of foot. *Nerve supply.* Tibial nerve.

**Soleus.** *Origin.* Posterior aspect of upper third of fibula, soleal line on tibia, fibrous arch between tibia and fibula. *Insertion.* Middle third of posterior aspect of calcaneus (common tendon with gastrocnemius). *Action.* Plantar flexor of foot. *Nerve supply.* Tibial nerve.

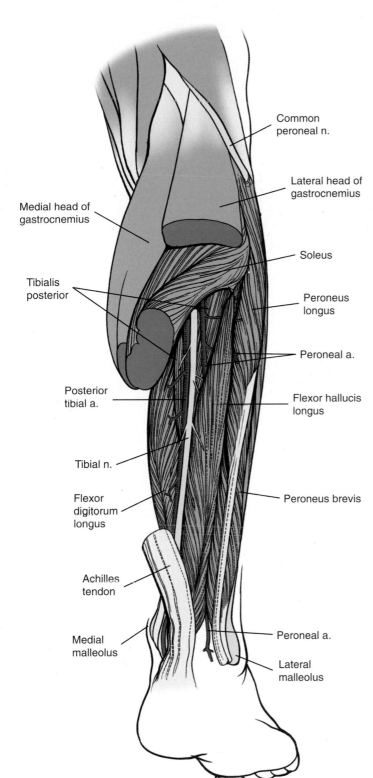

Common peroneal n.

Lateral head of gastrocnemius

Medial head of gastrocnemius

Soleus

Tibialis posterior

Peroneus longus

Peroneal a.

Posterior tibial a.

Flexor hallucis longus

Tibial n.

Flexor digitorum longus

Peroneus brevis

Achilles tendon

Medial malleolus

Peroneal a.

Lateral malleolus

**Figure 11-27**  The gastrocnemius and soleus muscles have been resected to reveal the deep flexor compartment and the neurovascular structures.

**Flexor Hallucis Longus.** *Origin.* Lower two thirds of posterior surface of fibula, interosseous membrane. *Insertion.* Base of distal phalanx of hallux. *Action.* Flexor of hallux and plantar flexor of foot. *Nerve supply.* Tibial nerve.

**Flexor Digitorum Longus.** *Origin.* Posterior surface of middle half of tibia and fascia covering tibialis posterior. *Insertion.* Distal phalanges of lateral four toes. *Action.* Flexor of toes and dorsiflexor of foot. *Nerve supply.* Tibial nerve.

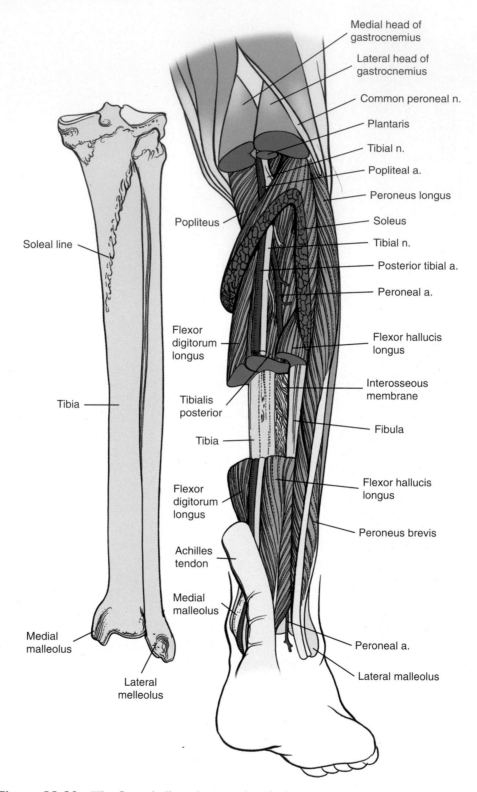

**Figure 11-28**   The flexor hallucis longus, the tibialis posterior, and the flexor digitorum longus have been resected to reveal the posterior aspect of the fibula, interosseous membrane, and tibia.

**Tibialis Posterior.** *Origin.* Lateral side of posterior aspect of tibia, upper two thirds of medial surface of fibula, interosseous membrane. *Insertion.* Tuberosity of navicular and via ligaments to all cuneiforms; second, third, and fourth metatarsals; and cuboid and sustentaculum tali. *Action.* Plantar flexor and invertor of foot. *Nerve supply.* Tibial nerve.

# Approach to the Fibula

## Landmarks and Incision

### Landmarks

The head and lower end of the *fibula* are palpable. The deep peroneal nerve can be rolled against the fibular neck. The nerve is vulnerable to direct pressure from bandaging, the upper end of a cast, or a bed; it also may be damaged by a careless skin incision. The shaft of the fibula is enclosed in muscles and is palpable only as a resistance felt on the lateral side of the leg.

### Incision

The longitudinal incision closely parallels the line of cleavage in the skin, and the resultant scar is not broad and unsightly. As is true for the tibia, incisions made directly over the lower and upper ends of the bone should be closed with special care to ensure sound primary healing.

## Superficial Surgical Dissection

Superficial surgical dissection consists of mobilizing the common peroneal nerve as it winds around the neck of the fibula and developing a plane between the peroneus and soleus muscles (Fig. 11-29).

The *common peroneal nerve* is the lateral portion of the tibial nerve; it is palpable at the neck of the fibula (Fig. 11-30).

## Deep Surgical Dissection

Deep surgical dissection consists of stripping off those muscles that originate from the fibula: the peroneus longus and peroneus brevis (lateral compartment); the extensor digitorum longus, peroneus tertius, and extensor hallucis longus (anterior compartment); and the flexor digitorum longus, flexor hallucis longus, and soleus (posterior compartment; see Figs. 11-25 and 11-30).

The *peroneal artery* arises from the posterior tibial artery soon after it leaves the popliteal artery.

Relatively small, it runs through the deep flexor compartment of the leg, close to the fibula. Its branches wind around the fibula to supply the peroneus longus muscle. The artery is close to the medial surface of the lower end of the fibula and may be damaged during operations on that part of the bone (see Fig. 11-27).

## Special Anatomic Points

### Compartment Syndromes

The muscles of the leg are enclosed in tight fibroosseous compartments. The fascial layers are tough and unyielding, and swelling within a particular compartment rapidly increases pressure. Pressure, in turn, leads to venous stasis, still more intercompartmental pressure, and, eventually, arterial ischemia. Increasing pressure after fractures occurs most commonly in the anterior compartment, even when the fracture is minor and not displaced, possibly because the fascia is so tight.

The fascial layers define four distinct muscle compartments: anterior (extensor), lateral (peroneal), superficial posterior (flexor), and deep posterior (flexor). All four can be affected by swelling, producing four distinct potential compartment syndromes. Fractures in this area may cause swelling in more than one compartment (see Fig. 11-23).

The cardinal physical sign of a compartment syndrome is inappropriate pain. Characteristically this pain is made worse by active or passive movements of the muscle in the affected compartments. Later on in the development of a compartment syndrome, compression lesions of the nerves may produce neurological signs and symptoms, and eventually arterial ischemia may occur.

The surgical treatment of a compartment syndrome is to decompress it. Decompression of the compartment reduces the intercompartmental compressure, which in turn relieves the muscle ischemia. Irreversible changes occur within the muscle if it has been subjected to ischemia for more than 4 to 6 hours. It follows that decompression must be carried out early in the development of a compartment syndrome to ensure a complete recovery. It is important to realize that neurological signs and symptoms develop late in the pathology of a compartment syndrome and that successful treatment depends on the diagnosis of a compartment syndrome at an early stage when the only physical sign is pain disproportionate to the underlying trauma. Compartment pressures can now be routinely measured, but in the conscious patient the diagnosis of a compartment syndrome still remains essentially clinical.

The compartment most commonly affected is the anterior compartment. It can be decompressed by incising the deep fascia that covers it along its entire length.

In cases of compartment syndrome, it is now accepted that all four compartments should be routinely decompressed. To achieve this, a two-incision technique is used. The anterolateral incision decompresses the anterior compartment and the peroneal compartment. The medial incision decompresses both the superficial and deep flexor compartments.

All compartments of the leg may be decompressed by excision of the fibula.

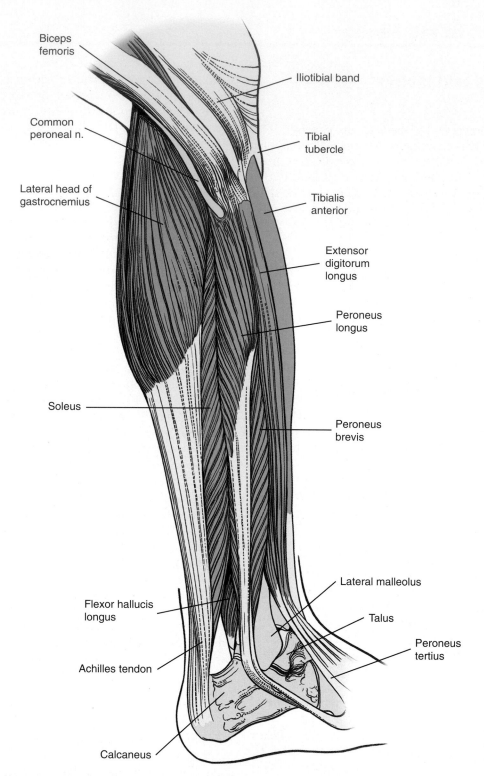

**Figure 11-29**  The superficial structures of the lateral aspect of the leg.

**Peroneus Brevis.** *Origin.* Lower two thirds of lateral aspect of fibula. *Insertion.* Base of fifth metatarsal. *Action.* Evertor and plantar flexor of foot. *Nerve supply.* Superficial peroneal nerve.

**Peroneus Longus.** *Origin.* Lateral tibial condyle, upper two thirds of lateral surface of fibula. *Insertion.* Lateral side of medial cuneiform and base of first metatarsal. *Action.* Evertor and plantar flexor of foot. *Nerve supply.* Superficial peroneal nerve.

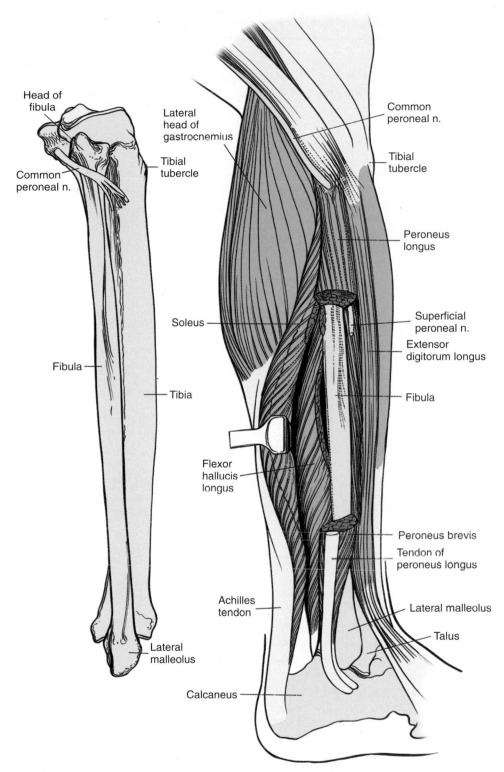

**Figure 11-30**   The peroneal muscles have been resected, and the soleus and flexor digitorum longus have been detached partially from the origin to expose the lateral aspect of the fibula.

# Minimal Access Approach to the Proximal Tibia

The minimal access approach to the proximal tibia is used for the insertion of intramedullary nails used in the treatment of the following:

1. Fresh tibial shaft fractures
2. Pathological tibial shaft fractures
3. Delayed union and nonunion of tibial shaft fractures

Tibial nails do not have the wide variability in design seen in femoral nails. All tibial nails are angled at their upper end to allow insertion via an anterior route, and all tibial nails are straight when viewed in the anterior-posterior plane.

## Position of the Patient

Two positions may be used for the insertion of tibial nails. Placing the patient on a traction table allows greater control of the fracture and easier distal locking. The free leg position allows greater knee flexion, which makes nail insertion easier.

### Traction Table

This is the most commonly used position. Place the patient supine on an operating table. Flex the hip to 60°. Place a support behind the posterior aspect of the distal thigh. Take care not to place the support in the popliteal fossa, where it will create pressure on the popliteal vein (Fig. 11-31; see Fig. 10-59).

Flex the knee to 100° to 120° of flexion, and apply traction by strapping the patient's foot to the sole of a traction boot or a Steinmann pin inserted through the os calcis. A conventional traction boot extends 5 to 8 cm above the heel. Use of this boot will prevent the insertion of distal locking bolts because the required skin incision will be covered by the boot. Again, ensure that the thigh support does not compress the structures within the popliteal fossa. To reduce the risk of thermal necrosis during the reaming of the medullary canal, do not use a tourniquet. Note that minimal traction is required to reduce a fresh tibial shaft fracture.

Place the contralateral leg in a support with the hip flexed and abducted and the knee flexed (see Fig. 11-31).

### Free Leg Position

Place the patient supine on an operating table. Remove the end of the table, and allow the injured knee to flex over the end of the table. Place the con-tralateral leg in a support with the hip flexed and abducted and the knee flexed. Do not use a tourniquet (Fig. 11-32).

## Landmarks and Incisions

### Landmarks

Palpate the *patella* on the anterior aspect of the knee. The *patellar tendon* is felt as a resistance extending from the inferior pole of the patella to the tibial tubercle.

### Incision

Make a 5-cm incision on the anterior aspect of the tibia, beginning at the inferior border of the patella and extending the incision down to just above the tibial tubercle (Fig. 11-33). This incision should overlie the medial border of the patellar tendon.

## Internervous Plane

There are no internervous planes involved in this approach.

## Superficial Surgical Dissection

Incise the subcutaneous fat and fibrous tissue arising from the medial aspect of the patellar tendon in the line of the skin incision. Numerous small arterial vessels are usually encountered and will need to be coagulated. Identify the medial border of the patellar tendon, and incise this fascia longitudinally along the border (Fig. 11-34).

## Deep Surgical Dissection

Retract and mobilize the patellar tendon laterally to expose a small bursa between the tendon and the anterior aspect of the tibia—the deep infrapatellar bursa (Fig. 11-35). The precise entry point of the nail into the medullary canal of the tibial shaft can be calculated preoperatively by overlaying a template of the nail on the anterior-posterior radiograph of the injured tibia. The entry point of the nail lies at the very proximal end of the tibia at the junction of the anterior and superior aspects of the bone. Note that this entry point, although on the superior aspect of the tibia, is extrasynovial (Fig. 11-37). The entry point for the nail must be confirmed radiographically (in the operating room) in both the anterior-

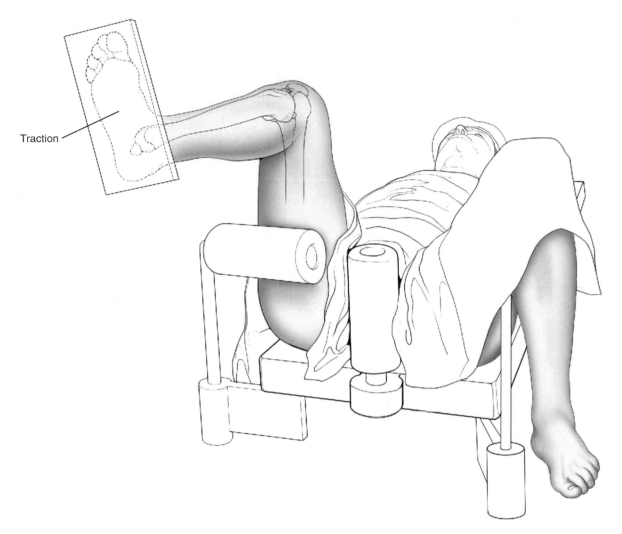

Traction

**Figure 11-31**  Traction table position. Flex the hip 60°. Flex the knee to 100° to 120° of flexion, and apply traction by strapping the foot to the sole of a traction boot. Place the opposite leg in a support with the hip flexed and abducted and the knee flexed.

posterior and lateral planes before entry is made (Fig. 11-36).

## Dangers

### Nerves and Vessels

The *infrapatellar branch of the saphenous nerve* is frequently damaged in this approach. It is impossible to preserve all the branches of the nerve, and patients should be warned that an area of numbness is likely following this surgical approach (see Fig. 10-32).

If a traction table is used and the thigh rest is placed within the popliteal fossa, compression of the *popliteal veins* can result. This can increase the risk of deep vein thrombosis.

### Ligaments and Meniscus

If the entry point is too far posterior, damage to the tibial insertion of the *anterior cruciate ligament* and the *anterior horn of the medial meniscus* may occur (see Fig. 11-37).

### Deformity

If the entry point is too far medial, a valgus deformity will be created at the fracture site in proximal fractures. If the entry point is too far lateral, a varus deformity will be created at the fracture site in proximal fractures.

### Bone

If the entry point is too far inferior on the anterior surface of the *tibia*, then splitting of the anterior cor-

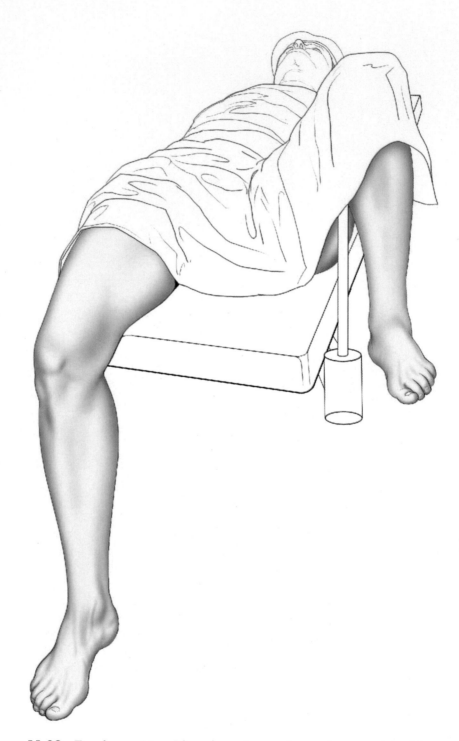

**Figure 11-32**   Free leg position. Place the patient supine on the operating table. Remove the end of the table. Allow the injured knee to flex over the end of the table. Place the contralateral leg in a support with the hip flexed and abducted and the knee flexed.

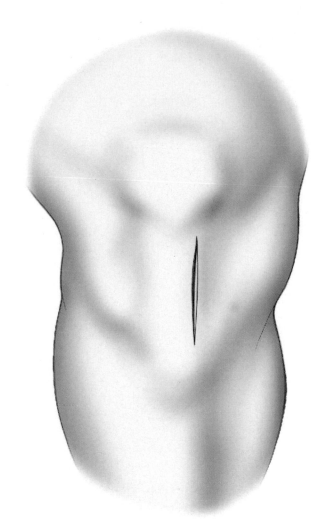

**Figure 11-33** Make a 5-cm long incision overlying the medial edge of the patella tendon.

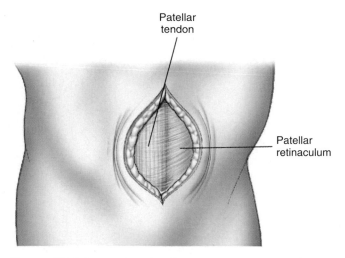

**Figure 11-34** Deepen the skin incision to expose the medial edge of the patella tendon.

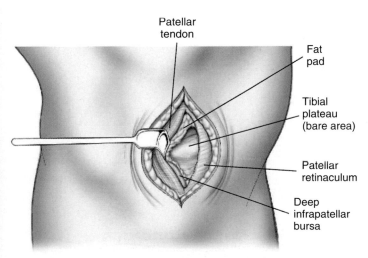

**Figure 11-35** Incise the fascia on the medial edge of the patella tendon and retract the tendon laterally.

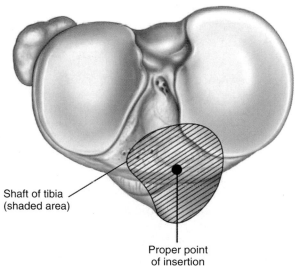

**Figure 11-36** View of the superior surface of the tibia, showing the entry point of the nail. The insertion point is extrasynovial, lying anterior to the tibial insertion of the anterior cruciate ligament and lateral to the anterior horn of the medial meniscus.

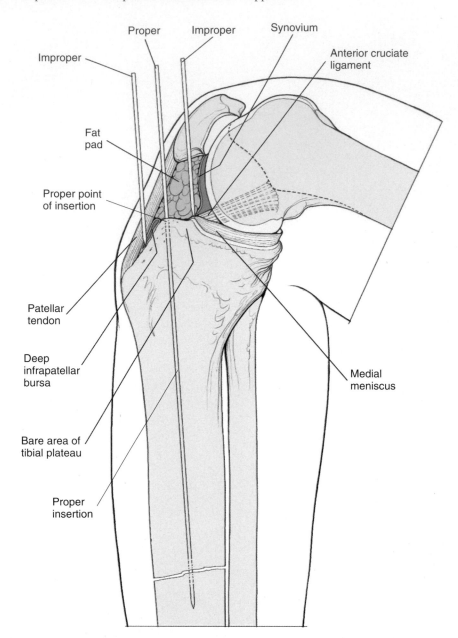

**Figure 11-37**   Correct and incorrect insertion points. Note that if the entry point is too far posterior then damage to the insertion of the anterior cruciate ligament on the tibia will occur. An entry point that is too far anterior will cause splintering of the anterior cortex of the tibia on nail insertion.

tex of the tibia may occur on nail insertion (see Fig. 11-37).

Nail insertion is very difficult if the knee is not flexed to beyond 90° due to pressure of the nail on the anterior aspect of the *patella*. Such pressure may be sufficient to produce a compression lesion of the patellofemoral joint or even transient subluxation of the patella, producing damage to the articular cartilage of the patella. For that reason, many surgeons

prefer a free leg position, which allows greater degrees of flexion than can be easily obtained using a traction table.

## How to Enlarge the Approach

This approach gives excellent visualization of the entry point of the nail but has no other uses. It cannot be usefully enlarged.

# REFERENCES

1. MULLER ME, ALLGOWER M, WILLENEGGER H: Manual of internal fixation. New York, Springer-Verlag, 1970
2. PHEMISTER DB: Treatment of ununited fractures by onlay bone grafts without screw or tie fixation and without breaking down of the fibrous union. J Bone Joint Surg 29:946, 1947
3. PATTERSON D, LEWIS GN, CASS CA: Clinical experience in Australia with an implanted bone growth stimulator (1976–1978). Orthop Transcripts 3:288, 1979
4. HARMON PH: A simplified surgical approach to the posterior tibia for bone grafting and fibular transference. J Bone Joint Surg 27:496, 1945
5. JONES KG, BARNETT HC: Cancellous-bone grafting for nonunion of the tibia through the postero-lateral approach. J Bone Joint Surg [Am] 37:1250, 1955
6. HENRY AK: Extensile exposure, 2nd ed. London, Churchill Livingstone, 1973
7. COVENTRY MB: Osteotomy about the knee for degenerative and rheumatoid arthritis: indications, operative technique and results. J Bone Joint Surg [Am] 55:234, 1973
8. BROWN PN, URBAN JG: Early weight bearing treatment of open fractures of the tibia. J Bone Joint Surg [Am] 51:59, 1969
9. SORENSON KH: Treatment of delayed union and nonunion of the tibia by fibular resection. Acta Orthop Scand 40:92, 1969
10. LEACH RE, HAMMOND G, STRIKER WS: Anterior tibial compartment syndrome: acute and chronic. J Bone Joint Surg [Am] 49:451, 1967
11. KIRGIS A, ALBRECHT S: Palsy of the deep peroneal nerve after proximal tibial osteotomy: an anatomical study. J Bone Joint Surg [Am] 74:1180, 1992

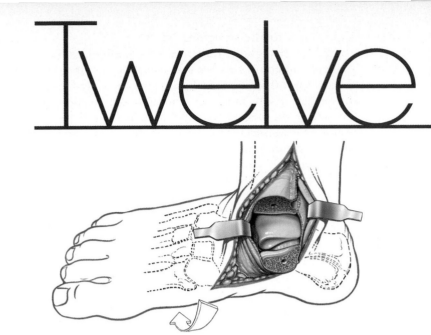

# Twelve

# The Ankle and Foot

Approaches to the structures of the ankle and foot usually are straightforward; the bones and joints that are explored commonly are superficial, if not subcutaneous. Apart from technical problems associated with the surgery itself, the most common complication in foot and ankle surgery is poor wound healing. For this reason, it is important to evaluate both the circulation and the sensation of the foot. Ischemic or neuropathic feet heal poorly and are a frequent contraindication to elective surgery. In patients with diabetes, ischemia and neuropathy may coexist; all feet of such patients must be evaluated carefully before any foot surgery is undertaken.

Wound healing also is affected by the thickness of the skin flaps that are cut; it is important to cut these flaps as thickly as possible and to avoid forceful retraction. Longer incisions require less forceful retraction to achieve identical exposure. As a result, they often are safer than are short incisions. (Remember that skin incisions heal from side to side and not from end to end.)

This chapter is divided into three sections. The first describes approaches to the ankle and the hindpart of the foot, because most provide access to both areas. The *anterior approach to the ankle* is used for arthrodesis; it offers excellent exposure of the anterior compartment of the ankle joint. The *approach to the medial malleolus* is a commonly used incision, providing access to the distal tibia in cases of fracture. A more extensive approach to the *medial side of the ankle joint* also exposes the distal tibia, but involves an osteotomy. The *posteromedial approach to the ankle* exposes the soft tissues of the area. It is used frequently for soft-tissue operations, including the surgical correction of clubfoot. The *posterolateral approach to the ankle joint* provides limited access to the back of the joint and the posterior facet of the subtalar joint.

The *lateral approach to the ankle and hindpart of the foot* exposes the ankle and the joints of the hindfoot. Finally, the *lateral approach to the hindpart of the foot* and the *posterolateral approach to the talocalcaneal joint* are used for surgery on the joints of the posterior part of the foot. The applied anatomy of the ankle and hindpart of the foot is considered in a separate section, following the description of the surgical approaches.

The second section of this chapter describes approaches to the midportion of the foot, the tarsometatarsal and midtarsal joints and those muscles that attach to them. Surgery in this area is relatively uncommon in general orthopaedic practice; it usually is associated with specific operative procedures designed for single pathologic states. Because these structures are very superficial, the approaches are dealt with mainly pictorially.

The final section comprises three of the most common approaches in surgery of the forepart of the foot. The *dorsal and dorsomedial approaches to the metatarsophalangeal joint of the great toe* are used in surgery for hallux valgus; the *dorsal approach to the metatarsophalangeal joints* of the second, third, fourth, and fifth toes provides safe access to these joints; and the *approach to the dorsal web spaces* can be used for the treatment of several conditions, including Morton's neuroma. The latter approach also can be used to reach the metatarsophalangeal joint.

The applied anatomy of the foot appears in two sections after this group of approaches. The first section deals with the applied anatomy of the approaches, that is, the applied anatomy of the dorsum of the foot. The second section, an account of the anatomy of the sole of the foot, should provide an understanding of those structures that may be damaged in severe foot trauma or infection.

# Anterior Approach to the Ankle

The anterior approach provides excellent exposure of the ankle joint for arthrodesis.[1] The decision to use this approach rather than the lateral transfibular approach, the medial transmalleolar approach, or the posterior approach depends on the condition of the skin and the surgical technique to be used. Its other uses include the following:

1. Drainage of infections in the ankle joint
2. Removal of loose bodies

3. Open reduction and internal fixation of comminuted distal tibial fractures (pilon fractures)

## Position of the Patient

Place the patient supine on the operating table. Partially exsanguinate the foot either by elevating it for 3 to 5 minutes or by applying a soft rubber bandage loosely to the foot and binding it firmly to the calf. Then, inflate a thigh tourniquet. Partial exsanguination allows the neurovascular bundle to be identified, because the venous structures will appear blue. Some continuous vascular oozing must be expected, however (Fig. 12-1).

## Landmarks and Incision

### Landmarks
The *medial malleolus* is the bulbous, subcutaneous, distal end of the medial surface of the tibia.

The *lateral malleolus* is the subcutaneous distal end of the fibula.

### Incision
Make a 15-cm longitudinal incision over the anterior aspect of the ankle joint. Begin about 10 cm proximal to the joint, and extend the incision so that it crosses the joint about midway between the malleoli, ending on the dorsum of the foot. Take great care to cut only the skin; the anterior neurovascular bundle and branches of the superficial peroneal nerve cross the ankle joint very close to the line of the skin incision (Fig. 12-2*A*). Alternatively, make a 15-cm longitudinal incision with its center overlying the anterior aspect of the medial malleolus (see Fig. 12-2).

## Internervous Plane

Although the approach uses no true internervous plane, the *extensor hallucis longus* and *extensor digito-*

*rum longus* muscles define a clear intermuscular plane. Both muscles are supplied by the deep peroneal nerve, but the plane may be used because both receive their nerve supplies well proximal to the level of the dissection. The plane must be used with great caution, however, because it contains the neurovascular bundle distal to the ankle (see Figs. 12-56 and 12-57).

## Superficial Surgical Dissection

Incise the deep fascia of the leg in line with the skin incision, cutting through the extensor retinaculum (see Fig. 12-2*B*). Find the plane between the extensor hallucis longus and extensor digitorum longus muscles a few centimeters above the ankle joint, and identify the neurovascular bundle (the anterior tibial artery and the deep peroneal nerve) just medial to the tendon of the extensor hallucis longus (see Fig. 12-2*C*). Trace the bundle distally until it crosses the front of the ankle joint behind the tendon of the extensor hallucis longus. Retract the tendon of the extensor hallucis longus medially, together with the neurovascular bundle. Retract the tendon of the extensor digitorum longus laterally. The tendons become mobile after the retinaculum has been cut, but the neurovascular bundle adheres to the underlying tissues and requires mobilization (Fig. 12-3*A*).

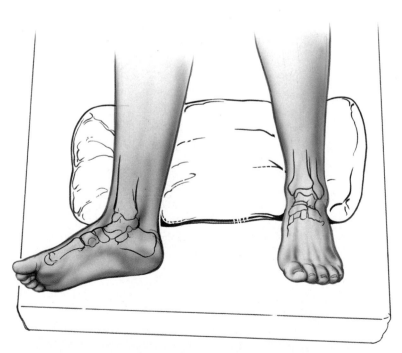

**Figure 12-1**  Position for the anterior approach to the ankle.

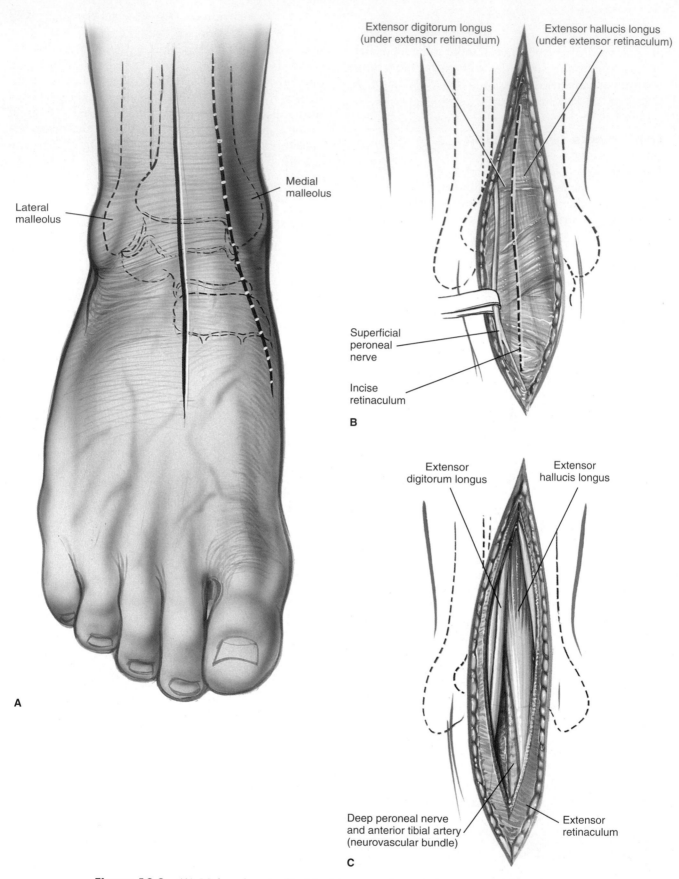

**Figure 12-2** **(A)** Make a longitudinal incision over the anterior aspect of the ankle joint. **(B)** Identify and protect the superficial peroneal nerve. Incise the extensor retinaculum in line with the skin incision. **(C)** Identify the plane between the extensor hallucis longus and the extensor digitorum longus, and note the neurovascular bundle between them.

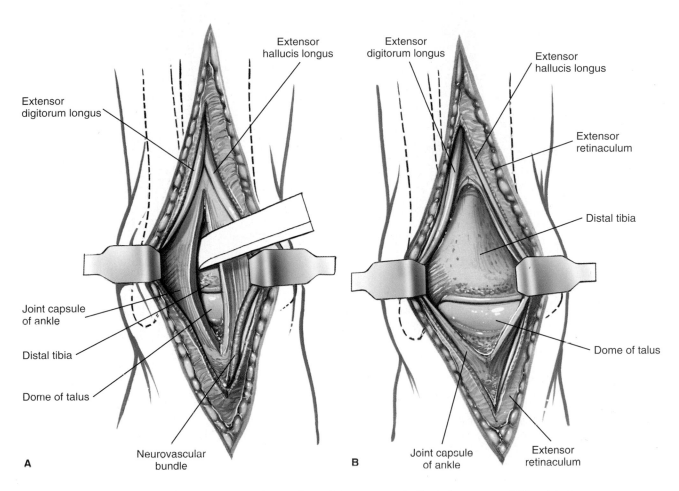

**Figure 12-3** **(A)** Retract the tendon of the extensor hallucis longus medially with the neurovascular bundle. Retract the tendon of the extensor digitorum longus laterally. Incise the joint capsule longitudinally. **(B)** Retract the joint capsule to expose the ankle joint.

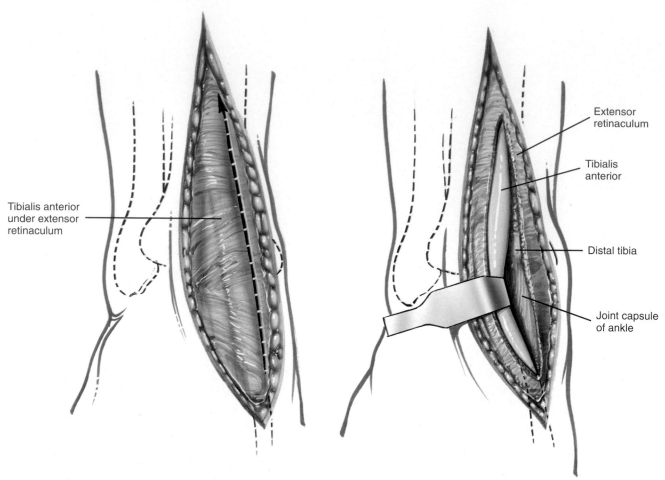

**Figure 12-4** **(A)** Alternately, incise the extensor retinaculum on the medial side of the tibialis anterior tendon. **(B)** Retract the tibialis anterior laterally to expose the anterior surface of the ankle joint.

Alternatively, in pillion fractures, incise the deep fascia to the medial side of the tibialis anterior tendon (Fig. 12-4), and expose the underlying surface of the tibia together with the anteromedial ankle joint capsule.

## Deep Surgical Dissection

Incise the remaining soft tissues longitudinally to expose the anterior surface of the distal tibia. Continue incising down to the ankle joint, then cut through its anterior capsule. Expose the full width of the ankle joint by detaching the anterior ankle capsule from the tibia or the talus by sharp dissection (see Fig. 12-3). Some periosteal stripping of the distal tibia may be required. Although the periosteal layer usually is thick and easy to define, the plane may be obliterated in cases of infection; the periosteum then must be detached piecemeal by sharp dissection.

## Dangers

### Nerves

Cutaneous branches of the **superficial peroneal nerve** run close to the line of the skin incision just under the skin. Take care not to cut them during incision of the skin (see Fig. 12-2*A*).

The **deep peroneal nerve** and **anterior tibial artery** (the anterior neurovascular bundle) must be identified and preserved during superficial surgical dissection. They are in greatest danger during the skin incision, because they are superficial and run close to the incision itself (see Figs. 12-56 and 12-57). Above the ankle joint, the neurovascular bundle lies between the tendons of the extensor hallucis longus and tibialis anterior muscles at the joint; the tendon of the extensor hallucis longus crosses the bundle. The plane between the tibialis anterior and the extensor hallucis longus can be used as long as the neurovascular bundle is identified and mobilized so as to preserve it (see Fig. 12-57).

## How to Enlarge the Approach

### Extensile Measures

Although this approach does not descend through an internervous plane, on occasion it can be extended proximally to expose the structures in the anterior compartment. To expose the proximal tibia, use the plane between the tibia and the tibialis anterior muscle (see Fig. 12-4). Distal extension to the dorsum of the foot is possible, but rarely, if ever, required (see Fig. 12-57).

---

# Anterior and Posterior Approaches to the Medial Malleolus

The anterior and posterior approaches are used mainly for open reduction and internal fixation of fractures of the medial malleolus.[2] The approaches provide excellent visualization of the malleolus.

## Position of the Patient

Place the patient supine on the operating table. The natural position of the leg (slight external rotation) exposes the medial malleolus well. Exsanguinate the limb by elevating it for 3 to 5 minutes, then inflate a tourniquet. Standing or sitting at the foot of the table makes it easier to angle drills correctly (Fig. 12-5).

## Incisions

Two skin incisions are available.

1. The *anterior incision* offers an excellent view of medial malleolar fractures. It also permits inspection of the anteromedial ankle joint and the anteromedial part of the dome of the talus.

   Make a 10-cm longitudinal curved incision on the medial aspect of the ankle, with its midpoint just anterior to the tip of the medial malleolus. Begin proximally, 5 cm above the malleolus and over the middle of the subcutaneous surface of the tibia. Then, cross the anterior third of the medial malleolus, and curve the incision forward to end some 5 cm anterior and distal to the malleolus. The incision should not cross the most prominent portion of the malleolus (Fig. 12-6).

2. The *posterior incision* allows reduction and fixation of medial malleolar fractures and visualization of the posterior margin of the tibia.

   Make a 10-cm incision on the medial side of the ankle. Begin 5 cm above the ankle on the posterior border of the tibia, and curve the incision downward, following the posterior border of the

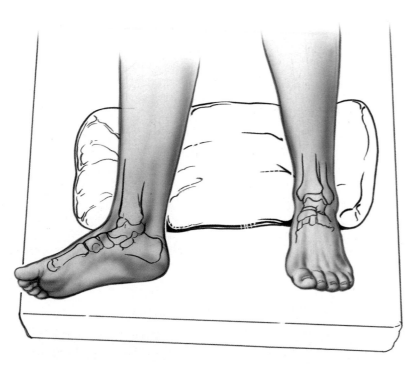

**Figure 12-5**   Position for the approach to the medial malleolus. The leg falls naturally into a few degrees of external rotation to expose the malleolus.

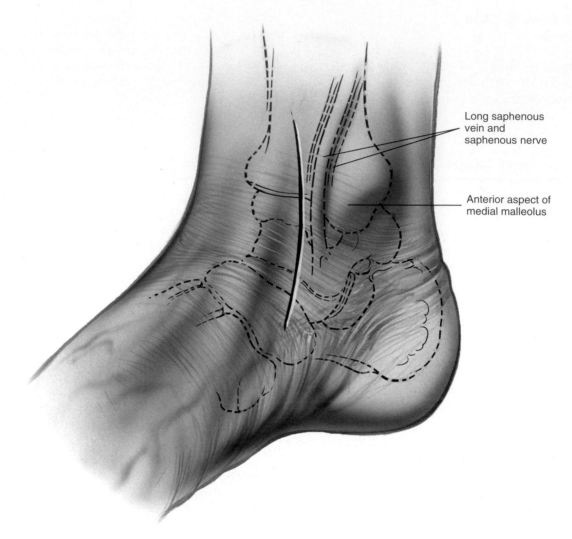

Long saphenous
vein and
saphenous nerve

Anterior aspect of
medial malleolus

**Figure 12-6**  Keep the incision just anterior to the tip of the medial malleolus.

medial malleolus. Curve the incision forward below the medial malleolus to end 5 cm distal to the malleolus (see Fig. 12-10).

## Internervous Plane

No true internervous plane exists in this approach, but the approach is safe because the incision cuts down onto subcutaneous bone.

## Superficial Surgical Dissection

### Anterior Incision
Gently mobilize the skin flaps, taking care to identify and preserve the long saphenous vein, which lies just anterior to the medial malleolus. Accurately locating the skin incision will make it unnecessary to mobilize

the skin flaps extensively. Next to the vein runs the saphenous nerve, two branches of which are bound to the vein. Take care not to damage the nerve; damage leads to the formation of a neuroma. Because the nerve is small and not easily identified, the best way to preserve it is to preserve the long saphenous vein, a structure that on its own is of little functional significance (Fig. 12-7).

### Posterior Incision
Mobilize the skin flaps. The saphenous nerve is not in danger (see Fig. 12-11).

## Deep Surgical Dissection

In cases of fracture, the periosteum already is breached. Protect as many soft-tissue attachments to

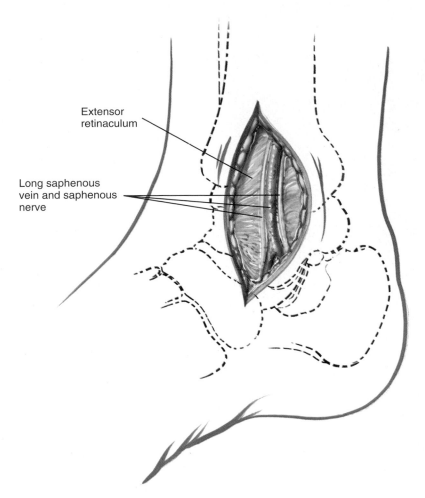

Extensor
retinaculum

Long saphenous
vein and saphenous
nerve

**Figure 12-7**   Widen the skin flaps.
Identify the long saphenous vein and the
accompanying saphenous nerve.

the bone fragment as possible to preserve its blood
supply.

### Anterior Incision

Incise the remaining coverings of the medial malleolus longitudinally to expose the fracture site. Make a
small incision in the anterior capsule of the ankle
joint so that the joint surfaces can be seen after the
fracture is reduced (Fig. 12-8). The superficial fibers
of the deltoid ligament run anteriorly and distally
downward from the medial malleolus; split them so
that wires or screws used in internal fixation can be
anchored solidly on bone, with the heads of the
screws covered by soft tissue (Fig. 12-9; see Fig.
12-54).

### Posterior Incision

Incise the retinaculum behind the medial malleolus
longitudinally so that it can be repaired (Figs. 12-10
and 12-11). Take care not to cut the tendon of the
tibialis posterior muscle, which runs immediately
behind the medial malleolus; the incision into the

retinaculum permits anterior retraction of the tibialis posterior tendon. Continue the dissection
around the back of the malleolus, retracting the
other structures that pass behind the medial malleolus posteriorly to reach the posterior margin (or
posterior malleolus) of the tibia. The exposure
allows reduction of some fractures of that part of
the bone.

Note that, although this approach will allow visualization of most fractures using appropriate reduction forceps, the angle of the approach is such that
the displaced fragments cannot be fixed internally
from this approach. Separate anterior approaches are
required to lag any posterior fragments back. It
always is advisable to obtain an intraoperative radiograph showing the displaced fragment fixed tem-
porarily with a K-wire before definitive fixation is
inserted. Reduction of these fragments is difficult
because of limited exposure, and inaccurate reduction may occur. To improve the view of the posterior
malleolus, externally rotate the leg still further (Fig.
12-12; see Figs. 12-53 and 12-54).

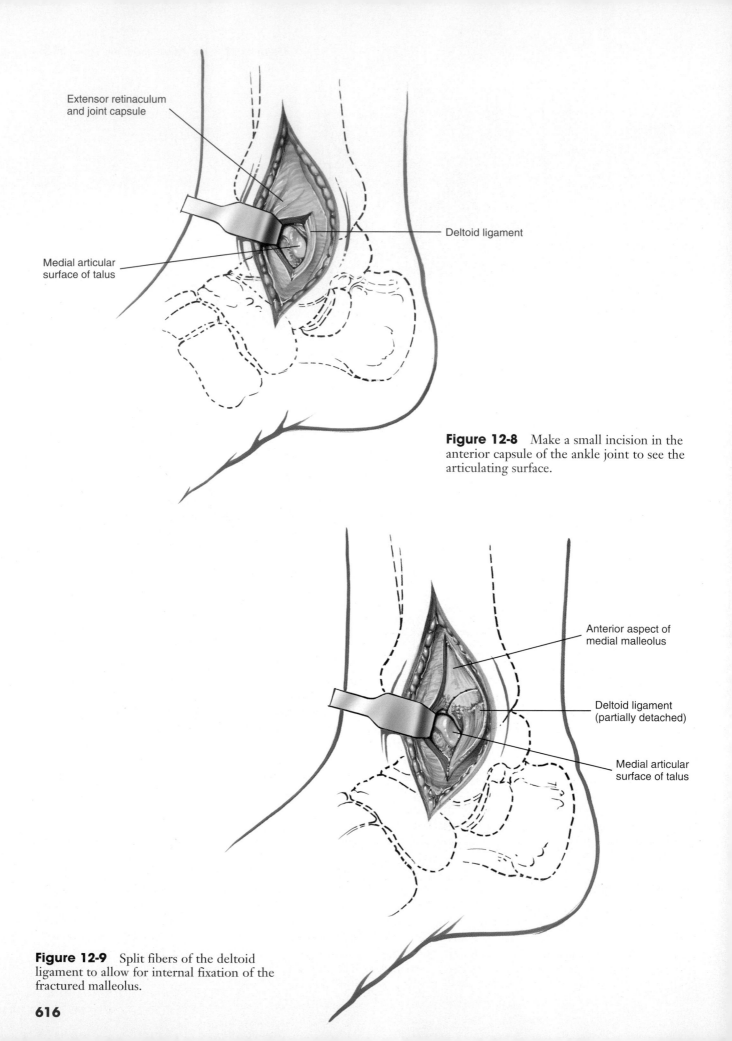

Extensor retinaculum
and joint capsule

Deltoid ligament

Medial articular
surface of talus

**Figure 12-8** Make a small incision in the anterior capsule of the ankle joint to see the articulating surface.

Anterior aspect of
medial malleolus

Deltoid ligament
(partially detached)

Medial articular
surface of talus

**Figure 12-9** Split fibers of the deltoid ligament to allow for internal fixation of the fractured malleolus.

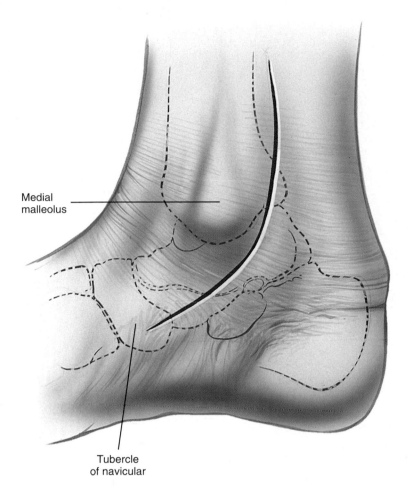

Medial
malleolus

Tubercle
of navicular

**Figure 12-10**   The posterior incision for the
approach to the medial malleolus follows the
posterior border of the medial malleolus.

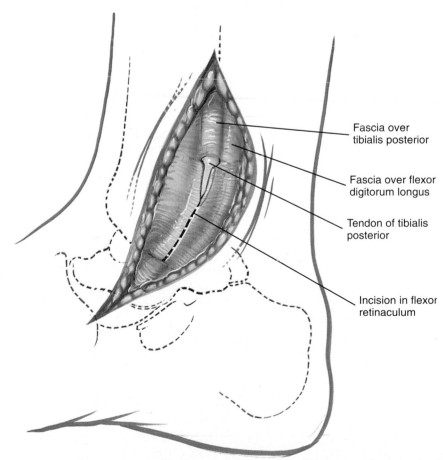

Fascia over
tibialis posterior

Fascia over flexor
digitorum longus

Tendon of tibialis
posterior

Incision in flexor
retinaculum

**Figure 12-11**   Retract the skin flaps
and begin to incise the retinaculum
behind the medial malleolus.

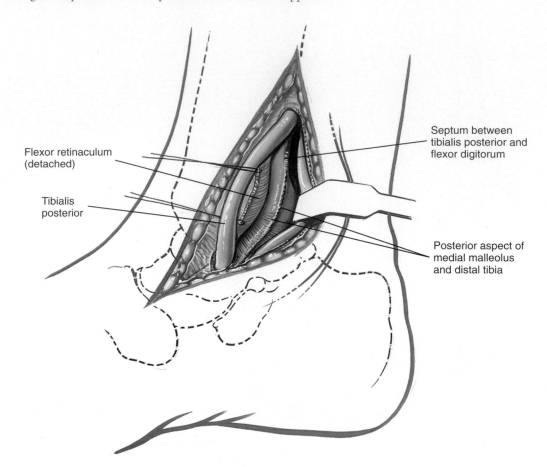

Flexor retinaculum
(detached)

Tibialis
posterior

Septum between
tibialis posterior and
flexor digitorum

Posterior aspect of
medial malleolus
and distal tibia

**Figure 12-12**    Anteriorly retract the tibialis posterior. Free up and retract the
remaining structures around the back of the malleolus posteriorly to expose the posterior
aspect of the medial malleolus.

## Dangers of the Anterior Incision

### Nerves
The **saphenous nerve,** if cut, may form a neuroma
and cause numbness over the medial side of the dorsum of the foot. Preserve the nerve by preserving the
long saphenous vein.

### Vessels
The **long saphenous** vein is at risk when the anterior skin flaps are mobilized. Preserve it if possible,
so that it can be used as a vascular graft in the future
(see Fig. 12-52).

## Dangers of the Posterior Incision

All the structures that run behind the medial malleolus (the tibialis posterior muscle, the flexor digitorum longus muscle, the posterior tibial artery and

vein, the tibial nerve, and the flexor hallucis longus
tendon) are in danger if the deep surgical dissection
is not carried out close to bone (see Figs. 12-52
through 12-54).

Leave as much soft tissue attached to fractured
malleolar fragments as possible; complete stripping
renders fragments avascular.

## How to Enlarge the Approach

### Extensile Measures
To enlarge both approaches proximally, continue the
incision along the subcutaneous surface of the tibia.
Subperiosteal dissection exposes the subcutaneous
and lateral surfaces of the tibia along its entire
length.

The exposure can be extended distally to expose
the deltoid ligaments and the talocalcaneonavicular
joint.

# Approach to the Medial Side of the Ankle

The medial approach exposes the medial side of the ankle joint.[3] Its uses include the following:

1. Arthrodesis of the ankle
2. Excision of osteochondral fragments from the medial side of the talus
3. Removal of loose bodies from the ankle joint

## Position of the Patient

Place the patient supine on the operating table. Exsanguinate the limb either by elevating it for 5 minutes or by applying a soft rubber bandage firmly; then inflate a tourniquet. The natural external rotation of the leg exposes the medial malleolus. The pelvis ordinarily does not have to be tilted to improve the exposure (see Fig. 12-5).

## Landmark and Incision

### Landmark
The *medial malleolus* is the palpable distal end of the tibia.

### Incision
Make a 10-cm longitudinal incision on the medial aspect of the ankle joint, centering it on the tip of the medial malleolus. Begin the incision over the medial surface of the tibia. Below the malleolus, curve it forward onto the medial side of the middle part of the foot (Fig. 12-13).

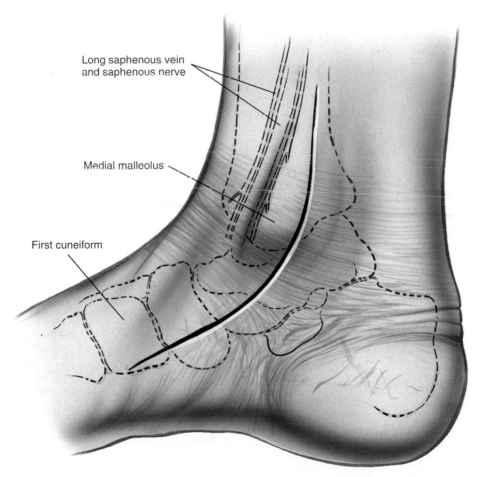

Long saphenous vein and saphenous nerve

Medial malleolus

First cuneiform

**Figure 12-13**   Make a 10-cm longitudinal incision on the medial aspect of the ankle joint, with its center over the tip of the medial malleolus. Distally, curve the incision forward onto the medial side of the middle part of the foot.

## Internervous Plane

The approach uses no internervous plane. Nevertheless, the surgery is safe because the tibia is subcutaneous and all dissection stays on bone.

## Superficial Surgical Dissection

Mobilize the skin flaps, taking care not to damage the long saphenous vein and the saphenous nerve, which run together along the anterior border of the medial malleolus (Fig. 12-14).

## Deep Surgical Dissection

To uncover the point at which the medial malleolus joins the shaft of the tibia, make a small longitudinal incision in the anterior part of the joint capsule.

Divide the flexor retinaculum and identify the tendon of the tibialis posterior muscle, which runs immediately behind the medial malleolus, grooving the bone (see Fig. 12-14). Retract the tendon posteriorly to expose the posterior surface of the malleolus (Fig. 12-15*A*).

Score the bone longitudinally to ensure correct alignment of the malleolus during closure. Then, drill and tap the medial malleolus so that it can be reattached (see Fig. 12-15*B*).

Using an osteotome or oscillating saw, cut through the medial malleolus obliquely from top to bottom; cut laterally at its junction with the shaft of the tibia, checking the position of the cut through the incision in the anterior joint capsule (see Fig. 12-15).

Retract the medial malleolus (with its attached deltoid ligaments) downward and forcibly evert the foot, bringing the dome of the talus and the articulating surface of the tibia into view (Figs. 12-16 and 12-17). Eversion is limited because of the intact fibula.

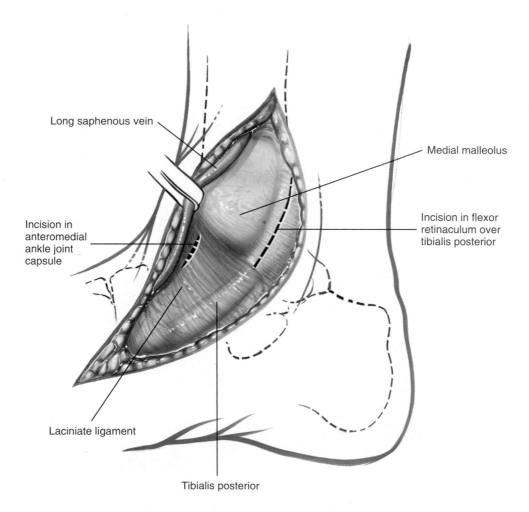

**Figure 12-14**  Carefully retract the skin flaps to protect the long saphenous vein and the accompanying saphenous nerve. Incise the posterior retinaculum, and make a small incision into the anterior joint capsule.

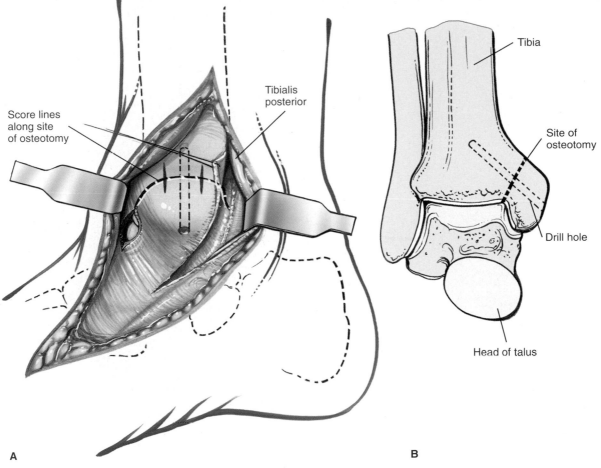

**Figure 12-15**  (**A**) Retract the tibialis tendon posteriorly. Drill and tap the medial malleolus, and score the potential osteotomy site for future alignment. (**B**) The line of the osteotomy and the score marks for the reattachment of the medial malleolus.

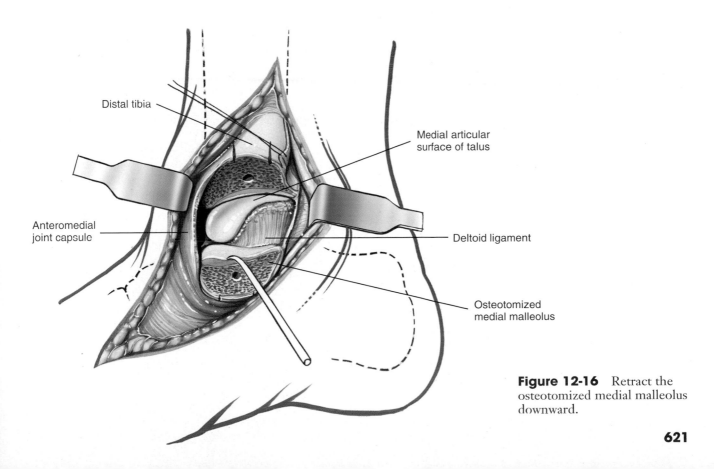

**Figure 12-16**  Retract the osteotomized medial malleolus downward.

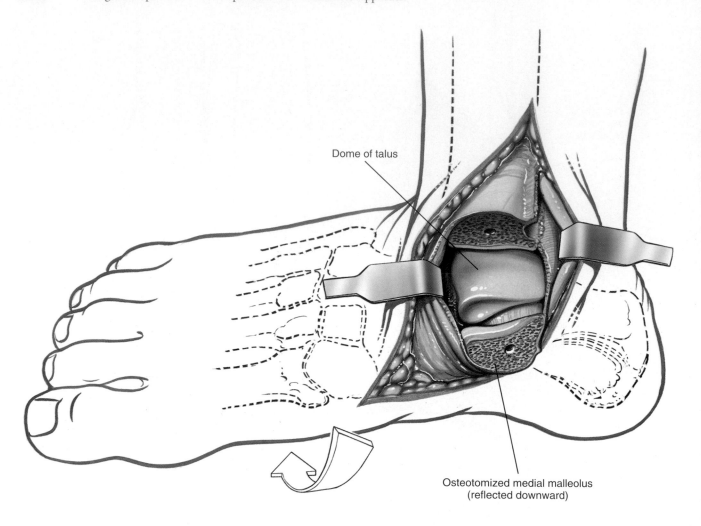

Dome of talus

Osteotomized medial malleolus
(reflected downward)

**Figure 12-17**    Forcefully evert the foot to bring the dome of the talus and the anterior surface of the tibia into view.

## Dangers

The **saphenous nerve** and the long saphenous vein should be preserved as a unit, largely to prevent damage to the saphenous nerve and subsequent neuroma formation.

The **tendon of the tibialis posterior muscle** is in particular danger during this approach, because it lies immediately posterior to the medial malleolus. Preserve the tendon by releasing and retracting it while performing osteotomy of the malleolus (see Figs. 12-14 and 12-15A). The tendons of the flexor hallucis longus and flexor digitorum longus muscle, together with the posterior neurovascular bundle, lie more posteriorly and laterally. They are in no danger as long as the osteotomy is performed carefully (see Figs. 12-53 and 12-55).

## Special Surgical Points

In cases of fracture, the interdigitation of the broken ends of bone prevents rotation between the two fragments when a screw is inserted and tightened. No such interdigitation exists in an osteotomy. Therefore, two Kirschner wires should be used in addition to a screw to prevent rotation when the screw is tightened. After the osteotomy has been stabilized with the screw, the two Kirschner wires can be removed. Tension band fixation also may be used. In any case, align the bones correctly by aligning the score marks made on the bone before the osteotomy.

## How to Enlarge the Approach

The approach usually is not enlarged either distally or proximally.

# Posteromedial Approach to the Ankle

The posteromedial approach to the ankle joint is routinely used for exploring the soft tissues that run around the back of the medial malleolus. This approach is used for the release of soft tissue around the medial malleolus in the treatment of club foot.

The approach can also be used to allow access to the posterior malleolus of the ankle joint, but gives limited exposure of the fracture site and is technically demanding. For this reason reduction and fixation of posterior malleolar fractures is usually achieved by indirect techniques.[4]

## Position of the Patient

Either of two positions are available for this approach. First, place the patient supine on the operating table. Flex the hip and knee, and place the lateral side of the affected ankle on the anterior surface of the opposite knee. This position will achieve full external rotation of the hip, permitting better exposure of the medial structures of the ankle (Fig. 12-18). Alternatively, place the patient in the lateral position with the affected leg nearest the table. Flex the knee of the opposite limb to get its ankle out of the way.

Exsanguinate the limb by elevating it for 3 to 5 minutes or applying a soft rubber bandage; then inflate a tourniquet.

## Landmarks and Incision

### Landmarks

The *medial malleolus* is the bulbous, distal, subcutaneous end of the tibia.

Palpate the *Achilles tendon* just above the calcaneus.

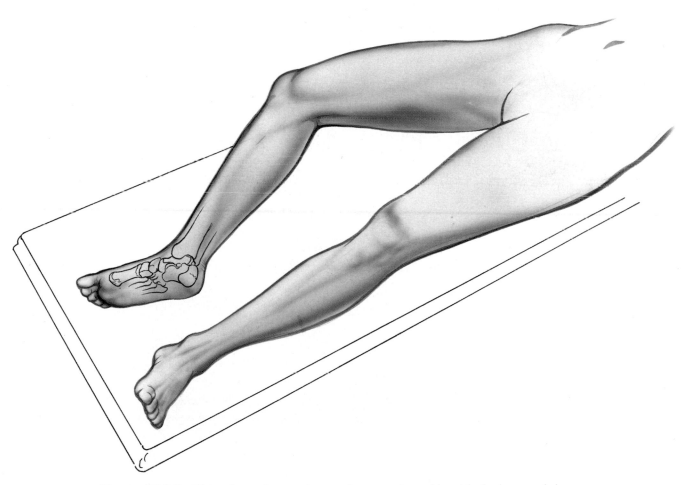

**Figure 12-18**   Place the patient supine on the operating table with the knee and the hip flexed to expose the medial structures of the ankle.

### Incision

Make an 8- to 10-cm longitudinal incision roughly midway between the medial malleolus and the Achilles tendon (Fig. 12-19).

## Superficial Surgical Dissection

Deepen the incision in line with the skin incision to enter the fat that lies between the Achilles tendon and those structures that pass around the back of the medial malleolus. If the Achilles tendon must be lengthened, identify it in the posterior flap of the wound and perform the lengthening now. Identify a fascial plane in the anterior flap that covers the remaining flexor tendons. Incise the fascia longitudinally, well away from the back of the medial malleolus (Figs. 12-20 and 12-21).

## Deep Surgical Dissection

There are three different ways to approach the back of the ankle joint.

First, identify the flexor hallucis longus, the only muscle that still has muscle fibers at this level (see Fig. 12-21). At its lateral border, develop a plane between it and the peroneal tendons, which lie just lateral to it (Fig. 12-22). Deepen this plane to expose the posterior aspect of the ankle joint by retracting the flexor hallucis longus medially (Fig. 12-23).

Second, identify the flexor hallucis longus and continue the dissection anteriorly toward the back of the medial malleolus. Preserve the neurovascular bundle by mobilizing it gently and retracting it and the flexor hallucis longus laterally to develop a plane between the bundle and the tendon of the flexor dig-

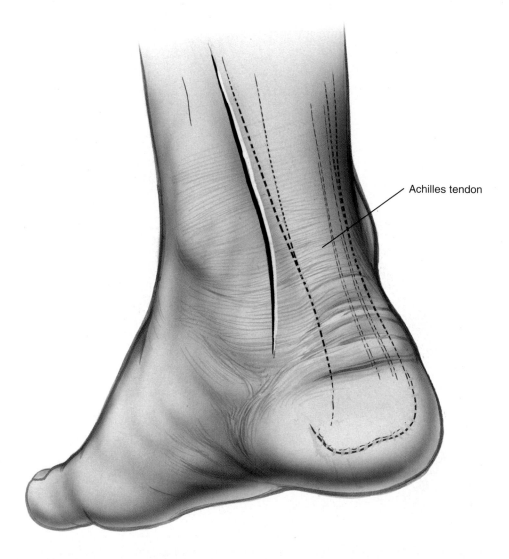

Achilles tendon

**Figure 12-19**   Make an 8- to 10-cm longitudinal incision roughly between the medial malleolus and the Achilles tendon.

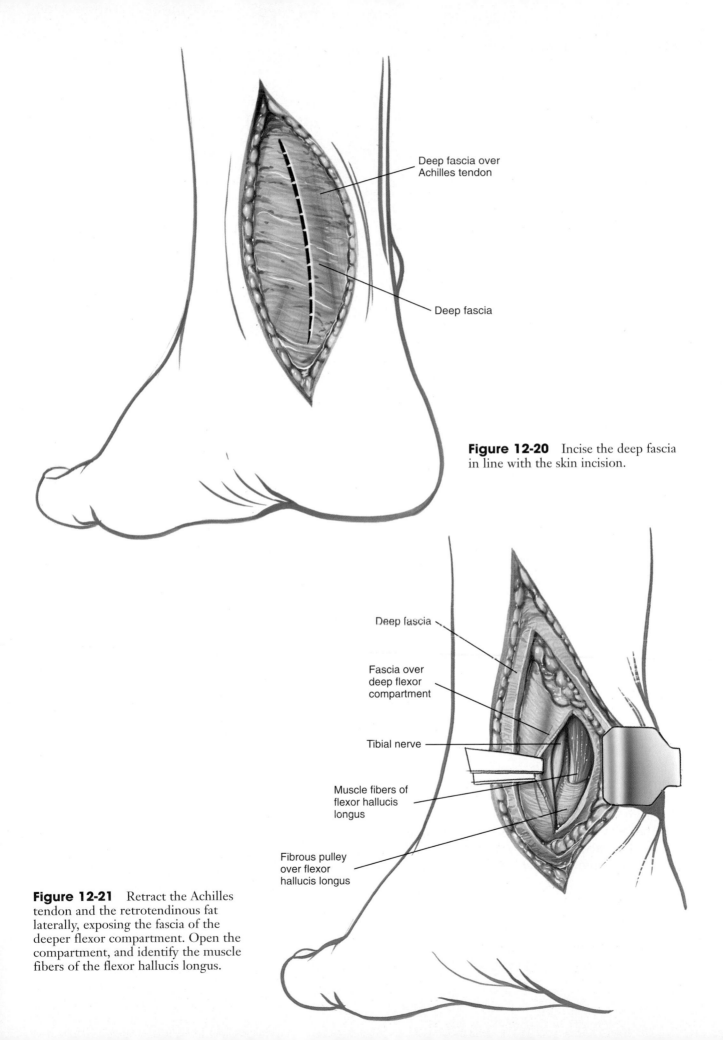

Deep fascia over
Achilles tendon

Deep fascia

**Figure 12-20**  Incise the deep fascia
in line with the skin incision.

Deep fascia

Fascia over
deep flexor
compartment

Tibial nerve

Muscle fibers of
flexor hallucis
longus

Fibrous pulley
over flexor
hallucis longus

**Figure 12-21**  Retract the Achilles
tendon and the retrotendinous fat
laterally, exposing the fascia of the
deeper flexor compartment. Open the
compartment, and identify the muscle
fibers of the flexor hallucis longus.

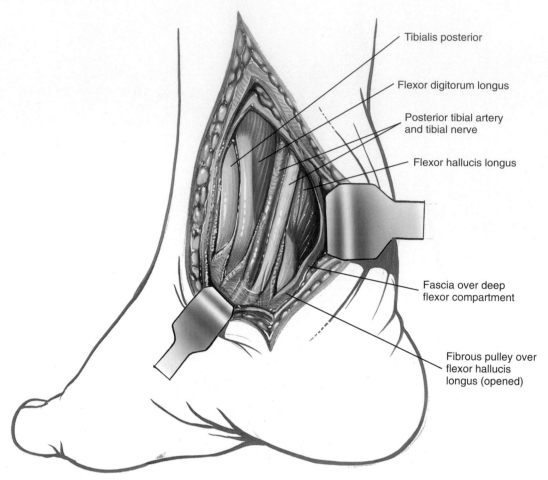

Tibialis posterior

Flexor digitorum longus

Posterior tibial artery and tibial nerve

Flexor hallucis longus

Fascia over deep flexor compartment

Fibrous pulley over flexor hallucis longus (opened)

**Figure 12-22**   Identify the posterior tibial artery and tibial nerve. Then, incise the fibro-osseous tunnel over the flexor hallucis longus tendon and the other medial tendons so that the structures can be mobilized and retracted medially.

itorum longus. This approach brings one onto the posterior aspect of the ankle joint rather more medially than does the first approach.

Third, when all the tendons that run around the back of the medial malleolus (the tibialis posterior, flexor digitorum longus, and flexor hallucis longus) must be lengthened, the back of the ankle can be approached directly, because the posterior coverings of the tendons must be divided during the lengthening procedure.

For all three methods, complete the approach by incising the joint capsule either longitudinally or transversely.

## Dangers

The posterior tibial artery and the tibial nerve (the posterior neurovascular bundle) are vulnerable dur-

ing the approach. Note that the tibial nerve is surprisingly large in young children and that the tendon of the flexor digitorum longus muscle is extremely small. Take care to identify positively all structures in the area before dividing any muscle tendons (see Figs. 12-52 and 12-53).

## How to Enlarge the Approach

### Extensile Measures
Extend the incision distally by curving it across the medial border of the ankle, ending over the talonavicular joint. This extension exposes both the talonavicular joint and the master knot of Henry. As is true for all long, curved incisions around the ankle, skin necrosis can result if the skin flaps are not cut thickly or if forcible retraction is applied.

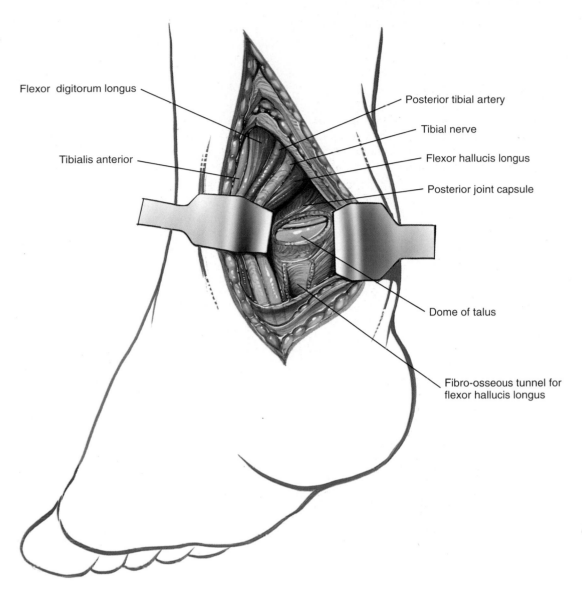

Flexor digitorum longus

Tibialis anterior

Posterior tibial artery

Tibial nerve

Flexor hallucis longus

Posterior joint capsule

Dome of talus

Fibro-osseous tunnel for flexor hallucis longus

**Figure 12-23**   Retract the posterior structures medially, exposing the posterior portion of the ankle joint.

# Posterolateral Approach to the Ankle

The posterolateral approach is used to treat conditions of the posterior aspect of the distal tibia and ankle joint. It is well suited for open reduction and internal fixation of posterior malleolar fractures. Because the patient is prone, however, it is not the approach of choice if the fibula and medial malleolus have to be fixed at the same time. In such cases, it is better to use either a posteromedial approach or a lateral approach to the fibula, and to approach the posterolateral corner of the tibia through the site of the fractured fibula. Neither of these approaches provides such good visualization of the bone as does the posterolateral approach to the ankle, but both allow other surgical procedures to be carried out without changing the position of the patient on the table halfway through the operation. Its other uses include the following:

1. Excision of sequestra
2. Removal of benign tumors
3. Arthrodesis of the posterior facet of the subtalar joint

4. Posterior capsulotomy and syndesmotomy of the ankle
5. Elongation of tendons

## Position of the Patient

Place the patient prone on the operating table. As always when the prone position is being used, longitudinal pads should be placed under the pelvis and chest so that the center portion of the chest and abdomen are free to move with respiration. A sandbag should be placed under the ankle so that it can be extended during the operation. Next, exsanguinate the limb by elevating it for 3 to 5 minutes or applying a soft rubber bandage; then inflate a tourniquet (Fig. 12-24).

## Landmarks and Incision

### Landmarks

The *lateral malleolus* is the subcutaneous distal end of the fibula.

The *Achilles tendon* is easily palpable as it approaches its insertion into the calcaneus.

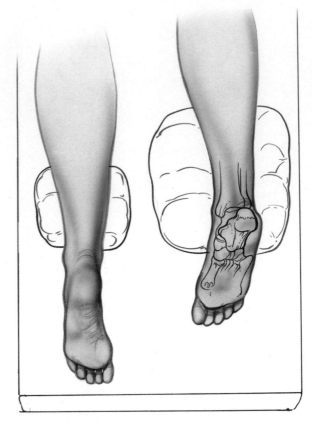

**Figure 12-24**   Position of the patient for the posterolateral approach to the ankle joint.

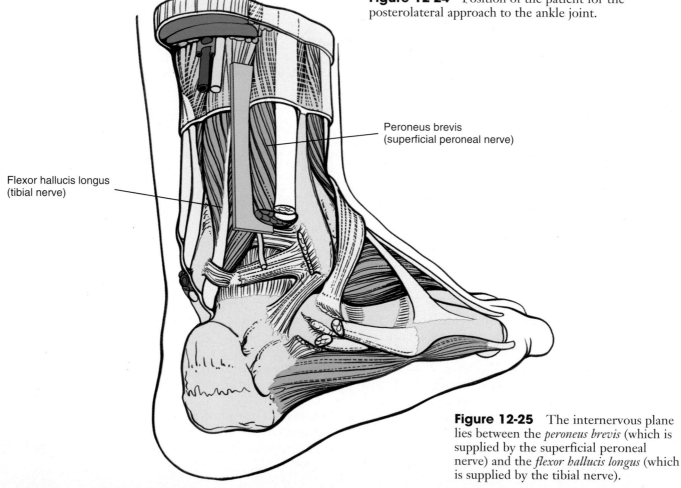

Peroneus brevis
(superficial peroneal nerve)

Flexor hallucis longus
(tibial nerve)

**Figure 12-25**   The internervous plane lies between the *peroneus brevis* (which is supplied by the superficial peroneal nerve) and the *flexor hallucis longus* (which is supplied by the tibial nerve).

## Incision

Make a 10-cm longitudinal incision halfway between the posterior border of the lateral malleolus and the lateral border of the Achilles tendon. Begin the incision at the level of the tip of the fibula and extend it proximally (Fig. 12-26).

## Internervous Plane

The internervous plane lies between the *peroneus brevis* muscle (which is supplied by the superficial peroneal nerve) and the *flexor hallucis longus* muscle (which is supplied by the tibial nerve; Fig. 12-25).

## Superficial Surgical Dissection

Mobilize the skin flaps. The short saphenous vein and sural nerves run just behind the lateral malleolus; they should be well anterior to the incision. Incise the deep fascia of the leg in line with the skin incision, and identify the two peroneal tendons as they pass down the leg and around the back of the lateral malleolus (Fig. 12-27). The tendon of the peroneus brevis muscle is anterior to that of the peroneus longus muscle at the level of the ankle joint and, therefore, is closer to the lateral malleolus. Note that the peroneus brevis is muscular almost down to the ankle, whereas the peroneus longus is tendinous in the distal third of the leg (see Figs. 12-62 and 12-63).

Incise the peroneal retinaculum to release the tendons, and retract the muscles laterally and anteriorly to expose the flexor hallucis longus muscle (Fig. 12-28). The flexor hallucis longus is the most lateral of the deep flexor muscles of the calf. It is the only one that is still muscular at this level (see Fig. 12-63).

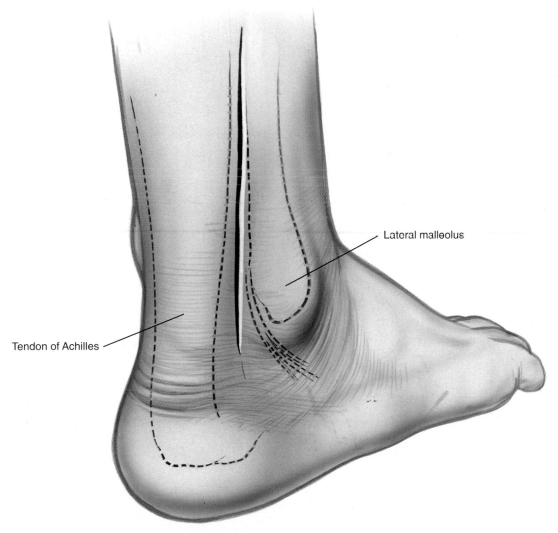

Lateral malleolus

Tendon of Achilles

**Figure 12-26** Make a 10-cm longitudinal incision halfway between the posterior border of the lateral malleolus and the lateral border of the Achilles tendon.

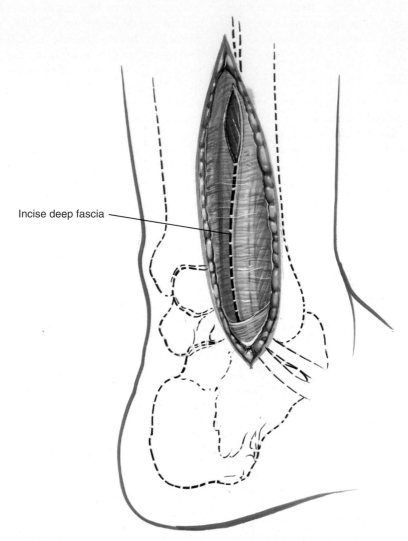

Incise deep fascia

**Figure 12-27**    Mobilize the skin flaps. Incise the deep fascia of the leg in line with the skin incision. Identify the two peroneal tendons as they pass around the ankle.

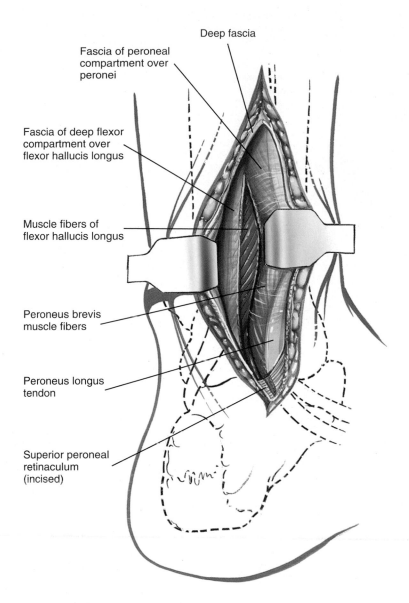

Deep fascia

Fascia of peroneal
compartment over
peronei

Fascia of deep flexor
compartment over
flexor hallucis longus

Muscle fibers of
flexor hallucis longus

Peroneus brevis
muscle fibers

Peroneus longus
tendon

Superior peroneal
retinaculum
(incised)

**Figure 12-28**   Incise the peroneal retinaculum to release the tendons. Retract them laterally and anteriorly. Incise the fascia over the flexor hallucis longus to expose its muscle fibers.

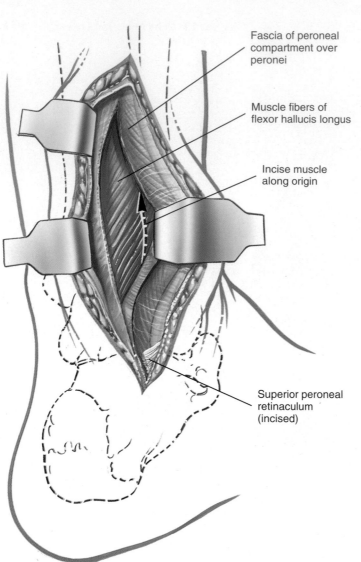

Fascia of peroneal
compartment over
peronei

Muscle fibers of
flexor hallucis longus

Incise muscle
along origin

Superior peroneal
retinaculum
(incised)

**Figure 12-29**  Make a longitudinal incision
through the lateral fibers of the flexor hallucis
longus as they arise from the fibula.

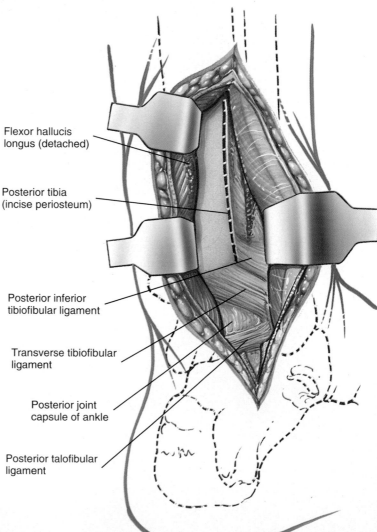

Flexor hallucis
longus (detached)

Posterior tibia
(incise periosteum)

Posterior inferior
tibiofibular ligament

Transverse tibiofibular
ligament

Posterior joint
capsule of ankle

Posterior talofibular
ligament

**Figure 12-30**  Retract the flexor hallucis
longus medially to reveal the periosteum
covering the posterior aspect of the tibia.

## Deep Surgical Dissection

To enhance the exposure, make a longitudinal incision through the lateral fibers of the flexor hallucis longus muscle as they arise from the fibula (Fig. 12-29). Retract the flexor hallucis longus medially to reveal the periosteum over the posterior aspect of the tibia (Fig. 12-30). If the distal tibia must be reached, incise the periosteum longitudinally and strip it medially and laterally to uncover the posterior aspect of the tibia (Fig. 12-31). To enter the ankle joint, follow the posterior aspect of the tibia down to the posterior ankle joint capsule and incise it transversely.

## Dangers

The **short saphenous vein** and the **sural nerve** run close together. They should be preserved as a unit, largely to prevent the formation of a painful neuroma (see Fig. 12-62).

## How to Enlarge the Approach

### Extensile Measures

To enlarge the approach proximally, extend the skin incision superiorly and identify the plane between the lateral head of the gastrocnemius muscle and the peroneus muscles. Develop this plane down to the soleus muscle; retract it medially with the gastrocnemius. Next, reflect the flexor hallucis longus muscle medially, detaching it from its origin on the fibula. Continue the dissection medially across the interosseous membrane to the posterior aspect of the tibia (see Posterolateral Approach to the Tibia in Chapter 11).

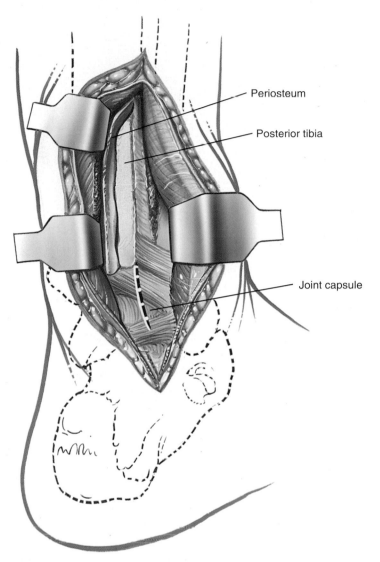

Periosteum

Posterior tibia

Joint capsule

**Figure 12-31**   Incise and elevate the periosteum to reveal the posterior aspect of the tibia. Enter the ankle joint by continuing the incision distally across the joint capsule.

# Approach to the Lateral Malleolus

The approach to the lateral malleolus is used primarily for open reduction and internal fixation of lateral malleolar fractures. It also offers access to the posterolateral aspect of the tibia.

## Position of the Patient

Place the patient supine on the operating table with a sandbag under the buttock of the affected limb. The sandbag causes the limb to rotate medially, bringing the lateral malleolus forward and making it easier to reach (Fig. 12-32). Operating with the patient on his or her side also provides excellent access to the distal fibula, but the medial malleolus cannot be reached unless the patient's position is changed, something that is necessary in the fixation of bimalleolar fractures (Fig. 12-33). Exsanguinate the limb by elevating it for 3 to 5 minutes, then inflate a tourniquet.

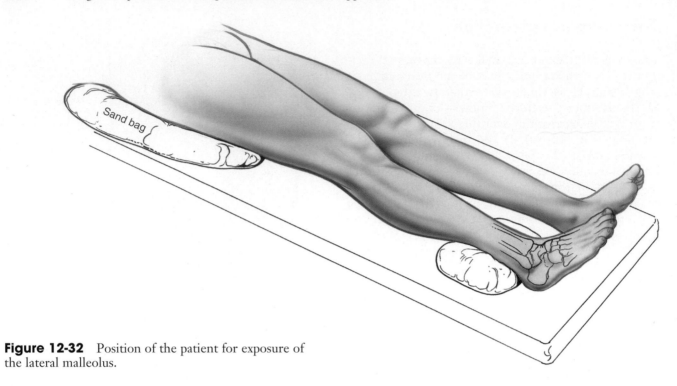

**Figure 12-32** Position of the patient for exposure of the lateral malleolus.

## Landmarks and Incision

### Landmarks

Palpate the subcutaneous surface of the fibula and the *lateral malleolus*, which lies at its distal end.

- The *short saphenous vein* can be seen running along the posterior border of the lateral malleolus before the limb is exsanguinated.

### Incision

Make a 10- to 15-cm longitudinal incision along the posterior margin of the fibula all the way to its distal end and continuing for a further 2 cm (Fig. 12-34*A*). In fracture surgery, center the incision at the level of the fracture.

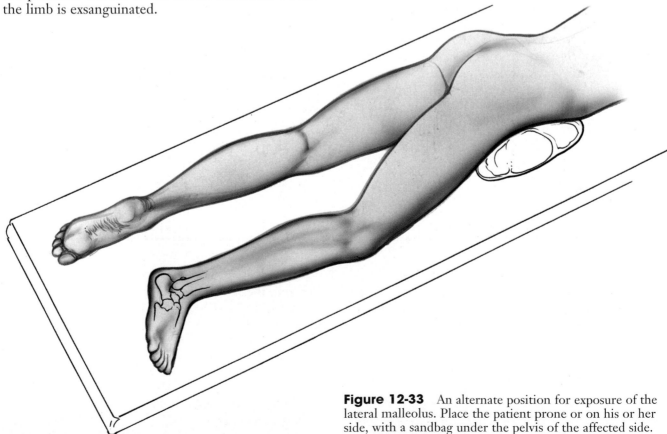

**Figure 12-33** An alternate position for exposure of the lateral malleolus. Place the patient prone or on his or her side, with a sandbag under the pelvis of the affected side.

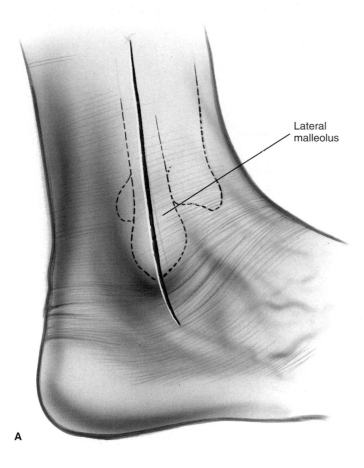

Lateral
malleolus

**Figure 12-34**  **(A)** Make a 10- to 15-cm incision along the posterior margin of the fibula all the way to its distal end. From there, curve the incision forward, below the tip of the lateral malleolus. **(B)** Incise the periosteum on the subcutaneous surface of the fibula longitudinally. **(C)** Expose the distal fibula subperiosteally.

A

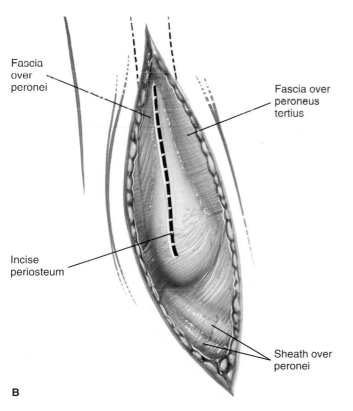

Fascia over peronei

Fascia over peroneus tertius

Incise periosteum

Sheath over peronei

B

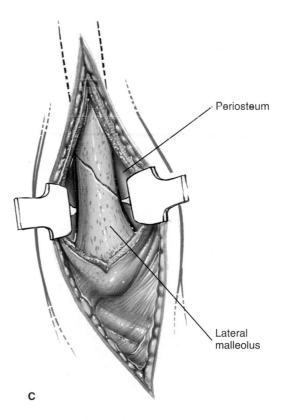

Periosteum

Lateral malleolus

C

## Internervous Plane

There is no internervous plane, because the dissection is being performed down to a subcutaneous bone. For higher fractures of the fibula, the internervous plane lies between the *peroneus tertius* muscle (which is supplied by the deep peroneal nerve) and the *peroneus brevis* muscle (which is supplied by the superficial peroneal nerve). (See Approach to the Fibula in Chapter 11.)

## Superficial Surgical Dissection

Elevate the skin flaps, taking care not to damage the short saphenous vein, which lies posterior to the lateral malleolus. The sural nerve, which runs with the short saphenous vein, also should be preserved.

## Deep Surgical Dissection

Incise the periosteum of the subcutaneous surface of the fibula longitudinally, and strip off just enough of it at the fracture site to expose the fracture adequately. Take care to keep all dissection strictly subperiosteal, because the terminal branches of the peroneal artery, which lie close to the lateral malleolus, may be damaged. Only strip off as much periosteum as is necessary for accurate reduction; periosteal stripping markedly reduces the blood supply of the bone in cases of fracture (Fig. 12-34B,C; see Fig. 12-62).

## Dangers

### Nerves

The sural nerve is vulnerable when the skin flaps are mobilized. Cutting it may lead to the formation of a painful neuroma and numbness along the lateral skin of the foot, which, although it does not bear weight, does come in contact with the shoe. The nerve also is valuable as a nerve graft. Preserve it if possible (see Fig. 12-59).

### Vessels

The terminal branches of the peroneal artery lie immediately deep to the medial surface of the distal fibula. They can be damaged if dissection does not remain subperiosteal. The damage may not be noticed during surgery because of the tourniquet, but a hematoma may form after the tourniquet is taken off. That is why it is best to deflate the tourniquet before closure to ensure hemostasis; then, the wound can be drained with a suction drain (see Fig. 12-62).

## How to Enlarge the Approach

### Extensile Measures

*Proximal Extension.* Extend the incision along the posterior border of the fibula, incising the deep fascia in line with the skin incision. Develop a new plane between the peroneal muscles (which are supplied by the superficial peroneal nerve) and the flexor muscles (which are supplied by the tibial nerve). The upper third of the fibula can be exposed if the common peroneal nerve can be identified near the knee and traced down toward the ankle. (For details of this approach, see Approach to the Fibula in Chapter 11.)

*Distal Extension.* To extend the approach distally, curve the incision down the lateral side of the foot. Identify the peroneal tendons and incise the peroneal retinacula. Detach the fat pad in the sinus tarsi and the origin of the extensor digitorum brevis muscle to expose the calcaneocuboid joint on the lateral side of the tarsus (see Figs. 12-59 and 12-60).

# Anterolateral Approach to the Ankle and Hindpart of the Foot

The full extent of the anterolateral approach to the ankle and hindpart of the foot allows exposure not only of the ankle joint, but also of the talonavicular, calcaneocuboid, and talocalcaneal joints. The approach is used commonly for ankle fusions, but also can be used for triple arthrodesis and even pantalar arthrodesis. In addition, it is possible to excise the entire talus through this approach, or to reduce it in cases of talar dislocation.

## Position of the Patient

Place the patient supine on the operating table; place a large sandbag underneath the affected buttock to rotate the leg internally and bring the lateral malleolus forward. Exsanguinate the limb either by elevating it for 3 to 5 minutes or by applying a soft rubber bandage; then inflate a tourniquet (see Fig. 12-32).

## Landmarks and Incision

### Landmarks

Palpate the *lateral malleolus* at the distal subcutaneous end of the fibula.

Palpate the *base of the fifth metatarsal*, a prominent bony mass on the lateral aspect of the foot.

### Incision

Make a 15-cm slightly curved incision on the antero-lateral aspect of the ankle. Begin some 5 cm proximal to the ankle joint, 2 cm anterior to the anterior border of the fibula. Curve the incision down, crossing the ankle joint 2 cm medial to the tip of the lateral malleolus, and continue onto the foot, ending some 2 cm medial to the fifth metatarsal base, over the base of the fourth metatarsal (Fig. 12-35).

## Internervous Plane

The internervous plane lies between the *peroneal muscles* (which are supplied by the superficial per-

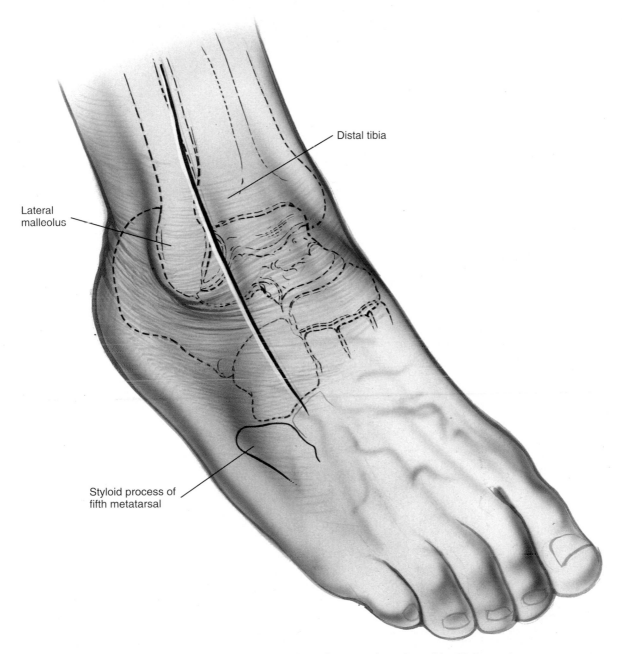

Distal tibia

Lateral malleolus

Styloid process of fifth metatarsal

**Figure 12-35**   Incision for the anterolateral approach to the ankle. Make a 15-cm slightly curved incision on the anterolateral aspect of the ankle. Begin approximately 5 cm proximal to the ankle joint and 2 cm anterior to the anterior border of the fibula. Curve the incision downward to cross the ankle joint 2 cm medial to the tip of the lateral malleolus, and continue onto the foot, ending about 2 cm medial to the fifth metatarsal.

**Figure 12-36** Incise the deep fascia and the superior and inferior retinacula in line with the incision. Take care to preserve the superficial peroneal nerve.

Superior extensor retinaculum

Inferior extensor retinaculum

Superficial peroneal nerve

Extensor retinaculum

Anterior inferior tibiofibular ligament

Tendons of extensor digitorum longus

Sinus tarsi fat pad

Tendon of peroneus tertius

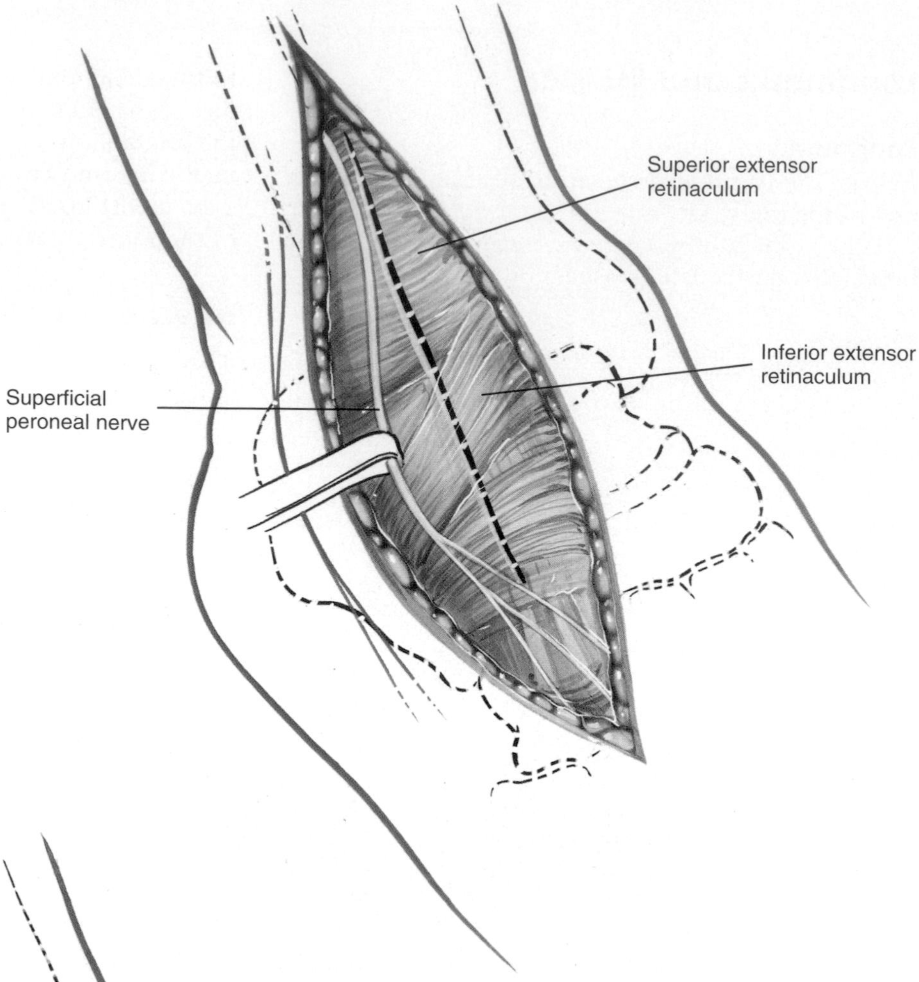

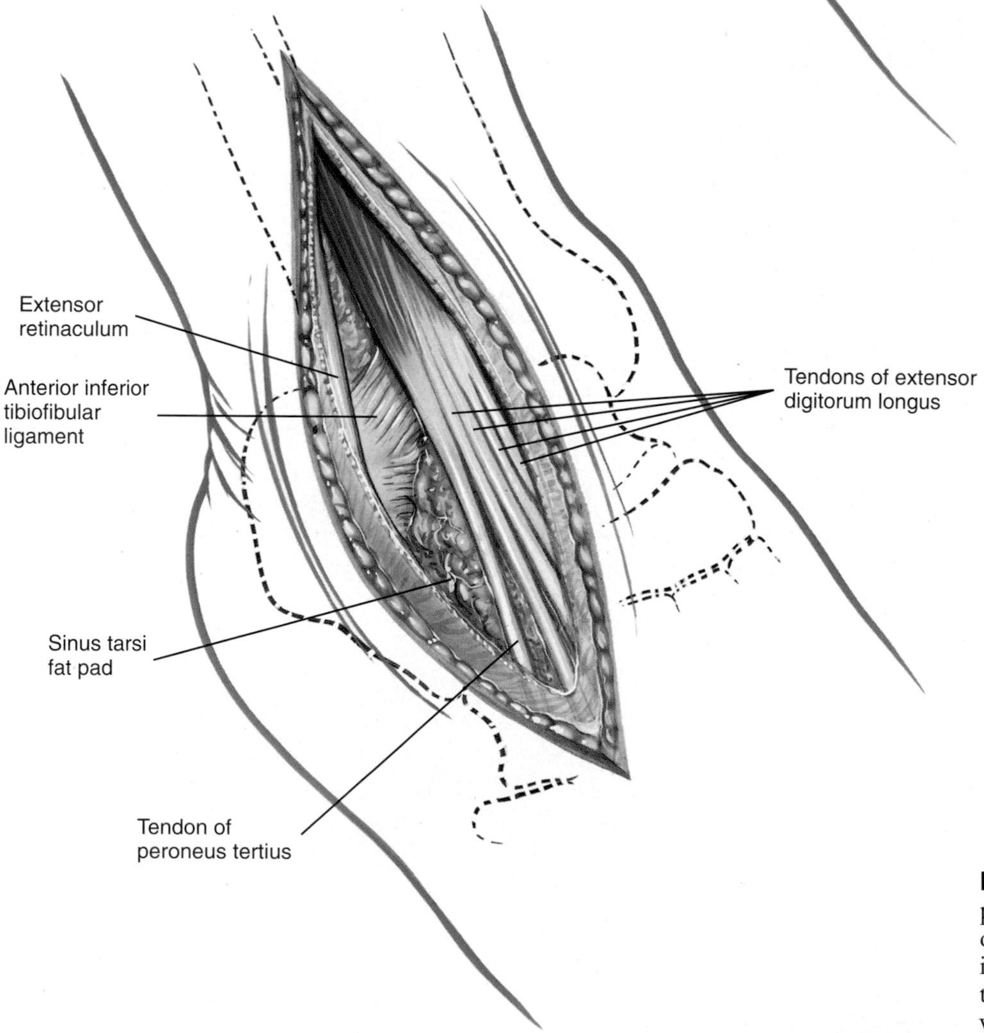

**Figure 12-37** Identify the peroneus tertius and the extensor digitorum longus muscles, and incise down to bone lateral to them in the upper half of the wound.

oneal nerve) and the *extensor muscles* (which are supplied by the deep peroneal nerve; see Figs. 12-56 and 12-59).

## Superficial Surgical Dissection

Incise the fascia in line with the skin incision, cutting through the superior and inferior extensor retinacula. Do not develop skin flaps. Take care to identify and preserve any dorsal cutaneous branches of the superficial peroneal nerve that may cross the field of dissection (Fig. 12-36). Identify the peroneus tertius and extensor digitorum longus muscles, and, in the upper half of the wound, incise down to bone just lateral to these muscles (Fig. 12-37).

## Deep Surgical Dissection

Retract the extensor musculature medially to expose the anterior aspect of the distal tibia and the anterior ankle joint capsule. Distally, identify the extensor digitorum brevis muscle at its origin from the calcaneus (Fig. 12-38), and detach it by sharp dissection. During dissection, branches of the lateral tarsal artery will be cut; cauterize (diathermy) these to prevent the formation of a postoperative hematoma. Reflect the detached extensor digitorum brevis muscle distally and medially, lifting the muscle fascia and the subcutaneous fat and skin as one flap. Identify the dorsal capsules of the calcaneocuboid and talonavicular joints, which lie next to each other across the foot, forming

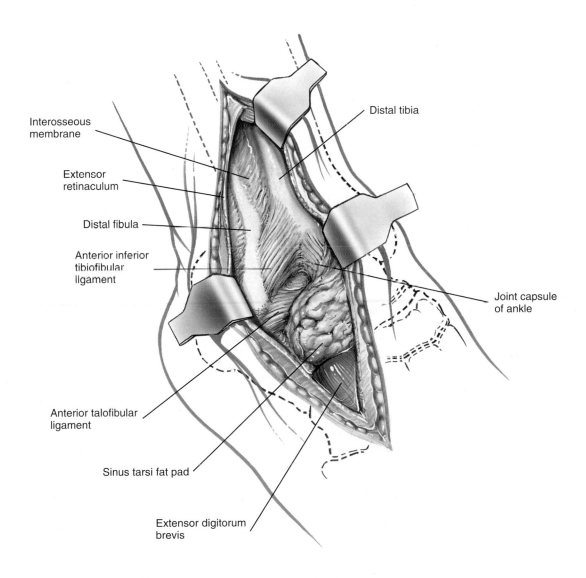

Interosseous membrane

Extensor retinaculum

Distal fibula

Anterior inferior tibiofibular ligament

Anterior talofibular ligament

Sinus tarsi fat pad

Extensor digitorum brevis

Distal tibia

Joint capsule of ankle

**Figure 12-38**    Retract the extensor musculature medially to expose the anterior aspect of the distal tibia and ankle joint. Identify the origin of the extensor digitorum brevis.

the clinical midtarsal joint (see Fig. 12-58). Next, identify the fat in the sinus tarsi and clear it away to expose the talocalcaneal joint, either by mobilizing the fat pad and turning it downward or by excising it. Preserving the fat pad prevents the development of a cosmetically ugly dimple postoperatively. Preserving the pad also helps the wound to heal (Fig. 12-39).

Finally, incise any or all the capsules that have been exposed. To open the joints, forcefully flex and invert the foot in a plantar direction (see Fig. 12-39).

## Dangers

The **deep peroneal nerve** and **anterior tibial artery** cross the front of the ankle joint. They are vulnerable if dissection is not carried out as close to the bone as possible (see Fig. 12-56).

## How to Enlarge the Approach

### Extensile Measures
The approach can be extended proximally to explore structures in the anterior compartment of the leg. Continue the incision over the compartment, and incise the thick deep fascia in line with the skin incision.

The approach also can be extended distally to expose the tarsometatarsal joint on the lateral half of the foot. Continue the incision over the fourth metatarsal, and expose the subcutaneous tarsometatarsal joints.

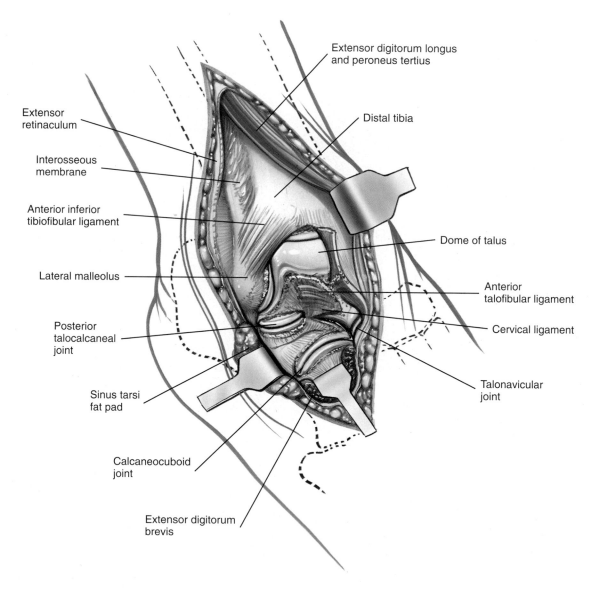

**Figure 12-39**  The extensor digitorum brevis has been detached from its origin and reflected distally. The fat pad covering the sinus tarsi has been detached and reflected downward. Incise the joint capsules that have been exposed.

# Lateral Approach to the Hindpart of the Foot

The lateral approach provides excellent exposure of the talocalcaneonavicular, posterior talocalcaneal, and calcaneocuboid joints. It permits arthrodesis of any or all these joints (triple arthrodesis).

## Position of the Patient

Position the patient supine on the operating table. Place a large sandbag beneath the affected buttock to rotate the leg internally, and bring the lateral portion of the ankle and hindpart of the foot forward. Exsanguinate the limb either by elevating it for 5 minutes or by applying a soft rubber bandage; then inflate a tourniquet (see Fig. 12-32).

## Landmarks and Incision

### Landmarks

The *lateral malleolus* is the palpable distal end of the fibula. The *lateral wall of the calcaneus* is subcutaneous. It is palpable below the lateral malleolus.

To palpate the *sinus tarsi*, stabilize the foot, holding the calcaneus with one hand, and place the thumb of the free hand in the soft-tissue depression just anterior to the lateral malleolus. The depression lies directly over the sinus tarsi.

### Incision

Make a curved incision starting just distal to the distal end of the lateral malleolus and slightly posterior to it. Continue distally along the lateral side of the hindpart of the foot and over the sinus tarsi. Then, curve medially, ending over the talocalcaneonavicular joint (Fig. 12-40).

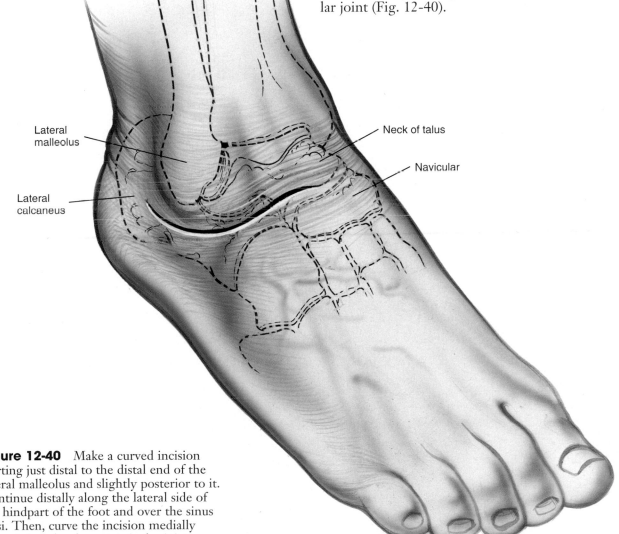

**Figure 12-40** Make a curved incision starting just distal to the distal end of the lateral malleolus and slightly posterior to it. Continue distally along the lateral side of the hindpart of the foot and over the sinus tarsi. Then, curve the incision medially toward the talocalcaneonavicular joint.

## Internervous Plane

The internervous plane lies between the *peroneus tertius tendon* (which is supplied by the deep peroneal nerve) and the *peroneal tendons* (which are supplied by the superficial peroneal nerve).

## Superficial Surgical Dissection

Do not mobilize the skin flaps widely, because large skin flaps may necrose. Ligate any veins that cross the operative field. Open the deep fascia in line with the skin incision, taking care not to damage the tendons of the peroneus tertius and extensor digitorum longus muscles, which cross the distal end of the incision (Figs. 12-41 and 12-42). Retract these tendons medially to gain access to the dorsum of the foot. Do not retract the peroneal tendons, which run through the proximal end of the wound, at this stage (Fig. 12-43).

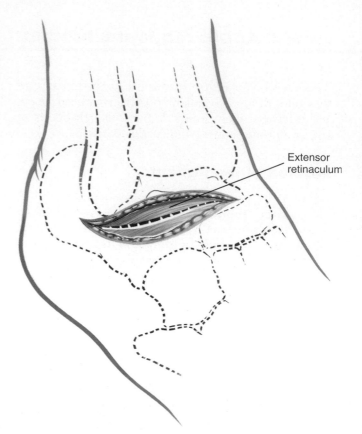

**Figure 12-41**    Incise and open the deep fascia in line with the skin incision.

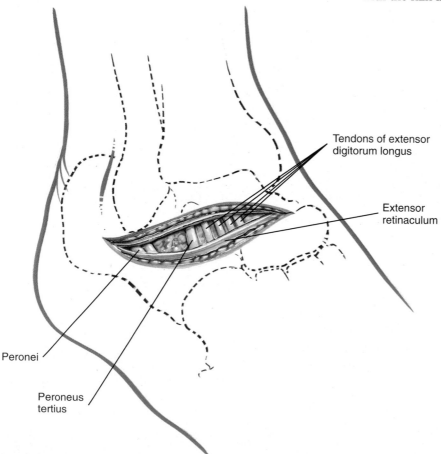

**Figure 12-42**    Take care not to damage the tendons of the peroneus tertius and the extensor digitorum longus, which cross under the distal end of the incision.

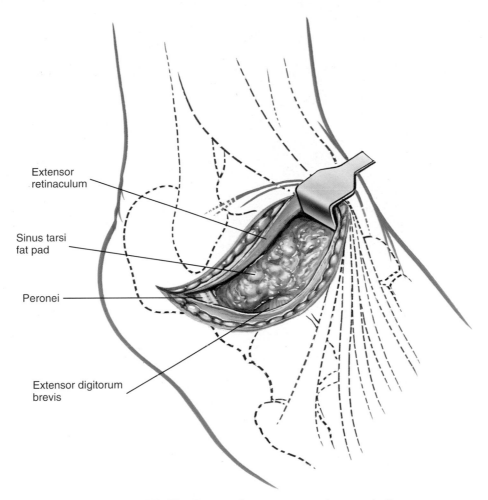

**Figure 12-43**  Retract the extensor tendons medially.

## Deep Surgical Dissection

Partially detach the fat pad that lies in the sinus tarsi by sharp dissection, leaving it attached to the skin flap; under it lies the origin of the extensor digitorum brevis muscle. Detach its origin by sharp dissection, and reflect the muscle distally to expose the dorsal capsule of the talocalcaneonavicular joint in the distal end of the wound and the dorsal capsule of the calcaneocuboid joint more laterally (Fig. 12-44). Incise these capsules and open their respective joints by inverting the foot forcefully (Fig. 12-45). Next, incise the peroneal retinacula and reflect the peroneal tendons anteriorly. Identify and incise the capsule of the posterior talocalcaneal joint. Open it by inverting the heel (Fig. 12-46).

The talocalcaneonavicular, posterior talocalcaneal, and calcaneocuboid joints now are exposed. Note that, in virtually all cases in which this approach is used, these joints are in abnormal posi-tion. The approach should remain safe as long as it stays on bone while the joints are being identified.

## Dangers

### Skin Flaps

Exposures in this area are notorious for producing necrosis of skin flaps. Therefore, skin flaps should be cut as thickly as possible, stripping and retraction should be kept to a minimum, and sharp curves in the skin incision should be avoided.

## How to Enlarge the Approach

### Local Measures

To open the calcaneocuboid, talocalcaneonavicular, and posterior subtalar joints, invert the foot. Note that *both* the talocalcaneonavicular joint and the pos-

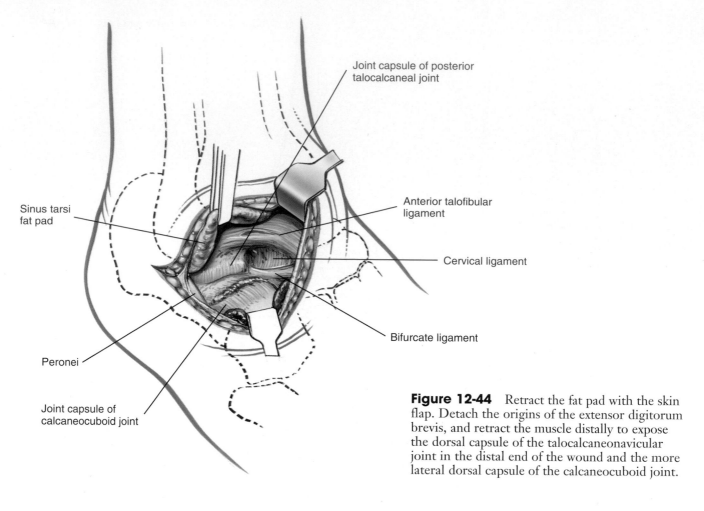

Sinus tarsi
fat pad

Peronei

Joint capsule of
calcaneocuboid joint

Joint capsule of posterior
talocalcaneal joint

Anterior talofibular
ligament

Cervical ligament

Bifurcate ligament

**Figure 12-44**   Retract the fat pad with the skin flap. Detach the origins of the extensor digitorum brevis, and retract the muscle distally to expose the dorsal capsule of the talocalcaneonavicular joint in the distal end of the wound and the more lateral dorsal capsule of the calcaneocuboid joint.

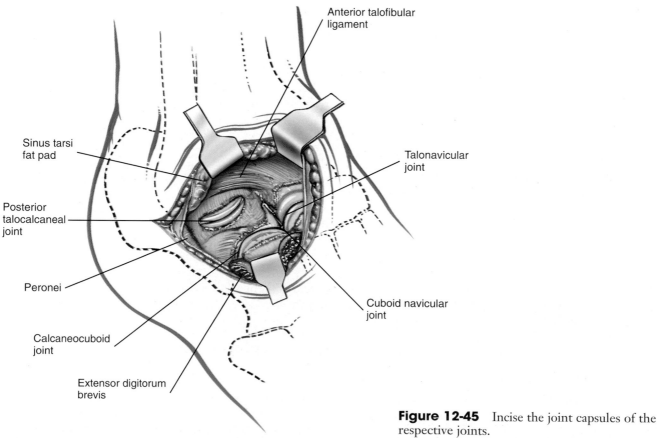

Sinus tarsi
fat pad

Posterior
talocalcaneal
joint

Peronei

Calcaneocuboid
joint

Extensor digitorum
brevis

Anterior talofibular
ligament

Talonavicular
joint

Cuboid navicular
joint

**Figure 12-45**   Incise the joint capsules of the respective joints.

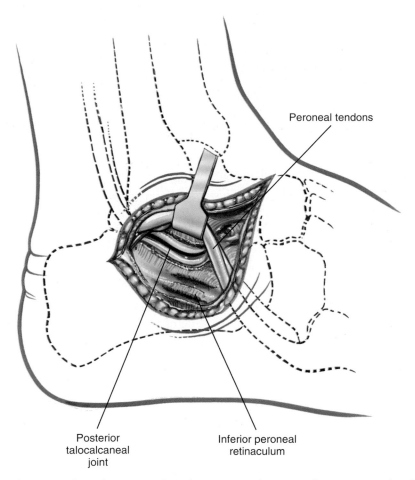

Peroneal tendons

Posterior talocalcaneal joint

Inferior peroneal retinaculum

**Figure 12-46**  Reflect the peroneal tendons anteriorly. Incise the joint capsule of the posterior talocalcaneal joint.

terior subtalar joint must be incised before inversion will open either one.

### Extensile Measures

To enlarge the approach proximally, continue the incision, curving it along the posterior border of the fibula. By developing a plane between the peroneal muscles and the flexor muscles, the entire length of the fibula can be exposed (see Approach to the Fibula in Chapter 11). In practice, however, this extension is required rarely, if ever.

The incision also may be extended posteriorly and proximally to reach the subcutaneous Achilles tendon.

## Lateral Approach to the Posterior Talocalcaneal Joint

The lateral approach to the posterior talocalcaneal joint exposes the posterior facet of the talocalcaneal joint more extensively than does the anterolateral approach. It also is used for open reduction and internal fixation of calcaneal fractures.

### Position of the Patient

Place the patient supine on the operating table with a sandbag under the buttock of the affected side to bring the lateral malleolus forward. Place a support on the opposite iliac crest, then tilt the table 20° to 30° away from the surgeon to improve access still further. Exsanguinate the limb either by elevating it for 3 to 5 minutes or by applying a soft rubber bandage; then inflate a tourniquet (see Fig. 12-32).

## Landmarks and Incision

### Landmarks
The *lateral malleolus* is the subcutaneous distal end of the fibula. The *peroneal tubercle* is a small protuberance of bone on the lateral surface of the calcaneus that separates the tendons of the peroneus longus and brevis muscles. It lies distal and anterior to the lateral malleolus.

### Incision
Make a curved incision 10 to 13 cm long on the lateral aspect of the ankle. Begin some 4 cm above the tip of the lateral malleolus on the posterior border of the fibula. Follow the posterior border of the fibula down to the tip of the lateral malleolus, and then curve the incision forward, passing over the peroneal tubercle parallel to the course of the peroneal tendons (Fig. 12-47).

## Internervous Plane

No internervous plane exists in this approach. The peroneus muscles, whose tendons are mobilized and retracted anteriorly, share a nerve supply from the superficial peroneal nerve. The approach is safe because the muscles receive their supply at a point well proximal to it.

## Superficial Surgical Dissection

Mobilize the skin flaps minimally, taking care not to damage the sural nerve as it runs just behind the lat-

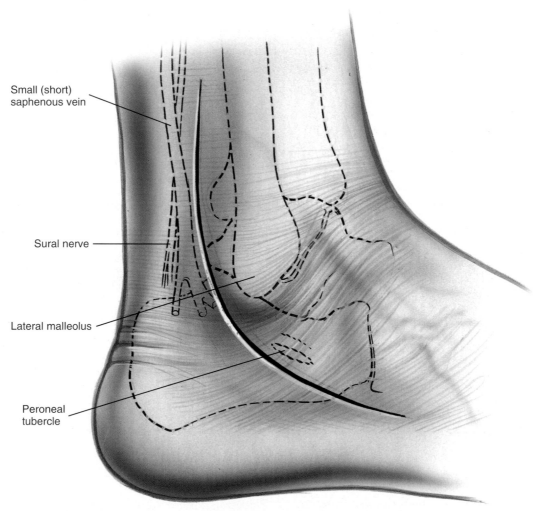

Small (short) saphenous vein

Sural nerve

Lateral malleolus

Peroneal tubercle

**Figure 12-47**    Make a curved incision 10 to 13 cm long on the lateral aspect of the ankle.

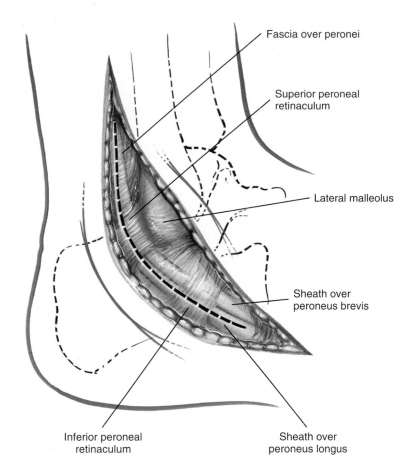

Fascia over peronei

Superior peroneal retinaculum

Lateral malleolus

Sheath over peroneus brevis

Inferior peroneal retinaculum

Sheath over peroneus longus

**Figure 12-48**   Incise the deep fascia in line with the upper part of the skin incision. Continue the fascial incision distally, following the course of the tendons. Incise the inferior peroneal retinaculum, and expose the peroneal tendons.

eral malleolus with the short saphenous vein. Begin incising the deep fascia in line with the upper part of the skin incision to uncover the two peroneal tendons. The tendons of the peroneus longus and peroneus brevis muscles curve around the back of the lateral malleolus. The peroneus brevis tendon, which is closest to the lateral malleolus, is muscular almost down to the level of the malleolus itself (see Fig. 12-59).

Continue incising the deep fascia, following the tendons. The peroneus brevis is covered by the inferior peroneal retinaculum distal to the tip of the fibula. Incise it in line with the tendon (Fig. 12-48). The peroneus longus is covered by a separate fibrous sheath of its own; incise that sheath in line with the tendon as well. These ligaments of the retinaculum must be repaired during closure to prevent tendon dislocation (Fig. 12-49). When both peroneal tendons have been mobilized, retract them anteriorly over the distal end of the fibula (Fig. 12-50).

**Figure 12-49**   Incise the deep fascia in line with the upper part of the skin incision. Continue the fascial incision distally, following the course of the tendons. Incise the inferior peroneal retinaculum and expose the peroneal tendons.

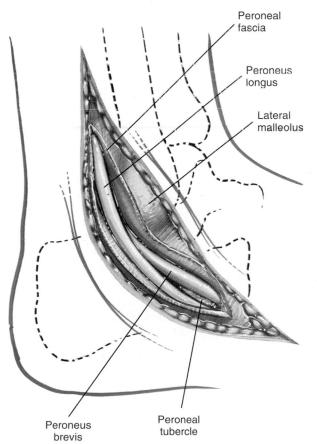

Peroneal fascia

Peroneus longus

Lateral malleolus

Peroneus brevis

Peroneal tubercle

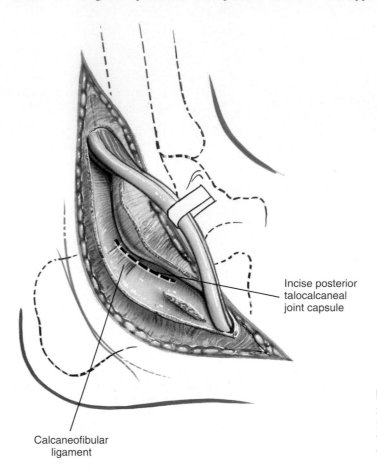

Incise posterior
talocalcaneal
joint capsule

Calcaneofibular
ligament

**Figure 12-50** Mobilize the peroneal tendons, and retract them anteriorly over the distal end of the fibula. Identify the calcaneofibular ligament. Incise it transversely to open the capsule of the posterior talocalcaneal joint.

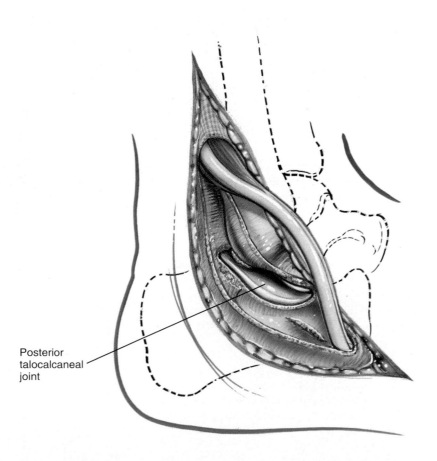

Posterior
talocalcaneal
joint

**Figure 12-51** Open the joint capsule to expose the posterior talocalcaneal joint.

## Deep Surgical Dissection

Identify the calcaneofibular ligament as it runs from the lateral malleolus down and back to the lateral surface of the calcaneus. The ligament is bound closely to the capsule of the talocalcaneal joint. The joint itself is difficult to palpate and identify, and a small amount of subperiosteal dissection on the lateral aspect of the calcaneus usually is required before the joint can be located. Having identified the joint, incise the capsule transversely to open it up (Fig. 12-51; see Figs. 11-50, 11-60, and 11-61).

## Dangers

### Nerves

For dangers pertaining to the **sural nerve**, see Approach to the Lateral Malleolus and Applied Surgical Anatomy of the Approaches to the Ankle in this chapter.

## How to Enlarge the Approach

### Local Measures

To expose the bare lateral surface of the calcaneus, incise the peritoneum over its lateral surface and strip it inferiorly by sharp dissection. To see the talus better, cut the calcaneofibular ligament and the capsule of the talocalcaneal joint superiorly to uncover its lateral border.

Exposure of the articular surfaces of the joint can be achieved only by inverting the foot. Forcible inversion does not open up the joint if the anterior part of the talocalcaneal (talocalcaneonavicular) joint remains intact.

# Applied Surgical Anatomy of the Approaches to the Ankle

## Overview

The key structures that cross the ankle joint fall into specific groups.

## Tendons

Three sets of tendons cross the ankle joint in addition to the Achilles and plantaris tendons, which lie posteriorly in the midline.

1. The flexor tendons—the tibialis posterior, flexor digitorum longus, and flexor hallucis longus (which are supplied by the tibial nerve)—pass behind the medial malleolus.
2. The extensor tendons—the tibialis anterior, extensor digitorum longus, extensor hallucis longus, and peroneus tertius (which are supplied by the deep peroneal nerve)—pass in front of the ankle joint.
3. The evertor tendons—the peroneus longus and peroneus brevis (which are supplied by the superficial peroneal nerve)—pass behind the lateral malleolus.

The tendons all are prevented from bowstringing around the ankle by thickened areas in the deep fascia of the leg, called the retinacula.

The different nerve supplies of the groups offer three potential internervous planes through which the ankle can be approached: medially, between flexors (tibialis posterior) and extensors (tibialis anterior); posterolaterally, between flexors (flexor hallucis longus) and evertors (peroneus brevis); and laterally, between extensors (peroneus tertius) and evertors (peroneus brevis).

### Neurovascular Bundles

Two major neurovascular bundles cross the ankle joint and supply the foot. They present the major surgical concerns for all approaches around the ankle.

1. The *anterior neurovascular bundle* crosses the front of the ankle roughly halfway between the malleoli. It lies between the tibialis anterior and extensor hallucis longus muscles proximal to the joint (see Fig. 12-57), and between the tendons of the extensor hallucis longus and extensor digitorum longus muscles distal to the joint. The tendon of the extensor hallucis longus crosses the bundle in a lateral to medial direction at the level of the ankle joint (see Fig. 12-56).

   The *anterior tibial artery*, which crosses the front of the ankle joint before becoming the dorsalis pedis artery, is palpable on the dorsum of the foot. It also communicates with the medial plantar artery through the first metatarsal space. Fractures through the base of the metatarsal bones and dislocations at the tarsometatarsal joint (Lisfranc's fracture/dislocation)* can damage both elements

---

*Lisfranc was one of Napoleon's surgeons, who is remembered best for his description of an amputation for trauma through the tarsometatarsal joint. The joint and injuries connected with it carry his name.

of this anastomosis and cause ischemia to the medial side of the distal portion of the foot.

The *deep peroneal nerve* accompanies the anterior tibial artery. It supplies two small muscles on the dorsum of the foot: the extensor digitorum brevis and the extensor hallucis brevis. It also supplies a sensory branch to the first web space. Anesthesia in this web space is one of the first clinical signs of anterior compartment compression. Ischemia of the deep peroneal nerve occurs before ischemic muscle damage (see Figs. 12-56 and 12-57).

2. The *posterior neurovascular bundle* runs behind the medial malleolus, between the tendons of the flexor digitorum longus and flexor hallucis longus muscles (Figs. 12-52 and 12-53).

The *posterior tibial artery* passes behind the flexor digitorum longus before entering the sole of the foot,

where it divides into medial and lateral plantar arteries (see Fig. 12-53).

The *tibial nerve* passes behind the medial malleolus with the posterior tibial artery. It gives off a calcaneal branch to the skin of the heel. After entering the sole of the foot, it divides into the medial and lateral plantar nerves, which supply motor power to the small muscles of the foot and sensation to the sole (see Fig. 12-53).

## Superficial Sensory Nerves

Three major sensory nerves cross the ankle joint superficially, all supplying the dorsum of the foot. Knowledge of their course is vital in planning skin incisions. The sensory supply to the sole and heel comes from the lateral and medial plantar nerves, which are branches of the tibial nerve that lies deep at the level of the ankle.

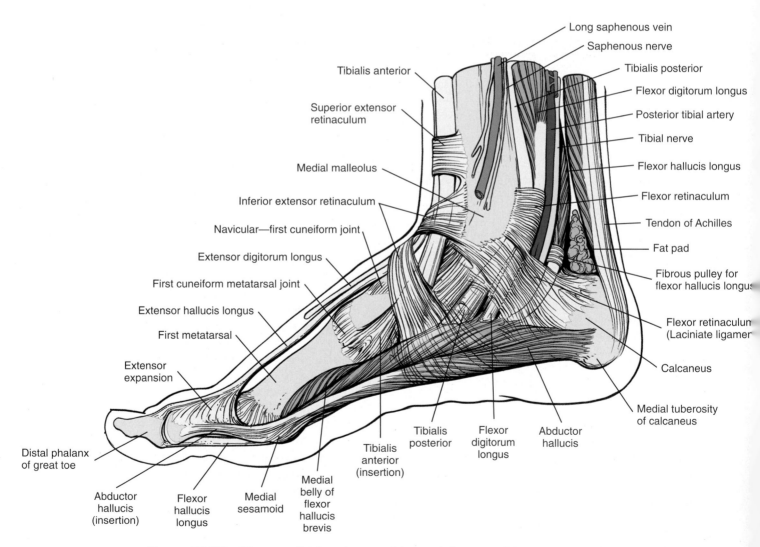

**Figure 12-52**   The superficial structures of the medial aspect of the foot and ankle. Fibers of the flexor retinaculum cross the neurovascular bundle, binding it to the medial side of the foot.

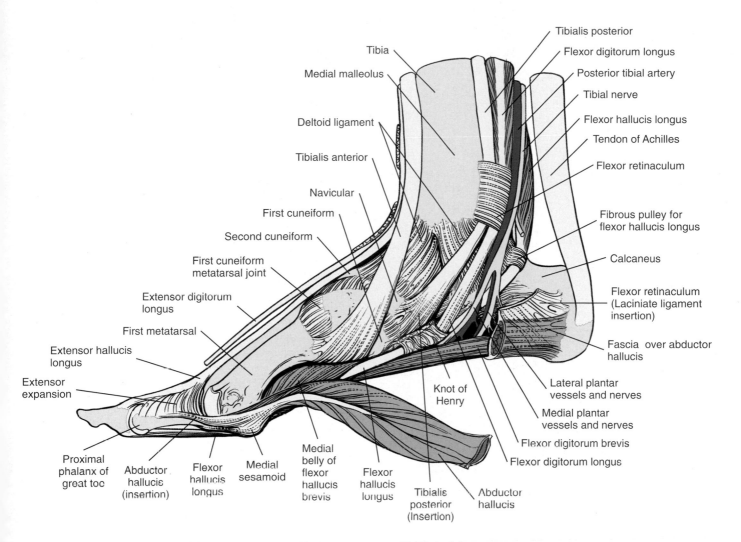

**Figure 12-53**   The extensor retinaculum and part of the flexor retinaculum have been removed to reveal the deeper tendons and the neurovascular bundle. The abductor hallucis has been detached from its origin to reveal the knot of Henry and the medial and lateral plantar arteries and nerves.

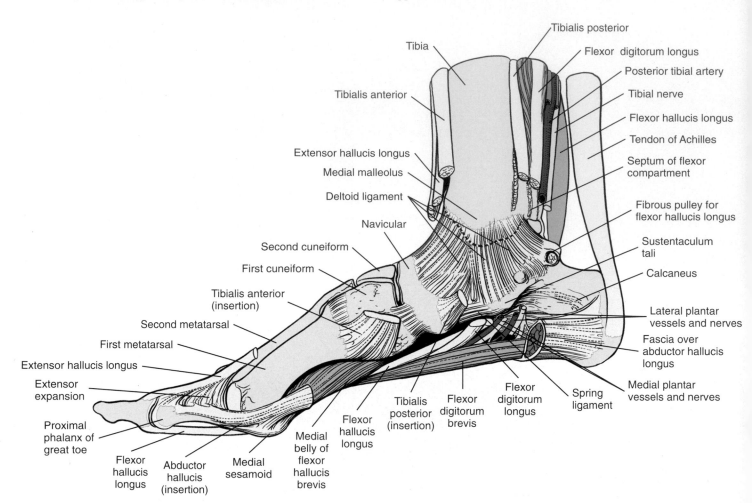

**Figure 12-54** The flexor and extensor tendons have been resected to expose the deltoid ligament of the ankle joint.

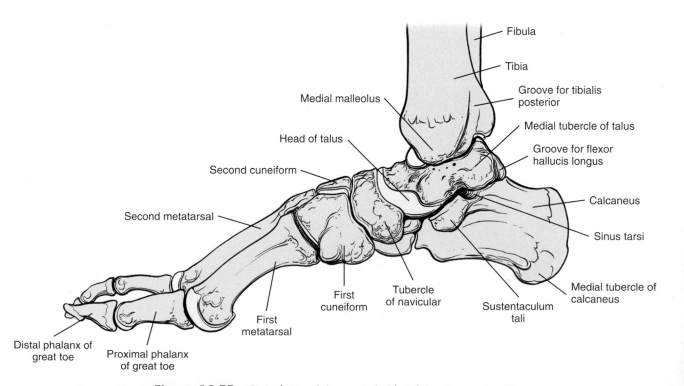

**Figure 12-55** Osteology of the medial side of the foot and ankle.

1. The *saphenous nerve* is the terminal branch of the femoral nerve. It runs with the long saphenous vein in front of the medial malleolus, where it usually divides into two branches that lie on either side of the vein and bind closely to it. It supplies the medial, non–weight-bearing side of the middle part and hindpart of the foot (see Fig. 12-52).

2. The *superficial peroneal nerve* is a terminal branch of the common peroneal nerve. It crosses the ankle joint roughly along the anterior midline,

where it usually divides into several branches. It supplies non–weight-bearing skin on the dorsum of the foot. The nerve is quite superficial at the level of the ankle joint; great care must be taken with skin incision in its area (Fig. 12-56; see Fig. 12-76).

3. The *sural nerve,* a terminal branch of the tibial nerve, runs with the short saphenous vein just behind the lateral malleolus. Similar to the saphenous nerve, the sural nerve binds very closely to

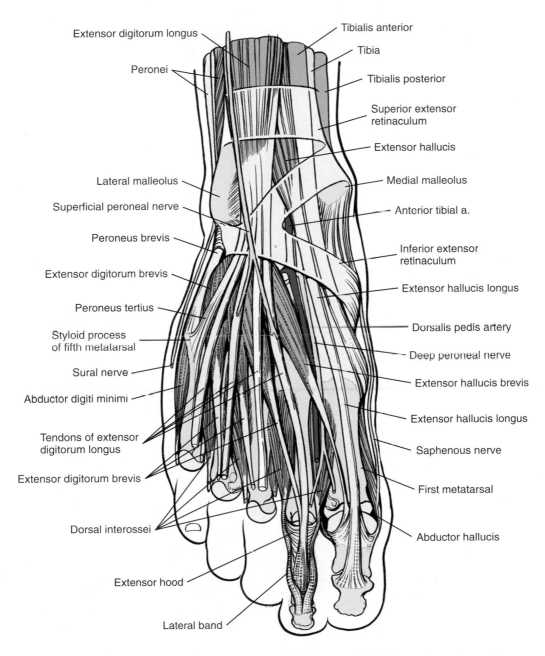

**Figure 12-56**   The anatomy of the superficial structures of the anterior portion of the ankle and the dorsum of the foot. At the level of the ankle joint, the neurovascular bundle lies immediately lateral to the extensor hallucis longus tendon.

its vein; preserving the vein is the key to preserving the nerve during surgery. The sural nerve supplies an area of non–weight-bearing skin on the lateral side of the foot (see Fig. 12-59).

## Landmarks

### Bony Structures of the Ankle

The dome of the talus and the inferior articular surface of the tibia form the articulation that bears weight in the ankle. The joint itself is stabilized by the medial and lateral malleoli, the bony landmarks of the area. The medial malleolus is both shorter and more anterior. It remains in contact with the medial

side of the talus throughout the range of motion (see Fig. 12-55).

The configuration of the malleoli causes the ankle mortise to point 15° laterally. During dorsiflexion, the widest portion of the talus (the anterior portion) is the ankle mortise, forcing the mortise itself to widen. The mortise narrows to accommodate the narrower part of the talus during plantar flexion. Hence, if an ankle must be immobilized, it must be put in the functional position, that is, dorsiflexion (Figs. 12-61; see Figs. 12-55 and 12-58, and 12-64). Note also that, if a screw is inserted between the fibula and the tibia (as in the reconstruction of a diastasis), then that screw should be inserted with the ankle placed in maximal dorsiflexion.

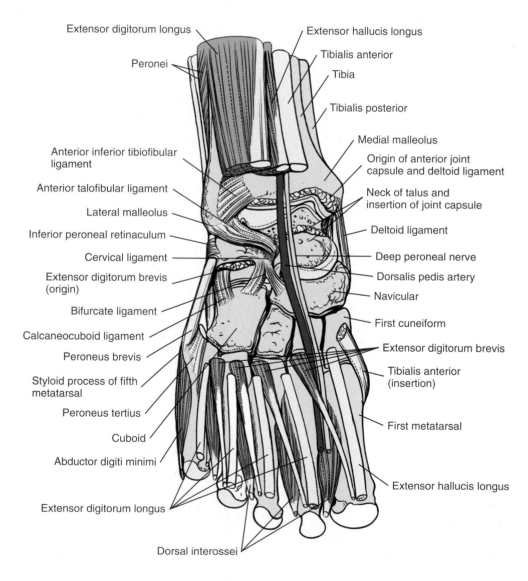

**Figure 12-57**   The extensor tendons have been resected to reveal the ligaments of the anterior portion of the ankle joint and the joints of the middle part of the foot.

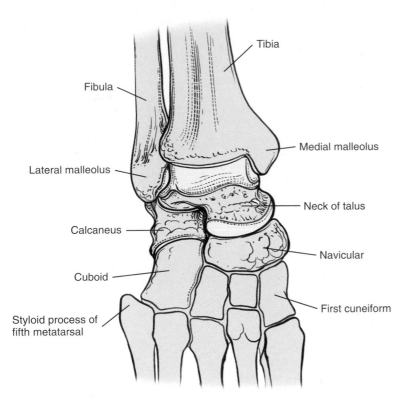

**Figure 12-58** Osteology of the anterior part of the ankle joint and middle part of the foot.

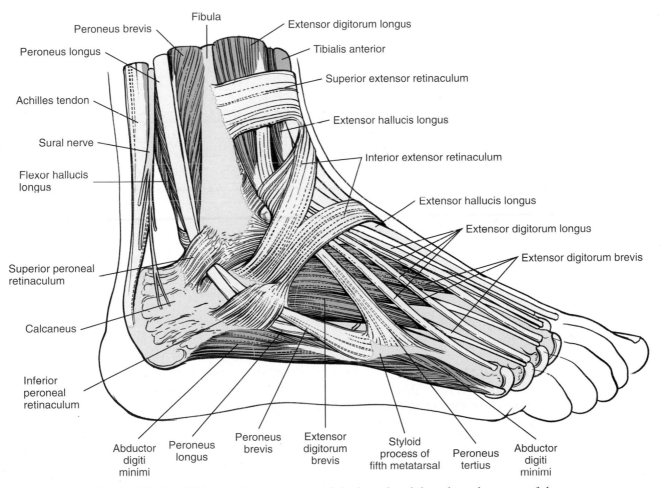

**Figure 12-59** The superficial anatomy of the lateral and dorsolateral aspects of the foot and ankle. The peroneal tendons are held in place by their superior and inferior retinacula.

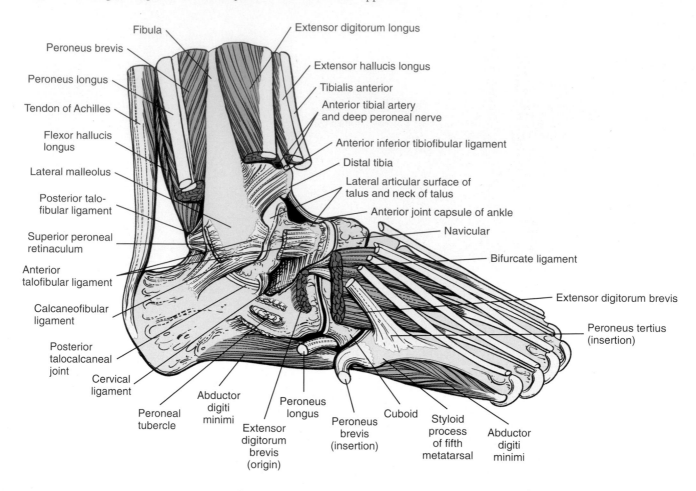

**Figure 12-60** The peroneal and extensor tendons have been resected to reveal the ligaments of the lateral and anterolateral ankle joint. Note the peroneal tubercle and the resected portion of the inferior peroneal retinaculum, which forms separate fibroosseous tunnels for the peroneal tendons. The calcaneofibular ligament is visible deep to the superior peroneal retinaculum.

## Medial Approaches to the Ankle

Two groups of flexors lie on the medial side of the ankle:

1. Three plantar flexors of the ankle and foot insert into the plantar surface of the foot and are supplied by the tibial nerve. Their positions behind the medial malleolus are remembered best in the form of the mnemonic "Tom, Dick, and Harry." The *t*ibialis posterior is closest to the medial malleolus; the flexor *d*igitorum longus is behind it; and the flexor *h*allucis longus is the most posterior and lateral of the three. A second mnemonic, "Timothy Doth Vex Nervous Housemaids," is older; it points out that the posterior *t*ibial vessels and *t*ibial *n*erve lie between the flexor *d*igitorum longus and

flexor hallucis longus muscles (see Figs. 12-52 and 12-53).

2. The three muscles that insert into the posterosuperior part of the os calcis (the gastrocnemius, soleus, and plantaris) do so via their common Achilles tendon. Supplied by the tibial nerve, they are the most powerful plantar flexors of the ankle. Because they insert more to the medial side of the posterior surface of the calcaneus than to the lateral side, they also invert the heel.

The Achilles tendon inserts into the middle third of the posterior surface of the calcaneus. The collagen fibers that comprise the tendon rotate about 90° around its longitudinal axis, between its origin and its insertion onto bone. Viewed from behind, the rotation is in a medial to lateral direction. Thus, fibers

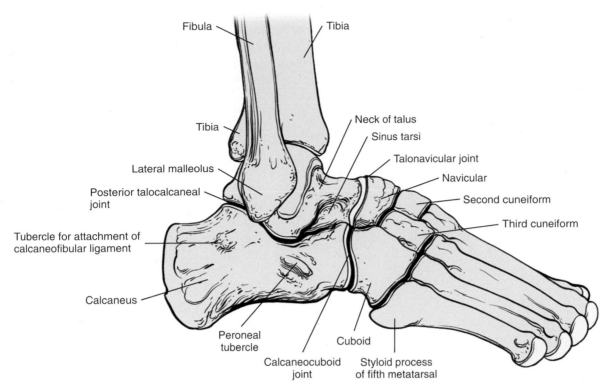

Fibula

Tibia

Tibia

Neck of talus

Sinus tarsi

Talonavicular joint

Lateral malleolus

Navicular

Posterior talocalcaneal
joint

Second cuneiform

Third cuneiform

Tubercle for attachment of
calcaneofibular ligament

Calcaneus

Peroneal
tubercle

Cuboid

Calcaneocuboid
joint

Styloid process
of fifth metatarsal

**Figure 12-61** Osteology of the lateral side of the foot and ankle.

that begin on the medial side of the tendon lie posteriorly, and those that begin on the lateral side lie anteriorly at the level of the insertion. This anatomic fact makes it possible to lengthen the Achilles tendon by dividing its anterior two thirds near the insertion and its medial two thirds 5 cm more proximally. Dorsiflexion of the foot lengthens the tendon, and no suture is required. The operation can be done either as an open or as a subcutaneous procedure.[5] This arrangement of the fibers can be remembered by thinking of this tendon lengthening as the "DAMP operation," which stands for *distal anterior medial proximal.*

A fat pad lies between the Achilles tendon and the bone, with a bursa that may become inflamed. A second bursa exists between the insertion of the tendon into the os calcis and the skin (see Fig. 12-52).

The *flexor retinaculum* is a thickening of the fascia that stretches from the medial malleolus to the back of the calcaneus. It covers the three flexor tendons that pass around the back of the tibial malleolus, as well as the neurovascular bundle.

The tibial nerve may be trapped by this retinaculum, producing pain and paresthesia in the distribution of the medial and lateral plantar nerves and their calcaneal branches. The syndrome is known as the tarsal tunnel syndrome (see Fig. 12-52).

## Anterior Approach to the Ankle

### Extensor Muscles
Four muscles cross the anterior aspect of the ankle joint. All are extensors of the ankle and are supplied by the deep peroneal nerve. The muscles, from medial to lateral, are the tibialis anterior, extensor hallucis longus, extensor digitorum longus, and peroneus tertius. The neurovascular bundle crosses the front of the ankle virtually under the tendon of the extensor hallucis longus (see Fig. 12-56).

### Extensor Retinacula
The *superior extensor retinaculum* is a thickening of the deep fascia above the ankle. It runs between the tibia and the fibula, and is split by the tendon of the tibialis anterior muscle, which lies in a synovial sheath just above the ankle (see Fig. 12-56).

The *inferior extensor retinaculum,* on the dorsum of the foot, is attached to the lateral side of the upper surface of the os calcis. The retinaculum is split medially; the upper part attaches to the medial malleolus, whereas the lower part travels across the foot, where it sometimes joins the plantar aponeurosis in the sole. The two retinacula prevent the anterior tendons from bowstringing; they should be repaired after any approach that cuts them (see Fig. 12-56).

## Lateral Approaches to the Ankle

The tendons of the *peroneal muscles* pass behind the lateral malleolus to reach the foot. Both evert the foot and are supplied by the superficial peroneal nerve (see Fig. 12-59).

The peroneus brevis tendon, which lies immediately behind the lateral malleolus, often is used in reconstruction of the lateral ligaments of the ankle. In cases of instability, maintain the distal insertion of the tendon intact; the proximal portion of the tendon is detached surgically, threaded through the fibula, and attached to the talus, calcaneus, or itself to substitute for the damaged ligaments. The peroneus brevis is recognizable both by its position immedi-ately behind the lateral malleolus and by its muscularity almost down to the level of the ankle joint.

The *superior peroneal retinaculum* is a thickening of the deep fascia extending from the tip of the lateral malleolus to the calcaneus (see Fig. 12-59).

The *inferior peroneal retinaculum* runs from the peroneal tubercle to the lateral side of the calcaneus (see Fig. 12-59).

The peroneal tendons are enclosed in a synovial sheath as they pass around the back of the lateral malleolus. The sheath encloses both tendons down to the peroneal tubercle. At this point, each tendon gains its own separate sheath (see Figs. 12-59 and 12-60). This also is the site of peroneal tendinitis, which commonly occurs in joggers.

# Applied Surgical Anatomy of the Approaches to the Hindpart of the Foot

Surgery performed on the hindpart of the foot is confined almost exclusively to three joints: the posterior part of the subtalar joint, the talocalcaneonavicular joint, and the calcaneocuboid joint. The anatomy of the approaches is the anatomy of the joints themselves, because they all are superficial structures (see Figs. 12-61 and 12-64).

The key to the anatomy is the tarsal canal, which runs obliquely across the foot, between the talus and the calcaneus. The canal is formed by two grooves, one on the inferior surface of the talus and the other on the superior surface of the calcaneus. The canal separates the talocalcaneonavicular joint from the talocalcaneal joint and acts as a landmark for surgical access to the two joints. At its lateral end, the canal widens considerably into the sinus tarsi.

The sinus tarsi contains a tough ligament, the ligamentum cervicis tali, and a large fat pad; the ligament must be divided and the fat pad mobilized for access to the sinus and joints. The extensor digitorum brevis muscle originates from the top of the anterior wall of the sinus. It must be detached for access to the calcaneocuboid joint.

Behind the tarsal canal lies the posterior part of the subtalar joint, which consists of a convex superior facet of the talus and a concave facet of the talus. The joint line is oblique when viewed from the lateral (operative) side. To see it better, the peroneal tendons that overlie it partially must be mobilized and retracted anteriorly.

Distal to the tarsal canal lies the anterior part of the subtalar joint, the talocalcaneonavicular joint. This complex joint consists of a ball (the head of the talus) articulating with a socket (the concave posterior aspect of the navicular, the concave anterior end of the superior surface of the calcaneus, and the spring ligament—short plantar calcaneonavicular ligament—that connects the two bony elements of the socket). From the lateral side, the talonavicular part of the joint appears nearly vertical. From a dorsal point of view, the joint runs transversely across the foot, in line with the calcaneocuboid joint.

Distal to the sinus tarsi lies the calcaneocuboid joint, formed by the anterior end of the calcaneus and the posterior aspect of the cuboid. From the lateral side, the joint looks vertical. A more dorsal view shows that it runs transversely across the foot in line with the talonavicular joint.

Once the sinus tarsi has been defined, all these joints become accessible if surgery remains on bone and the surgeon is aware of the different planes of the joints.

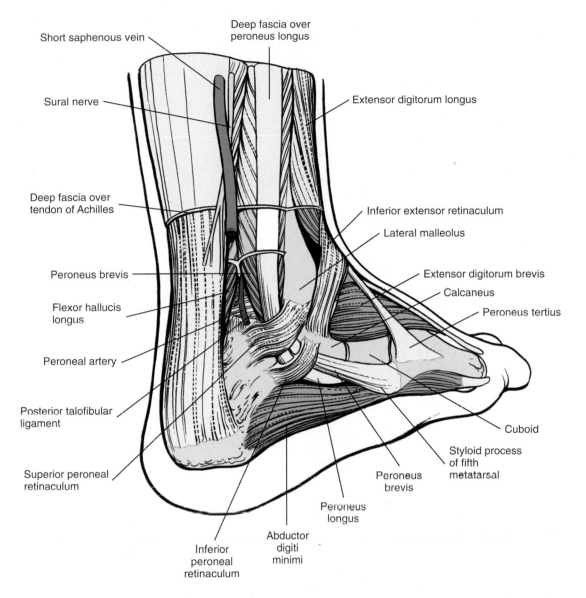

Short saphenous vein

Sural nerve

Deep fascia over peroneus longus

Deep fascia over tendon of Achilles

Peroneus brevis

Flexor hallucis longus

Peroneal artery

Posterior talofibular ligament

Superior peroneal retinaculum

Inferior peroneal retinaculum

Abductor digiti minimi

Peroneus longus

Peroneus brevis

Extensor digitorum longus

Inferior extensor retinaculum

Lateral malleolus

Extensor digitorum brevis

Calcaneus

Peroneus tertius

Cuboid

Styloid process of fifth metatarsal

**Figure 12-62** Superficial anatomy of the posterolateral aspect of the foot and ankle. Note that the muscle fibers of the peroneus brevis run all the way to the ankle joint and lie immediately posterior to the lateral malleolus.

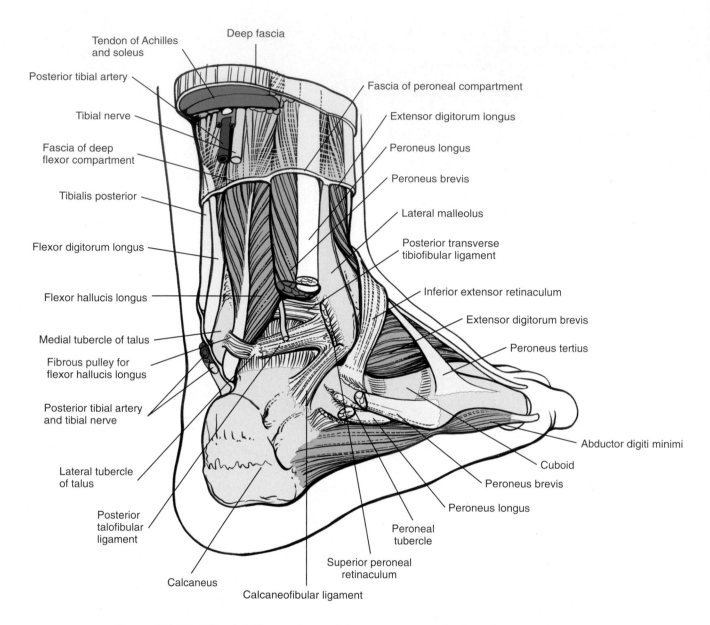

**Figure 12-63**    The Achilles tendon and the peroneus muscles have been resected to reveal the posterolateral aspect of the ankle joint and the deep flexor tendons of the foot. The flexor hallucis longus is immediately medial to the peroneus brevis. The fascia investing these muscles is deep to the deep fascia; it separates them into peroneal and deep flexor compartments. The flexor hallucis longus remains muscular down to the ankle joint.

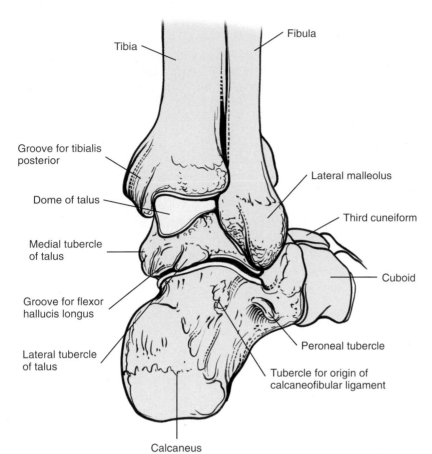

**Figure 12-64**   Osteology of the posterolateral aspect of the foot and ankle.

Tibia

Fibula

Groove for tibialis posterior

Lateral malleolus

Dome of talus

Third cuneiform

Medial tubercle of talus

Cuboid

Groove for flexor hallucis longus

Lateral tubercle of talus

Peroneal tubercle

Tubercle for origin of calcaneofibular ligament

Calcaneus

# Dorsal Approaches to the Middle Part of the Foot

The middle part of the foot extends from the calcaneocuboid and talonavicular joints to the tarsometatarsal Lisfranc's joints. All these bones and joints are superficial and can be approached directly by dorsal, medial, lateral, and plantar approaches. Operations in this area (which are performed rarely) usually involve surgery on the insertions of the four powerful muscles that, together, are responsible for controlling inversion and eversion of the foot. These muscles are the tibialis anterior, which inserts into the medial surface and undersurface of the medial cuneiform bone, and into the adjoining part of the base of the first metatarsal bone; the peroneus longus, which inserts into the lateral side of the medial cuneiform bone; the peroneus brevis, which inserts into the base of the lateral side of the metatarsal bone; and the tibialis posterior, which inserts into the tuberosity of the navicular bone, the inferior surface of the medial cuneiform bone, the intermediate cuneiform bone, and the bases of the second, third, and fourth metatarsal bones (see Figs. 12-53, 12-56, and 12-60).

The middle part of the foot is the target of various specialized procedures for the treatment of muscle imbalance, mobile flatfoot, and an accessory navicular bone. It also is approached for open reduction and internal fixation of fractures in and around Lisfranc's joint, and for local tarsal fusion. Only the general surgical approaches are considered here, because the details of operative technique and indications are beyond the scope of this book.

## Position of the Patient

Place the patient supine on the operating table. Dorsomedial approaches and medial approaches are carried out with the leg in its natural position of slight external rotation, whereas dorsolateral approaches require internal rotation of the limb, which is achieved by placing a sandbag under the buttock. For all procedures, exsanguinate the limb either by elevating it for 3 to 5 minutes or by applying a soft rubber bandage. Then, inflate a tourniquet (see Fig. 12-32).

## Landmarks and Incisions

### Landmarks

To palpate the *first metatarsal cuneiform joint*, feel along the medial border of the foot in a distal to proximal direction. The first metatarsal flares slightly at its base to meet the first cuneiform.

Continue moving proximally along the medial border of the foot to reach the *tubercle of the navicular*.

The medial side of the *talar head* is immediately proximal to the navicular. It can be located by inverting and everting the forepart of the foot. The motion that occurs between the talus and the navicular is palpable (Fig. 12-65).

Palpate the *base of the fifth metatarsal* by feeling along the lateral side of its shaft in a distal to proximal direction until its flared base is reached; this is the styloid process, into which the peroneus brevis muscle inserts (Fig. 12-67).

### Incisions

Make a longitudinal incision directly over the area to be exposed. Use a *dorsomedial* incision to expose the talonavicular joint, the navicular-medial cuneiform joint, and the first metatarsocuneiform joint, and to reveal the insertions of the tendons of the tibialis anterior and tibialis posterior muscles (see Fig. 12-65). Use a *dorsolateral incision* to expose the calcaneocuboid joint and the base of the fifth metatarsal (see Figs. 12-61 and 12-67).

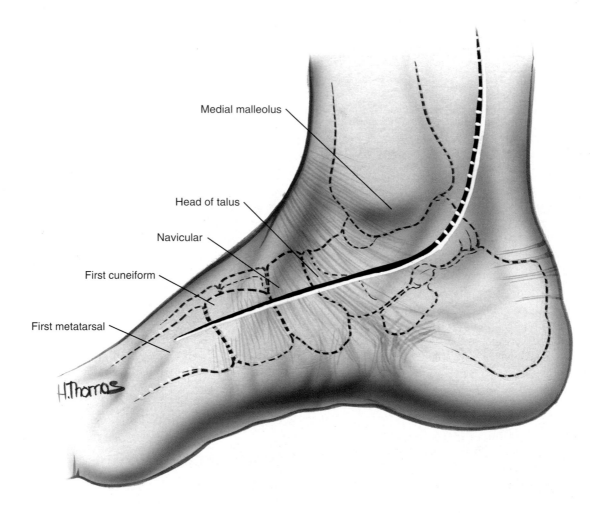

Medial malleolus

Head of talus

Navicular

First cuneiform

First metatarsal

H.Thomas

**Figure 12-65**    Incision for exposure of the middle part of the foot. Make a longitudinal incision directly over the area to be exposed. A dorsomedial incision exposes the talonavicular joint, the navicular-medial cuneiform joint, and the first metatarsocuneiform joint.

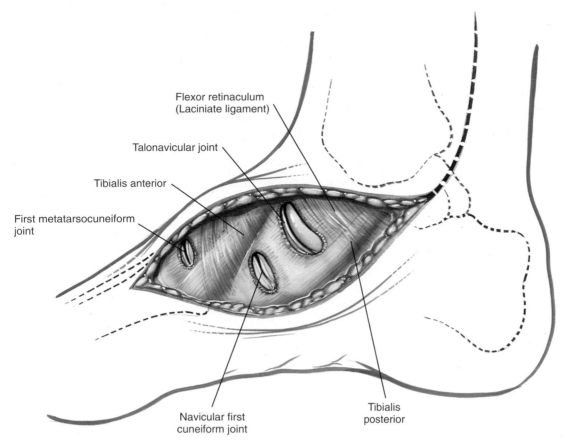

Flexor retinaculum
(Laciniate ligament)

Talonavicular joint

Tibialis anterior

First metatarsocuneiform
joint

Navicular first
cuneiform joint

Tibialis
posterior

**Figure 12-66** Develop the skin flaps. Note the insertions of the tibialis anterior and posterior muscles. Incise the joint capsules of the talonavicular joint, the navicular-medial cuneiform joint, and the first metatarsocuneiform joint according to the demands of the surgery.

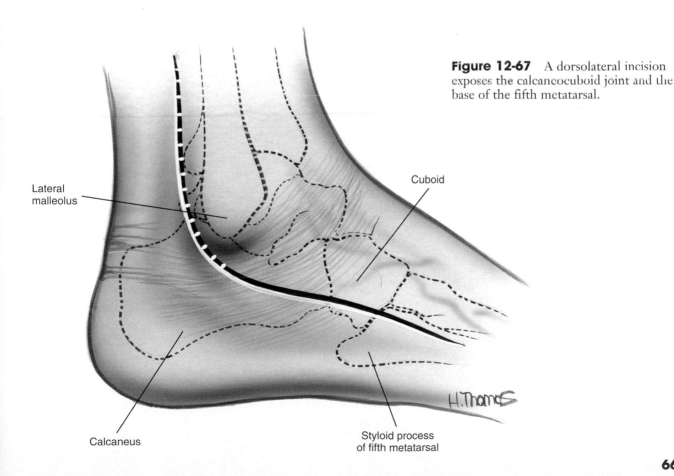

**Figure 12-67** A dorsolateral incision exposes the calcaneocuboid joint and the base of the fifth metatarsal.

Lateral
malleolus

Cuboid

Calcaneus

Styloid process
of fifth metatarsal

H.Thomas

If access to both the medial and lateral sides of the tarsus is required, it is better to make two separate longitudinal incisions centered over the structures to be explored. Separate incisions nearly always are required for the open reduction of fractures of Lisfranc's joint.

Transverse incisions are used best for wedge tarsectomy.

## Internervous Plane

There are no internervous planes in these approaches. Longitudinal incisions avoid damaging cutaneous nerves. Certain major reconstructive operations, such as wedge tarsectomy, necessarily cut cutaneous nerves, leaving portions of the dorsum of the foot partially anesthetic.

## Surgical Dissection

Cut down directly onto the structures that are to be exposed, taking care to avoid any cutaneous nerves that can be identified. Try to make sure that skin flaps are as thick as possible; minimize retraction as much as possible. The structures of the dorsum of the foot nearly all are subcutaneous. Take care to avoid damaging the insertions of the four powerful invertors and evertors of the foot (Figs. 12-66 and 12-68).

## How to Enlarge the Approach

These approaches can be extended proximally. On the *lateral side*, extend the incision posteriorly and then up behind the posterior border of the lateral

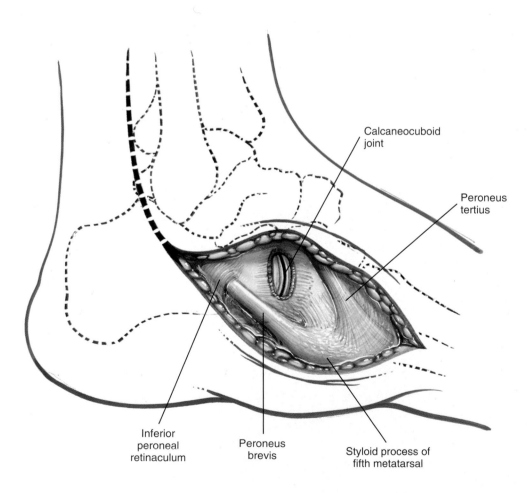

Calcaneocuboid joint

Peroneus tertius

Inferior peroneal retinaculum

Peroneus brevis

Styloid process of fifth metatarsal

**Figure 12-68**   Develop the skin flaps on the lateral side of the middle part of the foot. Note the tendon of the peroneus brevis as it inserts into the base of the fifth metatarsal. The joint capsule of the calcaneocuboid joint can be incised, if necessary.

malleolus; this exposes not only the lateral side of the ankle joint, but also the posterior part of the subtalar joint and the calcaneocuboid joint. (See sections describing the posterolateral approach to the ankle and lateral approach to the hindpart of the foot.)

On the *medial side*, extend the incision up behind the medial malleolus, curving it to a point midway between the medial malleolus and the Achilles tendon. This extension exposes those structures that pass around the back of the medial malleolus. It is used commonly in the treatment of clubfoot, but its safety is controversial; the neurovascular bundle must be protected. (See the section regarding the posteromedial approach to the ankle.)

# Dorsal and Dorsomedial Approaches to the Metatarsophalangeal Joint of the Great Toe

The dorsal and dorsomedial approaches make possible most surgery on the metatarsophalangeal joint of the great toe for the treatment of bunions or hallux rigidus. Their uses include the following:

1. Excision of the metatarsal head[6]
2. Excision of the proximal part of the proximal phalanx[7]
3. Excision of metatarsal exostosis (bunionectomy)
4. Distal metatarsal osteotomy[8,9]
5. Soft-tissue correction of hallux valgus, including reefing procedures, tenotomies, and muscle reattachments[10]
6. Arthrodesis of the metatarsophalangeal joint[11]
7. Insertion of joint replacements
8. Dorsal wedge osteotomy of the proximal phalanx in cases of hallux rigidus[12]

## Position of the Patient

Place the patient supine on the operating table. After exsanguination, use a tourniquet placed on the middle of the thigh. Alternatively, use a soft rubber bandage to exsanguinate the foot, and then wrap the leg tightly just above the ankle (see Fig. 12-1).

## Landmarks and Incisions

### Landmarks

The *head of the first metatarsal bone* and the *metatarsophalangeal joint* are palpable on the ball of the foot and on its medial border. In cases of bunion, the metatarsal head is medially prominent.

Palpate the *extensor hallucis longus tendon* on the dorsum of the foot. When it is tight, it stands out when the great toe is flexed passively in a plantar direction.

### Incisions

*Dorsomedial Incision.* The dorsomedial skin incision provides access to the exostosis on the metatarsal head without much skin retraction; it is by far the most commonly performed incision. It does have drawbacks, however. The bursa covering the exostosis may have become inflamed, complicating the surgery, and the skin on the medial aspect of the metatarsophalangeal joint is thinner than on the dorsum of the joint and may not heal as well.

Begin the dorsomedial incision just proximal to the interphalangeal joint on the dorsomedial aspect of the great toe. Curve it over the dorsal aspect of the metatarsophalangeal joint, remaining medial to the tendon of the extensor hallucis longus muscle. Then, curve the incision back by cutting along the medial aspect of the shaft of the first metatarsal, finishing some 2 to 3 cm from the metatarsophalangeal joint (Fig. 12-69).

*Dorsal Incision.* Begin the dorsal incision just proximal to the interphalangeal joint and just medial to the tendon of the extensor hallucis longus muscle. Extend the incision proximally, parallel and just medial to the tendon of the extensor hallucis longus. Finish about 2 to 3 cm proximal to the metatarsophalangeal joint. Note that the final incision is straight (Fig. 12-72).

## Internervous Plane

There is no true internervous plane. The bone is subcutaneous; the two tendons close to the dissection, the extensor hallucis longus and the abductor hallucis, receive their nerve supplies proximal to this approach and cannot be denervated by it.

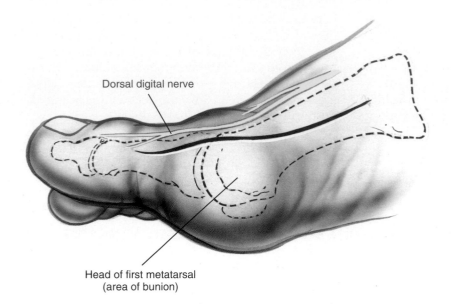

Dorsal digital nerve

Head of first metatarsal
(area of bunion)

**Figure 12-69**   Dorsomedial skin incision for the medial approach to the metatarsophalangeal joint of the great toe. Note the proximity of the dorsal digital nerve to the incision.

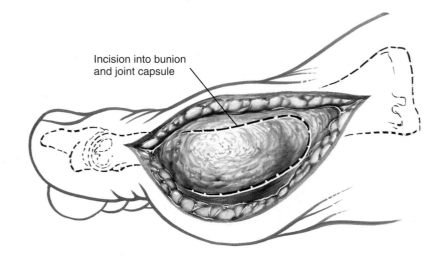

Incision into bunion and joint capsule

**Figure 12-70**   Incise the deep fascia. Develop a joint capsule flap. Protect the dorsal digital branch of the medial cutaneous nerve.

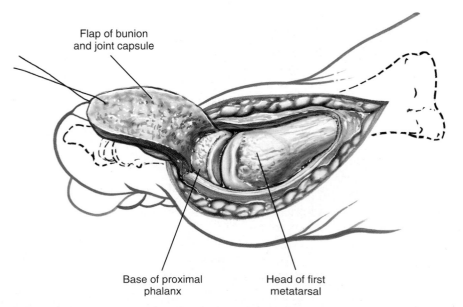

Flap of bunion and joint capsule

Base of proximal phalanx

Head of first metatarsal

**Figure 12-71**   Make a U-shaped incision into the joint capsule, leaving the capsule attached to the proximal end of the proximal phalanx.

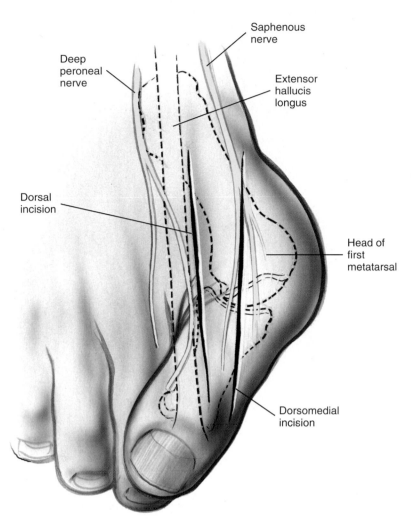

**Figure 12-72**   Dorsal incision for the approach to the metatarsophalangeal joint of the great toe. Note that the tendon of the extensor hallucis longus is displaced laterally and that the sensory nerve to the medial aspect of the great toe runs parallel to the incision. Note that the great toe is framed by branches of the saphenous nerve medially and the deep peroneal nerve laterally.

## Superficial Surgical Dissection

### Dorsomedial Incision

Incise the deep fascia in line with the incision. Then, cut down to the dorsomedial aspect of the metatarsophalangeal joint. The dorsal digital branch of the medial cutaneous nerve, which often is visible, is retracted laterally with the skin flap on the lateral edge of the wound. Make a U-shaped incision into the joint capsule, leaving the capsule attached to the proximal end of the proximal phalanx (Figs. 12-70 and 12-71).

### Dorsal Incision

Divide the deep fascia in line with the incision, and retract the tendon of the extensor hallucis longus muscle laterally. To enter the joint, incise the dorsal aspect of the joint capsule. Note that the type and position of the capsulotomy depend on the procedure to be performed (Figs. 12-73 and 12-74).

## Deep Surgical Dissection

For both incisions, incise the periosteum of the proximal phalanx and first metatarsal bones longitudinally. Using blunt instruments, strip the coverings off the bones, taking care not to damage the tendon of the flexor hallucis longus muscle, which lies in a fibro-osseous tunnel on the plantar surface of the proximal phalanx, between the sesamoid bones. The extent of the deep dissection depends on the procedure to be carried out. Strip only a minimum of periosteum off the bone. Do not strip all the soft-tissue attachments off the metatarsus if a distal osteotomy of that bone is to be performed, because the metatarsal head is rendered avascular by stripping.

## Dangers

The **tendon of the extensor hallucis longus** muscle, which lies in the lateral edge of the wound,

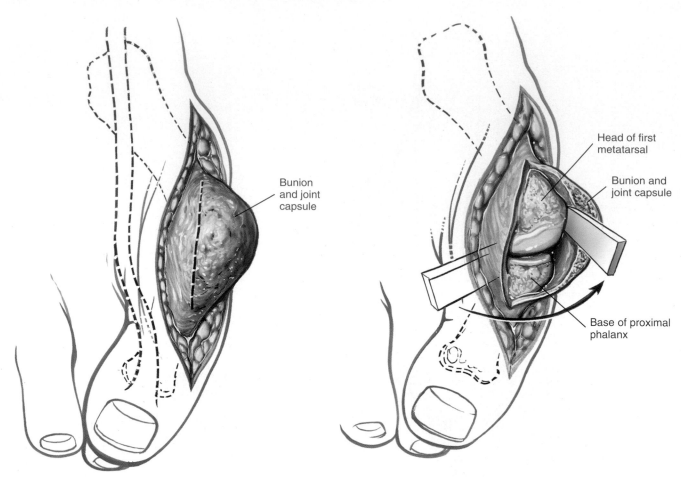

**Figure 12-73** Develop the skin flaps. Divide the deep fascia in line with the skin incision, and retract the tendon of the extensor hallucis longus laterally.

**Figure 12-74** Incise the joint capsule dorsally, and remove as much of the capsule as necessary depending on the procedure to be performed.

should not be cut during the approach. Indeed, in cases of bunion, the tendon bowstrings laterally across the metatarsophalangeal joint and is even more lateral to the incision than usual. Protect the dorsal digital nerve if it can be seen along the line of the incision (see Figs. 12-69 and 12-72).

The **tendon of the flexor hallucis longus** muscle is vulnerable as the base of the proximal phalanx is stripped. The tendon lies in a groove on the plantar surface of the proximal phalanx so close to the periosteum that, if care is not taken, it may be dam-

aged during stripping. The tendon often is displaced laterally in patients with hallux valgus (see Fig. 12-52).

## How to Enlarge the Approach

Careful and systematic stripping of the structures off the bones provides an adequate view of the joint. The approach cannot be extended usefully to other joints in the foot, but may be extended proximally for access to the shaft of the metatarsus.

# Dorsal Approach to the Metatarsophalangeal Joints of the Second, Third, Fourth, and Fifth Toes

The dorsal approach, which exposes the metatarsophalangeal joints of the second, third, fourth, and fifth toes, avoids incision of the plantar skin of the foot. Most plantar approaches scar the weight-bearing skin, violating a basic surgical principle.

The uses for the approach include the following:

1. Excision of metatarsal heads
2. Distal metatarsal osteotomy
3. Partial proximal phalangectomy
4. Fusion of metatarsophalangeal joints (rare)
5. Capsulotomy of metatarsophalangeal joints
6. Muscle tenotomy
7. Neurectomy

## Position of the Patient

Place the patient supine on the operating table. Position a bolster under the thigh to flex the knee and allow the foot to lie with its plantar surface on the table (Fig. 12-75).

## Landmarks and Incision

### Landmarks

To palpate each *metatarsal head*, place a thumb on the plantar surface and an index finger on the dorsal surface of the foot. Skin callosities under the heads indicate that the area concerned is bearing an unaccus-

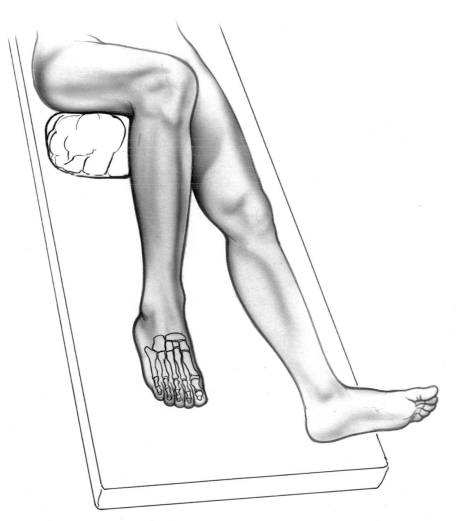

**Figure 12-75**   Position of the patient for approaches to the toes.

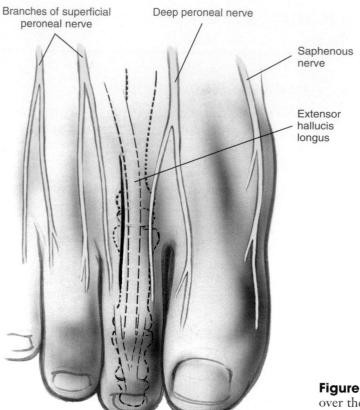

Branches of superficial peroneal nerve

Deep peroneal nerve

Saphenous nerve

Extensor hallucis longus

**Figure 12-76**  Make a 2- to 3-cm longitudinal incision over the dorsolateral aspect of the affected metatarsophalangeal joint.

tomed amount of weight, indicating pathology in the weight distribution around the foot.

Palpate the tendons of the *extensor digitorum longus* muscle on the dorsal aspect of the foot.

### Incision

Make a 2- to 3-cm longitudinal incision over the dorsolateral aspect of the affected metatarsophalangeal joint. The incision should run parallel with, but just lateral to, the long extensor tendon (Fig. 12-76). If two adjacent joints need to be exposed, make the incision between them. Alternatively, a transverse dorsal incision may be made over the joints.

### Internervous Plane

There is no true internervous plane for any of these metatarsophalangeal approaches. The approaches are well dorsal to the plantar nerves and vessels, the key neurovascular structures in this area. Take care to avoid cutting the dorsal digital nerves, branches of which may cross the operative field.

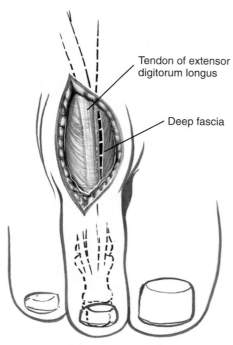

Tendon of extensor digitorum longus

Deep fascia

**Figure 12-77**  Incise the deep fascia in line with the incision on the medial side of the long extensor tendon.

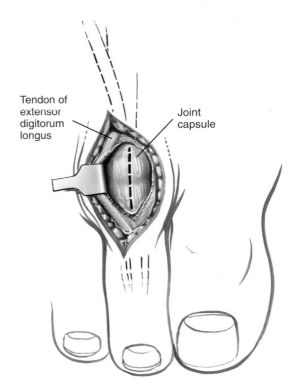

**Figure 12-78** Expose the dorsal capsule of the metatarsophalangeal joint. Make a longitudinal incision into the capsule.

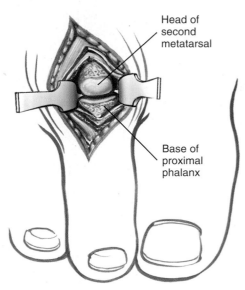

**Figure 12-79** Retract the joint capsule to expose the metatarsophalangeal joint.

## Deep Surgical Dissection

Incise the dorsal capsule of the metatarsophalangeal joint longitudinally to enter the joint (Figs. 12-78 and 12-79).

## Dangers

The **long extensor tendon** should be protected during the procedure.

At the level of the metatarsophalangeal joints, the **plantar nerves and vessel** lie between the metatarsal heads, beneath the deep transverse metatarsal ligament. As long as the dissection remains on the dorsal aspect of the ligaments, the nerves are safe. Dissection around the metatarsal heads and proximal phalanges must be carried out so as to avoid damage to the nerves and vessel that supply the weight-bearing skin of the toes (see Fig. 12-56).

## Superficial Surgical Dissection

Incise the deep fascia in line with the incision, and retract the long extensor tendon to reveal the dorsal aspect of the metatarsophalangeal joint (Fig. 12-77). Often, an extensor tenotomy or lengthening is performed at the same time as the operation on the joint. In this case, divide the extensor tendon in a "Z" fashion rather than retracting it. If two joints are being exposed, retract the tendon laterally to gain access to the adjacent joint.

# Approach to the Dorsal Web Spaces

The approach to the dorsal web spaces allows pathology of the web space to be explored, especially in cases of Morton's metatarsalgia, when it can be used to excise an interdigital "neuroma."[13] Other uses include drainage of web space infections, which, curiously, are much rarer in the foot than in the hand. The approach is used most often for exploration of the cleft between the third and fourth toes.

Dissection of the first web space exposes the sesamoid bones and is used for adductor tenotomy.

## Position of the Patient

Place the patient supine on the operating table. Apply a tourniquet either at the midpoint of the thigh or just above the ankle after the leg has been

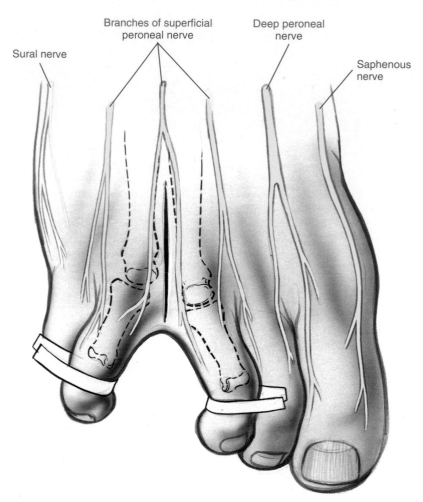

Sural nerve

Branches of superficial peroneal nerve

Deep peroneal nerve

Saphenous nerve

**Figure 12-80**   Make a longitudinal incision, centering it over the web space.

exsanguinated. Alternatively, use a soft rubber bandage to exsanguinate the foot, then use the bandage as a tourniquet at the ankle (see Fig. 12-75). Place a pillow under the patient's thigh to flex the knee, so that the sole of the foot lies flat on the operating table.

## Landmarks and Incision

Separate the two toes of the affected web space. Make a dorsal longitudinal incision over the center of the web space, starting at the distal end of the web and extending proximally some 2 to 3 cm (Fig. 12-80).

## Internervous Plane

There is no internervous plane.

## Superficial Surgical Dissection

Incise the deep transverse metatarsal ligament in line with the skin incision by blunt dissection, opening a pair of scissors with the blades in a longitudinal

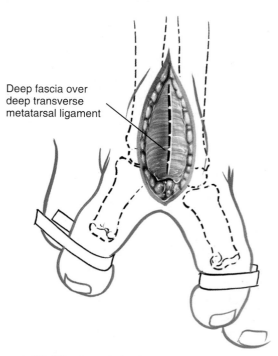

Deep fascia over deep transverse metatarsal ligament

**Figure 12-81**   Incise the fascia in line with the skin incision.

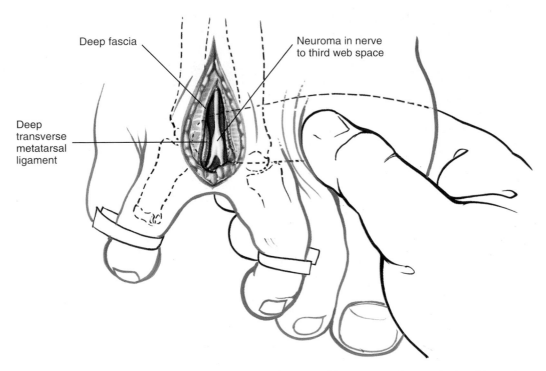

**Figure 12-82**   Incise the deep transverse metatarsal ligament in line with the skin and fascial incision to reveal the neurovascular bundle.

plane, to expose the neurovascular bundle (Figs. 12-81 and 12-82). The neuroma, if one is present, often bulges into the wound. It becomes more prominent if digital pressure is applied to the space between the metatarsal head on the plantar surface of the foot (see Fig. 12-82).

## Dangers

The only danger in an approach to a single cleft is to the digital nerve and vessel that usually are the target of the approach. Take care, however, to avoid cutting any dorsal cutaneous nerves that run under the incision. If more clefts must be explored, avoid disrupt-

ing the arterial supply to the toes. Accidental incision of one digital artery does not render a toe ischemic, but if the second digital artery to the same toe is incised in the next web space, ischemia may result (see Fig. 12-56).

Excising a neuroma from a web space usually leaves the weight-bearing surface of the affected toes at least partially anesthetic, but trophic changes do not occur.

## How to Enlarge the Approach

The approach rarely is enlarged and is used primarily for specific web space pathology.

# Applied Surgical Anatomy of the Foot

## Overview

Surgery of the foot often is undertaken to correct bony abnormalities. All the bones of the foot can be approached dorsally; dorsal approaches usually are better than plantar approaches for two major reasons:

1. The critical neurovascular structures in the forepart of the foot all are on the plantar side of the metatarsal bones, so they remain protected.
2. Dorsal incisions avoid cutting through the specialized weight-bearing skin of the sole of the foot.

In pathologic situations in which abnormal skin lies over bones that protrude (e.g., metatarsalgia), a plantar approach may have to be used and the abnormal skin excised.

Although the dorsal anatomy is the critical surgical anatomy of the foot, the plantar anatomy includes its key neurovascular structures. Knowledge of the latter allows the surgeon to explore wounds in the sole of the foot, which do not mimic any described surgical approach. For these reasons, the anatomy of the sole of the foot also is described in this section.

## Anatomy of the Dorsum of the Foot

The skin of the dorsum of the foot is comparatively thin and loose. Distally, the lines of cleavage run roughly transversely. The loose skin, which facilitates retraction, accounts for the enormous amount of dorsal swelling that can occur after foot trauma.

### Nerve Supply

Branches of three cutaneous nerves run right under the skin of the dorsum of the foot: the medial side houses the branches of the saphenous nerve; most of the dorsum of the foot is supplied by the dorsal cutaneous branches of the superficial peroneal nerve; and the lateral side of the foot is supplied by the sural nerve.

The first web space is supplied by branches of the deep peroneal nerve. Numbness in the first web space is the earliest sign of a deep peroneal nerve lesion in the anterior compartment of the leg (see Figs. 12-56, 12-69, 12-72, 12-76, and 12-80).

### Superficial Veins

The veins are arranged in a dorsal venous arch. The medial side drains into the long saphenous vein; the lateral side drains into the short saphenous vein. Superficial veins, of course, must be on the dorsum of the foot, because they would collapse under the force of ordinary weight bearing if they were on the sole.

### Tendons

Two sets of tendons lie immediately deep to the cutaneous nerves: those of the extensor digitorum longus and extensor digitorum brevis muscles, and those of the extensor hallucis longus and extensor hallucis brevis muscles. The extensor digitorum tendons insert into the dorsal extensor expansion of the lateral four toes, an arrangement that is identical to that in the fingers. Frequently, these tendons cross-communicate in the forepart of the foot. The great toe, similar to the thumb, has no dorsal extensor expansion (see Fig. 12-56).

### Deep Artery

The artery of the dorsum of the foot, the dorsalis pedis artery, runs forward beneath the tendon of the extensor hallucis brevis muscle before disappearing into the first intermetatarsal space (see Fig. 12-57).

## Sole of the Foot

### Skin

The skin of the sole of the foot is highly specialized, tough, and resilient. It responds to abnormal stresses by hypertrophying in the keratinized layer, forming callosities. In cases of severe metatarsalgia, the skin over the protruding metatarsal heads becomes thin and attenuated. In Fowler's procedure (a transverse incision), the lips of pathologic skin are removed, and the thicker, normal skin is sutured back into its correct position.[14,15] The skin also may atrophy in patients with ischemic or neuropathic conditions.

### Deep Fascia

The deep fascia of the sole is similar to the deep palmar fascia of the hand; it also may suffer Dupuytren's contracture. The fascia is much thicker in its central parts and thinner where it covers the intrinsic muscles of the hallux and little toe. Its central part, the plantar aponeurosis, originates from the medial tubercle of the calcaneus and runs forward to attach to the proximal phalanges of each of the toes.

The attachment of the plantar aponeurosis to the medial tubercle of the calcaneus often is a site for the inflammatory degeneration that produces a painful heel. The point of maximal tenderness in this condition corresponds to the anatomic insertion of the plantar aponeurosis. On rare occasions, this condition, which is known as plantar fasciitis ("policeman's heel"), may necessitate surgical detachment of the origin of the fascia.

Medial and lateral fibrous septa originate from the medial and lateral borders of the plantar fascia to attach to the first and fifth metatarsal bones. These septa divide the foot into three compartments, much as the septa do in the hand. The compartments may limit areas of infection within the foot.

### First Layer of Muscles

The superficial layer consists of three muscles: the flexor digitorum brevis, abductor hallucis, and abductor digiti minimi.

The flexor digitorum brevis arises mainly from the plantar aponeurosis and partly from the medial calcaneal tubercle. It divides into four tendons that insert into the middle phalanx of the lateral four toes and flexes the toes independent of the position of the ankle.

The abductor hallucis takes origin from the medial tubercle of the calcaneus, inserts into the medial side of the proximal phalanx of the great toe, and abducts the great toe. It is the only muscle whose action tends to oppose the deformity of hallux valgus (see Fig. 12-52).

### Superficial Nerves and Vessels

The medial and lateral plantar arteries and nerves lie between the first and second layers of muscle. They are relatively superficial, but, as in the hand, rarely are injured, because of the toughness of the overlying plantar fascia.

### Second Layer of Muscles

The second layer of muscles consists of the long flexor tendons (the flexor hallucis longus, flexor digitorum longus, and flexor accessorius), which are critical in maintaining the longitudinal arch of the foot (see Figs. 12-53 and 12-54). Helping these muscles are the lumbricals, which arise from the tendons of the flexor digitorum longus. As they do in the hand, the lumbricals flex the metatarsophalangeal joints while they keep the interphalangeal joint extended. Weakness results in clawing of the toes, producing the equivalent in the foot of the intrinsic minus hand. A persistent extension deformity of the metatarsophalangeal joint eventually causes this joint to undergo subluxation, and the metatarsal head has to bear weight that no longer is distributed to the displaced toe during toe-off in walking. Pain (metatarsalgia) is the result.

### Third Layer of Muscles

The third layer of muscles consists of the flexor hallucis brevis, adductor hallucis, and flexor digiti minimi brevis.

The flexor hallucis brevis inserts into the base of the proximal phalanx of the great toe via medial and lateral sesamoid bones. The medial sesamoid also receives slips from the abductor hallucis, and the lateral sesamoid from the adductor hallucis (see Fig. 12-54). The sesamoid bones may be displaced in cases of hallux valgus, with the lateral sesamoid moving to a position between the first and second metatarsal bones. If that happens, the lateral sesamoid can block mechanically the realignment of the first ray. The joint between the sesamoid bones and the metatarsal head may degenerate and become painful.

The adductor hallucis, which inserts into the proximal phalanx via the lateral sesamoid bone, is the most important deforming force in hallux valgus. Many operations for this condition involve detaching the muscle from its insertion and reinserting it into the head of the metatarsal so that it can act as a dynamic corrector of metatarsus varus.

### Fourth Layer of Muscles

The fourth and deepest layer of muscles consists of the interosseus muscles attached to the metatarsal bones, and two tendons, those of the peroneus longus and tibialis posterior muscles, which are major supports of the longitudinal arch of the foot.

## REFERENCES

1. COLONNA PC, RALSTON EL: Operative approaches to the ankle joint. Am J Surg 82:44, 1951
2. GATELLIER J, CHASTANG J: Access to the fractured malleolus with piece chipped off at back. J Chir [Paris] 24:5B, 1924
3. KOENIG F, SCHAEFER P: Osteoplastic surgical exposure of the ankle joint: 41st report of progress in orthopaedic surgery. Chir 215:196, 1929
4. RUEDI TP, MURPHY WM: AO principles of fracture management. Thieme, 2001
5. WHITE JW: Torsion of the Achilles tendon: its surgical significance. Arch Surg 46:784, 1943
6. MAYO CH: The surgical treatment of bunion. Ann Surg 48:30D, 1908
7. KELLER WL: Surgical treatment of bunions and hallux valgus. N Y Med J 80:741, 1904
8. MITCHELL CL, FLEMMING JL, ALLEN R ET AL: Osteotomy: bunionectomy for hallux valgus. J Bone Joint Surg 40-1:41, 1958
9. HAMMOND G: Mitchell osteotomy: bunionectomy for hallux valgus and metatarsus primus varus in America's Academy of Orthopaedic Surgeons. Instr Course Lect 21:1, 1972
10. MCBRIDE ED: A conservative operation for bunions. J Bone Joint Surg 10:735, 1928
11. MCKEEVER DC: Arthrodesis of the first metatarso-phalangeal joint for hallux valgus, hallux rigidus and metatarsus primus varus. J Bone Joint Surg [Am] 34:129, 1952
12. CITRON N, NEIL M: Dorsal wedge osteotomy of the proximal phalanx for hallux rigidus. J Bone Joint Surg [Br] 69B:835, 1987
13. BETTS LO: Morton's metatarsalgia, neuritis of fourth digital nerve. Med J Aust 1:514, 1940
14. FOWLER AW: A method of forefoot reconstruction. J Bone Joint Surg [Br] 41:507, 1959
15. KATES A, KESSEL L: Arthroplasty of the forefoot. J Bone Joint Surg [Br] 49:552, 1967
16. KLEIGER B: Disorders of the foot and ankle. In: Jahss M, ed: The ankle. 1983:776

# Thirteen

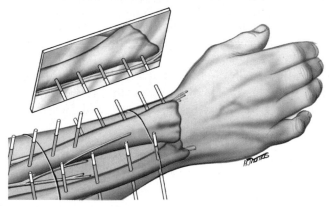

# Approaches for External Fixation

Although a wide variety of external fixators can be constructed, they all consist of only two elements. Pins are inserted into the bone to anchor the external fixator to the skeleton. These pins are then connected to provide stability. Pins may be inserted by transfixing the limb (transfixion pins), or they may stop just beyond the far cortex of the bone into which they are inserted (half pins). Transfixion pins can be connected at both their ends; therefore, external fixators that use these pins provide the greatest stability. Because transfixion pins transfix the soft tissues on both sides of the bone, however, they tether these soft tissues more than half pins do, often making it difficult to mobilize joints above and below the external fixator.

Skeletal pins are inserted through stab incisions in the skin in a "blind" fashion without dissection of the soft tissues that intervene between the skin and the bone except in the distal third of the radius. Studies of cross-sectional anatomy in cadaveric material reveal a large number of possible pin placements for any given bone in any given position. The most common indication for the use of an external fixator, however, is in open (compound) fractures. These injuries usually are associated with fracture displacements, and the normal anatomy frequently is distorted. When skeletal pins are used, nerves and vessels may be damaged as they course down the limb. Distortion of the normal anatomy or normal anatomic variation may make apparently safe routes hazardous. For this reason, only a few of the safest pin placements are discussed for each bone in this chapter. More specific information should be obtained from other sources if an external fixator is being used for a specialized procedure such as leg lengthening.

The rigidity of an external fixator system can be modified in many ways. As mentioned above, transfixion pins provide more stability than do half pins. Spreading the pins widely and increasing their number also adds to the rigidity of the system. Placement of the pins, therefore, is influenced not only by the underlying anatomy, but also by the biomechanical requirements of the fixation system. Finally, soft-tissue damage also may dictate pin position.

Skin incisions for pin insertion should be generous, because tight skin around a pin inevitably leads to low-grade sepsis, which in turn can cause pin loosening.

# The Humerus

Because of the intimate relationship of the neurovascular bundles to the bone, the humerus is one of the most difficult bones in which to apply external fixators safely.

The *median nerve* runs with the brachial artery. In the upper two thirds of the arm, it is almost exactly medial to the humerus, but in the distal third of the humerus, it crosses over laterally to lie anterior to the bone at the level of the elbow joint.

The *ulnar nerve* runs with the median nerve in the upper two thirds of the arm and then courses posteriorly to run in direct relationship to the posteromedial aspect of the humerus at the level of the elbow joint.

The *radial nerve* crosses the posterior aspect of the humerus in a medial to lateral direction roughly in the middle third of the bone. At the level of the elbow joint, it is anterolateral to the humerus.

## Proximal Third

In the proximal third of the bone, half pins may be inserted via a lateral route. These pins should not protrude very far beyond the medial cortex to avoid damage to the neurovascular bundle. Anterior insertion of half pins also is possible, although the biceps tendon may be damaged. Both anterior and laterally inserted half pins may damage the **axillary nerve** as it courses around the bone on the deep surface of the deltoid muscle.

## Middle Third

Anterior half pins may be inserted in the middle third of the humeral shaft. The **radial nerve** runs across the back of the humerus in the middle third of the bone, however, and its course is variable. Care should be taken that these pins do not penetrate the far cortex too deeply.

## Distal Third-Elbow Joint

At the level of the elbow joint, transfixion pins may be inserted in a lateral to medial direction, avoiding the neurovascular bundles that lie anterior and posterior to the epicondyles of the humerus (Fig. 13-1).

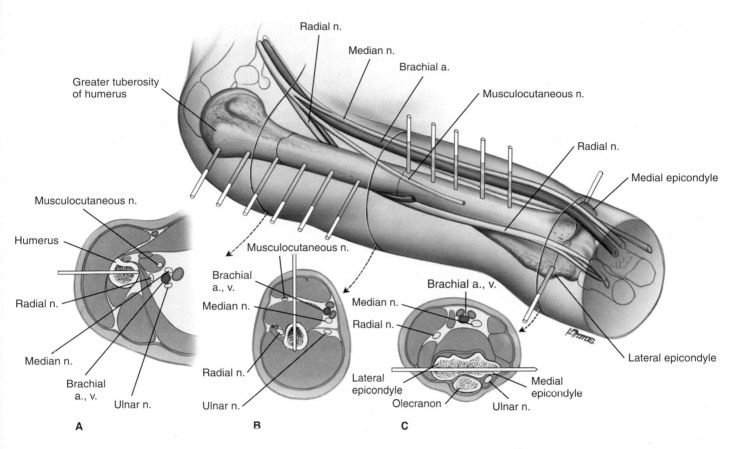

**Figure 13-1** The placement of skeletal pins in the humerus varies with anatomic site. The variable relationship of the neurovascular bundles to the bone dictates different pin placement for the proximal, middle, and distal thirds.

**(A) Proximal third:** Insert a half pin from the lateral side of the bone. Take care not to penetrate the medial cortex too far to avoid damage to the neurovascular bundle (brachial artery and median nerve).

**(B) Middle third:** Place a half pin anteriorly. Take care not to penetrate the far cortex too deeply to avoid damage to the radial nerve, which courses in a medial to lateral direction on the posterior aspect of the middle third of the bone.

**(C) Distal third:** Insert transfixion pins from the lateral to the medial point. Take care to avoid the ulnar nerve as it runs in the groove on the back of the medial humeral epicondyle, where the nerve is easily palpable.

# The Radius and Ulna

The relationships of the radius and ulna to the neurovascular structures are fundamentally different, and the pin placement required in each bone is distinct.

## Ulna

The ulna has an easily palpable subcutaneous surface throughout its entire length. The ulnar nerve enters the forearm on the anteromedial aspect of the ulna, but passes rapidly into the anterior compartment of the forearm to run down on the anterior aspect of the bone together with the ulnar artery.

Transfixion pins can be inserted throughout the entire length of the ulna from either side of the subcutaneous surface of that bone. In the proximal end of the ulna, the **ulnar nerve** is at risk, but it can be palpated easily as it crosses the back of the medial epicondyle of the humerus to allow safe pin placement posterior to the nerve.

## Radius

The radial artery and sensory branch of the radial nerve run down the forearm roughly on the anterolateral aspect of the radius.

### Proximal Third

The posterior interosseous nerve winds around the proximal third of the radius in an anterolateral to posteromedial direction and is very close to the bone. Because radial fractures nearly always involve a rotational deformity of the bone, the exact position of the **posterior interosseous nerve** in the proximal third of the radius cannot be predicted safely. For this reason, pin placement in the upper third of this bone is not recommended unless it is performed as an open procedure.

### Middle Third

In the middle third of the radius, dorsally inserted half pins can be used without risk.

### Distal Third

In the distal third of the radius, the lateral insertion of half pins is safe. The radial artery passes anterior to these pins. Because the branches of the **superficial radial nerve** are variable in position, it is important to make a small incision and dissect down to bone to avoid them, rather than inserting pins blindly (Fig. 13-2).

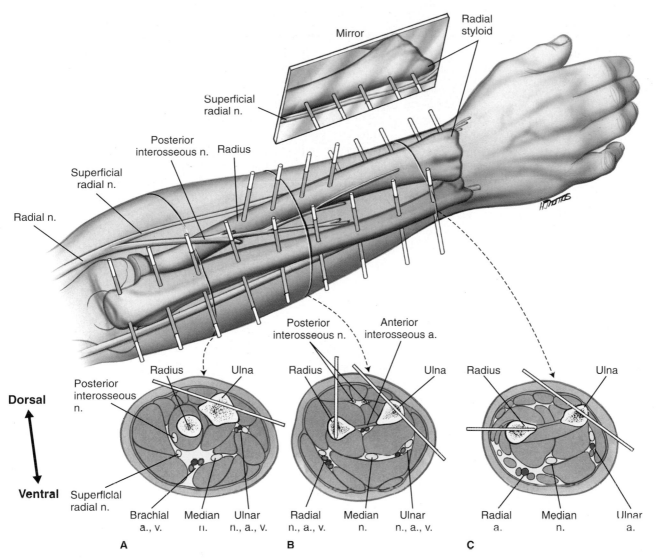

**Figure 13-2**   The position of pins in the radius and ulna is dictated by the presence of the neurovascular bundles in the forearm. Pin placements vary depending on the level of bone to be used. The degree of supination and pronation of the forearm will need to be varied to allow different pin placements in the radius.

**(A) Proximal third:** Because the posterior interosseous nerve winds around the neck of the radius and has a variable relationship to the bone, it is not possible to insert pins safely in the proximal third of the radius except under direct vision. In the ulna, use transfixion pins, taking care to avoid the ulna nerve in the region of the elbow joint.

**(B) Middle third:** Place anterior half pins into the radius. Take care not to penetrate the bone too deeply to avoid damage to the posterior interosseous nerve. Place transfixion pins through the subcutaneous surface of the ulna.

**(C) Distal third:** Place laterally inserted half pins into the distal radius. Take care to avoid the superficial branches of the radial nerve. Place transfixion pins through the ulna using its subcutaneous surface.

## The Femur

The femoral artery enters the thigh in direct anterior relationship to the head of the femur (the femoral pulse). The artery courses down the limb, passing to the medial side of the bone in its middle third, and crosses the knee joint in direct posterior relationship to the distal femur. The sciatic nerve enters the thigh posterior to the femoral head and maintains this posterior relationship as it runs distally. At a variable point in the thigh, the nerve splits into its tibial and common peroneal components. The tibial nerve joins the femoral artery in the back of the knee joint. The common peroneal nerve runs with the tendon of the biceps muscle posterolateral to the bone.

Half pins can be inserted laterally throughout the entire length of the femur without damage to any of the neurovascular structures. These pins do tether the fascia lata and vastus lateralis muscles, however, and it often is not possible to mobilize the knee successfully with them in position. In the distal third of the femur, laterally inserted half pins can be extended medially to transfix the limb. Be aware that these pins may penetrate the knee joint occasionally, resulting in leakage of synovial fluid and possible septic arthritis of the knee.

In the middle third of the bone, anteriorly inserted half pins also are safe. Care should be taken not to penetrate the posterior cortex too deeply, though, to avoid damage to the tibial nerve (Fig. 13-3).

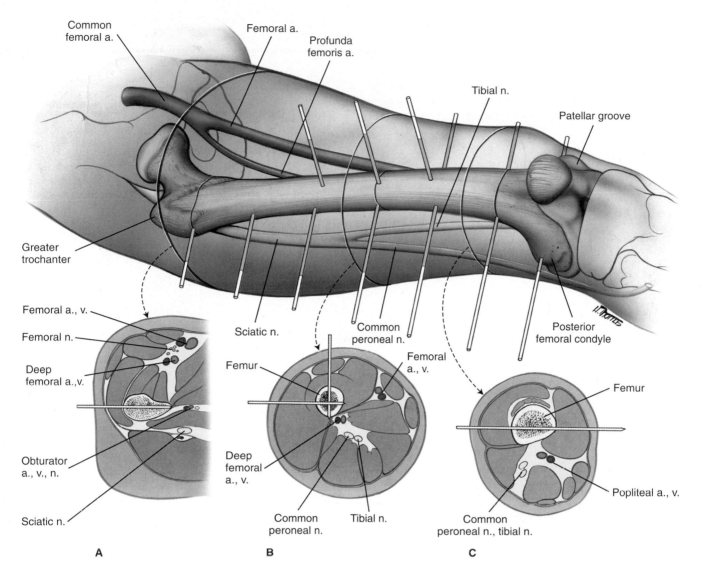

**Figure 13-3**   The variable relationship of the femoral artery to the femur dictates different pin positions depending on the level of pin placement.

**(A) Proximal third:** Insert half pins from the lateral surface of the bone. Avoid penetrating the medial cortex too deeply to avoid damage to the profunda femoris artery and its tributaries.

**(B) Middle third:** Place laterally inserted half pins. Avoid penetrating the medial cortex too far to avoid damage to the femoral artery. Alternatively, place anteriorly inserted half pins. Avoid penetrating the posterior cortex too deeply to prevent damage to the sciatic nerve.

**(C) Distal third:** Place transfixion pins through the bone in a lateral to medial direction. Be aware that transcondylar pins will penetrate the knee joint synovium.

## The Tibia and Fibula

The anterior and posterior neurovascular bundles course down the leg on either side of the interosseous membrane lying between the tibia and fibula.

### Fibula

The intimate relationship of the **common peroneal nerve** to the neck of the fibula makes pin insertion into the upper third of the fibula hazardous. Fortunately, this rarely is necessary.

### Tibia

The tibia has a broad subcutaneous surface throughout its entire length. Because the bone is triangular in shape, the middle of this surface lies anterior to both neurovascular bundles. The subcutaneous surface of the bone can be used throughout its entire length for the placement of half pins. This route allows good bony anchoring without the risk of soft-tissue tethering.

Transfixion pins can be inserted from the lateral side of the bone throughout the length of the tibia. At the level of the ankle joint, a pin may be inserted transversely in a posterolateral to anteromedial direction through both the fibula and the tibia. It must be realized, however, that this can damage the inferior tibiofibular joint (Fig. 13-4).

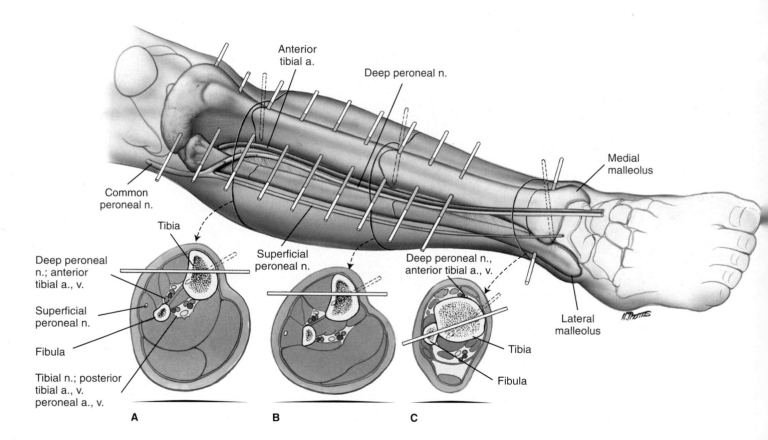

**Figure 13-4**    Because the neurovascular bundles lie largely posterior to the tibia, and it has a subcutaneous surface, pin placement is relatively straightforward.

**(A) Proximal third:** Insert anterior half pins through the subcutaneous surface of the bone. If half pins are used, avoid penetrating the bone too far to protect the anterior neurovascular bundle, the anterior tibial artery, and the peroneal nerve. Alternatively, insert transfixion pins in a lateral to medial direction.

**(B) Middle third:** Insert anterior half pins through the subcutaneous surface. Alternatively, use transfixion pins from lateral to medial points.

**(C) Distal third:** Insert anteriorly placed half pins. Alternatively, insert transfixion pins in a posterolateral to anteromedial direction. These pins will fix both the fibula and the tibia.

# Index

*Note:* Page numbers followed by *f* indicate figures.